NATIONAL ACADEMIES

Sciences
Engineering
Medicine

NATIONAL
ACADEMIES
PRESS
Washington, DC

A New Vision for Women's Health Research

Transformative Change at the National Institutes of Health

T0357812

Sheila P. Burke, Alina Salganicoff, and Amy Geller, *Editors*

Committee on the Assessment of NIH Research on Women's Health

Board on Population Health and Public Health Practice

Health and Medicine Division

Consensus Study Report

NATIONAL ACADEMIES PRESS 500 Fifth Street, NW Washington, DC 20001

This Project has been funded in whole with federal funds from the Office of Research on Women's Health, National Institutes of Health, Department of Health and Human Services, under Contract No. HHSN263201800029I, Task Order No. 75N98023F00005. Any opinions, findings, conclusions, or recommendations expressed in this publication do not necessarily reflect the views of any organization or agency that provided support for the project.

International Standard Book Number-13: 978-0-309-73139-3
International Standard Book Number-10: 0-309-73139-9
Digital Object Identifier: https://doi.org/10.17226/28586
Library of Congress Control Number: 2025931421

This publication is available from the National Academies Press, 500 Fifth Street, NW, Keck 360, Washington, DC 20001; (800) 624-6242 or (202) 334-3313; http://www.nap.edu.

Printed in the United States of America.

Suggested citation: National Academies of Sciences, Engineering, and Medicine. 2025. *A new vision for women's health research: Transformative change at the National Institutes of Health*. Washington, DC: The National Academies Press. https://doi.org/10.17226/28586.

The **National Academy of Sciences** was established in 1863 by an Act of Congress, signed by President Lincoln, as a private, nongovernmental institution to advise the nation on issues related to science and technology. Members are elected by their peers for outstanding contributions to research. Dr. Marcia McNutt is president.

The **National Academy of Engineering** was established in 1964 under the charter of the National Academy of Sciences to bring the practices of engineering to advising the nation. Members are elected by their peers for extraordinary contributions to engineering. Dr. John L. Anderson is president.

The **National Academy of Medicine** (formerly the Institute of Medicine) was established in 1970 under the charter of the National Academy of Sciences to advise the nation on medical and health issues. Members are elected by their peers for distinguished contributions to medicine and health. Dr. Victor J. Dzau is president.

The three Academies work together as the **National Academies of Sciences, Engineering, and Medicine** to provide independent, objective analysis and advice to the nation and conduct other activities to solve complex problems and inform public policy decisions. The National Academies also encourage education and research, recognize outstanding contributions to knowledge, and increase public understanding in matters of science, engineering, and medicine.

Learn more about the National Academies of Sciences, Engineering, and Medicine at **www.nationalacademies.org**.

Consensus Study Reports published by the National Academies of Sciences, Engineering, and Medicine document the evidence-based consensus on the study's statement of task by an authoring committee of experts. Reports typically include findings, conclusions, and recommendations based on information gathered by the committee and the committee's deliberations. Each report has been subjected to a rigorous and independent peer-review process and it represents the position of the National Academies on the statement of task.

Proceedings published by the National Academies of Sciences, Engineering, and Medicine chronicle the presentations and discussions at a workshop, symposium, or other event convened by the National Academies. The statements and opinions contained in proceedings are those of the participants and are not endorsed by other participants, the planning committee, or the National Academies.

Rapid Expert Consultations published by the National Academies of Sciences, Engineering, and Medicine are authored by subject-matter experts on narrowly focused topics that can be supported by a body of evidence. The discussions contained in rapid expert consultations are considered those of the authors and do not contain policy recommendations. Rapid expert consultations are reviewed by the institution before release.

For information about other products and activities of the National Academies, please visit www.nationalacademies.org/about/whatwedo.

CRYSTAL SCHILLER, Associate Professor, Department of Psychiatry; Associate Director, Center for Women's Mood Disorders, University of North Carolina at Chapel Hill School of Medicine

ANGELES ALVAREZ SECORD, Professor, Division of Gynecologic Oncology, Department of OB/GYN; Director, Gynecologic Oncology Clinical Trials; Associate Director, Clinical Research Gynecologic Oncology Program, Duke Cancer Institute, Duke University Health System

METHODIUS G. TUULI, Chace-Joukowsky Professor and Chair, Department of Obstetrics and Gynecology, The Warren Alpert Medical School of Brown University; Chief of Obstetrics and Gynecology, Women & Infants Hospital

BIANCA D. M. WILSON, Associate Professor, University of California, Los Angeles; Affiliate Faculty Member, the California Center for Population Research

National Academy of Medicine Fellows

2023–2025 Gant/American Board of Obstetrics and Gynecology Fellow

MICHELLE P. DEBBINK, Assistant Professor, Department of Obstetrics & Gynecology, Division of Maternal-Fetal Medicine; Vice Chair, Equity, Diversity, and Inclusion; Associate Program Director, Women's Health Equity Fellowship, University of Utah

2021–2023 American Board of Emergency Medicine Fellow

TRACY E. MADSEN, Associate Professor, Division of Sex and Gender, Department of Emergency Medicine, The Warren Alpert Medical School of Brown University; Associate Professor, Department of Epidemiology, School of Public Health, Brown University

Study Staff

AMY GELLER, Study Director
AIMEE MEAD, Program Officer
L. BRIELLE DOJER, Research Associate
MAGGIE ANDERSON, Research Assistant
RACHEL RILEY SORRELL, Senior Program Assistant (*until August 2024*)
ELLA CASTANIER, Senior Program Assistant (*from October 2024*)
Y. CRYSTI PARK, Program Coordinator
MISRAK DABI, Senior Finance Business Partner
ROSE MARIE MARTINEZ, Senior Board Director
SHARYL NASS, Senior Board Director

Consultants

HAMAD AL-IBRAHIM, Policy Tech Innovation LLC
JOE ALPER, Independent Consultant
YUDHIJIT BHATTACHARJEE, Independent Consultant
JULIANE KWONG, Cedars-Sinai Medical Center
BENJAMIN RENTON, Brown University School of Public Health
JEN SAUNDERS, Independent Consultant
NANCY SUN, Cedars-Sinai Medical Center
WASAY WARSI, Cedars-Sinai Medical Center

Reviewers

This Consensus Study Report was reviewed in draft form by individuals chosen for their diverse perspectives and technical expertise. The purpose of this independent review is to provide candid and critical comments that will assist the National Academies of Sciences, Engineering, and Medicine in making each published report as sound as possible and to ensure that it meets the institutional standards for quality, objectivity, evidence, and responsiveness to the study charge. The review comments and draft manuscript remain confidential to protect the integrity of the deliberative process.

We thank the following individuals for their review of this report:

RICHARD BRAMAN, Fly Health, LLC
PAMELA Y. COLLINS, Johns Hopkins University
SARAH K. ENGLAND, Washington University School of Medicine
BETHANY G. EVERETT, University of Utah
LEE FLEISHER, University of Pennsylvania
RICHARD G. FRANK, The Brookings Institution
BETH Y. KARLAN, University of California, Los Angeles
JOANN E. MANSON, Harvard Medical School
RICHARD NAKAMURA, National Institutes of Health (retired)
DAVID OUYANG, Cedars-Sinai Medical Center
JENNIFER R. RICHARDS, Johns Hopkins Center for
    Indigenous Health
NANETTE F. SANTORO, University of Colorado School of Medicine
JULIA F. SIMARD, Stanford University

OMAIDA C. VELAZQUEZ, University of Miami
ANUSHREE VICHARE, The George Washington University
NICOLE C. WRIGHT, Tulane University
RUTH ENID ZAMBRANA, University of Maryland

Although the reviewers listed above provided many constructive comments and suggestions, they were not asked to endorse the conclusions or recommendations of this report nor did they see the final draft before its release. The review of this report was overseen by SUSAN C. SCRIMSHAW, International Nutrition Foundation, and ERIC B. LARSON, University of Washington School of Medicine. They were responsible for making certain that an independent examination of this report was carried out in accordance with the standards of the National Academies and that all review comments were carefully considered. Responsibility for the final content rests entirely with the authoring committee and the National Academies.

Contents

Preface

More than 30 years after the passage of the landmark National Institutes of Health (NIH) Revitalization Act and the Congressional mandate to NIH to increase its investment and commitment to advancing the state of women's health research (WHR), Congress asked the National Academies of Sciences, Engineering, and Medicine to assess the status of WHR at NIH. The committee grappled with this broad charge by closely examining NIH's investments in WHR and workforce development and identifying research gaps and opportunities. In countless ways, NIH has made important advances, including implementing a policy requiring that NIH-funded research consider sex as a biological variable and investing in innovative and breakthrough research that has saved the lives of and improved treatment options for many women. Despite this progress, major gaps remain that must be addressed if our national research enterprise is to significantly drive progress to improve the health and well-being of women in this country.

After reviewing NIH's investments, structure, and priorities, the committee concluded that the nation needs a bold new approach. The status quo is not enough. Over the past decade, funding on WHR has stagnated and shrunk as a share of the overall NIH budget. Sex differences are not sufficiently studied or reported, and investments in women-specific research fall short. Many WHR training programs and grants have been reduced, and too few researchers have the knowledge base required to make the needed advances in WHR.

The committee was faced with the difficult task of making recommendations for whether and how the structure of NIH should change to advance this research priority and how to distribute the funding to fill the gaps. After months of careful deliberation, the committee concluded that in addition to doubling the NIH investment in WHR, three major structural elements are needed to address the persistent gaps in research: (1) a new WHR Institute to provide a home for the study of health conditions that predominantly or exclusively affect women and greatly impair the quality of millions of women's lives, including conditions such as endometriosis, uterine fibroids, the menopause transition, pelvic floor disorder, vulvodynia, and polycystic ovary syndrome, which no Institute or Center (IC) currently prioritizes; (2) a major new interdisciplinary WHR fund, modeled on NIH's Common Fund, to catalyze interdisciplinary research in women's health; and (3) a sustained commitment and prioritization by the current ICs to conduct research that examines sex and gender differences and women's health. The committee also proposes expanding programs to grow the WHR workforce to ensure that it reflects the rich diversity of the research field and the U.S. population.

The committee is composed of experts representing many of the disciplines and medical specialties critical to making needed research advances. A common thread among us is the belief that research can improve women's health, quality of life, and well-being. We were also cognizant of the importance of ensuring that future research includes an emphasis on the women who are disproportionately marginalized and discriminated against by society and the health system and experience the greatest challenges in achieving the good health and well-being to which we are all entitled. We also recognized the need to broaden the definition of WHR to include those with experiences as girls, women, and females at some point over the life course.

We are grateful for the many contributions of the committee members and their remarkable work on this study conducted under a compressed time frame. It was our pleasure to get to know and work with each of them. Their dedication to women's health and commitment to the task is unquestioned.

We would especially like to extend our deepest appreciation to the study staff. Amy Geller worked tirelessly to get us to completion. We benefited greatly from her nimble leadership and superb research and project management skills. She was skillfully supported by an exceptional, creative, and tirelessly dedicated study team—Aimee Mead, L. Brielle Dojer, Maggie Anderson, and Rachel Riley. This report would not have been possible without their dedicated effort and meticulous attention to detail. We would be remiss if we did not also extend our thanks to Rose Marie Martinez, who played a quiet but critical role in shepherding this report through its many stages. We also thank Crysti Park, Aisha Bhimla, Zarah Batulan, Elizabeth Boyle, Nicholas Murdock, and Dara Ancona for their additional support. We thank the National Academies and Health and Medicine Division communications staff, including Amber McLaughlin. This project received valuable assistance from Megan Lowry (Office of News and Public Information); Misrak Dabi (Office of the Chief Financial Officer); and Monica Feit, Samantha Chao, Leslie Sim, Taryn Young, and Lori Brenig (Health and Medicine Division Executive Office). We received important research assistance from Rebecca Morgan and Will Anderson (National Academies Research Center).

We also greatly benefited from the participation of two National Academy of Medicine Fellows, Michelle Debbink, 2023–2025 Gant/American Board of Obstetrics and Gynecology Fellow, and Tracy Madsen, 2021–2023 American Board of Emergency Medicine Fellow, who provided meaningful input to our deliberations and contributions to preparing this report. We also appreciate the insightful comments of the reviewers. This report is undoubtedly stronger because of their careful review.

Several consultants made critical contributions to this report. In particular, we would like to thank Hamad Al-Ibrahim, who devised a state-of-the-art, artificial intelligence–informed approach to analyze the research and funding investment that NIH has supported over the past decade. Nancy Sun provided essential data preparation and analytics, and we were further supported in this area by Juliane Kwong and Wasay Warsi. Joe Alper, Yudhijit Bhattacharjee, and Jennifer Saunders provided helpful background for and editing of the report. We also thank Benajmin Renton for his research support.

We also want to extend our heartful appreciation to the legion of scientists, clinicians, and advocates who shared their expertise and insights with us in open sessions and in writing. Their passion for generating research to improve women's health inspired us. We are especially grateful to the many women who candidly shared their sometimes very painful personal health experiences. Their perspectives enriched this study and movingly illustrated to us why NIH's work is so vital and why we as a nation must do more to improve women's lives. The following speakers provided their research, expertise, and perspectives at our information-gathering meetings: Madina Agénor, Victoria L. Bae-Jump, Lisa Barroilhet, Irina Burd, William Catherino, Evelina Cebotari, Janine Austin Clayton, Christos Coutifaris, Kristina M. Deligiannidis, Amanda Dennis, Angela Doyinsola, C. Neill Epperson, Lori Frank, Karen Freund, Jamie Hart, Irene Headen, Reshma Jagsi, Beth Y. Karlan, Kristin Kramer, Erica E. Marsh, Carolyn Mazure, Margaret M. McCarthy, Michele McGuirl, Lindsey Miltenberger, Eliseo J. Pérez-Stable, Tory Eisenlohr-Moul, Karen L. Parker, Vivian Pinn, Nancy Praskievicz, Karen Reue, Ayanna Robinson, George Santangelo, Jake Scholl, Danny J. Schust, Tara Schwetz, Carolyn W. Swenson, Sarah Temkin, Marina Volkov, Vivian Ota Wong, Steven Young, and Christopher M. Zahn. We also thank the following individuals who provided technical review of sections of the report: Nancy Praskievicz, Jake Scholl, Evelina Cebotari, Kristin Kramer, and Stephanie Constant (NIH); Danny J. Schust (Duke University); and Christos Coutifaris (University of Pennsylvania).

We offer our thanks to committee members' executive assistants and support staff, without whom scheduling meetings and conference calls would have been nearly impossible: Hannah Bagley, Kathy Farnum, Duane Haneckow, Lamia Pierre, Tamala Knox, Kathleen Prutting, Bryana Castillo Sanchez, Lidiana Sanvar, and Kisha Young.

Finally, the committee would like to thank the NIH Office of Research on Women's Health, the study sponsor, for its support of this work.

It is our hope that the road map the committee has laid out in this report will not only guide Congress and NIH but also inspire a new generation of researchers to embrace the challenge and address the urgent need to make new scientific breakthroughs to improve women's lives. This journey began at NIH over 30 years ago, and we believe this is the time to renew and expand this commitment with transformative change. To quote the late Nancy Adler, a leading researcher and passionate advocate for WHR, "to invest in the health of women is to invest in the well-being and progress of society."[1]

Alina Salganicoff and Sheila Burke, *Cochairs*
Committee on the Assessment of NIH Research on Women's Health

---

[1] Institute of Medicine. 2010. *Women's Health Research: Progress, Pitfalls, and Promise.* Washington, DC: The National Academies Press. https://doi.org/10.17226/12908.

Acronyms and Abbreviations

ACE	adverse childhood experience
ACRWH	Advisory Committee on Research on Women's Health
AD	Alzheimer's disease
ADR	autoimmune disease research
ADRD	Alzheimer's disease and Alzheimer's disease–related disorders
AHRQ	Agency for Healthcare Research and Quality
AIAN	American Indian or Alaska Native
AMA	American Medical Association
AMH	anti-Mullerian hormone
APOE	apolipoprotein E
BIRCWH	Building Interdisciplinary Research Careers in Women's Health
BRAIN	Brain Research through Advancing Innovative Neurotechnologies
CAD	coronary artery disease
CC	Clinical Center
CCRWH	Coordinating Committee on Research on Women's Health
CDC	Centers for Disease Control and Prevention
CEE	conjugated equine estrogen
CIT	Center for Information Technology
CRH	corticotropin-releasing hormone

CSR	Center for Scientific Review
CVD	cardiovascular disease
DALY	disability-adjusted life-year
DPCPSI	Division of Program Coordination, Planning, and Strategic Initiatives
DSCA	Division of Scientific Categorization and Analysis
ECR	early-career reviewer
FCG	Four Core Genotypes
FDA	Food and Drug Administration
FIC	Fogarty International Center
FSH	follicle-stimulating hormone
FY	fiscal year
GABA	gamma-aminobutyric acid
GAO	Government Accountability Office
GBD	global burden of disease
GD	gestational diabetes
GPC	Gender Policy Council
GWAS	genome-wide association studies
HD	Huntington's disease
HHS	Department of Health and Human Services
HMD	Health and Medicine Division
HOA	hip osteoarthritis
HPA	hypothalamic-pituitary-adrenal
HPG	hypothalamic-pituitary-gonadal
IC	Institute or Center
ICO	Institute, Center, or Office
IPV	intimate partner violence
KO	knee osteoarthritis
LGBTQIA+	Lesbian, gay, bisexual, transgender, queer/questioning, intersex, asexual and all other identities not encompassed in the acronym
LH	luteinizing hormone
LLM	large language model
LRP	Loan Repayment Program

MHT	menopausal hormone therapy
MMRC	maternal mortality review committee
MPA	medroxyprogesterone acetate
MS	multiple sclerosis
NAM	National Academy of Medicine
NCATS	National Center for Advancing Translational Sciences
NCCIH	National Center for Complementary and Integrative Health
NCI	National Cancer Institute
NEI	National Eye Institute
NHGRI	National Human Genome Research Institute
NHLBI	National Heart, Lung, and Blood Institute
NHPI	Native Hawaiian and Pacific Islander
NIA	National Institute on Aging
NIAAA	National Institute on Alcohol Abuse and Alcoholism
NIAID	National Institute of Allergy and Infectious Diseases
NIAMS	National Institute of Arthritis and Musculoskeletal and Skin Diseases
NICHD	*Eunice Kennedy Shriver* National Institute of Child Health and Human Development
NIDA	National Institute on Drug Abuse
NIDCD	National Institute on Deafness and Other Communications Disorders
NIDCR	National Institute of Dental and Craniofacial Research
NIDDK	National Institute of Diabetes and Digestive and Kidney Diseases
NIEHS	National Institute of Environmental Health Sciences
NIH	National Institutes of Health
NIMH	National Institute of Mental Health
NIMHD	National Institute on Minority Health and Health Disparities
NINDS	National Institute of Neurological Disorders and Stroke
NOSI	Notice of special interest
OA	osteoarthritis
OADR	Office of Autoimmune Diseases Research
OAR	Office of AIDS Research
OBSSR	Office of Behavioral and Social Sciences Research
OCP	oral contraceptive pills
OCRP	Ovarian Cancer Research Program
OD	Office of the Director

ODP	Office of Disease Prevention
OER	Office of Extramural Research
OIR	Office of Intramural Research
OMB	Office of Management and Budget
OPA	Office of Portfolio Analysis
ORRA	Office of Research Reporting and Analysis
ORWH	Office of Research on Women's Health
PARP	poly(adenosine diphosphate-ribose) polymerase
PCOS	polycystic ovary syndrome
PD	Parkinson's disease
PI	principal investigator
PMDD	premenstrual dysphoric disorder
PND	perinatal depression
PO	program official
PTB	preterm birth
QALY	quality-adjusted life-year
RA	rheumatoid arthritis
RCDC	Research, Condition, and Disease Categorization
RePORT	Research Portfolio Online Reporting Tools
RePORTER	RePORT Expenditures and Results
RFA	Request for Applications
RNA	ribonucleic acid
RNP	ribonucleoprotein
RPG	research project grant
RPL	recurrent pregnancy loss
RSDP	Reproductive Scientist Development Program
SABV	sex as a biological variable
SAMHSA	Substance Abuse and Mental Health Services Administration
SCORE	Specialized Centers of Research Excellence on Sex Differences
SDOH	social determinants of health
SEP	special emphasis panel
SGM	sexual and gender minority
SGMRO	Sexual & Gender Minority Research Office
SNP	single nucleotide polymorphism
SPI	super principal investigator
SRG	scientific review group
SRO	scientific review officer

SSRI	selective serotonin reuptake inhibitor
STEMM	Science, technology, engineering, mathematics, and medicine
TNB	transgender and nonbinary
WHI	Women's Health Initiative
WHR	women's health research
WRHR	Women's Reproductive Health Research Career Development Program
YLD	years lived with disability
YLL	years of life lost

Key Terms

The committee strived to use language that is respectful, accurate, and maximally inclusive. This relies on attempting to reflect preferences for how individuals and groups wish to be addressed, but there is not always consensus on preferred terms, and these preferences may evolve. These terms are defined for the purposes of this report and adapted or informed by other National Academies of Sciences, Engineering, and Medicine reports and other reports.[1]

---

[1] Canadian Institutes of Health Research. 2022. *National women's health research initiative.* https://cihr-irsc.gc.ca/e/53095.html (accessed August 27, 2024); Jones, C. P. 2002. Confronting institutionalized racism. *Phylon (1960-), 50(1/2),* 7–22; NASEM. 2024. *Advancing research on chronic conditions in women.* Washington, DC: The National Academies Press; NASEM. 2023. *Federal policy to advance racial, ethnic, and tribal health equity.* Washington, DC: The National Academies Press; NASEM. 2022. *Measuring sex, gender identity, and sexual orientation.* Washington, DC: The National Academies Press; NASEM. 2020. *Understanding the well-being of LGBTQI+ populations.* Washington, DC: The National Academies Press; NASEM. 2022. *Measuring sex, gender identity, and sexual orientation.* Washington, DC: The National Academies Press; NIH Office of Equity, Diversity, and Inclusion. n.d. *Terms and definitions.* https://www.edi.nih.gov/people/sep/lgbti/safezone/terminology (accessed July 12, 2024); ORWH. n.d. *Sex and gender.* https://orwh.od.nih.gov/sex-gender (accessed July 12, 2024); SGMRO. 2024. *About SGMRO.* https://dpcpsi.nih.gov/sgmro (accessed August 20, 2024); WHO. n.d. *Gender and health.* https://www.who.int/health-topics/gender/strengthening-health-sector-response-to-gender-based-violence-in-humanitarian-emergencies#tab=tab_1 (accessed July 30, 2024).

Women's Health Research Terms

Female: An individual (human or animal) whose sex traits (see definition of "sex") include features typically associated with or assigned as female; females typically have any of the following organs or characteristics:

- External genitalia including a vulva, vagina, and/or clitoris; or
- Internal sex organs and gonads including a cervix, uterus, fallopian tubes, or ovaries; or
- Sex chromosome complement that consists of a predominantly X configuration (typically two X chromosomes) in the absence of an active *Sry* gene.

Human females can include individuals who were assigned female at birth and identify as women, men, nonbinary, transgender, genderfluid, and/or Two-Spirit. This definition should not be conflated with the definition of women; though most women are assigned female at birth, many are not. Furthermore, the definition is not proscriptive, exhaustive, or immutable, as indicated in the definition of sex.

Women: The terms "female" and "woman" are used differently according to context and perspective, which may cause confusion. In this report, the definition of women goes beyond the sex and gender binary and includes all people who identify as a woman or girl, solely or in addition to other gender identities and regardless of biological sex traits. This inclusive definition recognizes individuals who have been or may be affected by a set of biological and/or social variables that influence women differently than men across the life course.

Women's health: Includes physical, biological, reproductive, psychological, emotional, and cultural/spiritual health and wellness across the life course, for more than those identifying as women or girls. It includes the experiences and needs of all people who identify as a woman, girl, female, nonbinary, transgender (men or women), genderfluid, or Two-Spirit or were assigned female at birth.

Women's health research: The scientific study of the range of and variability in women's health as defined and the mechanisms and outcomes in disease and non-disease states across the life course. It considers both sex and gender and how these affect women's health and well-being, disease risk, pathophysiology, symptoms, diagnosis, and treatment. This work also addresses interacting concerns related to women's bodies and roles and social and structural determinants and systems.

Sexual Orientation, Gender Identity and Expression, and Sex Characteristics Terms

Sex: A multidimensional construct that refers to a person's biological status, based on a cluster of anatomical and physiological traits that include external genitalia, secondary sex characteristics, gonads, chromosomes, and hormones. It is typically categorized as male, female, or intersex and determined at birth. Some notable characteristics about sex include

- Usually assigned as female or male;
- Most often defined at birth based on visual inspection of external genitalia;
- Sex traits are usually assumed to be unambiguous, but may not be;
- Sex traits are usually assumed to correspond to the same sex, but may not;
- Some sex traits can change or be altered over time.

Intersex: People whose sex traits do not all correspond to a single sex.

Gender: A multidimensional construct that links gender identity, gender expression, and social and cultural expectations about status, characteristics, and behavior that are associated with sex traits. It influences how people perceive themselves and each other, how they act and interact, and the distribution of power and resources in society. Gender identity is not confined to a binary (girl/woman, boy/man), nor is it static; it exists along a continuum and can change over time. There is considerable diversity in how individuals and groups understand, experience, and express gender through the roles they take on, the expectations placed on them, relations with others, and the complex ways that gender is institutionalized in society.

Gender identity refers to a person's deeply felt, internal, and individual experience of gender, which may or may not correspond to their physiology or designated sex at birth.

Gender identities include

- **"Cisgender"** (**"cis"**) refers to a person whose current gender identity aligns with the sex they were assigned at birth.
- **"Transgender"** (**"trans"; not "transgendered"**) refers to a person whose current gender identity differs from the sex assigned at birth.
- **"Nonbinary"** is often used to describe a gender identity that is neither exclusively man nor woman (i.e., outside the gender binary).
- **"Genderqueer"** describes a person who does not follow gender norms.

- "Genderfluid" refers to a person who does not identify with a fixed gender.
- "Two-Spirit" is a placeholder term for specific gender and sexual orientation identities that are centered in Indigenous tribal worldviews, practices, and knowledges.

Gender binary refers to the concept that there are only two genders, male and female, and that everyone must be one or the other. The concept is also often misused to assert that gender is biologically determined and reinforces the idea that men and women are opposites and have different roles in society.

Gender expression is how an individual signals their gender to others through behavior and appearances (e.g., clothing, appearance, mannerisms). This may be conscious or subconscious and may or may not reflect their gender identity or sexual orientation.

Sexual orientation is a multidimensional construct encompassing emotional, romantic, and sexual attraction, identity, and behavior. Categories of sexual orientation include heterosexual (straight), lesbian/gay (homosexual), bisexual, queer, pansexual, and questioning.

- "Heterosexual" ("straight") refers to people whose attraction and behavior are oriented toward people of a different, usually binary, gender.
- "Lesbian/Gay" ("homosexual") refers to people whose attraction and behavior are oriented toward people of the same, usually binary, gender.
- "Bisexual" refers to people whose attraction and behavior are oriented toward people of both the same and different genders.
- "Queer" is an umbrella term for belonging to the LGBTQIA+ community and also used to refer to a person whose attraction and behavior are oriented toward people of more than one gender.
- "Pansexual" refers to people whose attraction and behavior are oriented toward people of any gender.
- "Questioning" refers to someone who is uncertain about sexual orientation and identity.

Sexual and gender minorities (SGM): SGM populations include but are not limited to individuals who identify as lesbian, gay, bisexual, asexual, transgender, Two-Spirit, queer, and/or intersex. Individuals with same-sex or -gender attractions or behaviors and those with a difference in sex development are also included. These populations also encompass those who do not self-identify with one of these terms but whose sexual orientation, gender identity or expression, or reproductive development is characterized by nonbinary constructs of sexual orientation, gender, and/or sex.

Social and Structural Determinants of Health

Social determinants of health (SDOH): The conditions and environments in which people live, learn, work, play, worship, and age that affect a wide range of health, functioning, and quality-of-life outcomes and risks. SDOH can both promote and harm health. For the purposes of this report, SDOH are organized by the Healthy People 2030 domains: economic stability, education access and quality, health care access and quality, neighborhood and built environment, and social and community context.

Structural determinants of health: Macrolevel factors, such as institutional practices, governance processes, and social norms, that shape the distribution or maldistribution of SDOH, including housing, income, employment, exposure to environmental toxins, and interpersonal discrimination, across and within social groups. Structural determinants of health, also referred to as the "determinants of the determinants of health," include structural racism and other structural inequities and thus impact not only population health but also health equity.

Summary[1]

In 1993, Congress passed the National Institutes of Health (NIH) Revitalization Act, a landmark law codifying the importance of including women in research and formally establishing NIH's Office of Research on Women's Health (ORWH). Thirty years later, many questions about women's health remain unaddressed, women's health research (WHR) remains underfunded, and breakthroughs to improve health and well-being for half the population in the United States—women and girls—have lagged. This gap is partly attributable to a lack of baseline understanding of basic sex-based differences in physiology and gender-based discriminatory practices that have resulted in a failure to prioritize and fund research into conditions and factors specific to, more common among, or that affect women and girls differently. Girls, women, families, society, and the economy all pay a price for this gap.

The committee concluded that the nation needs a comprehensive approach to develop a robust WHR agenda and establish a supportive NIH infrastructure. Augmented funding for WHR, while crucial, needs to go hand-in-hand with greater accountability, rigorous oversight, agency-wide prioritization, and seamless integration of WHR across NIH Institutes, Centers, and Offices (ICOs). This multifaceted approach is essential to fully capitalize on both existing and future funding and resources.

---

[1] This summary does not include references. Citations for the information presented herein are provided in the main text.

WHY STUDY WOMEN'S HEALTH?

There are multiple reasons for the vast gaps in knowledge regarding women's health prevention, diagnosis, and treatment and the need to prioritize WHR now, including the past exclusion of women in clinical trials arising from concerns about potential risks to fertility and pregnancy; a lack of prioritization of research on women's physiology, given that the focus of human health research has been adult male anatomy and physiology; and lack of support for and development of the WHR workforce. Although women are now enrolled in clinical trials at the same rate as men overall, underrepresentation of women as research subjects still persists among certain subgroups, and most studies enrolling men and women do not study or analyze sex or gender differences, representing missed opportunities to advance health. Intentionally studying underlying sex and gender differences would lead to stronger science and a better understanding of sex- and gender-specific health issues and interventions that will benefit the health of the whole population.

Despite having a longer life expectancy than men, women spend more years living with a disability and in poor health. On average, a woman will spend 9 years in poor health, 25 percent more time than men, affecting quality of life and productivity. Conditions affecting both women and men have disparities in outcomes and treatment success. For example, although women have a lower prevalence of cardiovascular disease (CVD) than men, they have worse prognoses after experiencing an acute cardiovascular event, and research on the underlying pathophysiology of why this occurs is limited. Further, data show a gender disparity in the allocation of NIH research funding across different diseases, with those disproportionately affecting women being underfunded relative to their burden compared to diseases that disproportionately affect men.

Starting in adolescence, there are conditions specific to the experiences of women and girls, and the knowledge gap regarding them fails both women and their health care providers. For example, gynecologic conditions, such as endometriosis, polycystic ovary syndrome (PCOS), and premature ovarian insufficiency, generally require a chronic management approach, yet physicians lack clear guidance and innovative tools to address these costly and debilitating conditions. Significant knowledge gaps exist regarding the health effects of the menopause transition and complications during pregnancy associated with increased risk of developing chronic conditions later in life.

Women who are racially and ethnically minoritized, are economically disadvantaged, live in rural areas, or identify as belonging to sexual and gender minority groups experience a disproportionate burden

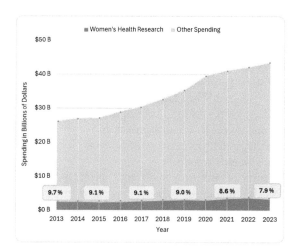

FIGURE S-1 Overall National Institutes of Health (NIH) grant funding and the proportion of NIH funding on women's health research, fiscal year 2013–2023.

of disease and adverse outcomes, including violence, autoimmune diseases, mental illness, maternal morbidity and mortality, and cancer. These inequities are in large part a result of structural factors and lack of access to positive social determinants of health that remain largely understudied and underreported in biomedical research, which is discussed in the report.

The committee found in its analysis that on average just 8.8 percent of NIH spending from fiscal year (FY) 2013 to FY 2023 across all ICOs focused on WHR, and funding has decreased as a share of overall NIH funding during this period despite steady increases in the NIH budget and total projects (see Figure S-1).

COMMITTEE STATEMENT OF TASK

As part of the Consolidated Appropriations Act of 2023, Congress requested the National Academies of Sciences, Engineering, and Medicine assemble an ad hoc committee to assess the state of WHR at NIH. ORWH sponsored the study. The committee was asked to assess NIH research on women's health, including knowledge gaps and the proportion of NIH-funded research on women's health conditions, including those that are female specific, are more common among women, or affect women differently.

The committee was tasked with providing recommendations regarding the following:

- Research priorities for NIH-supported research on women's health.
- NIH training and education efforts to build, support, and maintain a robust women's health research workforce.
- NIH structure (extra- and intramural), systems, and review processes to optimize women's health research.
- NIH-wide workforce to effectively solicit, review, and support women's health research.
- Allocation of funding such that NIH women's health funding reflects the burdens of disease among women.

Women's Health at NIH

NIH is the largest U.S. government research body, with a budget of $47.1 billion in FY 2024. NIH comprises 21 Institutes and six Centers (ICs), each with its own focus and role to advance biomedical research and public health, and most provide grants to extramural researchers. The purview of most ICs includes aspects of women's health. For example, most female-specific cancers primarily fall within the scope of the National Cancer Institute. However, many female-specific conditions, such as fibroids, endometriosis, and PCOS, are not prioritized by any specific IC.[2]

NIH also has offices that support and coordinate various functions across the agency. NIH established ORWH to strengthen research on women's health conditions, improve representation of women in clinical trials, and increase the number of women in biomedical careers. ORWH is the hub for women's health at NIH, developing and leading programs and initiatives and directing the development of the NIH-Wide Strategic Plan for Research on the Health of Women. ORWH's role, however, is largely coordination, and it only has a small budget to co-fund research with ICs.

RECOMMENDATIONS

The committee identified five steps Congress and NIH should take to advance WHR:

1. Create pathways to facilitate and support innovative and transformative research for women's health;
2. Strengthen oversight, prioritization, and coordination for WHR across NIH;
3. Expand, train, support, and retain the WHR workforce;

---

[2] This sentence was changed after release of the report to clarify the scope of NIH ICs.

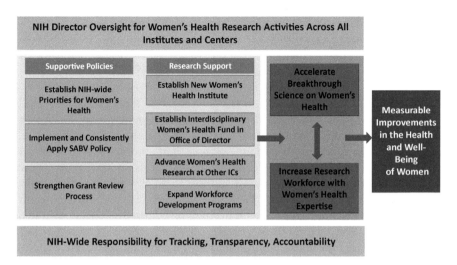

FIGURE S-2 Recommended organization, structure, and actions to improve women's health research at the National Institutes of Health (NIH).
NOTE: ICs = Institutes and Centers; SABV = sex as a biological variable.

4. Optimize NIH programs and policies to support WHR; and
5. Increase NIH investment in WHR.

Figure S-2 provides a high-level overview of the committee's recommendations.

CREATE PATHWAYS TO FACILITATE AND SUPPORT INNOVATIVE AND TRANSFORMATIVE RESEARCH FOR WOMEN'S HEALTH

NIH is underspending on research to support women's health, leading to significant scientific and clinical gaps on conditions that do not fall within the primary expertise of existing ICs. Furthermore, funding levels for WHR have stagnated and decreased as a share of the NIH budget over the past decade.

NIH Organizational Structure

The organizational structure of NIH limits its ability to effectively address gaps in WHR. ORWH is a small, inadequately funded office without the authority to require ICs to conduct WHR or oversee compliance with the NIH policy on sex differences research. This has left a considerable gap in the coverage of and investment in WHR across the agency. NIH has not provided the level of oversight at the director and IC level to ensure women's health is studied comprehensively. Furthermore, many women's health conditions and women-specific life stages are not prioritized by of any of the 27 existing ICs and remain understudied despite millions of women experiencing the burdens of these conditions.[3]

> Recommendation 1: The National Institutes of Health (NIH) should form a new Institute to address the gaps in women's health research (WHR) and create a new interdisciplinary research fund. Furthermore, NIH leadership should expand its oversight and support for WHR across the Institutes and Center (IC)s. Congress should appropriate additional funding to adequately support these new efforts. Specifically,
>
> 1a. Congress should elevate the Office of Research on Women's Health (ORWH) to an Institute with primary responsibility to lead, conduct, and support research on female physiology and chromosomal differences, reproductive milestones across the life course, and female-specific conditions that do not fall under the purview of other ICs.
>   • Certain programs currently housed in ORWH, such as women's health workforce development programs, and their corresponding budget will be part of the new WHR Institute.
>   • The new WHR Institute should have a dedicated independent budget comparable to that of other NIH Institutes with similar scope, amounting to at least $4 billion over the first 5 years.
> 1b. Congress should establish a new fund for WHR in the Office of the Director to support interdisciplinary women's health and sex differences research with a focus on innovation and accelerating biomedical discoveries. The fund should have a dedicated independent budget comparable to that of other major NIH initiatives, such as the Common Fund, Cancer Moonshot, and BRAIN Initiative. The fund will ramp up over the first 2 years, achieving full funding of $3 billion in Year 3, with a total investment of $11.4 billion over the initial 5 years.
> 1c. The NIH director and IC directors should prioritize WHR. The NIH director should assume oversight and responsibility for the WHR portfolio across NIH with respect to funding allocations and implementation of priorities, such as sex as a biological variable, and policies relevant to women's health. IC directors should increase support for WHR that falls under their purview.
>   • The NIH director, in collaboration with IC directors, should set annual benchmarks in the year-to-year proportion of extramural and intramural funding to be granted for WHR, following a comprehensive analysis of research needs (see Recommendation 3).

---

[3] This sentence was updated after release of the report to clarify the scope of NIH ICs.

- The NIH director should evaluate progress on addressing WHR gaps and associated funding levels across NIH and should submit an annual report to Congress and to the public on the year-to-year trends by IC. The Office of the Director should receive additional funds to support NIH-wide programmatic evaluation and increased administrative responsibilities.
- The Director of the National Institute on Minority Health and Health Disparities (NIMHD) should expand the Institute's role to include women, girls, and females among the populations that experience disparities. Congress should increase NIMHD's budget to adequately support including women's health disparities research into its portfolio and coordinate this research with other ICs.

Implementing Recommendation 1a would require a statutory change by Congress or a reorganization of ICs, since the NIH Reform Act limits the number of NIH ICs to 27. See Chapter 9 (and Table 9-1) on the roles and responsibility of the new WHR Institute.

STRENGTHEN OVERSIGHT, PRIORITIZATION, AND COORDINATION FOR WHR ACROSS NIH

Tracking NIH Investments in WHR

The Research, Condition, and Disease Categorization system—designed to track NIH-funded projects for reporting to the public—is inadequately designed to guide budget allocations and inform Congress and the public on how much is spent in distinct research areas.

Recommendation 2: The National Institutes of Health (NIH) should reform its process for tracking and analyzing its investments in research funding to improve accuracy for reporting to Congress and the public on expenditures on women's health research (WHR).
2a. The new process should improve accuracy of grants coded as Women's Health and eliminate duplicate or multiplicative counting of grants across Research, Condition, and Disease Categorization (RCDC) categories. This may be achieved by applying proportionate accounting of grants to generate more accurate estimates for categories related to WHR.
2b. NIH should update its process for reviewing, revising, and adding new RCDC categories that pertain to WHR.
2c. NIH should make transparent and accessible the process and data used for portfolio analysis so researchers, analysts, and the public can examine and replicate NIH investments into research for women's health.

Recommendation 2, and retrospective funding analyses, should be facilitated by expanding the use of modern data analysis methods, such as large language models, that can efficiently identify and categorize grant content.

Priority Setting for WHR

Most NIH ICs have a strategic plan to inform its research priorities—women's health is rarely mentioned in these plans, and they often do not reflect elements of the NIH-Wide Strategic Plan for Research on the Health of Women. In addition, the time frames for the IC plans vary significantly and do not align with the timeline of the agency-wide plan, limiting NIH's ability to set, implement, and oversee cohesive and cross-agency priorities for WHR. To address these issues, a comprehensive NIH-wide prioritization process is needed.

> **Recommendation 3: The Director of the National Institutes of Health (NIH) should develop and implement a transparent, biennial process to set priorities for women's health research (WHR). The process should be data driven and include input from the scientific and practitioner communities and the public. Priorities of the director and the Institutes and Centers (ICs) should respond to the gaps in the evidence base and evolving women's health needs. To inform research priorities for women's health, NIH should**
>
> 3a. **Employ data-driven methods, such as epidemiologic studies and disability or quality-adjusted life years, to assess the public health effect of conditions that are female specific, disproportionately affect women, or affect women differently. NIH should report this assessment publicly and use it, in combination with other analyses as needed (e.g., of expected return on investment), to identify research priorities and direct funding for WHR.**
>
> 3b. **To ensure priorities for WHR are implemented, ICs should issue Requests for Applications, Notices of Special Interest, Program Announcements, and similar mechanisms, in addition to current funding activities.**

EXPAND, TRAIN, SUPPORT, AND RETAIN THE WHR WORKFORCE

To address WHR, a robust and productive NIH intramural and extramural research workforce with broad expertise in biomedical research, clinical trials, and implementation science is essential. NIH support of the WHR workforce falls short of what is needed to address the unmet needs of women's health. Investment is needed to develop a cadre of the next generation of women's health researchers. In addition to intramural and extramural researchers, IC program staff need expertise in women's health for effective prioritization and coordination. Inadequate funding of WHR has led to an insufficient number of WHR investigators and even fewer with interest and expertise in studying women's health at the intersection of other important social identities, including race, ethnicity, and disability.

WHR Career Pathways

A coordinated approach is needed to attract and support researchers (those who study WHR, not only researchers who are women) across their careers to make meaningful discoveries in women's health. Existing grant mechanisms are insufficiently funded and structured to support career trajectories in WHR. Increased funding and expanded numbers of career support grants for WHR investigators are needed, coupled with support for sponsorship, mentorship, and protected research time, such as through training grants. Mentorship and career development are vital to developing a WHR workforce, but NIH grants do not generally fund mentor time. In addition, many institutions do not have the funding to support early-career clinician-scientists, particularly in surgical subspecialties, including obstetrics and gynecology.

Gender-based bias and sexism persist in the United States, including in its health and research systems. For NIH, these biases affect the grant-review and award processes. Bias related to race and ethnicity are independent and intersectional contributors to gaps in health research generally and WHR specifically. NIH has acknowledged these issues and implemented initiatives to address them. However, research suggests that significant disparities remain, and further structural changes are necessary to achieve equity in the grant-making process.

> **Recommendation 4: The National Institutes of Health (NIH) should augment existing and develop new programs to attract researchers and support career pathways for scientists through all stages of the careers of women's health researchers.**
>
> 4a. NIH should create a new subcategory within the Loan Repayment Program (LRP) for investigators conducting research in women's health or sex differences. K awardees who study women's health or sex differences should be automatically considered for an LRP grant. For every year in the program, awardees should receive loan repayment assistance up to $50,000 for up to 5 years, allowing up to $250,000 in loan repayments.

4b. NIH should create new and expand existing early-career grant mechanisms (K, T, and F grants) that specifically support growing and developing the women's health research workforce. Appropriate models for new mechanisms are the Stephen I. Katz and Grants for Early Medical/Surgical Specialists' Transition to Aging Research awards. These grants should prioritize early-career investigators with innovative approaches focused on women's health.

4c. NIH should create new and expand existing mid-career investigator awards to support and promote the mid-career women's health research workforce (e.g., K24, R35, U, P, and administrative supplement grants).

4d. NIH should allow financial support of up to 10 percent, as a line-item component, for mentors (primary or designee mentor) on all mentored grants, such as F31, K01, K99, and T32 grants, that support careers of early and midcareer investigators in women's health and sex differences research.

4e. All early-career mentored institutional K-awards should be supported up to 5 years to increase the likelihood of retaining a workforce to study women's health.

Expand WHR Workforce Development Programs

Several WHR workforce development programs have been effective at launching and supporting researchers' careers. However, NIH needs to expand these programs to accelerate growth of the workforce.

Recommendation 5: The National Institutes of Health (NIH) should augment existing and develop new grant programs specifically designed to promote interdisciplinary science and career development in areas related to women's health. NIH should prioritize and promote participation of women and investigators from underrepresented communities.

5a. NIH should double the Building Interdisciplinary Research Careers in Women's Health (BIRCWH) program to achieve a total of 40 centers, with 6 new centers awarded in the next fiscal year and 5 centers each of the following 3 fiscal years. NIH should augment funding for each center to $1.5 million annually, amounting to a total of $60 million per year for the enhanced BIRCWH program.

5b. NIH should expand the Specialized Centers of Research Excellence (SCORE) on Sex Differences program by engaging Institutes and Centers (ICs) to add 5 additional centers to achieve a total of 17 centers over the next 3 to 5 fiscal years. At least three of these centers should reside in the new Women's Health Research

Institute (see Recommendation 1). The NIH director should provide incentives for other ICs to participate in this program, which could include the provision of matching funds from the Office of the Director. NIH should augment funding for each SCORE to $2.5 million annually, amounting to a total of $42.5 million annually for the enhanced SCORE program, with long-term commitment of funds to renew SCORE programs that meet their goals.

5c. NIH should fund additional multi-project program grants, with or without built-in training components, that focus on women's health research (e.g., P and U grants) to both expand research on these topics and to support researchers studying women's health across the career spectrum.

5d. NIH should expand the Women's Reproductive Health Research (WRHR) program to include 5 additional centers to achieve a total of 20 centers over the next 2 fiscal years. Existing centers that have demonstrated successful metrics should receive funding to host additional scholars. The funding for each center should be augmented to $500,000 annually, amounting to a total of $10 million annually for the enhanced WRHR program.

5e. NIH should expand the Research Scientist Development Program (RSDP) to support 10 scholars with full support, including salary, supplies, and travel, for a total of 5 years amounting to $1.25 million annually for the enhanced RSDP program.

However, any expansion should include new funding to ensure that existing research budgets are not reduced. These programs should be distributed across the country, and grantee institutions should collaborate with other disciplines within their organization to offer mentees a comprehensive and multidisciplinary research experience.

OPTIMIZE NIH PROGRAMS AND POLICIES TO SUPPORT WHR

Peer Review

Representation of women's health expertise—including of staff in the Center for Scientific Review, IC program officers and council members, and peer reviewers—is essential during the NIH peer review process. Despite progress in this area, special emphasis panels, not standing study sections, evaluate a large proportion of WHR-related grants, indicating that standing study sections lack the required expertise to review such grants. While NIH has been working to improve representation of expertise throughout the grant peer review process, NIH needs to expand these important efforts to accelerate progress.

Recommendation 6: The National Institutes of Health (NIH) should continue and strengthen its efforts to ensure balanced representation and appropriate expertise when evaluating grant proposals pertaining to women's health and sex differences research in the peer review process.

6a. NIH should sustain and broaden its efforts to systematically employ data science methods to identify experts, use professional networks, and recruit recently funded investigators.

6b. The NIH Center for Scientific Review (CSR) should expand the Early-Career Reviewer program to enroll qualified individuals from underrepresented areas of expertise in women's health and include women's health, sex differences, and sex as a biological variable training for participants.

6c. CSR should work with NIH-funded institutions to identify qualified individuals with expertise in women's health. Institutions would provide rosters of trained reviewers to CSR to enrich the pool of reviewers.

6d. In the immediate term, special emphasis panels should be used more often to ensure that applications for women's health and sex differences research receive expert and appropriate reviews.

Sex as a Biological Variable (SABV) Policy

Addressing the persistent and extensive gaps in knowledge about how conditions disproportionately affect, present in, and progress differently in women requires that SABV be meaningfully factored into research designs, analyses, and reporting in vertebrate animal and human studies. NIH's SABV policy represents an important advancement, and the number of grants addressing SABV has increased since NIH instituted it. However, overall uptake and application of SABV in practice has not been optimal. This is in part due to a lack of practical, field-specific SABV knowledge and experience among investigators and limited NIH oversight and assurance of implementation. Although guidance and trainings on the SABV policy outline distinctions between sex and gender and indicate in some ways that studies of gender satisfy adherence to the policy, the policy's language and implementation is not clearly geared toward studies of gender, gender identity, and intersex status. In addition, although SABV is a scorable review criterion in the peer review process, NIH has no cross-agency mechanism for assessing how SABV in grants is evaluated or tracking appropriateness and completeness of SABV implementation.[4] Furthermore, grantees face no

---

[4] This sentence was updated after release of the report to clarify that SABV is a scorable review criterion.

consequences if they do not implement their plans for SABV and are not incentivized to do so.

> Recommendation 7: The National Institutes of Health (NIH) should revise how it supports and implements its sex as a biological variable (SABV) policy to ensure it fulfills the intended goals. For its intramural and extramural review processes, where applicable:
>
> 7a. NIH should expand education and training resources for investigators on how to implement SABV, with separate programs that are more effectively tailored for scientists in distinct fields (e.g., basic, preclinical, clinical, translational, and population research).
>
> 7b. NIH should ensure that SABV is consistently and systematically reviewed. Reviewers should be required to undergo training to enable them to assess SABV in proposals and grant applications.
>
> 7c. The NIH Center for Scientific Review should, as part of the competitive renewal applications process, include an evaluation of grantee efforts and publications relating to previously proposed studies of SABV as it applies to the project funded in the last cycle, as well as that proposed in the current renewal application.
>
> 7d. To strengthen and foster research designed to rigorously examine sex, gender, or gender identity differences aimed at providing new insights into women's health, that research should:
> - Be protected from across-the-board budget cuts to protect the sample sizes and analyses needed to study sex differences.
> - Have access to administrative supplements to ensure sex, gender, and gender identity differences can be studied rigorously and with adequate sample size.
> - Have priority for funding when such projects fall in the discretionary range of the payline.
> - Undergo a streamlined process for requesting higher budgets than those allowed by the program announcement or request for proposal.
>
> 7e. NIH should expand the SABV policy in human studies to explicitly factor the effect of biological sex, gender, and gender identity in research designs, analyses, and reporting to promote research on sex and gender diversity, including intersex status, gender expression, and nonbinary-identified populations. This expansion may involve adapting the policy language.[5]

Although Recommendation 7d would afford a unique status to grants that focus on SABV, the committee believes these actions are needed to incentivize and support investigators to address SABV in a meaningful way.

---

[5] Recommendation 7 was changed after release of the report to clarify that it applies to both extramural and intramural research.

When sex is completely accounted for in study designs and analyses, the resulting discoveries benefit the entire population. After the study of sex differences becomes more consistently incorporated into NIH-funded research, these protections can be revisited.

PRIORITY RESEARCH AREAS

Given the breadth of conditions that are female specific, are more common in women, or affect women differently, and the need to support innovation for new lines of inquiry over time, the committee does not provide specific priority women's health conditions to study. Instead, it has identified types of research needed along the research continuum (see Recommendation 8 in Chapter 9). Progress in these domains will advance the field's understanding of the etiology of multiple conditions. For example:

- Basic research that rigorously assesses hormonal profiles and basic female physiology to understand the mechanisms of biological sex differences in risk factors, disease prevalence, pathology, and progression;
- Preclinical research to understand basic etiology of female-specific and gynecologic chronic conditions;
- Clinical research that collects and analyzes data separately for women and men to identify sex and gender differences in treatment efficacy, side effects, and overall effects, with attention to hormonal, genetic, epigenetic, and metabolic factors that might influence pharmacokinetics, pharmacodynamics, and efficacy of drugs and biologic therapies;
- Population-level research that studies how policies at the system, payor, local, state, and national levels affect women's health and whether these have a disparate effect on women at greater risk for marginalization and poorer health outcomes, including racially and ethnically minoritized women, women with disabilities, sexual and gender minority populations, and those who are low income;
- Implementation science research that develops and tests strategies for implementing innovative health care services delivery approaches, focusing particularly on communities experiencing health disparities; and
- Considerations across the research continuum, such as prioritizing conditions that affect a woman's quality of life (e.g., depressive disorder, endometriosis, fibroids, irritable bowel syndrome, osteoarthritis, osteoporosis, and PCOS), to reduce the amount of time women live with painful or debilitating conditions, as well as conditions that cause early mortality, such as CVD and female-specific cancers.

Research on the role of sex, gender, gender identity, and sex beyond the binary within each type of research will improve health of the whole population by improving understanding of the mechanisms through which these factors play a role in disease prevention, development of health conditions, and treatment outcomes. Within these areas, funding should be allocated by a process like that described in Recommendation 3.

INCREASE NIH INVESTMENT IN WHR

The committee was asked to "determine the appropriate level of funding that is needed to address gaps in women's health research at NIH" and recommend "the allocation of funding needed to address gaps in women's health research at NIH." The committee interpreted this as a request to identify the level of funding necessary to catapult new efforts and bolster existing investments in NIH-supported WHR over the next 5 years and into the future.

Since researchers have barely begun to understand the complexities of sex differences in health and neglected research on many female-specific conditions, including the effect of gender and society on women's health, the funding needed to bring the WHR knowledge base up to par with that of conditions for which science has contributed to a deep understanding of prevention, diagnosis, and treatment is significant, and the effort will take decades even with appropriate funding.

The committee recommends that Congress appropriate $15.71 billion in new funding over the next 5 years to invest in women's health and sex differences research and workforce development (see Table S-1). This would approximately double the average NIH annual investment in women's health ($3.41 billion on average over the past 5 years based on the committee funding analysis), with additional funds needed to cover operational costs, increased oversight by the NIH director, and increased funding for the National Institute on Minority Health and Health Disparities.

These investments are only a first step. Putting the United States on a path to improve women's quality of life and decrease morbidity and mortality resulting from conditions that are female specific, are more common in women, or affect women differently requires sustained commitment to WHR, accountability, and integrating and coordinating WHR across all NIH structures and processes. In an ideal world, the nation would invest far more than this amount in the short term, as the need is urgent and the weight of neglecting WHR falls on not only half of the population but society as a whole.

TABLE S-1 New Funding Needed to Accelerate Progress to Fill the Women's Health Research (WHR) Knowledge Gap

Action	New Funding (in Millions of Dollars)					Total 5-Year Funding (New)	Total 5-Year Funding (New and Existing)
	Year 1	Year 2	Year 3	Year 4	Year 5		
New Institute	$800.000	$800.000	$800.000	$800.000	$800.000	$4,000.000	$4,000.000
New Fund	$900.000	$1,500.000	$3,000.000	$3,000.000	$3,000.000	$11,400.000	$11,400.000
Expanded Workforce Programs*	$42.770	$56.795	$66.795	$74.295	$74.295	$314.950	$314.950
Total New Funding	**$1,742.770**	**$2,356.795**	**$3,866.795**	**$3,874.295**	**$3,874.295**	**$15,714.950**	**$15,714,950**
Existing Research Funding for WHR^	$3,405.000	$3,405.000	$3,405.000	$3,405.000	$3,405.000	–	$17,025.000
Total Funding	**$5,147.770**	**$5,761.795**	**$7,271.795**	**$7,279.295**	**$7,279.295**	**$15,714.950**	**$32,739,950**

NOTES: *Expanded workforce programs are: BIRCWH (Building Interdisciplinary Research Careers in Women's Health), RSDP (Reproductive Scientist Development Program), SCORE (Specialized Centers of Research Excellence on Sex Differences), WRHR (Women's Reproductive Health Research Career Development Program). ^Existing research funding is the estimated average spending on WHR 2019–2023 based on the committee's funding analysis and includes the historical workforce investments; assumes no change in years 1 to 5, although this number should increase each year as NIH Institutes and Centers prioritize WHR. New funding calculations are based on Recommendation 5 in this report, with initial ramp up of BIRCWH in years 1 through 4, SCORE in years 1 through 3, and WRHR in years 1 and 2. Current funding for workforce programs was subtracted from the total recommended amount in years 1–5 to calculate expanded workforce program funding.

1

Statement of Task and Approach

INTRODUCTION

While the health and well-being of a population drives its vibrancy and potential, individuals in the United States suffer from many health problems—both acute and chronic—that hamper the overall population's ability to most effectively work, care for their families, and contribute to society. At the same time, the United States is a leader in research innovation and health discoveries for basic, clinical, and translational science, leading to breakthrough treatments, such as vaccines, cancer therapies, regenerative medicine, and various community-based initiatives that have improved the health of the population. However, the biomedical and social scientific enterprises have not yielded the anticipated breakthroughs that contribute to improved health and well-being for half the population in the United States—women and girls.[1] This gap appears, in part, attributable to a lack of baseline understanding of basic sex-based differences in physiology and the lack of attention and support for research into conditions and factors specific to, more common among, or that affect women and girls differently.

---

[1] The terms "female" and "woman" are used differently according to context and perspective, which may cause confusion. For the purpose of this report, the definition of women goes beyond the sex and gender binary and includes all people who identify as a woman or girl, solely or in addition to other gender identities and regardless of biological sex traits. This inclusive definition recognizes individuals who have been or may be affected by a set of biological or social variables that influence women differently than men across the life course (see later in this chapter for a discussion of report definitions).

Advances in women's health research (WHR) contribute to overall scientific progress and innovation by unveiling insights that would be relevant to all. However, it is well documented that WHR is inadequate to meet the needs of women and girls (Baird et al., 2021a; IOM, 2001, 2010; NASEM, 2020, 2022a, 2024b; World Economic Forum, 2024). Data that can help advance health are lost when studied in the aggregate or without sex- and gender-specific analyses. Intentionally studying the underlying sex and gender differences and related mechanisms that shape the evolution of disease and disability leads to stronger science. Furthermore, investments in research to better understand the gender-specific health issues and corresponding interventions will benefit the health of the whole population, enhance the economy, and position the United States as a global leader as it is in other areas of research (World Economic Forum, 2024).

The result of inadequate prioritization of and investment in women's health and sex differences research has perpetuated persistent gaps in our understanding of conditions that are female specific, such as reproductive cancers and fibroids; disproportionately affect women, such as autoimmune disorders and osteoporosis; or affect women differently than men, such as heart disease and diabetes. The inadequate attention paid to women's health and sex differences has created disparities in the diagnosis, prevention, treatment, and outcomes in many conditions that affect women. Girls, women, families, society, and the economy all pay a price for this gap.

Despite having a longer life expectancy than men, women spend more years living with a disability and in poor health—on average, a woman will spend 9 years in poor health, 25 percent more time relative to men, affecting her quality of life and productivity (World Economic Forum, 2024). Conditions that affect both women and men have disparities in outcomes and treatment success. For example, a lifetime invasive cancer diagnosis is more common among men, but recent declines in cancer incidence and mortality have been larger in men (Siegel et al., 2024). Although women have a lower prevalence of cardiovascular disease (CVD)—4.2 percent versus 7.0 percent in men—they have worse prognoses after an acute cardiovascular event, and research on the underlying pathophysiology of why this occurs is limited (CDC, 2023; Gao et al., 2019).

Starting in adolescence, there are conditions specific to the experiences of women and girls, such as menarche and premenstrual dysphoric disorder (PMDD), and several intersex conditions present during the onset of puberty. Many conditions specific to women, such as endometriosis, polycystic ovary syndrome (PCOS), and cervical and uterine cancers, lead to significant morbidity and mortality. Complications during pregnancy, such as gestational diabetes and preeclampsia, are associated with increased risk of developing chronic conditions, such as diabetes and CVD, later in life (ORWH, 2024). On the other end of the life course, more than 1 million U.S. women experience menopause each year (Peacock et al., 2023), but significant gaps in knowledge about its health effects—and the health effects of perimeno-pause—remain (Davis et al., 2023; Moreau and Hildreth, 2014; Samargandy et al., 2022; see Chapters 5 and 7 for more information on research gaps), in large part because of a lack of preclinical research on aging that considers it.[2] Moreover, less than 15 percent of women receive evidence-based treatment for menopausal symptoms, leading to considerable effects on quality of life. The menopause transition can also increase the risk of certain health conditions, including CVD and osteoporosis (Davis et al., 2023). See Chapters 5 and 7 for more examples of women's health outcomes.

Women who are racially and ethnically minoritized, are economically disadvantaged, live in rural areas, or identify as belonging to sexual and gender minority groups, experience a disproportionate burden of disease and adverse outcomes over the life course, including autoimmune diseases, cancer, mental illness, maternal morbidity and mortality, and violence (ORWH, 2024). These inequities are in large part a result of structural factors and lack of access to beneficial social determinants of health (SDOH) (see Chapter 6 for a detailed discussion of this topic) (NASEM, 2023; ORWH, 2024). The women in these populations, and the structural and social factors that contribute to their poor health outcomes, remain largely understudied, underrepresented, and underreported in biomedical research (ORWH, 2024). Moreover, the existing data on health outcomes predominantly reflect the experiences of White patients. In many cases, the data lack disaggregation by race, ethnicity, geography, and other relevant factors, leading to the omission of certain populations—such as American Indian and Alaska Native and Native Hawaiian and Pacific Islander individuals—from both data collection and analysis, masking or misrepresenting their health experiences and challenges (NASEM, 2023). Consequently, the findings presented, including those in this report, may not accurately represent the health realities of all demographic groups. This data gap requires alternative methods for analyzing small samples (see NASEM 2023 and 2024b for more information).

Advances in women's health are absent in many areas, resulting in a lack of prevention, diagnosis, and treatment options for many conditions (Howard et al., 2017; Kuehner, 2017; McHugh et al., 2018; Piccinelli and Wilkinson, 2000):

- Women live longer than men, which is one potential risk factor putting them at double the risk of Alzheimer's disease (AD)—1 in 5 versus 1 in 10 for men.[3] Although women are enrolled at equal rates

---

[2] This sentence was changed after release of the report to update the references cited.

[3] This sentence was changed after release of the report to clarify that life-span is not the only risk factor for AD.

to men in dementia-related clinical trials, the outcomes of those trials infrequently report sex-disaggregated efficacy and safety data (NASEM, 2022b; ORWH, n.d.-a).

- Research on substance misuse and substance use disorders has focused on men, even though sex and gender influence risk, severity, and outcomes (McHugh et al., 2018).
- The cause and risk factors for endometriosis, which can cause severe pain, fatigue, depression, anxiety, and infertility, remain obscure, with little progress over the past 30 years on understanding its pathophysiology (NASEM, 2024b). It has no nonsurgical diagnosis method or cure and frequently recurs even after surgery.
- Fibroids are the leading cause of hysterectomy in the United States, but it takes years from the onset of symptoms to receive a diagnosis (NASEM, 2024b). Although millions are affected by this condition, treatments are limited.
- Eighty percent of people with autoimmune diseases are women, but diagnosis is often delayed due to a lack of understanding of the fundamental mechanisms for most of these diseases (Angum et al., 2020).
- With regard to mental health, research on girls and women for decades has demonstrated that mental health disorders, such as depression and anxiety, are more common than among boys and men. However, limited evidence explains the mechanisms and risk factors producing these gendered differences (Howard et al., 2017; Kuehner, 2017; McHugh et al., 2018; Piccinelli and Wilkinson, 2000).

Data point to a gender disparity in the allocation of National Institutes of Health (NIH) research funding across different diseases, with those that disproportionately affect women underfunded relative to their burden compared to those that disproportionately affect men (see Chapters 4 and 7). Based on an analysis of 2019 NIH funding data and burden of disease data (disability adjusted life-years), one study found that, of 34 conditions that have a disproportionate effect based on gender, 25 are male-favored in that they either disproportionately affect women and are underfunded or disproportionately affect men and are overfunded (Mirin, 2021) (see Figure 1-1). In Figure 1-1, the conditions are arranged by greatest to least burden (panel A) and greatest to least amount of NIH funding (panel B). Disease burden is indicated by the size of the circle representing the condition, and which gender is disproportionately affected is indicated by the circle's color. HIV/AIDS in the United States, for example, is male dominant and a receives a high level of funding relative to its burden.[4]

---

[4] This sentence was changed after release of the report to clarify that the data are based on the U.S. population.

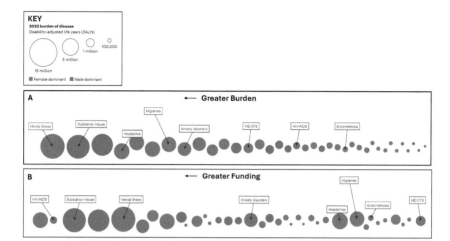

FIGURE 1-1 Female- and male-dominant diseases ranked by burden versus National Institutes of Health (NIH) funding.

NOTES: Mirin (2021) uses burden of disease and funding data provided by NIH. Due to differences between NIH's Research, Condition, and Disease Categorization System and the burden of disease data based on the work of GBD 2015 DALYs and HALE Collaborators, 2016, NIH provides information only for disease categories that it can successfully align. This matching has limitations (i.e., some categories are supersets of others—such as headaches and migraines).

SOURCE: Smith, 2023. © 2023 Springer Nature Limited. All rights reserved.

The funding analysis overseen by this committee identified just 8.8 percent of all NIH spending from fiscal year (FY) 2013–2023 as WHR. It also found that funding for WHR and the number of projects on women's health have remained flat during this period despite steady increases in the NIH budget and total projects (see Chapter 4 and Appendix A for more on the funding analysis and methodology).

To address the disparities in women's health outcomes, Congress requested as part of the Consolidated Appropriations Act of 2023[5] that the National Academies of Sciences, Engineering, and Medicine (National Academies) assemble an ad hoc committee to conduct a study to assess the state of WHR at NIH. The Office of Research on Women's Health (ORWH) at NIH sponsored the study. Specifically, the committee was asked to assess NIH research on women's health, including knowledge gaps and the proportion of NIH-funded research on women's health conditions, including those that are female specific, are more common among women, or affect

---

[5] *Consolidated Appropriations Act of 2023*, Public Law 117–328, §772, 117th Cong., 2d sess. (December 29, 2022).

women differently. The committee was also asked to capture conditions across the life-span, evaluate both sex differences and racial and ethnic health disparities, determine the appropriate level of funding needed to address the identified gaps, and identify metrics to track progress toward closing these gaps (see Box 1-1 for the full committee statement of task).

BOX 1-1
Committee Statement of Task

The National Academies of Sciences, Engineering, and Medicine (National Academies) will convene an ad hoc committee with specific scientific, ethical, regulatory, and policy expertise to develop a framework for addressing the persistent gaps that remain in the knowledge of women's health research across all NIH Institutes and Centers (ICs). Specifically, the study should be designed to analyze the proportion of research that the NIH funds on conditions that are female-specific and/ or more common amongst women or that differently impact women (e.g., different pathophysiology or course of disease), establish how these conditions are defined and ensure that it captures conditions across the lifespan, evaluates sex differences and racial and ethnic health disparities. The committee should define women's health for the purpose of the report, taking into account today's social and cultural climate. Ultimately, the study should determine the appropriate level of funding that is needed to address gaps in women's health research at NIH.

The National Academies consensus committee, as a first step, will conduct an analysis and develop a matrix of identified NIH research on conditions that are female-specific, more common amongst women or that differently impact women, investigating sex differences, and centered on the unique health needs of women.

The committee will make recommendations for the following:

- Research priorities for NIH-supported research on women's health
- NIH training and education efforts to build, support, and maintain a robust women's health research workforce
- NIH structure (extra- and intramural), systems, review processes to optimize women's health research
- NIH-wide workforce to effectively solicit, review and support women's health research
- Allocation of funding needed to address gaps in women's health research at NIH.

The committee will identify metrics to ensure that research is tracked to meet the continuing health needs of women.

In addition, the committee was tasked with making recommendations regarding the following:

- Research priorities for NIH-supported research on women's health;
- NIH training and education efforts to build, support, and maintain a robust WHR workforce;
- NIH structure (extra- and intramural), systems, and review processes to optimize WHR;
- NIH-wide workforce to effectively solicit, review, and support WHR; and
- Allocation of funding such that NIH women's health funding reflects the burdens of disease among women.

URGENCY OF ADDRESSING WHR

Improving women's health through targeted research not only benefits individual women but also has broader societal implications. Healthy women contribute to healthier families, communities, and future generations, and addressing women's health needs can reduce health care costs associated with undiagnosed or improperly managed conditions. Increased health care costs can stem from misdiagnosis or delayed diagnosis resulting from a lack of knowledge in women's health, leading to unnecessary tests, treatments, and hospitalizations. In addition, women often respond differently to treatments compared to men because of biological differences. Therefore, research conducted primarily on male subjects can lead to prescribing medications, dosages, or therapies that are less effective or cause more side effects in women. For example, one recent study found that women are at greater risk for implant failure after a total hip replacement, in part because women tend to have smaller joints and bones than men (Inacio et al., 2013). See Chapter 2 for more information on the history of male-focused research.

Women-specific health conditions, such as those related to reproductive health, or female-dominant conditions, such as autoimmune diseases, often require ongoing management—without proper management, women may have higher health care use rates. Recent data suggest that anxiety and depression, both more prevalent in women than men, accelerate the development of cardiometabolic risk factors, such as hypertension and diabetes (Civieri et al., 2024; COVID-19 Mental Disorders Collaborators, 2021; Goodwin et al., 2022). Civieri and colleagues (2024) noted significant age and sex effects—the association was greater in younger women. The McKinsey Health Institute estimates that addressing the women's health gap could "add years to life and life to years" and that "addressing the 25 percent more time that women spend in 'poor health' relative to men not only would improve the health and lives of millions of women but also could boost the global economy by at least $1 trillion annually by 2040" (World Economic Forum, 2024).

Addressing the women's health gap could improve the quality of life for women and the health of future generations. The McKinsey report found that sex-specific conditions affect women and girls most frequently between the ages of 15 and 50, so although health conditions affect them over the life course, nearly half of this burden falls during their working years, affecting their ability to earn money and support themselves and their families (World Economic Forum, 2024). The authors also looked at 183 of the most widely used interventions across 64 health conditions (e.g., asthma, lower respiratory infections, diabetes mellitus, stroke, and cardiovascular disease) representing roughly 90 percent of the health burden for women. Of the more than 650 academic papers on these conditions, they found that only 50 percent of the interventions studied reported sex-disaggregated data, and when these were available, 64 percent of the interventions studied were found to put women at a disadvantage resulting from lower efficacy, access, or both; for men, this was the case for only 10 percent of interventions (see Figure 1-2) (World Economic Forum, 2024).

Women's health issues, such as chronic conditions, can lead to absenteeism from work, reduced productivity, increased health care-related absences, and reduced economic productivity both at the individual and societal levels (Whiteley et al., 2013; World Economic Forum, 2024). Failure to prioritize women's health can reinforce gender disparities, limiting opportunities for women. Women experiencing poor health may face barriers in accessing education or pursuing career opportunities, affecting their own and their children's future prospects. Furthermore, when a woman is a caregiver, her

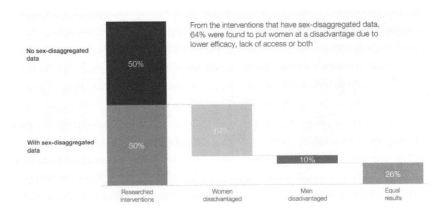

FIGURE 1-2 Effectiveness of and access to interventions vary between men and women.
SOURCE: World Economic Forum, 2024. CC BY-NC-ND 4.0.

own poor health can strain relationships within her family, affecting emotional well-being and family cohesion (see Chapter 6 for more information) (Caputo et al., 2016; CDC, n.d.; DePasquale et al., 2016, 2019).

Investing in WHR is essential to ensure that health care systems can effectively address the diverse and specific health needs of women, leading to better outcomes, improved quality of life, and the ability to lead healthier and more fulfilling lives, participate fully in economic and social activities, and contribute actively to their families, communities, and societies as a whole.

PAST AND ONGOING EFFORTS IN WHR

A robust history of reports and actionable recommendations aimed at enhancing women's health was set against an evolving landscape as this report was written. During the development of this report, notable entities, such as NIH, the White House, and Congress, have introduced programs, legislation, and initiatives, and the private sector has published insightful reports and provided funding for innovative initiatives in women's health. The committee sought to build upon this foundation of work, integrating key insights and initiatives summarized in this section.

Relevant National Academies Reports

This report adds to and builds from numerous past and ongoing efforts to improve women's health (see Table 1-1). Reports from the National Academies and other organizations have provided important background, evidence, and recommendations to advance women's health that this report builds on. Several are summarized next.

The 2001 Institute of Medicine (IOM) report *Exploring the Biological Contributions to Human Health: Does Sex Matter?* explored the knowledge base on and research priorities for animal and cellular models that could be used to determine when sex and gender differences exist and their effect at the cellular, developmental, organ, organismal, and behavioral levels (IOM, 2001). The report concluded that sex and gender differences are an important human variable and recommended considering sex as a biological variable across the life-span in all biomedical and health-related research and promoting research across different life stages to understand the effect of sex differences on health, illness, and longevity.

Building on that 2001 report, in 2010, IOM released *Women's Health Research: Progress, Pitfalls, and Promise.* This report observed that investing in WHR has led to significant advancements in treating conditions such as cancer and heart disease, and continued efforts should integrate women's health into all research while focusing on genetic, behavioral, and social determinants (IOM, 2010). It also concluded there was a lack of accounting for sex and gender differences in the design and analysis

TABLE 1-1 Major Events and Milestones in Federal Women's Health Research (WHR)

Year	Event
1962	After the thalidomide crisis, FDA requires evidence that drugs are "safe and effective," but women of childbearing age are banned from clinical trials.
1975	Pregnant women are designated a vulnerable population in clinical research due to the risks that treatments or interventions may pose to both them and the developing fetus.
1977	NIH prohibits including women of childbearing age in all Phase I/II trials.
1985	*Women's Health: Report of the Public Health Service Task Force on Women's Health Issues* concludes that "the historical lack of research focus on women's health concerns had compromised the quality of health information available to women as well as the health care they receive."
1986	NIH enacts the Inclusion of Women and Minorities in Clinical Research policy, urging NIH funding applicants to include women in human studies.
1987	NIH issues guidelines urging inclusion of women for the first time in NIH Guide to Grants and Contracts.
1990	A GAO review of inclusion of women in clinical research concludes that • NIH policy on inclusion of women in clinical trials was not well communicated or understood within NIH or the research community, applied inconsistently among Institutes, and applied only to extramural research; and • There was "no readily accessible source of data on the demographics of NIH study populations," so it was impossible to determine whether NIH was enforcing its own recommendations. The Women's Health Equity Act is passed. The NIH ORWH is established and requires including women in clinical research.
1991	WHI, the largest clinical study in women, is launched by NIH. NIH ORWH launches strategic planning process to define research priorities for WHR.
1993	The NIH Revitalization Act is signed into law. It requires including women in all clinical research and analyzing results by sex for Phase III clinical trials and formalizes NIH ORWH in law.
1994	NIH guidelines on including women and minority-group members as participants in clinical research (first issued in 1990 and supported by the 1993 NIH Revitalization Act) become effective on publication in *Federal Register* of March 28, 1994; they state that NIH must • Ensure that women and members of minorities and their subpopulations are included in all human subjects research; • For Phase III clinical trials, ensure that women and minorities and their subpopulations must be included such that valid analysis of differences in intervention effect can be accomplished; • Not allow cost as an acceptable reason for excluding these groups; and • Initiate programs and support for outreach efforts to recruit these groups into clinical studies.

TABLE 1-1 Continued

Year	Event
1998	NIH ORWH launches second strategic planning process to define research priorities for WHR and releases *Agenda for Research on Women's Health for the 21st Century.*
2000	GAO issues follow-up audit of NIH that concludes that although women are in clinical trials at rates proportional to their numbers in general population, "NIH has made less progress in implementing the requirement that certain clinical trials be designed and carried out to permit valid analysis by sex, which could reveal whether interventions affect women and men differently."
	NIH ORWH initiates the Building Interdisciplinary Research Careers in Women's Health program to support research career development of junior faculty members (Interdisciplinary WHR scholars) who have recently completed clinical training or postdoctoral fellowships and are commencing basic, translational, clinical, or health services research relevant to women's health.
2002	The Specialized Centers of Research on Sex Differences program, which aims to translate scientific knowledge about how diseases differently impact men and women into new treatments that improve clinical care, is launched.
2006	The NIH Reform Act is reauthorized and directs NIH to "establish an electronic system to uniformly code research grants and activities of the Office of the Director and of all the national research institutes and national centers."
2007	The Working Group on Women in Biomedical Careers is established.
2008	NIH implements the RCDC system for tracking spending. The Working Group on Women in Biomedical Careers launches the Research on Causal Factors and Interventions That Promote and Support Women in Biomedical Careers Initiative.
2009	NIH ORWH launches third strategic planning process to identify research priorities in women's health.
2010	The Patient Protection and Affordable Care Act (Public Law 111–148) formally codifies the Offices of Women's Health within HHS and establishes an Office of Women's Health in the director's office of the Agency for Healthcare Research and Quality, Centers for Disease Control and Prevention, Food and Drug Administration, Health Resources and Services Administration, and Substance Abuse and Mental Health Services Administration. It formally establishes an HHS Coordinating Committee on Women's Health and the National Women's Health Information Center. Each agency is appropriated such sums as are necessary for FY 2010–2014.
2012	NIH ORWH and the National Institute on Aging create the Women of Color Research Network to provide women of color and supporters of their advancement in biomedicine with information about the NIH grants process, advice on career development, and a forum for networking and sharing information.
2014	NIH enacts new policies to address sex differences by requiring applicants to report their cell and animal inclusion plans as part of preclinical experimental design.

(continued)

TABLE 1-1 Continued

Year	Event
2016	The Sex as a Biological Variable policy for NIH-funded research on vertebrate animals and humans becomes effective for applications due on or after January 25, 2016.
	NIH ORWH and the FDA Office of Women's Health launch the Diverse Women in Clinical Trials Initiative to raise awareness about the importance of participation of diverse groups of women in clinical research and share best practices about clinical research design, recruitment, and subpopulation analyses.
2017	NIH updates its policy on the inclusion of women and minorities in clinical research, requiring that NIH-defined Phase 3 clinical trials report results of analyses conducted by sex or gender and race and ethnicity in ClinicalTrials.gov (NOT-OD-18-014).
	NIH launches the U3 Administrative Supplement Program, its only program focused on researching health disparities among populations of women that have been understudied, underrepresented, and underreported (U3) in biomedical research.
2018	The Specialized Centers of Research program is expanded to become the Specialized Centers of Research Excellence on Sex Differences, which establishes 11 new centers, each serving as a national resource for translational research on the role of sex differences in the health of women. It also adds a vital Career Enhancement Core.
2019	NIH offers its first R01 (via RFA-OD-19-029) focused on studying the intersection of sex and gender in health and disease.
2020	In their FY 2021 reports, the House and Senate appropriations committees request that NIH convene a conference to evaluate research underway related to women's health.
2021	*Advancing NIH Research on the Health of Women: A 2021 Conference* is held in response to the 2020 request from the House and Senate appropriations committees.
2023	Congress mandates *Assessment of NIH Research on Women's Health* in the Consolidated Appropriations Act of 2023/Public Law 117–328.
	The Office of the Vice President convenes the White House Roundtable on Maternal Health.
	White House Initiative on Women's Health Research is launched.
2024	ARPA-H Sprint for Women's Health is launched.
	The president issues an Executive Order on Advancing Women's Health Research and Innovation, outlining new mandates on women's health for federal agencies.

NOTES: ARPA-H = Advanced Research Projects Agency for Health; FDA = Food and Drug Administration; FY = fiscal year; GAO = Government Accountability Office; HHS = Department of Health and Human Services; NIH = National Institutes of Health; ORWH = Office of Research on Women's Health; RCDC = Research, Condition, and Disease Categorization; WHI = Women's Health Initiative. Table 1-1 was updated after release of the report to correct the descriptions of four milestones (1986, 2016, 2017, 2019).
SOURCES: Adapted from IOM, 2010; additional information from: FDA, 2024; NASEM, 2022b; ORWH, n.d.-c; Society for Women's Health Research, n.d.

of studies and of reporting on sex and gender differences, problems that persist in research today. The report discussed how disadvantaged women require targeted research to address their disproportionate health burdens. In addition, it concluded that women's quality of life needs more attention from researchers, emphasizing wellness and non-mortality outcomes, and recommended that cross-institute NIH initiatives should explore the common factors influencing multiple diseases in women.

Ovarian Cancers: Evolving Paradigms (NASEM, 2016) and *Enhancing NIH Research on Autoimmune Disease* (NASEM, 2022a) focused on health conditions that are female specific or disproportionately affect women. These two reports concluded that sex differences remain a gap in health research and highlighted the need for more women-centric research. *Advancing Research on Chronic Conditions in Women*, released in July 2024, reviewed the evidence on select chronic conditions, including female-specific and gynecologic conditions and chronic conditions that predominantly affect women or affect them differently. Referencing many reports on related topics in WHR, it concluded that significant gaps persist across the research continuum, from basic science to population health, and continue to hinder prevention, diagnosis, treatment, and management of chronic conditions in women (NASEM, 2024b).

Improving Representation in Clinical Trials and Research: Building Research Equity for Women and Underrepresented Groups (NASEM, 2022b) and *Advancing Clinical Research with Pregnant and Lactating Populations: Overcoming Real and Perceived Liability Risks* (NASEM, 2024a) both highlight the gaps in scientific knowledge about the applicability and effectiveness of medical treatments for women, including pregnant women, resulting from a lack of investment in and inclusion of them in clinical trials. Furthermore, several reports over the past several decades have identified gaps in knowledge about health outcomes, health predictors, and effective translational research for multiple relevant subgroups, such as ethnically minoritized women, lesbian and sexually minoritized women, gender minorities, and intersex populations (IOM, 2001; NASEM, 2020, 2022b,c). These reports, including *Understanding the Well-Being of LGBTQI+ Populations; Measuring Sex, Gender Identity, and Sexual Orientation; and Lesbian Health: Current Assessment and Directions for the Future*, provide recommendations that highlight the ways sex, gender, and gender identity are relevant to effective population research and indicate multiple gaps in our understanding and financial investment, including parenting and pregnancy, aging, and menopause (IOM, 1999; NASEM, 2020, 2022c).

While the United States has made some progress in addressing the research gaps identified in these reports concerning women's health, and some of these recommendations have been put into action, both this report and recent others on autoimmune diseases and chronic conditions in women underscore that substantial progress is still required. The historical and ongoing investment in consensus studies and reports that assess, respond to, and seek to increase WHR provide an important foundation to this report. Moreover, the consistency in their recommendations and calls to action over the years indicate that significant changes are needed to move the needle on increasing and improving science to benefit women's and girls' health.

Recent Relevant Actions and Reports by Nonprofits and Research Institutes

Recently, women's health has garnered a great deal of attention from a variety of organizations. This work has identified research gaps, exploring the depth of the gap in women's health, analyzing the cost of addressing women's health needs, and newly funded activities aimed at advancing women's health.

In 2022, RAND released a series of reports analyzing the effect of increased funding for WHR, focusing on brain health, immune and autoimmune diseases, and CVD (WHAM, n.d.). Using microsimulation models, the study assessed the societal cost of increased funding in rheumatoid arthritis (RA), coronary artery disease (CAD), and AD and AD-related dementias (ADRD) (Baird et al., 2021b,c, 2022). RAND calculated the potential benefits of doubling NIH funding over 30 years, with the assumption that current investments start yielding benefits after 10 years. The reports found that investing in WHR yields higher returns than general research and that small health improvements from increased funding lead to significant savings, such as increased life years, reduced disease years, and enhanced work productivity. It estimates that investing in research in each of these disease areas could generate significant returns in terms of cost savings: $930 million for AD/ADRD, $1.9 billion for CAD, and $10.5 billion for RA (Baird et al., 2021b,c, 2022). The study underscores the potential for significant societal benefits from increased investment in WHR, suggesting that such investments can yield greater gains compared to general research. By using extensive national data on the costs of care and the impact on labor force participation of patients and caregivers and making extremely conservative estimations of the impact of increased investment in research on age prevalence of disease, disease trajectories, and health-related quality of life (a 0.01 percent improvement in each for CAD and ADRD), the study was designed to estimate whether investments in research on women's health would pay for themselves over 30 years by improving survival, reducing disability, and reducing health care and associated costs. For high-impact diseases, these investments greatly exceed that bar. Choosing to only look at return on investment makes it unlikely that the full benefits of improving women's health are realized in the analysis and does not take into account women's other contributions to the economy or the nonmedical costs of these diseases beyond caregiver labor force participation.

The Women's Health Innovation Opportunity Map 2023, developed by the Bill & Melinda Gates Foundation and NIH, identifies 50 critical opportunities to drive innovation and improve women's health. The Innovation Equity Forum calls on stakeholders across the research and development ecosystem to act on these opportunities for equitable, high-return innovations (see Box 1-2 for a summary of the recommended research areas) (Bill & Melinda Gates Foundation and NIH, 2023).

The McKinsey report *Closing the Women's Health Gap: A $1 Trillion Opportunity to Improve Lives and Economies* highlights the significant disparities in women's health and outlines the potential economic and social benefits of addressing these gaps (World Economic Forum, 2024). Despite living longer than men, women spend more years in poor health, leading to considerable losses in productivity and quality of life. The report estimates that addressing this gap could boost the global economy by at least $1 trillion annually by 2040. This can be achieved by investing in women-centric research to fill knowledge gaps about conditions specific to women and understanding

---

BOX 1-2
Recommendations from the Innovation Equity Forum:
Women's Health Innovation Opportunity Map Opportunities

1. **Data and Modeling**
   Data collection and use, capacity building, disease metrics, return on investment data gaps, incorporating qualitative data
2. **Research Design and Methodologies**
   Sex- and gender-intentional research, resource sharing in low-resource settings, computational modeling, translational models
3. **Regulatory and Science Policy**
   Sex- and gender-intentional policies, legal frameworks, outcome reporting, data standardization
4. **Innovation Introduction**
   Data Repositories, innovation hubs, market pathways, innovations in funding, market shaping
5. **Social and Structural Determinants**
   Inclusive agendas, global reviews, intersectional research, grant review representation, cultural practices
6. **Training and Careers**
   Educational resources, educational advocacy, investigating barriers to and enablers of women's careers, enhancing support from men

SOURCE: Bill & Melinda Gates Foundation and NIH, 2023.

sex-based differences in diseases. This report notes that systematic collection and analysis of sex-, ethnicity-, and gender-specific health data are crucial for accurately representing women's health burdens and evaluating intervention impacts. To enhance access to gender-specific care, the report emphasized that it is essential to improve access to prevention, diagnosis, and treatment tailored to women's needs. Establishing policies and financial incentives that support women's health initiatives can further these efforts.

Many organizations are calling for or investing in WHR. In May 2024, for example, the American Cancer Society announced the launch of the largest-ever study of cancer risk and outcomes among Black women, enrolling over 100,000 participants. It will span 30 years and follow Black women aged 25–55 who have not been diagnosed with cancer, aiming to understand the factors contributing to cancer incidence, mortality, and resilience in this high-risk group. The study will survey participants from diverse backgrounds in 20 states about their behavioral, environmental, and lived experiences, without involving medication, clinical testing, treatment, or lifestyle changes. This research is critical because U.S. Black women face the highest cancer death rates and shortest survival times compared to other racial or ethnic groups, with the reasons for these disparities often remaining unclear (American Cancer Society, 2024).

The Commonwealth Fund's 2024 *State Scorecard on Women's Health and Reproductive Care* also highlights wide disparities in women's health and reproductive care. The report offers an examination of women's health care across the United States, reviewing each state on health care access, affordability, quality of care, and health outcomes. The report further notes the need for more rigorous collection of self-reported data on race and ethnicity in medical records and additional research on Black, Hispanic, and American Indian and Alaska Native women, which could improve understanding of the disparities in cancer outcomes in underrepresented communities (Collins et al., 2024).

U.S. GOVERNMENT ACTIONS

The WHR gap is gaining significant recognition by the federal government, including Congress, government agencies, and the White House. Several key actions are described next.

Recent White House Initiatives

White House Roundtable on Maternal Health

In December 2023, building on the White House Blueprint for Addressing the Maternal Health Crisis announced the previous year, the Office of the Vice President convened private-sector leaders for a conversation on improving maternal and infant health. At the roundtable, administration officials and representatives from health start-ups, insurance groups, digital health technology, investors, and others focused on women's health and maternal mortality, discussing how the private-sector and public–private partnerships could address these issues to advance equity and improve access to high-quality care.

As part of the convening, the Centers for Medicare & Medicaid Services announced a new model, Transforming Maternal Health, to support state Medicaid agencies in developing and implementing a whole-person approach to maternal health for women with Medicaid and Children's Health Insurance Program coverage. In addition, Department of Health and Human Services (HHS) officials announced a new maternal health collaborative that would build on efforts across HHS, focusing on data-driven quality improvement in maternal morbidity and mortality postpartum. HHS also announced a Notice of Funding Opportunity for the State Maternal Health Innovation Program aimed to reduce maternal mortality and severe maternal morbidity (White House, 2023b).

White House Initiative on Women's Health Research

In November 2023, the White House launched its Initiative on Women's Health Research, led by the First Lady and White House Gender Policy Council (GPC), which the White House established in 2021 to coordinate with its other policy councils and across all federal agencies to support a strategic approach to advancing gender equality and equity (White House, 2023a). Recognizing that women have been understudied and underrepresented in health research, the initiative aims to spur investment and innovation in WHR, close research gaps, and improve women's health. It involves departments, agencies, and offices across the federal government (see Box 1-3). In February 2024, the First Lady announced its first major output, an investment of $100 million from the Advanced Research Projects Agency for Health for its Sprint for Women's Health, for work from women's health researchers and start-up companies unable to secure private funding (White House, 2023a).

Executive Order on Advancing Women's Health Research and Innovation

In March 2024, the president issued an executive order on Advancing Women's Health Research and Innovation, outlining new mandates for federal agencies. It calls on all agencies to further integrate WHR in federal research programs and prioritize federal investments in it. It calls specifically for ORWH to create and "co-chair a subgroup of the Initiative to promote interagency alignment and consistency in the development of agency research and data standards to enhance the study of women's health," in

---

BOX 1-3
Federal Departments, Agencies, and Offices Involved in the
White House Initiative on Women's Health Research

In addition to its chair, the initiative involves the heads of the following executive departments, agencies, and offices or their designees:

1. The Office of the Vice President
2. The Department of Defense
3. The Department of Agriculture
4. The Department of Health and Human Services
5. The Department of Veterans Affairs
6. The Environmental Protection Agency
7. The Office of Management and Budget
8. The Domestic Policy Council
9. The Office of Science and Technology Policy
10. The National Science Foundation
11. The National Institutes of Health
12. The Food and Drug Administration
13. The Centers for Disease Control & Prevention
14. The Indian Health Service
15. The Centers for Medicare & Medicaid Services
16. The Health Resources and Services Administration
17. The Substance Abuse and Mental Health Services Administration
18. The Agency for Healthcare Research and Quality
19. The Advanced Research Projects Agency for Health
20. The National Institutes of Health Office of Research on Women's Health

The initiative chair may designate involvement from the heads of other agencies and offices.

SOURCE: White House, 2023a.

---

collaboration with the chair of the initiative and the director of the Office of Management and Budget (OMB) (White House, 2024a).

As part of this work, the executive order directs OMB and GPC to identify gaps in federal funding for WHR and submit recommendations to the White House for additional funding and programming needed to advance this research. OMB is also tasked with annually reporting on progress made on these recommendations and consulting with federal agencies on funding needed for WHR (White House, 2024a).

TABLE 1-2 NIH Actions on Women's Health Research (WHR) Related to White House Executive Order

Executive Order Goal	NIH Action
Prioritize and increase investments in WHR	Launch an NIH crosscutting effort to transform women's health throughout the life-span
	Create a dedicated, one-stop shop for NIH funding opportunities on women's health
Foster innovation and discovery in women's health	Support private-sector innovation through additional federal investments in WHR
	Use biomarkers to improve the health of women through early detection and treatment of conditions, such as endometriosis
Expand and leverage data collection and analysis related to women's health	Help standardize data to support research on women's health
Improve women's health across the life-span	Create a comprehensive research agenda on menopause

NOTE: This table is not comprehensive; it lists only NIH actions on WHR that were announced concurrently with the Executive Order on Advancing Women's Health Research and Innovation issued in March 2024.
SOURCE: Information from White House, 2024b.

NIH and Other Agency Actions to Advance WHR

Concurrently with the executive order, agencies also announced new actions in support of WHR (Table 1-2 lists actions announced by NIH). To prioritize and increase investments in WHR, NIH is launching an Institute-wide effort to close gaps in WHR across the life course. It will allocate $200 million of existing NIH funding to this effort beginning in FY 2025, noting that it is "a first step towards the transformative central Fund on Women's Health" at NIH "to advance a cutting-edge, interdisciplinary research agenda and to establish a new nationwide network of research centers of excellence and innovation in women's health" across the life-span (White House, 2024b). The NIH Office of the Director (OD), ORWH, and directors of multiple other NIH Institutes will cochair this effort, which will allow for interdisciplinary projects that cut across the Institutes and Centers (ICs), including research on the effect of perimenopause and postmenopause on heart, brain, and bone health (White House, 2024b). In addition, NIH has created a "one-stop shop" where researchers can find all of its current, open funding WHR opportunities rather than having to search across all Institutes (White House, 2024b).[6]

---

[6] See https://orwh.od.nih.gov/research/funded-research-and-programs/funding-opportunities-and-notices (accessed July 26, 2024).

To foster innovation and discovery in women's health, NIH's Small Business Innovation Research Program and the Small Business Technology Transfer Program[7] will increase their investments supporting research and development in women's health by 50 percent, funding proposals that will help "bridge the gap between performance of basic science and commercialization of resulting innovations" (White House, 2024b). Additionally, NIH is launching a new initiative focused on biomarker discovery and validation research that aims to improve the prevention, diagnosis, and treatment of "conditions that affect women uniquely, including endometriosis" (White House, 2024b).

To expand and leverage data collection and analysis related to women's health, NIH is launching an effort to standardize these data. NIH will bring together data and scientific experts from across the federal government to develop common data elements that will "help researchers share and combine datasets, promote interoperability, and improve the accuracy of datasets when it comes to women's health" (White House, 2024b).

NIH will also develop a research agenda on menopause. This effort will use its Pathways to Prevention Program to summarize the current state of research of menopause, identify gaps, and devise a path forward. The program identifies research gaps in areas of broad public health importance, holding workshops to advance knowledge in these areas (ODP, n.d.). NIH anticipates this effort "will help guide innovation and investments in menopause-related research and care across the federal government and research community" (White House, 2024b).

Other federal agencies have also directed funding to advancing women's health issues as part of the White House Initiative. For example, in July 2024, the Substance Abuse and Mental Health Services Administration announced notices of funding opportunities totaling $27.5 million aimed at improving women's behavioral health. These opportunities include $15 million for the Community-Based Maternal Behavioral Health Services Program, which aims to improve access to evidence-based maternal mental health and substance use treatment. The Women's Behavioral Health Technical Assistance Center, funded at $12.5 million, works to build the capacity of women's behavioral health providers, general health care providers, and others involved in the holistic care of women with or at risk for mental health and substance use conditions (HHS, 2024).

Since the White House Women's Health Initiative and Executive Order on Advancing Women's Health Research and Innovation were launched at the start of the committee's work, with concurrent implementation, this report does not build on or assess these efforts, as the administration's initiatives were in early stages of development.

---

[7] Small Business Innovation Research Program and Small Business Technology Transfer Program are collectively the Small Business Programs. NIH provides funding to early-stage small businesses through these programs. More information can be found at https://seed.nih.gov/small-business-funding/small-business-program-basics/understanding-sbir-sttr.

Recent Congressional Actions

Several recent Congressional actions have also focused on expanding research related to women's health. For example, in 2021, the House and the Senate appropriations committees requested that NIH develop a conference to assess WHR; Advancing NIH Research on the Health of Women focused on chronic debilitating conditions, maternal morbidity and mortality, and stagnant cervical cancer survival rates as its focus areas related to women's health (Temkin et al., 2022). The conference report, *Perspectives on Advancing NIH Research to Inform and Improve the Health of Women*, highlighted the need for clear definitions of chronic debilitating conditions specific to women (ORWH, 2022). It also noted the lack of an NIH Research, Condition, and Disease Categorization (RCDC) code for identifying female-specific research topics in NIH-funded studies. Without a code, it is challenging to quantify research on chronic conditions in women.

The Reproductive Empowerment and Support through Optimal Restoration Act was introduced in June 2024 and is intended to "expand and promote research and data collection on reproductive health conditions" and "provide training opportunities for medical professionals to learn how to diagnose and treat reproductive health conditions."[8] The act directs HHS to collect data and issue reports on women's access to restorative reproductive medicine and infertility care through proper testing, diagnosis, and treatment. It also highlights the use of funding through Title X and the HHS Office of Population Affairs to promote medical training for medical students and professionals to support women with reproductive health conditions and infertility.

In May 2024, 17 senators cosponsored the Advancing Menopause Care and Mid-Life Women's Health Act,[9] which authorized $275 million over 5 years to strengthen and expand federal research on menopause, focusing on workforce training, awareness and education, and health promotion and prevention (gillibrand.senate.gov, 2024). The act calls for establishing new RCDC codes for chronic or debilitating conditions related to menopause and midlife women's health and strengthening coordination within NIH and across HHS to expand research into menopause and midlife women's health (Murray et al., 2024).

While not directly relevant to women's health, in May 2024, Senator Bill Cassidy, M.D. (R-LA), ranking member of the Senate Health, Education, Labor, and Pensions Committee, released a white paper with recommendations about how to modernize NIH. The paper recommends that

---

[8] *RESTORE Act of 2023*, HR 3479, 118th Cong., 1st sess. (May 18, 2023).
[9] Advancing Menopause Care and Mid-Life Women's Health Act, S.4246, 118th Congress (2023–2024). *[This footnote was changed after release of the report to correct the cited House bill HR6749 to Senate Bill 4246.]*

NIH increase its focus on maintaining a balanced portfolio, so all stages of medical research and other public health priorities are funded adequately. This includes "prioritizing work to address diseases of significant unmet need." The white paper also offers recommendations to improve biomedical research within the agency by streamlining peer review of research, addressing challenges in recruiting and maintaining the biomedical workforce, and expanding collaboration between NIH, other public health institutions, and the private sector (Cassidy, 2024). The paper does not mention women's health or sex differences research.

In June 2024, House Energy and Commerce Committee Chair Cathy McMorris Rodgers (R-WA) also released a proposal to reform NIH that included several policy and structural recommendations (Rodgers, 2024). A key recommendation for structural change was reorganizing the 27 ICs into 15, with a realignment intended to improve coordination around research goals, agendas, and constituencies. This realignment proposes consolidating the *Eunice Kennedy Shriver* National Institute of Child Health and Human Development (NICHD)—which studies certain aspects of pregnancy—with the National Institute on Deafness and Other Communication Disorders into a new Institute for Disability Focused Research, which could significantly impact research on women's health, in addition to child health and development. The proposal does not mention women's health or sex differences research. Other policy recommendations include limiting IC leadership terms to 5 years, with two consecutive terms if approved by the NIH director, and limiting grants and awards to primary investigators with no more than three ongoing concurrent NIH engagements.

Summary of Government Actions on Women's Health

It is encouraging to see increased effort and attention on women's health in the United States (see Table 1-1). However, such attention has come and gone over time, with many summative reports noting similar conclusions—more research that will expand and improve the knowledge base in women's and girls' health is urgently needed. To ensure that current efforts stimulate essential interest and investment in WHR and can create real impact, systemic changes are needed to bring parity to the understanding of and ability to address women's health with that of men's health. This report focuses on the pivotal role NIH can play in accomplishing this goal.

WOMEN'S HEALTH AT NIH

The aim of this consensus study was to identify ways NIH could continue to build upon current initiatives and structures and identify needed changes in the interest of optimizing women's and girls' health in the United States. NIH is the largest U.S. government research body, with a budget of $47.1 billion in FY 2024. NIH comprises 27 ICs, each with its own focus and role to advance biomedical research and public health, most of which provide grants to extramural researchers. Though none focuses specifically on WHR, the focus of most ICs includes aspects of women's health. For example, the National Cancer Institute would have women-specific cancers within its purview. NIH also has Offices that support and coordinate various functions across NIH. Some of these Offices support coordination on specific research topics, and while they do not fund extramural research, they can supplement grants from ICs. (See Chapter 3 for an overview of NIH structure and policies and programs related to women's health.)[10]

In 1990, NIH established ORWH to strengthen research on women's health conditions, improve representation in clinical trials, and increase the number of women in biomedical careers (Kirschstein, 1991; Pinn, 1992, 1994). Since then, efforts to improve WHR have been ongoing. ORWH continues to be the hub for women's health at NIH, developing and leading programs and initiatives, such as Building Interdisciplinary Research Careers in Women's Health and Specialized Centers of Research Excellence on Sex Differences, and overseeing important policies, such as sex as a biological variable (ORWH, n.d.-d). NIH-wide, there is a Strategic Plan for Research on the Health of Women that includes goals such as advancing research on the biological, behavioral, social, structural, and environmental factors affecting women's health; supporting research on the biology of how sex influences health and disease; and, through training and education, developing a workforce prepared to advance research on women's health and the science of sex and gender (ORWH, n.d.-b).

THE COMMITTEE'S APPROACH

Definitions and Terms

Terms such as "women," "sex," "female," gender," and other related concepts are used differently across the population and sometimes misused. Therefore, the committee has defined such terms for the purpose of this report. The definitions for "sex," "gender," "women," "women's health," "WHR" (and terms related to these) are discussed next. A full list of report definitions is available in the key terms at the beginning of the report (additional definitions include sexual orientation, sexual and gender minority populations, and structural and social determinants of health).

---

[10] This paragraph was updated after release of the report to clarify the scope of NIH ICs.

Sex and Gender

Sex is a multidimensional construct that refers to biological status, based on a cluster of anatomical and physiological traits that include external genitalia, secondary sex characteristics, gonads, chromosomes, and hormones (NASEM, 2022c). It is typically categorized as male, female, or intersex and determined at birth. Some notable characteristics about sex include

- Usually assigned as female or male;
- Most often defined at birth based on visual inspection of external genitalia;
- Traits usually assumed to be unambiguous but may not be;
- Traits usually assumed to correspond to the same sex but may not; and
- Some traits that can change or be altered over time (NASEM, 2022c).

Intersex refers to people whose sex traits do not all correspond to a single sex (NASEM, 2022c).

A female is an individual whose sex traits (see definition of "sex") include features typically associated with or assigned as female; they typically have any of the following organs or characteristics:

- External genitalia including a vulva, vagina, and/or clitoris; or
- Internal sex organs and gonads including a cervix, uterus, fallopian tubes, or ovaries; or
- Sex chromosome complement that consists of a predominantly X configuration—typically two X chromosomes—in the absence of an active SRY gene.

Female individuals include those who were assigned female at birth and identify as women, men, nonbinary, transgender, genderfluid, and/or Two-Spirit. This definition should not be conflated with that of women; though most women are assigned female at birth, many are not. Furthermore, the definition is not proscriptive, exhaustive, or immutable, as indicated in the definition of sex.

Gender is a multidimensional construct that links gender identity, gender expression, and social and cultural expectations about status, characteristics, and behavior associated with sex traits (NASEM, 2022c). "It influences how people perceive themselves and each other, how they act and interact, and the distribution of power and resources in society. Gender identity is not confined to a binary (girl/woman, boy/man), nor is it static; it exists along a continuum and can change over time. There is considerable diversity in how individuals and groups understand, experience, and express gender through the roles they take on, the expectations placed on them, relations with others, and the complex ways that gender is institutionalized in society" (CIHR, 2023). Gender identity "refers to a person's deeply felt, internal and individual experience of gender, which may or may not correspond to the person's physiology or designated sex at birth" (WHO, n.d.). Gender identities include the following (NASEM, 2022c):

- "Cisgender" ("cis") refers to a person whose current gender identity aligns with the sex they were assigned at birth.
- "Transgender" ("trans"; not "transgendered") refers to a person whose current gender identity differs from the sex assigned at birth.
- "Nonbinary" is often used to describe a gender identity that is neither exclusively man nor woman (i.e., outside the gender binary).
- "Genderqueer" describes a person who does not follow gender norms.
- "Genderfluid" describes a person who does not identify with a fixed gender.
- "Two-Spirit" is a placeholder term for specific gender and sexual orientation identities that are centered in Indigenous tribal worldviews, practices, and knowledges.

Gender binary "refers to the concept that there are only two genders, male and female, and that everyone must be one or the other. The concept is also often misused to assert that gender is biologically determined. This concept also reinforces the idea that men and women are opposites and have different roles in society" (NIH Office of Equity, n.d.). Gender expression is how an individual signals gender to others through behavior and appearance, such as clothing and mannerisms. This may be conscious or subconscious and may or may not reflect gender identity or sexual orientation (NASEM, 2022c; NIH Office of Equity, n.d.).

Race and Ethnicity

In discussions of race and ethnicity, this report refers to "racially and ethnically minoritized" individuals and populations rather than "minorities," recognizing that being minoritized is not about the number of individuals in a population but rather about power and equity (NASEM, 2023).

When referring to specific racial and ethnic populations, this report strives to use language that reflects the preferences of these groups and individuals. However, there is not always consensus on preferred terms, and these preferences may evolve. This report strives to be consistent in its use of the following terms: "American Indian or Alaska Native," "Asian," "Black," "Hispanic or Latino/a/x/e," "Native Hawaiian or Pacific Islander," and "White" (NASEM, 2023). When describing data from cited studies, however, terminology from source papers is used, introducing differences in language throughout the report.

Women, Women's Health, and WHR

As noted, the committee's definition of women goes beyond the sex and gender binary and includes all people who identify as a woman or girl, solely or in addition to other gender identities, regardless of biological sex traits. This inclusive definition recognizes individuals who have been or may be affected by a set of biological and social variables that influence women differently than men across the life course (NASEM, 2022c, 2024b).

Women's health includes physical, biological, reproductive, psychological, emotional, cultural/spiritual health and wellness across the life course for more than those identifying as women or girls. It includes the experiences and needs of all people who identify as a woman, girl, female, nonbinary, transgender (men or women), genderfluid, or Two-Spirit or were assigned female at birth (CIHR, 2022).

WHR is the scientific study of the range of and variability in women's health as defined and the mechanisms and outcomes in disease and non-disease states across the life course. It considers both sex and gender and how these affect women's health and well-being, disease risk, pathophysiology, symptoms, diagnosis, and treatment. This work also addresses interacting concerns related to women's bodies and roles and social and structural determinants and systems (CIHR, 2022).

Approach to Recommendations

Given the scope of WHR, the committee could not review every condition that is female specific, is more common in women, or affects women differently. Instead, the committee reviewed a range of women's health conditions in these categories to identify the types of research gaps across WHR. These examples provided insight into the research enterprise and allowed the committee to identify types of research NIH should prioritize. The committee also leveraged recent evidence-based reports that reviewed the state of WHR and identified gaps, such as the 2022 National Academies report that reviewed autoimmune diseases and the 2024 report on chronic conditions in women (NASEM, 2022a, 2024b). The recommendations were also informed by the committee's funding analysis of WHR at NIH (see Chapter 4 and Appendix A) and review of the NIH WHR structures, policies, and programs.

Report Guiding Principles

The committee's makeup reflects a variety of disciplines and perspectives, as does the approach it took to understand the mechanisms that shape women's health and research. It was guided by a broad range of considerations, including of sex and biology, the sex-gender system, and the role of gender on social position. The gender system and health framework in Figure 1-3 reflects this variety of perspectives the committee brought to its task (Heise et al., 2019).

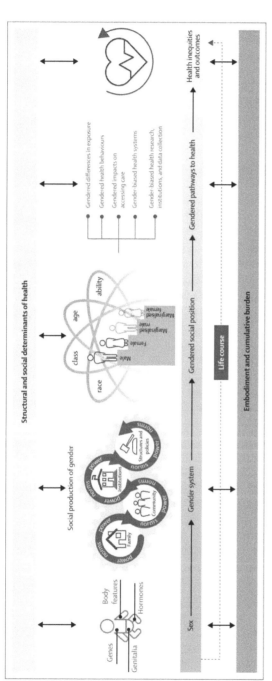

FIGURE 1-3 Heise conceptual framework of the gender system and health.

NOTES: Infants enter the world with a specific biological endowment—ie, male or female genes, body features, genitalia, and hormones. They are immediately immersed into the gender system, depicted as a set of interlocking cogs, representing the domains of the family, community, institutions, and structures and policies, through which power is distributed and norms are created, instilled, and enforced. The system interacts with other axes of power and privilege to shape an individual's overall social position in relation to others. Gender inequalities and restrictive gender norms translate into differential patterns of health and wellbeing for people with different social positions through multiple pathways. Some consequences for health are a function solely of sex and are not mediated through the gender system (dotted arrow). Two additional direct pathways through which social processes condition health-related outcomes across the life course include structural and social determinants of health (top bar) and embodiment and cumulative burden (bottom bar).

SOURCE: Heise et al., 2019. Reprinted from *The Lancet*, 393(10189):2440–2454. Gender inequality and restrictive gender norms: Framing the challenges to health, with permission from Elsevier.

Heise Framework

The Heise sociological framework on the gender system and health provides a comprehensive conceptualization of the profound hierarchy of sex and gender and how these systems are associated with health inequities and outcomes (Heise et al., 2019). It includes the distinction between health differences arising from biological sex, including sex-linked cancers, such as ovarian versus prostate cancer, compared to health inequities that originate from gender inequity and other social hierarchies, not sex.

Sequentially, the framework begins with the biological basis for sex, including the genetic, hormonal, and phenotypic characteristics with which every human is born (Heise et al., 2019). After birth, humans operate in a gender system that includes interlocking levels of society that socially produce gender. These levels include the family, community, institutions, and structures and policies that both formulate and reflect power and norms in societies. The structural inequities at each of these levels co-occur with the social production of gender and have been similarly characterized in several National Academies reports, such as *Communities in Action: Pathways to Health Equity* (NASEM, 2017) and *Federal Policy to Advance Racial, Ethnic and Tribal Health Equity* (NASEM, 2023). These reports describe how structural inequities, biases, and socioeconomic and political drivers impact health equity and SDOH, including education, neighborhood/built environment, social/community context, economic stability, and health care access and quality.

Once gendered, humans are subject to a social position, where intersecting identities such as race, ethnicity, class, sexual orientation and gender identity, age, disability status, immigration status, and sex establish a hierarchy. These gendered social positions produce differential positive and negative exposures leading to health or disease and gendered health behaviors, access to care, health systems, research, institutions, and data collection. These multiple and gendered pathways occur and evolve over the life course and are embodied cumulatively, resulting in poor health and health inequities. Embodiment may refer to the cumulative burden of gender over the life course that may be measured, for example, in the form of stress and allostatic load as a precursor to autoimmune diseases (Krieger, 2001; Mair et al., 2011; Petteway et al., 2019; Rodriquez et al., 2019). The framework also acknowledges the interaction between each of the five main model components and structural and social determinants of health. Each SDOH is gendered, as socioeconomic status, food insecurity, and housing, for example, differentially affect women at the population level, and contribute to health outcomes (WHO, 2008).

The domains detailed in this framework identify the range of women's health issues and factors affecting women's health in the United States, provide a road map for the areas of research needing support from NIH, and highlight factors, particularly structural ones, that may affect participation in the scientific workforce.

Sex and Biology

Sex-specific factors, such as genetics, hormones, organs, biology, and physiology, are important contributors to disease. Basic science in this domain would include studying the normal hormonal changes occurring over the life-span across the types of factors the Heise framework details—genes, hormones, genitals, and body features, for example—and associated with puberty, menstruation, perimenopause, and menopause as physiological stages universally affecting approximately half of all humans (see Chapter 5 for more information on hormones over the life course in women). Similarly, fertility-related issues, such as contraception and fecundity, abortion, pregnancy, lactation, biological mechanisms underlying the onset of labor, and breastfeeding, are commonly experienced phenomena among women and contribute to a significant burden of morbidity.

Hormone therapy, including estrogen and testosterone use, and surgical procedures related to transgender health care are crucial dimensions of women's health. Other important lines of inquiry in this domain include breast, uterine, vaginal, ovarian and cervical cancer, endometriosis, PCOS, vulvodynia, pelvic inflammatory disease, and pregnancy-related conditions, such as preeclampsia, preterm birth, and other contributors to morbidity and mortality in women. In addition to conditions such as these that are primarily sex specific, biological research in this domain includes basic science research on conditions that predominantly affect women or girls, such as myalgic encephalomyelitis and chronic fatigue syndrome, RA, osteoporosis, migraines, and fibromyalgia (Al-Hassany et al., 2020; Alpizar-Rodriguez et al., 2017; Arout et al., 2018; Deumer et al., 2021; Zhang et al., 2024).

The study of sex differences is another aspect of research on the biological components of women's health (Galea et al., 2020; McCarthy, 2024; Reue, 2024). For example, research has found sex differences in the role of estrogen in neuropsychiatric disorders, diabetes and its complications, physiological responses to cardiovascular pathophysiology, and CVD outcomes (Corbi et al., 2024; Gao et al., 2024; Iqbal et al., 2024; Merone et al., 2022; Ndzie Noah et al., 2021). Research that includes and examines differences between male, female, and intersex populations would help with understanding variations in physiological, epigenetic, and other biological pathways producing differences in health outcomes.

Sex-Gender System

It is important to distinguish between sex and gender in understanding risk factors and precursors to health inequities for women (see Figure 1-4). As noted, sex refers to biology, based on a cluster of anatomical and physiological traits that include external genitalia, secondary sex characteristics, gonads, chromosomes, and hormones (NASEM, 2022c). Gender, on the other hand, refers to the social status and power ascribed to people based

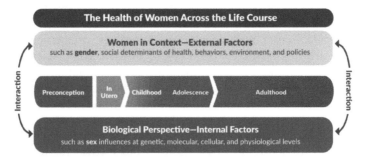

FIGURE 1-4 Dimensions of sex (biological variable) and gender (social and cultural variable).
SOURCE: ORWH, 2022.

on actual and assumed sex characteristics, including norms, behaviors, and associated roles. Both sex and gender are critical to WHR but play different roles. The locus of power lies with the creation of a hierarchy of gender, and this extends to those who do not ascribe to traditional binary sex-gender identities and expressions. These norms and power structures operate at the family, community, institutional, and structural/policy levels. Marginalization of women and gender minorities needs to be addressed to ultimately improve health. This includes social and structural factors, such as gender-based violence, employment policies/norms, parental and caregiving leave, representation of women in government and leadership, and equal pay.

Gendered Social Position

Intersectionality describes how different dimensions of social status and positioning overlap and interact (see Figure 1-5). Several National Academies reports have relied on intersectionality frameworks to ground an analysis of how the impact of a central social status (in this case, woman or female) on health is impacted by the multiple other social statuses held by a person (NASEM, 2020, 2023). The general concept of intersectionality and what it represents in the United States is rooted in the writings of Black and Chicana feminist activists from the 1970s and 1980s, many of them lesbian identified (Combahee River Collective, 1977; Moraga and Anzaldúa, 1983; Smith, 1983). As an academic term, "intersectionality" was initially coined in critical race studies to describe the position of Black women in U.S. culture and specifically employment settings (Crenshaw, 1989). Intersectionality and similar concepts have been further explicated by multiple authors across several disciplines (Battle and Ashley, 2008; Collins and Moyer, 2008; Comas-Díaz and Greene, 1994). It can be applied across multiple dimensions of social status and positioning, including LGBTQIA+ identity

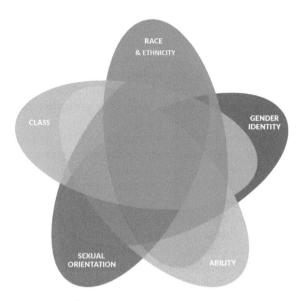

FIGURE 1-5 Intersectionality.
NOTES: This figure illustrates the concept of intersectionality using select examples. Other dimensions of social status and positioning include immigration status and geography.
SOURCE: Adapted from NASTAD, n.d. *Inequities and intersectionality*. https://nastad.org/inequities-and-intersectionality (accessed August 1, 2024). Image designed by Rashad Muhammad.

and status (Agenor et al., 2019; Bowleg, 2012; Lett et al., 2020), disability (Brown and Moloney, 2018; Warner and Brown, 2011), age (Holman and Walker, 2021; Thomas Tobin et al., 2023), weight (Latner et al., 2014; Panza et al., 2020; Reece, 2018; Wilson et al., 2011), and class or socio-economic status (Homan et al., 2021; Iyer et al., 2008). The concept is an important consideration for women's health and WHR, since the health of women and female individuals is affected by not only their sex and/or gender but also these other various aspects of social status.

STUDY PROCESS AND REPORT OVERVIEW

Information-Gathering Process

The committee gathered information in a variety of ways (committee biosketches are available in Appendix D). It held five information-gathering sessions between December 2023 and May 2024 (agendas are available in Appendix C; meetings were virtual or hybrid) on a range of topics, including the state of women's health; an overview of relevant NIH processes, programs, and structures; the state of the science on several areas of WHR; and workforce issues. In addition, the committee heard from interested members of the public at its meetings (see next section for more information). Proceedings of a workshop in brief were developed for the 2-day information-gathering meetings in January and March 2024 (NASEM, 2024c,d). The study's online activity page also informed the public about its work.[11]

The committee examined the literature on WHR to identify research gaps and barriers to such research. The committee was not charged with undertaking a systematic review but to identify research gaps and mechanisms to advance WHR at NIH. The committee conducted a review to gather such information from the peer-reviewed and grey literature (i.e., materials such as government reports, technical reports, white papers), and drew from comprehensive reviews of the evidence and recent National Academies reports. In addition, the committee used data from the NIH RePORTER[12] database to identify funding on WHR at NIH (see Chapter 4 and Appendix A for a description of this process).

Summary of Public Comments

Over the course of the study, the committee received input from patients, clinicians, researchers, advocacy organizations, philanthropies, and others, in both writing and verbal presentations.[13] The committee solicited public comments via the project website and listserv and heard from individuals at its information-gathering meetings. It asked for input on the following and any other aspect of its charge, with a focus on how NIH could better meet the needs of women, per its purview (see summary of comments received in the next section):

- What does "women's health" mean to you? What are important considerations for how to define women's health and WHR?
- What are the knowledge and research gaps in women's health and WHR? What are the barriers to filling these gaps?
- What should be the most important considerations NIH should use in prioritizing the research on women's health it supports?
- From an equity perspective, what improvements can be made to NIH processes to advance health and gender equity in its research investments?

---

[11] See https://www.nationalacademies.org/our-work/assessment-of-nih-research-on-womens-health (accessed June 19, 2024).

[12] See https://reporter.nih.gov/exporter (accessed June 19, 2024).

[13] Public access materials can be requested from PARO@nas.edu.

- How can NIH training and education systems and programs be improved to build and maintain a robust WHR workforce? What are the barriers and opportunities within the current programs?
- How do the structure, systems, and review processes of NIH affect the type of and level of investments in WHR? How could these systems be strengthened and improved to better support advances in women's health?

The committee received over 90 written and verbal responses that covered many topics and included background information on the state of women's health. Many expressed concern about the lack of a clear definition of women's health, leading to misunderstandings of terms such as "more common among women" or "differently impact women." Commentors also raised concerns that among conditions that affect both men and women, sex differences are not communicated.

The comments highlighted the gap in knowledge on women's health, specifically in areas such as major life stages, including puberty, pregnancy, menopause, and aging; perinatal mental health; maternal mortality; endometrial cancer; pelvic floor disorders; menstrual pain; migraines; lung cancer; shifts in estrogen during the life course; postpartum depression; PMDD; vulvodynia; PCOS; endometriosis; and fibroids. Another concern expressed was the underrepresentation of women in clinical trials for certain health conditions, resulting in a lack of gender-specific details in evaluated outcomes. A large proportion of the public comments (39) addressed the lack of funding for WHR. Many expressed that the research gaps will not be resolved if funding levels are not increased.

Commentors also raised critical needs of the women's health workforce. They discussed how the NIH WHR workforce is not adequately supported, and researchers interested in women's health are instead turning to other areas of study that have a steadier stream of funding. They also noted the need to increase funding and diversity of the workforce. Regarding the intramural NIH workforce, commentors noted the lack of development internally, lack of training on women's health and sex differences, and need to hire and retain people with women's health expertise. An additional highlighted challenge was the lack of alignment between priorities and research needs across Institutes and study sections for women's health, such as at the National Institute on Aging, NICHD, and National Institute of Diabetes and Digestive and Kidney Diseases. Suggestions to advance the workforce included recruiting more experts in women's health, particularly in obstetrics, to NIH by expanding fellowship opportunities and ensuring that grant mechanisms prioritize WHR. Others recommended expanding funding and mentorship opportunities for early- and mid-career researchers, integrating research training in postgraduate medical education, and investing in a physician-scientist workforce specializing in women's health conditions, such as pelvic floor disorders.

In addition, the committee received many comments regarding the structure of NIH and how to improve it to advance women's health. Commentors suggested addressing structural barriers, promoting interdisciplinary collaboration, and investing in a dedicated research infrastructure aimed at enhancing research capacity and improving women's health outcomes. Commentors also suggested NIH's structure and review processes should better reflect women's health concerns, including establishing dedicated ICs, transparent funding tracking, and experts who would be better able to appreciate the innovation and methodology in women's health applications on study sections. Several commentors emphasized the need to address the scientific scope of study sections and their performance to ensure the identification of the most impactful applications.

Many commentors highlighted areas of women's health that lack funding to meet research needs and have a substantial effect on quality of life. For example, one noted that endometriosis research funding, which affects about 10 percent of females, is $2 per patient for women, girls, and nonbinary individuals, in comparison to diabetes funding, which affects about 3–7 percent of reproductive age women, which is $31 per patient, or 1,500 percent more, for the same peer group (Azeez et al., 2019; Ellis et al., 2022). Another noted that while chronic vulvovaginal pain significantly impacts quality of life of U.S. women and chronic pelvic pain accounts for 10 percent of all gynecology office visits, both are understudied (Carter, 1999). A patient advocate described how, although many "women in the United States will develop chronic vulvovaginal pain in their lifetime, these conditions are understudied, underfunded, and generally misunderstood and ignored by medical research institutions."

A large proportion of comments highlighted how the knowledge gap on women's health conditions leads to suffering, noting that a "lack of effective treatment options combined with diagnostic delay takes a toll on our hospital systems when patients show up repeatedly with the same symptoms and their gynecologists aren't prepared to treat them" and "women's health has suffered due to historical underinvestment and persistent bias that favored the study of male research subjects." Many comments were sobering, emphasizing the impact of these conditions and the gaps in knowledge and treatment on the lives of patients. Several of these examples are presented throughout the report.

Report Overview

In this report, the committee reviews the state of WRH and NIH structures, systems, policies, and processes that could be improved to ensure a robust WHR infrastructure; assesses NIH's investment in WHR over the past 11 years; and reviews the state of research on women's health. The committee highlights women's health research-related activities at NIH throughout the report as examples; however, due to the breadth of its mandate, the report does not attempt to enumerate every relevant funding opportunity, program, or policy.[14] Chapter 2 provides an overview of why research on women's health is needed. Chapter 3 discusses the NIH structure, policies, and programs that are relevant to WHR, such as the Sex as a Biological Variable policy and peer review process. Next, the committee reviews the process NIH uses to track funding on conditions and diseases and presents the findings of its funding analysis (Chapter 4). The biological basis for women's health through the lens of chromosomes and hormones is reviewed in Chapter 5, and the structural and social drivers of women's health outcomes are discussed in Chapter 6. While it was not possible for the committee to review every condition in depth, in Chapter 7, it presents a framework for quantifying and categorizing health conditions that affect women's morbidity, mortality, and quality of life in different ways and selects exemplars to illustrate pressing needs for further investment in WHR. Chapter 8 provides an overview of the NIH extra- and intramural workforce and discusses barriers and opportunities to growing a robust WHR workforce. The report ends with the committee's conclusions and recommendations based on its findings in Chapters 2–8 (Chapter 9). The committee identified five steps Congress and NIH should take to advance WHR:

1. Create pathways to facilitate and support innovative and transformative research for women's health;
2. Strengthen oversight, prioritization, and coordination for women's health research across NIH;
3. Expand, train, support, and retain the women's health research workforce;
4. Optimize NIH programs and policies to support women's health research; and
5. Increase NIH investment in women's health research.

CONCLUDING OBSERVATIONS

Advancing women's health has far-reaching benefits for families, communities, and society. Healthy women are pivotal for nurturing strong family units, thriving communities, and economic growth. However, the gaps in WHR underscore the urgent need for a concerted and sustained investment and efforts to advance this research. By prioritizing and investing in WHR and improving our understanding of the chromosomal, hormonal,

---

[14] This sentence was added after release of the report to clarify the content of the report.

and gendered impacts on health, better prevention, diagnosis, and treatment interventions to support women's health and well-being can be offered. This is needed to inform and empower women to make decisions about their health, leading to better outcomes and improved quality of life. This collective action is essential for achieving health equity and ensuring that all individuals, regardless of gender, can thrive and contribute actively to society.

REFERENCES

Agenor, M., A. E. Perez, J. W. Koma, J. A. Abrams, A. J. McGregor, and B. O. Ojikutu. 2019. Sexual orientation identity, race/ethnicity, and lifetime HIV testing in a national probability sample of U.S. women and men: An intersectional approach. *LGBT Health* 6(6):306–318.

Al-Hassany, L., J. Haas, M. Piccininni, T. Kurth, A. Maassen Van Den Brink, and J. L. Rohmann. 2020. Giving researchers a headache—sex and gender differences in migraine. *Frontiers in Neurology* 11:549038.

Alpizar-Rodriguez, D., R. B. Mueller, B. Möller, J. Dudler, A. Ciurea, P. Zufferey, D. Kyburz, U. A. Walker, I. von Mühlenen, P. Roux-Lombard, M. Mahler, C. Lamacchia, D. S. Courvoisier, C. Gabay, and A. Finckh. 2017. Female hormonal factors and the development of anti-citrullinated protein antibodies in women at risk of rheumatoid arthritis. *Rheumatology* 56(9):1579–1585.

American Cancer Society. 2024. *To Drive a Deeper Understanding of Cancer Disparities, American Cancer Society Launches Largest U.S. Population Study of Black Women.* https://pressroom.cancer.org/releases?item=1322 (accessed October 21, 2024).

Angum, F., T. Khan, J. Kaler, L. Siddiqui, and A. Hussain. 2020. The prevalence of autoimmune disorders in women: A narrative review. *Cureus* 12(5):e8094.

Arout, C. A., M. Sofuoglu, L. A. Bastian, and R. A. Rosenheck. 2018. Gender differences in the prevalence of fibromyalgia and in concomitant medical and psychiatric disorders: A national Veterans Health Administration study. *Journal of Women's Health* 27(8):1035–1044.

Azeez, O., A. Kulkarni, E. V. Kuklina, S. Y. Kim, and S. Cox. 2019. Hypertension and diabetes in non-pregnant women of reproductive age in the United States. *Preventing Chronic Disease* 16(146).

Baird, M. D., M. A. Zaber, A. Chen, A. W. Dick, C. E. Bird, M. Waymouth, G. Gahlon, D. D. Quigley, H. Al-Ibrahim, and L. Frank. 2021a. *The WHAM report: The case to fund women's health research: An economic and societal impact analysis.* Santa Monica, CA: RAND Corporation.

Baird, M. D., M. A. Zaber, A. W. Dick, C. E. Bird, A. Chen, M. Waymouth, G. Gahlon, D. D. Quigley, H. Al-Ibrahim, and L. Frank. 2021b. *Research funding for women's health: A modeling study of societal impact: Findings for coronary artery disease.* Santa Monica, CA: RAND Corporation.

Baird, M. D., M. A. Zaber, A. W. Dick, C. E. Bird, A. Chen, M. Waymouth, G. Gahlon, D. D. Quigley, H. Al-Ibrahim, and L. Frank. 2021c. *Societal impact of research funding for women's health in Alzheimer's disease and Alzheimer's disease-related dementias.* Santa Monica, CA: RAND Corporation.

Baird, M. D., M. A. Zaber, A. W. Dick, C. E. Bird, A. Chen, M. Waymouth, G. Gahlon, D. D. Quigley, H. Al-Ibrahim, and L. Frank. 2022. *Research funding for women's health: A modeling study of societal impact: Findings for rheumatoid arthritis.* Santa Monica, CA: RAND Corporation.

Battle, J., and C. Ashley. 2008. Intersectionality, heteronormativity, and Black lesbian, gay, bisexual, and transgender (LGBT) families. *Black Women, Gender + Families* 2(1):1–24.

Bill & Melinda Gates Foundation, and NIH. 2023. *Women's health innovation opportunity map 2023: 50 high-return opportunities to advance global women's health R&D.* Seattle, WA: Bill & Melinda Gates Foundation.

Bowleg, L. 2012. The problem with the phrase women and minorities: Intersectionality—an important theoretical framework for public health. *American Journal of Public Health* 102(7):1267–1273.

Brown, R. L., and M. E. Moloney. 2018. Intersectionality, work, and well-being: The effects of gender and disability. *Gender & Society* 33(1):94–122.

Caputo, J., E. K. Pavalko, and M. A. Hardy. 2016. The long-term effects of caregiving on women's health and mortality. *Journal of Marriage and Family* 78(5):1382–1398.

Carter, J. E. 1999. A systematic history for the patient with chronic pelvic pain. *Journal of the Society of Laparoscopic & Robotic Surgeons* 3(4):245–252.

Cassidy, B. 2024. *NIH in the 21st century: Ensuring transparency and American biomedical leadership.* Washington, DC: Senate Committee on Health, Education, Labor, and Pensions.

CDC (Centers for Disease Control and Prevention). n.d. *Caregiving for Family and Friends— a Public Health Issue.* https://www.cdc.gov/aging/caregiving/pdf/caregiver-brief-508.pdf (accessed August 9, 2024).

CDC. 2023. *Heart Disease Prevalence.* https://www.cdc.gov/nchs/hus/topics/heart-disease-prevalence.htm (accessed October 21, 2024).

CIHR (Canadian Institutes of Health Research). 2022. *National Women's Health Research Initiative.* https://cihr-irsc.gc.ca/e/53095.html (accessed August 23, 2024).

CIHR. 2023. *What Is Gender? What Is Sex?* https://cihr-irsc.gc.ca/e/48642.html (accessed October 21, 2024).

Civieri, G., S. Abohashem, S. S. Grewal, W. Aldosoky, I. Qamar, E. Hanlon, K. W. Choi, L. M. Shin, R. P. Rosovsky, S. C. Bollepalli, H. C. Lau, A. Armoundas, A. V. Seligowski, S. M. Turgeon, R. K. Pitman, F. Tona, J. H. Wasfy, J. W. Smoller, S. Iliceto, J. Goldstein, C. Gebhard, M. T. Osborne, and A. Tawakol. 2024. Anxiety and depression associated with increased cardiovascular disease risk through accelerated development of risk factors. *JACC Advances* 3(9):101208.

Collins, S. R., D. C. Radley, S. Roy, L. C. Zephyrin, and A. Shah. 2024. *2024 State Scorecard on Women's Health and Reproductive Care.* https://www.commonwealthfund.org/publications/scorecard/2024/jul/2024-state-scorecard-womens-health-and-reproductive-care (accessed July 19, 2024).

Collins, T., and L. Moyer. 2008. Gender, race, and intersectionality on the federal appellate bench. *Political Research Quarterly* 61(2):219–227.

Comas-Díaz, L., and B. Greene, editors. 1994. *Women of color: Integrating ethnic and gender identities in psychotherapy.* New York: The Guilford Press.

Combahee River Collective. 1977. *The Combahee River Collective statement.* United States, 2015. Web Archive. https://www.loc.gov/item/lcwaN0028151/ (accessed October 30, 2024)

Corbi, G., M. Comegna, C. Vinciguerra, A. Capasso, L. Onorato, A. M. Salucci, A. Rapacciuolo, and A. Cannavo. 2024. Age and sex mediated effects of estrogen and β3-adrenergic receptor on cardiovascular pathophysiology. *Experimental Gerontology* 190:112420.

COVID-19 Mental Disorders Collaborators. 2021. Global prevalence and burden of depressive and anxiety disorders in 204 countries and territories in 2020 due to the COVID-19 pandemic. *Lancet* 398(10312):1700–1712.

Crenshaw, K. 1989. Demarginalizing the intersection of race and sex: A Black feminist critique of antidiscrimination doctrine, feminist theory and antiracist policies. *University of Chicago Legal Forum* 1989(1):139–167.

Davis, S. R., J. Pinkerton, N. Santoro, and T. Simoncini. 2023. Menopause—biology, consequences, supportive care, and therapeutic options. *Cell* 186(19):4038–4058.

DePasquale, N., K. D. Davis, S. H. Zarit, P. Moen, L. B. Hammer, and D. M. Almeida. 2016. Combining formal and informal caregiving roles: The psychosocial implications of double- and triple-duty care. *Journal of Gerontology, Series B* 71(2):201–211.

DePasquale, N., M. J. Sliwinski, S. H. Zarit, O. M. Buxton, and D. M. Almeida. 2019. Unpaid caregiving roles and sleep among women working in nursing homes: A longitudinal study. *Gerontologist* 59(3):474–485.

Deumer, U. S., A. Varesi, V. Floris, G. Savioli, E. Mantovani, P. López-Carrasco, G. M. Rosati, S. Prasad, and G. Ricevuti. 2021. Myalgic encephalomyelitis/chronic fatigue syndrome (ME/CFS): An overview. *Journal of Clinical Medicine* 10(20).

Ellis, K., D. Munro, and J. Clarke. 2022. Endometriosis is undervalued: A call to action. *Frontiers in Global Women's Health* 3:902371.

FDA (Food and Drug Administration). 2024. *OWH History—from the FDA Office of Women's Health.* https://www.fda.gov/consumers/owh-historical-information/owh-history (accessed July 19, 2024).

Galea, L. A. M., E. Choleris, A. Y. K. Albert, M. M. McCarthy, and F. Sohrabji. 2020. The promises and pitfalls of sex difference research. *Frontiers in Neuroendocrinology* 56:100817.

Gao, L., X. Wang, L. Guo, W. Zhang, G. Wang, S. Han, and Y. Zhang. 2024. Sex differences in diabetes-induced hepatic and renal damage. *Experimental and Therapeutic Medicine* 27(4):148.

Gao, Z., Z. Chen, A. Sun, and X. Deng. 2019. Gender differences in cardiovascular disease. *Medicine in Novel Technology and Devices* 4:100025.

GBD 2015 DALYs and HALE Collaborators. 2016. Global, regional, and national disability-adjusted life-years (DALYs) for 315 diseases and injuries and healthy life expectancy (HALE), 1990–2013: A systematic analysis for the Global Burden of Disease Study 2015. *Lancet* 388(10053):1603–1658.

Gillibrand.senate.gov. 2024. *Gillibrand, Other Women Senators Rally to Introduce Historic New Bipartisan Legislation to Boost Menopause Research, Expand Training and Awareness Around Menopause.* https://www.gillibrand.senate.gov/news/press/release/gillibrand-other-women-senators-rally-to-introduce-historic-new-bipartisan-legislation-to-boost-menopause-research-expand-training-and-awareness-around-menopause/ (accessed October 30, 2024).

Goodwin, R. D., L. C. Dierker, M. Wu, S. Galea, C. W. Hoven, and A. H. Weinberger. 2022. Trends in U.S. depression prevalence from 2015 to 2020: The widening treatment gap. *American Journal of Preventive Medicine* 63(5):726–733.

Heise, L., M. E. Greene, N. Opper, M. Stavropoulou, C. Harper, M. Nascimento, D. Zewdie, G. L. Darmstadt, M. E. Greene, S. Hawkes, L. Heise, S. Henry, J. Heymann, J. Klugman, R. Levine, A. Raj, and G. Rao Gupta. 2019. Gender inequality and restrictive gender norms: Framing the challenges to health. *Lancet* 393(10189):2440–2454.

HHS (Department of Health and Human Services). 2024. *Biden-Harris Administration Announces $27.5 Million in Funding Opportunities Enhancing Women's Behavioral Health.* https://www.hhs.gov/about/news/2024/07/08/biden-harris-administration-announces-funding-opportunities-enhancing-women-behavioral-health.html (accessed August 2, 2024).

Holman, D., and A. Walker. 2021. Understanding unequal ageing: Towards a synthesis of intersectionality and life course analyses. *European Journal of Ageing* 18(2):239–255.

Homan, P., T. H. Brown, and B. King. 2021. Structural intersectionality as a new direction for health disparities research. *Journal of Health and Social Behavior* 62(3):350–370.

Howard, L. M., A. M. Ehrlich, F. Gamlen, and S. Oram. 2017. Gender-neutral mental health research is sex and gender biased. *Lancet Psychiatry* 4(1):9–11.

Inacio, M. C. S., C. F. Ake, E. W. Paxton, M. Khatod, C. Wang, T. P. Gross, R. G. Kaczmarek, D. Marinac-Dabic, and A. Sedrakyan. 2013. Sex and risk of hip implant failure: Assessing total hip arthroplasty outcomes in the United States. *JAMA Internal Medicine* 173(6):435–441.

IOM (Institute of Medicine). 1999. *Lesbian health: Current assessment and directions for the future*. Washington, DC: National Academy Press.

IOM. 2001. *Exploring the biological contributions to human health: Does sex matter?* Washington, DC: National Academy Press.

IOM. 2010. *Women's health research: Progress, pitfalls, and promise*. Washington, DC: The National Academies Press.

Iqbal, J., G. D. Huang, Y. X. Xue, M. Yang, and X. J. Jia. 2024. Role of estrogen in sex differences in memory, emotion and neuropsychiatric disorders. *Molecular Biology Reports* 51(1):415.

Iyer, A., G. Sen, and P. Östlin. 2008. The intersections of gender and class in health status and health care. *Global Public Health* 3(sup1):13–24.

Kirschstein, R. L. 1991. Public health policy forum: Research on women's health. *American Journal of Public Health* 81(3):291–293.

Krieger, N. 2001. Theories for social epidemiology in the 21st century: An ecosocial perspective. *International Journal of Epidemiology* 30(4):668–677.

Kuehner, C. 2017. Why is depression more common among women than among men? *Lancet Psychiatry* 4(2):146–158.

Latner, J. D., J. P. Barile, L. E. Durso, and K. S. O'Brien. 2014. Weight and health-related quality of life: The moderating role of weight discrimination and internalized weight bias. *Eating Behaviors* 15(4):586–590.

Lett, E., N. L. Dowshen, and K. E. Baker. 2020. Intersectionality and health inequities for gender minority Blacks in the U.S. *American Journal of Preventive Medicine* 59(5):639–647.

Mair, C. A., M. P. Cutchin, and M. Kristen Peek. 2011. Allostatic load in an environmental riskscape: The role of stressors and gender. *Health & Place* 17(4):978–987.

McCarthy, M. M. 2024. *Science of Sex Differences—Session 3. Presentation to the NASEM Committee on the Assessment of NIH Research on Women's Health, Meeting 3 (March 7, 2024)*. https://www.nationalacademies.org/documents/embed/link/LF2255DA3DD1C41C0A42D3BEF0989ACAECE3053A6A9B/file/D742EE187634F09559D108E4A9EF4805B6A5C0D86737?noSaveAs=1 (accessed March 29, 2024).

McHugh, R. K., V. R. Votaw, D. E. Sugarman, and S. F. Greenfield. 2018. Sex and gender differences in substance use disorders. *Clinical Psychology Review* 66:12–23.

Merone, L., K. Tsey, D. Russell, and C. Nagle. 2022. Sex inequalities in medical research: A systematic scoping review of the literature. *Women's Health Reports* 3(1):49–59.

Mirin, A. A. 2021. Gender disparity in the funding of diseases by the U.S. National Institutes of Health. *Journal of Women's Health* 30(7):956–963.

Moraga, C., and G. E. Anzaldúa. 1983. *This bridge called my back: Writings by radical women of color*. Saline, MI: Third Women Press.

Moreau, K. L., and K. L. Hildreth. 2014. Vascular aging across the menopause transition in healthy women. *Advances in Vascular Medicine* 2014:204390.

Murray, P., L. Murkowski, T. Baldwin, S. Collins, A. Klobuchar, and S. Capito. 2024. *Advancing Menopause Care and Mid-Life Women's Health Act*. https://www.murray.senate.gov/wp-content/uploads/2024/05/One-Pager_Menopause-Bill_Final-1.pdf (accessed July 30, 2024).

NASEM (National Academies of Sciences, Engineering, and Medicine). 2016. *Ovarian cancers: Evolving paradigms in research and care*. Washington, DC: The National Academies Press.

NASEM. 2017. *Communities in action: Pathways to health equity*. Washington, DC: The National Academies Press.

NASEM. 2020. *Understanding the well-being of LGBTQI+ populations*. Washington, DC: The National Academies Press.

NASEM. 2022a. *Enhancing NIH research on autoimmune disease*. Washington, DC: The National Academies Press.

NASEM. 2022b. *Improving representation in clinical trials and research: Building research equity for women and underrepresented groups.* Washington, DC: The National Academies Press.

NASEM. 2022c. *Measuring sex, gender identity, and sexual orientation.* Washington, DC: The National Academies Press.

NASEM. 2023. *Federal policy to advance racial, ethnic, and tribal health equity.* Washington, DC: The National Academies Press.

NASEM. 2024a. *Advancing clinical research with pregnant and lactating populations: Overcoming real and perceived liability risks.* Washington, DC: The National Academies Press.

NASEM. 2024b. *Advancing research on chronic conditions in women.* Washington, DC: The National Academies Press.

NASEM. 2024c. *Discussion of policies, systems, and structures for research on women's health at the National Institutes of Health: Proceedings of a workshop—in brief.* Washington, DC: The National Academies Press.

NASEM. 2024d. *Overview of research gaps for selected conditions in women's health research at the National Institutes of Health: Proceedings of a workshop—in brief.* Washington, DC: The National Academies Press.

NASTAD (National Alliance of State and Territorial AIDS Directors). n.d. *Inequities and Intersectionality.* https://nastad.org/inequities-and-intersectionality (accessed August 1, 2024).

Ndzie Noah, M. L., G. K. Adzika, R. Mprah, A. O. Adekunle, J. Adu-Amankwaah, and H. Sun. 2021. Sex-gender disparities in cardiovascular diseases: The effects of estrogen on ENOS, lipid profile, and NFATS during catecholamine stress. *Frontiers in Cardiovascular Medicine* 8:639946.

NIH Office of Equity, Diversity, and Inclusion. n.d. *Terms and Definitions.* https://www.edi.nih.gov/people/sep/lgbti/safezone/terminology (accessed July 12, 2024).

ODP (Office of Disease Prevention). n.d. *Pathways to Prevention (P2P) Program.* https://prevention.nih.gov/research-priorities/research-needs-and-gaps/pathways-prevention (accessed July 30, 2024).

ORWH (Office of Research on Women's Health). n.d.-a. *NIH Fact Sheets on Women's Health Research.* Washington, DC: National Institutes of Health.

ORWH. n.d.-b. *NIH-Wide Strategic Plan for Research on the Health of Women.* https://orwh.od.nih.gov/about/strategic-plan#:~:text=Forging%20into%20the%20Future:%20 Research,objectives%20of%20the%20strategic%20plan (accessed July 30, 2024).

ORWH. n.d.-c. *Office of Research on Women's Health: Historical Timeline—30 Years of Advancing Women's Health.* https://orwh.od.nih.gov/sites/orwh/files/docs/ORWH21_Timeline_508C.pdf (accessed July 30, 2024).

ORWH. n.d.-d. *ORWH Research Programs & Initiatives.* https://orwh.od.nih.gov/our-work (accessed July 30, 2024).

ORWH. 2022. *Perspectives on Advancing NIH Research to Inform and Improve the Health of Women.* Washington, DC: NIH.

ORWH. 2024. *Health of women of U3 populations data book.* Washington, DC: National Institutes of Health.

Panza, E., K. Olson, C. M. Goldstein, E. A. Selby, and J. Lillis. 2020. Characterizing lifetime and daily experiences of weight stigma among sexual minority women with overweight and obesity: A descriptive study. *International Journal of Environmental Research and Public Health* 17(13).

Peacock, K., K. Carlson, K. M. Ketvertis, and C. Doerr. 2023. Menopause (nursing). In *Statpearls.* Treasure Island, FL: StatPearls Publishing.

Petteway, R., M. Mujahid, and A. Allen. 2019. Understanding embodiment in place-health research: Approaches, limitations, and opportunities. *Journal of Urban Health* 96(2):289–299.

Piccinelli, M., and G. Wilkinson. 2000. Gender differences in depression: Critical review. *British Journal of Psychiatry* 177(6):486–492.

Pinn, V. W. 1992. Women's health research: Prescribing change and addressing the issues. *Journal of the American Medical Association* 268(14):1921–1922.

Pinn, V. W. 1994. The role of the NIH's Office of Research on Women's Health. *Academic Medicine* 69(9):698–702.

Reece, R. L. 2018. Coloring weight stigma: On race, colorism, weight stigma, and the failure of additive intersectionality. *Sociology of Race and Ethnicity* 5(3):388–400.

Reue, K. 2024. *Mechanisms Underlying Sex Differences in Cardiometabolic Disease. Presentation to the NASEM Committee on the Assessment of NIH Research on Women's Health, Meeting 3.* https://www.nationalacademies.org/documents/embed/link/LF2255DA3DD1C41C0A42D3BEF0989ACAECE3053A6A9B/file/D6CD67C8F77A41DD29AD85ABA5F56A4A95B87EC8C535?noSaveAs=1 (accessed July 30, 2024).

Rodgers, C. M. 2024. *Reforming the National Institutes of Health: Framework for discussion.* Washington, DC: House Committee on Energy and Commerce.

Rodriquez, E. J., E. N. Kim, A. E. Sumner, A. M. Nápoles, and E. J. Pérez-Stable. 2019. Allostatic load: Importance, markers, and score determination in minority and disparity populations. *Journal of Urban Health* 96(1):3–11.

Samargandy, S., K. A. Matthews, M. M. Brooks, E. Barinas-Mitchell, J. W. Magnani, R. C. Thurston, and S. R. El Khoudary. 2022. Trajectories of blood pressure in midlife women: Does menopause matter? *Circulation Research* 130(3):312–322.

Siegel, R. L., A. N. Giaquinto, and A. Jemal. 2024. Cancer statistics, 2024. *CA* 74(1):12–49.

Smith, B. 1983. *Home girls: A Black feminist anthology.* New York: Kitchen Table—Women of Color Press.

Smith, K. 2023. *Women's Health Research Lacks Funding – These Charts Show How.* https://www.nature.com/immersive/d41586-023-01475-2/index.html (accessed February 1, 2024).

Society for Women's Health Research. n.d. *The Role of Women's Health Research.* https://swhr.org/about/the-role-of-womens-health-research/ (accessed July 18, 2024).

Temkin, S. M., S. Noursi, J. G. Regensteiner, P. Stratton, and J. A. Clayton. 2022. Perspectives from advancing National Institutes of Health research to inform and improve the health of women: A conference summary. *Obstetrics and Gynecology* 140(1):10–19.

Thomas Tobin, C. S., Á. Gutiérrez, H. R. Farmer, C. L. Erving, and T. W. Hargrove. 2023. Intersectional approaches to minority aging research. *Current Epidemiology Reports* 10(1):33–43.

Warner, D. F., and T. H. Brown. 2011. Understanding how race/ethnicity and gender define age-trajectories of disability: An intersectionality approach. *Social Science & Medicine* 72(8):1236–1248.

WHAM (Women's Health Access Matters). n.d. *The WHAM Report.* https://whamnow.org/the-report/ (accessed July 30, 2024).

White House. 2023a. *Memorandum on the White House Initiative on Women's Health Research.* https://www.whitehouse.gov/briefing-room/presidential-actions/2023/11/13/memorandum-on-the-white-house-initiative-on-womens-health-research/ (accessed October 20, 2024).

White House. 2023b. *Readout of White House Roundtable on Innovation in Maternal Health.* https://www.whitehouse.gov/briefing-room/statements-releases/2023/12/15/readout-of-white-house-roundtable-on-innovation-in-maternal-health/ (accessed April 4, 2024).

White House. 2024a. *Executive Order on Advancing Women's Health Research and Innovation.* https://www.whitehouse.gov/briefing-room/presidential-actions/2024/03/18/executive-order-on-advancing-womens-health-research-and-innovation/ (accessed March 28, 2024).

White House. 2024b. *Fact Sheet: President Biden Issues Executive Order and Announces New Actions to Advance Women's Health Research and Innovation.* https://www.whitehouse.gov/briefing-room/statements-releases/2024/03/18/fact-sheet-president-biden-issues-executive-order-and-announces-new-actions-to-advance-womens-health-research-and-innovation/ (accessed March 25, 2024).

Whiteley, J., M. DiBonaventura, J. S. Wagner, J. Alvir, and S. Shah. 2013. The impact of menopausal symptoms on quality of life, productivity, and economic outcomes. *Journal of Women's Health* 22(11):983–990.

WHO (World Health Organization). n.d. *Gender and Health.* https://www.who.int/health-topics/gender/strengthening-health-sector-response-to-gender-based-violence-in-humanitarian-emergencies#tab=tab_1 (accessed July 30, 2024).

WHO. 2008. *Closing the gap in a generation: Health equity through action on the social determinants of health—final report of the Commission on Social Determinants of Health.* Geneva, Switzerland: World Health Organization.

Wilson, B. D., C. Okwu, and S. A. Mills. 2011. Brief report: The relationship between multiple forms of oppression and subjective health among Black lesbian and bisexual women. *Journal of Lesbian Studies* 15(1):15–24.

World Economic Forum. 2024. *Closing the women's health gap: A $1 trillion opportunity to improve lives and economies.* Cologny, Switzerland: World Economic Forum.

Zhang, Y. Y., N. Xie, X. D. Sun, E. C. Nice, Y. C. Liou, C. Huang, H. Zhu, and Z. Shen. 2024. Insights and implications of sexual dimorphism in osteoporosis. *Bone Research* 12(1):8.

2

The Need for Women's Health Research

INTRODUCTION

This chapter details the many compelling reasons for the nation's research enterprise to prioritize women's health. During its review, the committee identified a clear need for additional funding for women's health research (WHR). However, this need may not be self-evident, as some may point to the existence of the National Institutes of Health (NIH) Office of Research on Women's Health (ORWH) and its successes as an indication that WHR has been prioritized sufficiently. However, decades after NIH established ORWH, several lines of evidence suggest WHR remains under-funded and clinical outcomes for women lag behind men. Women represent 50.5 percent of the U.S. population, and although they live nearly 6 years longer than men, they live longer in poor health and with higher rates of disabilities (Census Bureau, n.d.; Di Lego et al., 2020; Yan et al., 2024).

This chapter illustrates how the factors outlined later in this report—research gaps and social and biological factors—underscore the urgent need for addressing WHR. It describes the centrality of women's health to a healthy society, the exclusion and subsequent underrepresentation of women in health research, the benefits of WHR for the entire population, why female biology requires sex-specific research, and examples of funding opportunities for conditions that are female specific, are more common in women, or affect women differently.

HEALTHY WOMEN ARE VITAL TO A HEALTHY
SOCIETY AND GROWING ECONOMY

Women represent 50.5 percent of the U.S. population and 56.8 percent of the workforce, with their participation in the workforce serving as a key driver of entrepreneurialism and economic growth (BLS, 2023; Bovino and Gold, 2018; Census Bureau, n.d.). Those assigned female at birth are solely responsible for gestation, childbirth, and lactation and the majority of the unpaid caregiving roles in society, including caring for children and older adults (Stall et al., 2023). The health, longevity, and well-being of women is critical to well-functioning families, the U.S. economy, and society at large.

Conditions that are female specific or more common in women affect women's ability to fully participate in society. For example, 10 percent of U.S. menopausal women reported missing work because of menopausal transition symptoms in the past year, which accrued to $1.8 billion in lost days of work (Faubion et al., 2023). Similarly, individuals with recurrent migraines, a condition more common in women than men and most common in women of childbearing age, are more likely to miss work and to do so for extended periods than those without migraine (Bonafede et al., 2018a; Burch et al., 2021). Migraine is estimated to cost employers $13 billion per year resulting from missed workdays and impaired work function (Hu et al., 1999). One study found that approximately 40 percent of adults with migraine were unemployed and 18 percent had no health insurance (Burch et al., 2021). See Box 2-1 for input from a patient regarding how migraines have affected her life.

Women are also more likely than men to engage in volunteerism, through which they contribute to social services, education, and health initiatives (Brown, 2020). Women are essential to the health care workforce. More women than men are nurses, doctors, and other health care workers (Cheeseman Day and Christnacht, 2019). Women also serve as the chief medical officers of their homes, promoting healthy behaviors and ensuring that family members access medical care (Williamson, 2024). Women are overrepresented in the education workforce and so play a critical role in educating the next generation (Superville, 2023). Considering women's central roles to both the workforce and families, research investments to improve women's health, and thereby reduce disability, stand to have a large economic impact (Baird et al., 2021).

WHR: STILL OVERLOOKED, UNDERSTUDIED

The inclusion of women as participants in health research and the study of female animals and tissues have evolved over the past few decades. During the 1970s, few women worked in medicine or science, and women's

---

BOX 2-1
Excerpts from a Patient Advocate During
Public Comments at a Committee Meeting

I started getting migraines when I was five. I only got one or two a year until I was 13. At age 13, I got migraines every day. At age 16, I became debilitated every day until I was 22. From 16 to 22, I was either hospitalized. . . . for inpatient IV therapy or outpatient 3-day IV therapy. Then, from that time, once I went through puberty, things slowed down, but since that time, my migraines are still more than 15 days per month, which is what a normal migraine patient would have. In addition to having normal pain migraines, I also have migraines that have brainstem aura, and I become fully paralyzed. I also have allodynia, which is like having a migraine on my skin.

Most migraine research is done on White males who are of an upper socioeconomic class, however one in five women get migraines. It's much more prevalent in women. And so, that is what I'm asking for, is more migraine research for women, and across racial and ethnic groups . . . and rural regions as well. Native and Indigenous people have the highest prevalence of migraines and severe headaches in the United States.

I grew up in a very rural community. That was part of the reason why it took so long for me to be able to get help. I had to drive 3 hours away in order to get headache access care. And this was back in the '90s. So, one of the things we definitely need to have is better headache research on how to train doctors and nurse practitioners on how to work with migraine patients.

---

health was a low priority in both the scientific and medical fields (ORWH, n.d.-b). Adult male anatomy and physiology were the primary focal point of the study of human health, and women were usually excluded from clinical research studies over concerns about potential risks to fertility and pregnancy and the variability of ovarian hormones and the menstrual cycle. These concerns reflected societal interests in protecting vulnerable populations, which emerged at least in part from discoveries of birth defects resulting from fetal exposure to certain drugs, including thalidomide and diethylstilbestrol (FDA, 2018; ORWH, n.d.-b). Responding to possibility of fetal harm from experimental drug research, the Food and Drug Administration (FDA) issued a 1977 guideline excluding "any premenopausal female capable of becoming pregnant" from participating in Phase I and early Phase II clinical trials (FDA, 2018). Inherent in this guidance was the assumption that women cannot avoid becoming pregnant, that potential risks to fertility and the fetus supersede the benefits to women of participation, and that it is acceptable to refrain from building an evidence base from which to care for women whether or not they are pregnant.

The Belmont Report, published by the National Commission for the Protection of Human Subjects of Biomedical and Behavioral Research in 1977, advanced the conviction that the autonomy of individuals should be respected (National Commission for the Protection of Human Subjects of Biomedical and Behavioral Research, 1979). Scientific, policy, and advocacy communities raised concerns about the practice of excluding women with childbearing potential from research regardless of their desire to participate or the relative potential benefits (IOM, 1994; ORWH, 2021, n.d.-b). Women's health organizations protested this exclusion, stating the FDA guidance had a chilling effect on including women in later-phase clinical trials and prevented women with life-threatening diseases from participating in early-phase trials, regardless of its explicit exception for these circumstances (BLS, 1973; FDA, 2018; IOM, 1994; Liu and Mager, 2016). Despite these concerns, FDA did not explicitly reverse its recommendation until 1993 (FDA, 2018). The new guidelines it issued called for investigators to analyze clinical data to assess the effects of sex on clinical outcomes and highlighted the growing recognition that medications may need to be dosed or administered differently for women (Liu and Mager, 2016).

Simultaneously, NIH was considering policies regarding the inclusion of women in research. Since the establishment of ORWH and the NIH Revitalization Act of 1993, which directed NIH to develop guidance on including women and racially and ethnically minoritized populations in clinical trials, representation of women has improved (Liu and Mager, 2016; ORWH, n.d.-b; Sosinsky et al., 2022). Girls and women made up 57.2 percent of enrollment in NIH-defined clinical research in fiscal year 2014 (ORWH, n.d.-a). However, underrepresentation persists among certain disciplines and conditions, and, among women, pregnant and lactating individuals, sexual- and gender-minority populations, and some racial and ethnic groups remain underrepresented in clinical trials. Moreover, even when research has included underrepresented groups, investigators have not conducted, reported, or published results and analyses specific to these groups (NASEM, 2022, 2023b; Sosinsky et al., 2022).

This history of exclusion is central to understanding the extensive gaps in the evidence base on women's health and the rationale for prioritizing WHR now. Because research conducted in men was assumed to generalize to women and women were viewed as a vulnerable population, systematically excluding them from biomedical research was seen as protective and assumed not to create significant barriers to their health and health care. However, this assumption has turned out to be incorrect in many ways. One striking example is cardiovascular disease (CVD). Early research on heart attack symptoms was based on male participants, which led to a focus on chest pain as the cardinal symptom. Women, however, are less likely than men to experience chest pain and more likely to have other symptoms, including shortness of breath, nausea, and pain between the shoulder blades during a heart attack (van Oosterhout et al., 2020). Differences in symptom presentation have led to misdiagnosis and delayed diagnosis of heart attacks in women, delayed treatment, and worse outcomes. Thus, the weaker evidence base on CVD in women, and differences in male and female physiology and disease course, have confounded care in women (Keteepe-Arachi and Sharma, 2017).

Pharmacologic responses to medications represent a second example of how research conducted in male participants may not generalize to females. Because many drugs were originally tested solely on male participants, dosing recommendations did not account for sex differences in how the body metabolizes different drugs (Courchesne et al., 2024; Huang et al., 2023; Soldin and Mattison, 2009). While one medication, the sleep medicine zolpidem (Ambien), has different dosages for men and women, this dosage is not necessarily supported by scientific evidence (Greenblatt et al., 2019; Zhao et al., 2023). Additional evidence-based research is needed to determine which sex differences in drug metabolism are linked to differences in clinically significant outcomes.

Depression treatment is another example of lack of generalizability from men to women. Although depression is twice as prevalent in women than men and certain reproductive-related hormone changes, especially during and after pregnancy, place women at increased risk of depression, antidepressant clinical trials historically underrepresented women or did not study sex differences and excluded pregnant women (Lee et al., 2023; Soares and Zitek, 2008; Trost et al., 2022; Weinberger et al., 2010). Perinatal depression, for instance, affects more than 15 percent of women and, along with other mental health conditions, is the leading cause of maternal mortality, accounting for 23 percent of pregnancy-related deaths in the United States (Dagher et al., 2021; Payne and Maguire, 2019; Sayres Van Niel and Payne, 2020; Trost et al., 2022).

In the United States, antidepressant medications are more accessible and affordable than other forms of treatment, including psychotherapy, so many women are prescribed these during pregnancy and lactation. Yet, because pregnant women were excluded from the clinical trials, physicians have been left to weigh the risks and benefits based on epidemiologic and observational studies that are considered less compelling and conclusive and offer a lower level of evidence and confidence for informing clinical decisions. Many physicians abruptly stopped antidepressants for women who became pregnant or refused to treat depression in their pregnant patients, causing acute psychiatric crisis. This practice and associated concerns about legal liability continues today (Coffman and Ash, 2019; NASEM, 2023b).

The early underrepresentation of women in mental health research has also affected the management of depression during perimenopause and postmenopause. Drugs in the most common class of antidepressant medication, selective serotonin reuptake inhibitors (SSRIs), were tested primarily in men but prescribed to women across the reproductive life-span. More recent research has shown, however, that SSRIs work less well in women over age 50. Adding estrogen therapy to SSRI treatment appears to restore its efficacy, though many women are ineligible for estrogen therapy because of their age and other health conditions. Moreover, this "solution" has only been tested in small clinical studies (Thase et al., 2005), pointing to the need for research to establish best practices in caring for women experiencing depression over the female life course (Cho et al., 2023; NAMS 2022 Hormone Therapy Position Statement Advisory Panel, 2022).

These and many other gaps in knowledge about women's health fail women and their health care providers, who cannot provide informed care to the degree they can for men. Of the female-specific conditions, gynecologic conditions, such as endometriosis, polycystic ovary syndrome, and premature ovarian insufficiency, generally require a chronic management approach, yet physicians lack clear guidance and state-of-the-art tools to address these costly and debilitating conditions (NASEM, 2024a).

> *The gaps in women's health research are large and at times feel overwhelming. My personal experiences are exacerbated by the frustrations of not being able to help my patients in more meaningful ways, by witnessing my peers and their daughter(s) suffering from so many gynecological conditions that remain with the same ineffective treatments that I offered to patients as an OB/GYN resident over 30 years ago.*
>
> —*Participant at committee information-gathering meeting*

In summary, the medical research gap in gender- and sex-based differences is multifactorial, attributable in some part to sexism, the relative complexity of female physiology, and persistent lack of prioritization of women's health by researchers and the institutions in which they work (Galea et al., 2020; IOM, 2010; Plevkova et al., 2020). The specific examples provided here are merely three among many. However, progress in science is made by building new avenues of investigation on the foundation of existing knowledge of anatomy, physiology, and disease. Many areas of science fail to appreciate the missed opportunities for breakthroughs caused by exclusion of women or female animals and whether the basic understanding of anatomy, physiology, or disease is correct when applied to them (see Chapter 5 for more information). The historical exclusion and subsequent underrepresentation of women in health research and the lack of focus on both sex-specific and non-sex-specific aspects of women's health have limited the understanding of human development, health, and disease and systematically created gaps in knowledge of conditions that are female specific, are more common in women, or affect women differently, including their diagnosis and treatment (Galea et al., 2020; Temkin et al., 2022, 2023).

Unfortunately, including female research participants has not been accompanied by systematic efforts to understand diseases in women—that is, such inclusion alone is insufficient for progress. The range and nature of basic development of female physiology, wide-ranging effects of hormones, and types of chronic diseases and conditions prevalent in women are still poorly understood. As a result, work that includes women is often largely informed by theories and measures that were developed by studying men. This work often continues to rely on the assumption that research findings would be generally similar among women, as though they were smaller versions of men, or that any significant differences would somehow have been identified already. In other words, current research often assumes that past limitations in science no longer affect the quality or applicability of today's findings. Unless these assumptions are systematically discarded, scientific breakthroughs in women's health remain stalled.

Today, research focused on conditions and illnesses that only affect women, are more common in women, and progress differently in women, are lagging and lacking (Temkin et al., 2022, 2023). These knowledge gaps translate into missed opportunities to prevent, diagnose, and treat many conditions and avoid prolonged suffering, disability, or death. As a result, gaps in the evidence base on women's health drive up the costs of care; increased funding to address these gaps can produce a striking return on investment for society as a whole in terms of improved outcomes, savings in health care expenditures, and reductions in potential years of labor force participation lost to disability (Baird et al., 2021).

INTERSECTING BARRIERS TO HEALTH CARE

Substantial barriers, including economic, geographic, institutional, social, and cultural barriers, discrimination and bias, lack of education and health literacy, and stigma, prevent women from accessing and receiving appropriate, acceptable, and effective health care (Long et al., 2023; Vohra-Gupta et al., 2023). While each of these barriers also affect men, they have a different effect on women, and they adversely affect health.

The high cost of health care in the United States is a significant barrier. Costs include insurance premiums, deductibles, and out-of-pocket expenses. Twenty-eight percent of women, compared to 21 percent of men, report they delayed or went without needed care because of the cost (Lopes et al., 2024). Twenty-seven percent of women aged 18–64 report they or a household member had trouble paying medical bills in 2022, compared with

23 percent of men; this includes 42 percent of women who were uninsured, 32 percent each of Hispanic and Black women, and 42 percent of women who report being in fair or poor health (Long et al., 2022). Women aged 19–64 with employer-sponsored coverage experience higher annual out-of-pocket health care costs than men, even when excluding maternity claims, totaling $15 billion more per year; women also derive less actuarial value from each dollar spent on health care premiums (Deloitte, 2023).

Systemic and institutional barriers to care include the shortage of health care providers, lack of workforce diversity, complexity of the health care system, and administrative burden associated with health care (NASEM, 2023a, 2024b). The shortage of health care providers such as primary care physicians and obstetrician-gynecologists is well documented and differentially affects women (AAMC, 2024; Raman and Cohen, 2023). Furthermore, structural care issues and the lack of diversity in the health care workforce also lead to disparities in care, particularly for racially and ethnically minoritized women and those belonging to marginalized groups adversely affected by discrimination, cultural misunderstandings, and language barriers (Chambers et al., 2022; Chauhan et al., 2020; Lange et al., 2017; Prather et al., 2016; Salsberg et al., 2021; Shamsi et al., 2020).

Systemic racism and discrimination, compounded by social and cultural barriers to health care, result in persistent disparities in treatment and outcomes for racially and ethnically minoritized women. Providers' implicit bias leads to poor care access and quality (Chambers et al., 2022; Prather et al., 2016). Black women continue to experience increased risk for pregnancy-related adverse events, including mortality, compared with their White counterparts (Liese et al., 2019; Prather et al., 2016). A recent systematic review demonstrated that a combination of implicit biases, race-based assumptions, and lack of cultural competence in maternity care and medical treatment is associated with adverse birth outcomes for Black women (Montalmant and Ettinger, 2024). Black women are less likely than White women to receive epidural analgesia during labor, be assessed for pain and receive pain treatment after cesarean delivery, and receive episiotomies to reduce the risk of painful vaginal and perianal ruptures (Badreldin et al., 2019; Friedman et al., 2015; Glance et al., 2007; Guglielminotti et al., 2024; Johnson et al., 2019).

Discrimination adversely affects cisgender lesbian and bisexual women and transgender people in a variety of ways (Gioia and Rosenberger, 2022). A recent study reported that 18 percent of LGBTQ adults avoided health care because of anticipated discrimination, including 22 percent of transgender adults (Casey et al., 2019). Trans-identified people and bisexual people were about two times as likely to report an unmet need for mental health care compared with cisgender heterosexual women (Steele et al., 2017). Thus, adverse consequences of health care discrimination faced by these communities contribute to poorer health outcomes, which then go untreated because of fear of discrimination, making for a vicious cycle.

Stigma is another barrier to care that affects health outcomes differently in women because of variations in societal roles, health behaviors, and the types of stigma focused on women. Women face stigma related to mental health issues and substance use, and those experiencing either issue are often perceived as neglectful or irresponsible mothers (Dennis and Chung-Lee, 2006; Nichols et al., 2021; Schofield et al., 2024). Women also face stigma regarding reproductive health issues, including seeking sexual health services, undergoing abortions, and dealing with infertility (Cutler et al., 2021; Öztürk et al., 2021; Valentine et al., 2022). Finally, women are more likely to experience weight-related discrimination and stigma than men, with women at higher weights reporting they experience more discrimination, including medical discrimination ("denied or provided inferior care"), at higher rates than men (45 vs. 28 percent) (Puhl et al., 2008).

Identifying new ways to overcome the disproportionate effect of the systemic and intersecting barriers to health care women experience is an important area for NIH research investment. The structural barriers to health care that NIH-funded research needs to address include employing implementation science to identify ways to overcome economic and geographic barriers to care, including high-quality telehealth services; developing novel service delivery methods to promote collaborative, coherent women's health care across the life-span; identifying evidence-based strategies to reduce stigma and discrimination; and engaging in community-led research to improve the acceptability of treatment alongside efficacy. This research has the potential to not only directly affect and improve women's health and well-being but also increase their overall contributions to productivity in the workplace and at home.

However, this research needs to be effectively translated into practice, with new findings communicated to relevant medical associations and other organizations so they can inform medical guidelines, physician decision making, and policy. One striking example of evidence not being translated is the failure of primary care physicians and internal medicine specialists to incorporate clinical science about women's heart disease into screening and other healthy heart activities (Bairey Merz et al., 2017; Garcia et al., 2016, Isiadinso et al., 2022). NIH has a crucial role in actively disseminating such results, beyond providing the data on its website. NIH could engage with medical journals and associations and facilitate discussions and collaborations to ensure that the latest research informs clinical practice and guidelines. It could also offer enhanced grant support to enable researchers to disseminate their findings more effectively. This could include funding for translating research into lay language, covering open access publication costs in journals, hosting webinars, and supporting other outreach activities to facilitate greater understanding and engagement with the research.

BREAKTHROUGHS IN WOMEN'S HEALTH BENEFIT EVERYONE

Studying sex differences and women independently of men has led to an improved understanding of health for everyone. Two examples of breakthroughs in women's health that benefited men are bone health and cancer treatment (Chapter 5 provides more information on both). One additional research area that holds great promise for men's health is longevity.

Bone Health

Women experience bone loss earlier than men due to changes in hormone levels during the menopause transition (Karlamangla et al., 2021). The porous component of bone that gives bones their strength is what most rapidly declines with age. Thus, as bone loss proceeds, women are at higher risk of fractures, which are associated with premature mortality and significant morbidity and disability, including loss of independence (Kling et al., 2014; McPhee et al., 2022); a nonhormonal class of medications called "bisphosphonates" were developed and approved by FDA to prevent bone loss in women (Karlamangla et al., 2021). Additional research on the mechanisms by which bisphosphonates prevent bone loss resulted in the development of two additional classes of medications and increased knowledge to guide evidence-based screening for bone loss in women. Findings from the studies in women were then tested in men. Based on studying how men did not experience the rapid loss experienced by women during the menopause transition, current guidelines recommend waiting until age 70 to screen men for osteoporosis, if no risk factors are present (Adler, 2000; Bello et al., 2024). Thus, medications developed to combat bone loss in women also benefit men, and surveillance guidelines based on research on women were adapted for men's unique bone loss timeline (see Chapter 5 for more details).

Cancer Treatment

After women undergo surgery for early-stage, estrogen receptor–positive breast cancer, they receive hormone therapy to prevent it from returning. One type, aromatase inhibitors, prevents the body from making estrogen, which is important in the growth of breast cancer (Chumsri et al., 2011). However, just as in the first example of the menopause transition causing bone loss, estrogen depletion caused by aromatase inhibitors causes bone loss, placing women at higher risk of fractures, and research identified nonhormonal treatments to maintain bone health. The American Society of Clinical Oncology set forth recommendations for assessing and preserving bone health for women treated with anti-estrogenic therapies in 2003

(Hillner et al., 2003). Seventeen years later, once testosterone-depleting treatments became the standard of care for prostate cancer, these screening and treatment standards, so well established in women's health, were applied to men (Saylor et al., 2020).

More recently, a new class of medicines, poly(adenosine diphosphate-ribose) polymerase (PARP) inhibitors, were developed to treat metastatic ovarian cancer with *BRCA* mutations in women (Wang et al., 2023). These drugs are effective at reducing cancer progression (MD Anderson Cancer Center, 2023; Taylor et al., 2021). Research examined whether PARP inhibitors could be used to treat breast cancer, and FDA has approved two for breast cancer with *BRCA* mutations (Robson et al., 2017). These discoveries have also benefited men with *BRCA*-mutated prostate cancer, and PARP inhibitors, either alone or in combination with other agents, are now used for certain prostate cancers, including those with *BRCA* mutations (Drew, 2015).

Taken together, these examples demonstrate how studying female-specific physiology and disease can lead to breakthroughs in the understanding of disease mechanisms and help identify new treatments for women. However, these examples also highlight how the breakthroughs that emerge from female-specific research can be tested in male-specific diseases to determine their relevance, thereby benefiting males as well.

Longevity

Although U.S. women generally live in poorer health and with more pain than men, they live 6 percent longer than men. Across nonhuman mammalian species, females live over 18 percent longer than males in the wild, suggesting that sex differences in longevity are at least in part related to biology (Lemaître et al., 2020). Recent research has begun examining the mechanisms contributing to longevity in women compared with men. Some hypothesize that sex chromosomes may be a cause, such as via X-linked mitochondrial inheritance, although these theories are under investigation (Hägg and Jylhävä, 2021). Others hypothesize that sex differences in longevity are related to differences in sex hormones (Hägg and Jylhävä, 2021). For example, castration (and associated testosterone withdrawal) is associated with longer male life-span; however, in mid-life and older men, lower circulating testosterone levels are associated with higher risk of all-cause mortality (Muehlenbein et al., 2022). In women, greater exposure to estrogen across the life-span (measured as a longer reproductive life-span, endogenous estrogen exposure, or total estrogen exposure) was associated with a lower risk of cardiovascular events, which in turn, is related to longer life-span (Mishra et al., 2021). Despite these potential lines of evidence, mechanisms explaining the longer life-span in women (and nonhuman female mammals) has not been clearly identified. Research identifying the mechanisms underlying extended longevity in women may unlock new approaches to extending the life-span for both women and men.

FEMALE-SPECIFIC BIOLOGY AND PHYSIOLOGY

As described in more detail in Chapter 5, certain biological factors—chromosomes and hormones—determine sex and sex characteristics. Differences begin at conception with the sex chromosomes, with most female fetuses having two X chromosomes and most male fetuses having one X and one Y chromosome. To prevent a double dose of X chromosome effects in females, one of the X chromosomes is silenced in every cell in the female body through a variety of mechanisms that have an effect on women's health (Lu et al., 2020).

Most chromosomal research has focused on the Y chromosome (see Chapter 5), and as a result, the effects of X-silencing on women's health are only beginning to be understood. In addition, genome-wide association studies (GWAS), which provide a way to compare the DNA of thousands of people to identify genetic markers for a disease, have typically excluded sex chromosomes (Dou et al., 2024; Lu et al., 2020). To capture the full potential of these methods to identify genetic markers of health and disease in both women and men, it will be essential to include sex chromosomes in GWAS. Some researchers are now beginning to appreciate the need to study these differences, and animal studies have revealed that a protein responsible for X-silencing interacts with myriad other proteins to drive autoimmune diseases more common in women (Dou et al., 2024). This recent breakthrough underscores the role of basic science in helping to explain the disproportionately high number of women compared to men who suffer from autoimmune disorders. Discovering the role of X-linked proteins in contributing to autoimmune disorders may lead to discoveries in other conditions as well.

Fully understanding the biological mechanisms that cause diseases that affect women requires a more extensive understanding of female physiology, which is more dynamic because of hormonal fluctuations during the reproductive life-span. Understanding the complexity of normal physiology in females can help inform how such natural fluctuations contribute to physical and mental health. During puberty, the ovaries mature and begin producing the hormones estrogen and progesterone (Bulun, 2016). Hormonal changes cause the development of secondary sex characteristics, including breasts, ovulation, and menses. Simultaneously, the adrenal glands produce more adrenal hormones, including testosterone (Bulun, 2016). As puberty progresses, ovarian hormone release begins to follow a daily and monthly pattern, the menstrual cycle. As shown

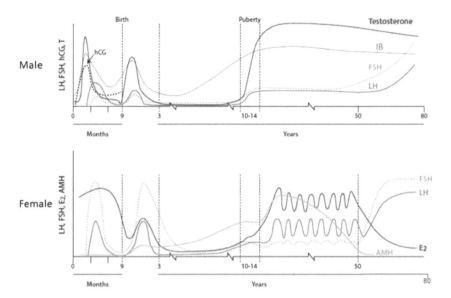

FIGURE 2-1 The HPG axis during prenatal and postnatal life.

NOTES: Circulating concentrations of gonadotropins (hCG, FSH, LH), testosterone, and inhibin B during the prenatal and postnatal period in male individuals (top panel), and gonadotropins, estradiol, and anti-Müllerian hormone in female individuals (lower panel). AMH = Anti-Müllerian hormone; E2 = estradiol; FSH = follicle-stimulating hormone; hCG = human chorionic gonadotropin; HPG = hypothalamic–pituitary–gonadal; IB = inhibin B; LH = luteinizing hormone; T = testosterone.

SOURCE: Adapted from Howard, 2021; licensed under CC BY 4.0 (https://creativecommons.org/licenses/by/4.0/deed.en).

in Figure 2-1, the hormonal changes of female puberty are distinct from those of male puberty (E2 is estradiol, a form of estrogen that varies regularly during the reproductive years) (Bulun, 2016). Many other hormones also follow predictable patterns during the female reproductive life-span in ways that are distinct from hormone changes in men. All organ systems have receptors for female sex hormones, so they powerfully regulate female physiology (Bulun, 2016).

These patterns continue throughout a woman's life until she becomes pregnant or postmenopausal. During pregnancy, the cyclic pattern of change in these hormones stops, and a different pattern emerges (see Figure 2-2); estrogens have multiple roles across many organ systems, including increasing blood flow to the developing fetus, preparing the breasts for lactation, changing metabolism, regulating the cardiovascular system, and modulating the immune system (Delgado and Lopez-Ojeda, 2023; Mauvais-Jarvis et al., 2013). Thus, the effects of estrogen across multiple biological systems are

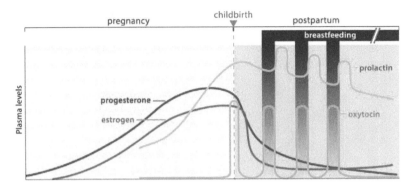

FIGURE 2-2 Estrogen, progesterone, prolactin, and oxytocin levels circulating in the female body during pregnancy and lactation.
SOURCE: Kohl et al., 2017; licensed under CC BY 4.0 (https://creativecommons. org/licenses/by/4.0/deed.en).

necessary to sustain pregnancy, trigger childbirth, and support lactation. While Figure 2-1 does not show the lifetime hormonal patterns for progesterone, that plays a critical role in the menstrual cycle and maintenance of pregnancy (see Figure 2-2), as detailed in Chapter 5.

Menopause marks the end of cyclical menstrual periods resulting from the loss of ovarian function and the end of the reproductive phase of the female life course; the final menstrual period can only be determined retrospectively after 1 year without menses (El Khoudary et al., 2019; Harlow et al., 2012). The menopause transition may occur naturally from aging, as ovaries stop producing eggs and ovarian secretion of estradiol becomes erratic, declines, and then stabilizes at a lower level postmenopause (El Khoudary et al., 2019; Harlow et al., 2012). Declining estrogen levels during this transition, either naturally or prematurely from surgical removal of the ovaries or some drugs used to treat cancer, are associated with a variety of symptoms, including hot flashes, night sweats, bone loss, insomnia, depression, vaginal atrophy and dryness, and weight gain. In addition, the menopause transition is associated with increased risk of Type 2 diabetes, osteoporosis, musculoskeletal symptoms, and cardiovascular disease (Bulun, 2016; Jiang et al., 2019; OASH, 2023; Opoku et al., 2023). The health changes and variety of biological systems affected by the hormonal changes of the menopause transition provide more evidence of the powerful regulation of female physiology by ovarian hormones. Chapter 5 discusses hormonal changes from puberty to postmenopause and their regulation of female biological systems in greater detail.

The field does not know a great deal about how hormones affect health outcomes in females, but studies have shown, for example, that ovarian hormones regulate depression in women across the reproductive years. Fifty-seven percent of adolescent girls (vs. 29 percent of adolescent boys) and 24 percent of women experience depression each year in the United States, and women are about twice as likely as men to do so (CDC, 2023; Lee et al., 2023). This increased risk begins during puberty and persists through the menopause transition, coinciding with ovarian secretion of hormones. Research suggests that ovarian hormone instability during puberty, combined with the stress of adolescence, triggers depression in girls.

Hormonal changes during the menstrual cycle trigger emotional and behavioral changes in some people. Individuals with premenstrual dysphoric disorder, for example, have severe symptoms occurring in the week before menses triggered by changes in estradiol and progesterone levels (Eisenlohr-Moul, 2024). Similarly, research that administered and then withdrew pregnancy-level doses of estrogen and progesterone to women with a history of postpartum depression showed that these hormone changes alone, absent the stress of childbirth and parenting, triggered depression (Bloch et al., 2000). Finally, research on the hormonal changes of peri- and postmenopause has shown that depression symptoms begin as estrogen levels decline during the transition, and short-term treatment with estrogen reverses them (Schmidt et al., 2000). However, recent scientific advances in the understanding of how hormones may regulate mood across the reproductive life cycle have not yet translated into novel treatments or improved access to clinical care, except for perinatal depression. Chapter 5 offers more information about hormone regulation of mood and the need for new treatments and improved access to existing treatments.

In summary, understanding of women's physiology is still limited because of insufficient research specifically focused on how women's bodies function differently from men's. This gap in knowledge means that many aspects of women's health and how women's bodies respond to various conditions and treatments are not well understood. Without well-funded, sustained efforts that focus on women and female model systems, the hormonal and chromosomal contributions to disease pathophysiology and potential therapeutic targets in improving human health represent a missed opportunity.

SYNERGISTIC IMPACT OF BIOLOGICAL AND SOCIAL FACTORS ON WOMEN'S HEALTH

Research often examines biological and social factors influencing women's health in separate studies. However, investigators have begun examining the complex interplay between the biological, social, and environmental factors that shape biology, health, and disease. For example, social and environmental factors have been shown to account for as much as 50 percent of the variability in health outcomes for both women and men, so they are powerful determinants of health (Braveman and Gottlieb, 2014; Magnan, 2021; Whitman et al., 2022; WHO, n.d.). Menarche and the menopause transition provide clear examples of these interacting forces. For example, data suggest that age of menarche may be influenced by social and environmental factors, such as race, ethnicity, financial instability, family stressors, and nutrition (Srikanth et al., 2023; Yermachenko and Dvornyk, 2014). Similarly, social and environmental factors, such as chronic stress, trauma, and early life adversity, are associated with differences in age of menopausal transition onset and symptoms (Cortés and Marginean, 2022). Race is also a factor; compared with White women, Black women in the United States transition to peri- and postmenopause earlier and experience worse symptoms, including hot flashes, depression, and sleep disturbances (Harlow et al., 2022).

Black women are also 3 times more likely than White women to have fibroids, benign growths of uterine muscle that cause excessive menstrual bleeding, pelvic pain, and poor quality of life (Eltoukhi et al., 2014; Marsh et al., 2024). In the United States, fibroids account for over 30 percent of all hysterectomies and up to $9.4 billion in annual health care costs (Bonafede et al., 2018b; Eltoukhi et al., 2014). Rates of inpatient hospitalization for fibroids are highest during the years women begin the menopause transition, ages 40–49. Over 80 percent of Black women experience fibroids by age 50, and over 50 percent of them have fibroids that are clinically significant (they affect quality of life or require treatment) (Eltoukhi et al., 2014). While the source of the increased risk for developing fibroids is unclear, they are thought to be driven by ovarian hormones, genetics, and impaired wound healing. The latter is a hallmark symptom of exposure to both chronic and acute stressors, both from stress's effects on the immune system and the adoption of health-damaging coping behaviors (Gouin and Kiecolt-Glaser, 2011). Because of structural inequities, Black women in the United States are exposed to more stressful and traumatic life experiences than White women and show increased stress hormones following stress exposure (Harlow et al., 2022; Schreier et al., 2016). Thus, while the racial disparity in fibroid incidence is commonly thought to be solely driven by biological factors, the interaction of social and biological factors likely plays a major role.

Furthermore, Black women are more likely to experience comorbid health conditions, including diabetes and heart disease, that are exacerbated by ovarian hormone shifts during the menopause transition (Harlow et al., 2022; Still et al., 2020). Simultaneously, they experience significant disparities in health care, including less access to care, less timely access to care, and care discrimination (Braveman and Gottlieb, 2014; Okoro et al., 2020). Thus, the increased pain and burden of illness in Black women during the transition to menopause are met with a lower likelihood of receiving treatment and poor pain management.

These are just some examples among many of the complex interaction of biological and social factors in women's health outcomes. Similar examples exist for Latina and American Indian or Alaska Native women and women whose bodies do not conform to social expectations for weight and gender expression and those who are immigrants, have differences in physical abilities, are neurodivergent, suffer with mental illness, or have lower socioeconomic status. All of these factors can intersect with racism, sexism, and one another to create unique biological and social interaction effects on health (NASEM, 2017, 2019). Studying the interaction between biological and social factors is therefore critically important to improve diagnosis, optimize treatments, increase access to care, improve care quality, reduce disability, and improve well-being.

CONCLUDING OBSERVATIONS

As summarized in this chapter and detailed throughout the report, the committee identified significant research gaps for women's health and WHR across a number of domains, including a lack of understanding of basic female physiology (Chapter 5), insufficient study of certain conditions (Chapter 7), and inattention to the social determinants of women's health outcomes (Chapter 6), including social and environmental factors that result in health inequities, and the need for research on the interaction of these factors. These gaps provide an opportunity for a concerted and coordinated effort to include more women in clinical trials, increase funding for WHR, and focus on both biological and social determinants of health. With the commitment of essential resources, infrastructure, and accountability, WHR will improve the quality of life of women and their families, benefit the economy, and promote a strong and healthy society.

REFERENCES

AAMC (Association of American Medical Colleges). 2024. *The complexities of physician supply and demand: Projections from 2021 to 2036.* Washington, DC: Association of American Medical Colleges.

Adler, R. A. 2000. Osteoporosis in men. In *Endotext*, edited by K. R. Feingold, B. Anawalt, M. R. Blackman, A. Boyce, G. Chrousos, E. Corpas, W. W. de Herder, K. Dhatariya, K. Dungan, J. Hofland, S. Kalra, G. Kaltsas, N. Kapoor, C. Koch, P. Kopp, M. Korbonits, C. S. Kovacs, W. Kuohung, B. Laferrère, M. Levy, E. A. McGee, R. McLachlan, M. New, J. Purnell, R. Sahay, A. S. Shah, F. Singer, M. A. Sperling, C. A. Stratakis, D. L. Trence, and D. P. Wilson. South Dartmouth, MA: MDText.com, Inc.

Badreldin, N., W. A. Grobman, and L. M. Yee. 2019. Racial disparities in postpartum pain management. *Obstetrics and Gynecology* 134(6):1147–1153.

Baird, M. D., M. A. Zaber, A. Chen, A. W. Dick, C. E. Bird, M. Waymouth, G. Gahlon, D. D. Quigley, H. Al-Ibrahim, and L. Frank. 2021. *Research funding for women's health: Modeling societal impact.* Santa Monica, CA: WHAM and RAND Coorporation.

Bairey Merz, C. N., H. Andersen, E. Sprague, A. Burns, M. Keida, M. Norine Walsh, P. Greenberger, S. Campbell, I. Pollin, C. McCullough, N. Brown, M. Jenkins, R. Redberg, P. Johnson, and B. Robinson. 2017. Knowledge, attitudes, and beliefs regarding cardiovascular disease in women. *Journal of the American College of Cardiology* 70(2):123–132.

Bello, M. O., L. Rodrigues Silva Sombra, C. Anastasopoulou, and V. V. Garla. 2024. Osteoporosis in males. In *Statpearls*. Treasure Island, FL: StatPearls Publishing.

Bloch, M., P. J. Schmidt, M. Danaceau, J. Murphy, L. Nieman, and D. R. Rubinow. 2000. Effects of gonadal steroids in women with a history of postpartum depression. *American Journal of Psychiatry* 157(6):924–930.

BLS (Bureau of Labor Statistics). 2023. *Labor Force Participation Rate for Women Highest in the District of Columbia in 2022.* https://www.bls.gov/opub/ted/2023/labor-force-participation-rate-for-women-highest-in-the-district-of-columbia-in-2022.htm (accessed August 12, 2024).

Bonafede, M., S. Sapra, N. Shah, S. Tepper, K. Cappell, and P. Desai. 2018a. Direct and indirect healthcare resource utilization and costs among migraine patients in the United States. *Headache* 58(5):700–714.

Bonafede, M. M., S. K. Pohlman, J. D. Miller, E. Thiel, K. A. Troeger, and C. E. Miller. 2018b. Women with newly diagnosed uterine fibroids: Treatment patterns and cost comparison for select treatment options. *Population Health Management* 21(S1):S13–s20.

Bovino, B. A., and J. Gold. 2018. *The key to unlocking U.S. GDP growth: Women.* Washington, DC: S&P Global.

Braveman, P., and L. Gottlieb. 2014. The social determinants of health: It's time to consider the causes of the causes. *Public Health Reports* 129(Suppl 2):19–31.

Brown, M. 2020. *Civic Engagement Benefits All of Us. So Why Are Women More Involved Than Men?* https://www.forbes.com/sites/civicnation/2020/03/17/civic-engagement-benefits-all-of-us-so-why-are-women-more-involved-than-men/ (accessed October 3, 2024).

Bulun, S. 2016. Physiology and pathology of the female reproductive axis. In *Williams Textbook of Endocrinology*, 13th ed., edited by S. Melmed, K. S. Polonsky, P. R. Larsen, and H. M. Kronenberg. Philadelphia, PA: Elsevier Health Sciences. Pp. 589–663.

Burch, R., P. Rizzoli, and E. Loder. 2021. The prevalence and impact of migraine and severe headache in the United States: Updated age, sex, and socioeconomic-specific estimates from government health surveys. *Headache* 61(1):60–68.

Casey, L. S., S. L. Reisner, M. G. Findling, R. J. Blendon, J. M. Benson, J. M. Sayde, and C. Miller. 2019. Discrimination in the United States: Experiences of lesbian, gay, bisexual, transgender, and queer Americans. *Health Services Research* 54(S2):1454–1466.

CDC (Centers for Disease Control and Prevention). 2023. *U.S. Teen Girls Experiencing Increased Sadness and Violence.* https://www.cdc.gov/media/releases/2023/p0213-yrbs.html (accessed September 4, 2024).

Census Bureau. n.d. *Quickfacts: United States.* https://www.census.gov/quickfacts/fact/table/US/PST045219 (accessed August 8, 2024).

Chambers, B. D., B. Taylor, T. Nelson, J. Harrison, A. Bell, A. O'Leary, H. A. Arega, S. Hashemi, S. McKenzie-Sampson, K. A. Scott, T. Raine-Bennett, A. V. Jackson, M. Kuppermann, and M. R. McLemore. 2022. Clinicians' perspectives on racism and Black women's maternal health. *Women's Health Reports* 3(1):476–482.

Chauhan, A., M. Walton, E. Manias, R. L. Walpola, H. Seale, M. Latanik, D. Leone, S. Mears, and R. Harrison. 2020. The safety of health care for ethnic minority patients: A systematic review. *International Journal for Equity in Health* 19(1):118.

Cheeseman Day, J., and C. Christnacht. 2019. *Women Hold 76% of All Health Care Jobs, Gaining in Higher-Paying Occupations*. https://www.census.gov/library/stories/2019/08/your-health-care-in-womens-hands.html (accessed October 3, 2024).

Cho, L., A. M. Kaunitz, S. S. Faubion, S. N. Hayes, E. S. Lau, N. Pristera, N. Scott, J. L. Shifren, C. L. Shufelt, C. A. Stuenkel, and K. J. Lindley. 2023. Rethinking menopausal hormone therapy: For whom, what, when, and how long? *Circulation* 147(7):597–610.

Chumsri, S., T. Howes, T. Bao, G. Sabnis, and A. Brodie. 2011. Aromatase, aromatase inhibitors, and breast cancer. *Journal of Steroid Biochemistry and Molecular Biology* 125(1–2):13–22.

Coffman, K. L., and P. Ash. 2019. Medicating during pregnancy. *Focus* 17(4):380–381.

Cortés, Y. I., and V. Marginean. 2022. Key factors in menopause health disparities and inequities: Beyond race and ethnicity. *Current Opinion in Endocrine and Metabolic Research* 26:100389.

Courchesne, M., G. Manrique, L. Bernier, L. Moussa, J. Cresson, A. Gutzeit, J. M. Froehlich, D.-M. Koh, C. Chartrand-Lefebvre, and S. Matoori. 2024. Gender differences in pharmacokinetics: A perspective on contrast agents. *ACS Pharmacology & Translational Science* 7(1):8–17.

Cutler, A. S., L. S. Lundsberg, M. A. White, N. L. Stanwood, and A. M. Gariepy. 2021. Characterizing community-level abortion stigma in the United States. *Contraception* 104(3):305–313.

Dagher, R. K., H. E. Bruckheim, L. J. Colpe, E. Edwards, and D. B. White. 2021. Perinatal depression: Challenges and opportunities. *Journal of Women's Health* 30(2):154–159.

Delgado, B. J., and W. Lopez-Ojeda. 2023. Estrogen. In *Statpearls*. Treasure Island, FL: StatPearls Publishing.

Deloitte. 2023. *Hiding in plain sight: The health care gender toll*. London: Deloitte.

Dennis, C.-L., and L. Chung-Lee. 2006. Postpartum depression help-seeking barriers and maternal treatment preferences: A qualitative systematic review. *Birth* 33(4):323–331.

Di Lego, V., P. Di Giulio, and M. Luy. 2020. Gender differences in healthy and unhealthy life expectancy. In *International Handbook of Health Expectancies*. Cham: Springer. Pp. 151–172.

Dou, D. R., Y. Zhao, J. A. Belk, Y. Zhao, K. M. Casey, D. C. Chen, R. Li, B. Yu, S. Srinivasan, B. T. Abe, K. Kraft, C. Hellström, R. Sjöberg, S. Chang, A. Feng, D. W. Goldman, A. A. Shah, M. Petri, L. S. Chung, D. F. Fiorentino, E. K. Lundberg, A. Wutz, P. J. Utz, and H. Y. Chang. 2024. Xist ribonucleoproteins promote female sex-biased autoimmunity. *Cell* 187(3):733–749.e716.

Drew, Y. 2015. The development of PARP inhibitors in ovarian cancer: From bench to bedside. *British Journal of Cancer* 113(Suppl 1):S3–S9.

Eisenlohr-Moul, T. 2024. *The Menstrual Cycle and Mental Health: Progress, Gaps, and Barriers. Presentation to the NASEM Committee on the Assessment of NIH Research on Women's Health, Meeting 3 (March 7, 2024)*. https://www.nationalacademies.org/documents/embed/link/LF2255DA3DD1C41C0A42D3BEF0989ACAECE3053A6A9B/file/D200E053FE7DBEC81160D764F44F8C5682FD9C162A7A?noSaveAs=1 (accessed August 7, 2024).

El Khoudary, S. R., G. Greendale, S. L. Crawford, N. E. Avis, M. M. Brooks, R. C. Thurston, C. Karvonen-Gutierrez, L. E. Waetjen, and K. Matthews. 2019. The menopause transition and women's health at midlife: A progress report from the study of Women's Health Across the Nation (SWAN). *Menopause* 26(10):1213–1227.

Eltoukhi, H. M., M. N. Modi, M. Weston, A. Y. Armstrong, and E. A. Stewart. 2014. The health disparities of uterine fibroid tumors for African American women: A public health issue. *American Journal of Obstetrics and Gynecology* 210(3):194–199.

Faubion, S. S., F. Enders, M. S. Hedges, R. Chaudhry, J. M. Kling, C. L. Shufelt, M. Saadedine, K. Mara, J. M. Griffin, and E. Kapoor. 2023. Impact of menopause symptoms on women in the workplace. *Mayo Clinic Proceedings* 98(6):833–845.

FDA (Food and Drug Administration). 2018. *Gender Studies in Product Development: Historical Overview.* https://public4.pagefreezer.com/content/FDA/16–06–2022T13:39/https:/www.fda.gov/science-research/womens-health-research/gender-studies-product-development-historical-overview (accessed August 8, 2024).

Friedman, A. M., C. V. Ananth, E. Prendergast, M. E. D'Alton, and J. D. Wright. 2015. Variation in and factors associated with use of episiotomy. *JAMA* 313(2):197–199.

Galea, L. A. M., E. Choleris, A. Y. K. Albert, M. M. McCarthy, and F. Sohrabji. 2020. The promises and pitfalls of sex difference research. *Frontiers in Neuroendocrinology* 56:100817.

Garcia, M., S. L. Mulvagh, C. N. Merz, J. E. Buring, and J. E. Manson. 2016. Cardiovascular disease in women: Clinical perspectives. *Circulation Research* 118(8):1273–1293.

Gioia, S. A., and J. G. Rosenberger. 2022. Sexual orientation-based discrimination in U.S. healthcare and associated health outcomes: A scoping review. *Sexuality Research and Social Policy* 19(4):1674–1689.

Glance, L. G., R. Wissler, C. Glantz, T. M. Osler, D. B. Mukamel, and A. W. Dick. 2007. Racial differences in the use of epidural analgesia for labor. *Anesthesiology* 106(1):19–25; discussion 16–18.

Gouin, J.-P., and J. K. Kiecolt-Glaser. 2011. The impact of psychological stress on wound healing: Methods and mechanisms. *Immunology and Allergy Clinics of North America* 31(1):81–93.

Greenblatt, D. J., J. S. Harmatz, and T. Roth. 2019. Zolpidem and gender: Are women really at risk? *Journal of Clinical Psychopharmacology* 39(3):189–199.

Guglielminotti, J., A. Lee, R. Landau, G. Samari, and G. Li. 2024. Structural racism and use of labor neuraxial analgesia among non-Hispanic Black birthing people. *Obstetrics and Gynecology* 143(4):571–581.

Hägg, S., and J. Jylhävä. 2021. Sex differences in biological aging with a focus on human studies. *eLife* 10:e63425.

Harlow, S. D., M. Gass, J. E. Hall, R. Lobo, P. Maki, R. W. Rebar, S. Sherman, P. M. Sluss, and T. J. de Villiers. 2012. Executive summary of the Stages of Reproductive Aging workshop + 10: Addressing the unfinished agenda of staging reproductive aging. *Menopause* 19(4):387–395.

Harlow, S. D., S.-A. M. Burnett-Bowie, G. A. Greendale, N. E. Avis, A. N. Reeves, T. R. Richards, and T. T. Lewis. 2022. Disparities in reproductive aging and midlife health between Black and White women: The study of Women's Health Across the Nation (SWAN). *Women's Midlife Health* 8(1):3.

Hillner, B. E., J. N. Ingle, R. T. Chlebowski, J. Gralow, G. C. Yee, N. A. Janjan, J. A. Cauley, B. A. Blumenstein, K. S. Albain, A. Lipton, and S. Brown. 2003. American Society of Clinical Oncology 2003 update on the role of bisphosphonates and bone health issues in women with breast cancer. *Journal of Clinical Oncology* 21(21):4042–4057.

Howard, S. R. 2021. Interpretation of reproductive hormones before, during and after the pubertal transition—identifying health and disordered puberty. *Clinical Endocrinology* 95(5):702–715.

Hu, X. H., L. E. Markson, R. B. Lipton, W. F. Stewart, and M. L. Berger. 1999. Burden of migraine in the United States: Disability and economic costs. *Archives of Internal Medicine* 159(8):813–818.

Huang, Y., Y. Shan, W. Zhang, A. M. Lee, F. Li, B. E. Stranger, and R. S. Huang. 2023. Deciphering genetic causes for sex differences in human health through drug metabolism and transporter genes. *Nature Communications* 14(1):175.

IOM (Institute of Medicine). 1994. *Women and health research: Ethical and legal issues of including women in clinical studies: Volume 2: Workshop and commissioned papers.* Washington, DC: National Academy Press.

IOM. 2010. *Women's health research: Progress, pitfalls, and promise.* Washington, DC: The National Academies Press.

Isiadinso, I., P. K. Mehta, S. Jaskwhich, and G. P. Lundberg. 2022. It takes a village: Expanding women's cardiovascular care to include the community as well as cardiovascular and primary care teams. *Current Cardiology Reports* 24(7):785–792.

Jiang, J., J. Cui, A. Wang, Y. Mu, Y. Yan, F. Liu, Y. Pan, D. Li, W. Li, G. Liu, H. Y. Gaisano, J. Dou, and Y. He. 2019. Association between age at natural menopause and risk of Type 2 diabetes in postmenopausal women with and without obesity. *Journal of Clinical Endocrinology & Metabolism* 104(7):3039–3048.

Johnson, J. D., I. V. Asiodu, C. P. McKenzie, C. Tucker, K. P. Tully, K. Bryant, S. Verbiest, and A. M. Stuebe. 2019. Racial and ethnic inequities in postpartum pain evaluation and management. *Obstetrics & Gynecology* 134(6):1155–1162.

Karlamangla, A. S., A. Shieh, and G. A. Greendale. 2021. Hormones and bone loss across the menopause transition. *Vitamins and Hormones* 115:401–417.

Keteepe-Arachi, T., and S. Sharma. 2017. Cardiovascular disease in women: Understanding symptoms and risk factors. *European Cardiology Review* 12(1):10–13.

Kling, J. M., B. L. Clarke, and N. P. Sandhu. 2014. Osteoporosis prevention, screening, and treatment: A review. *Journal of Women's Health* 23(7):563–572.

Kohl, J., A. E. Autry, and C. Dulac. 2017. The neurobiology of parenting: A neural circuit perspective. *BioEssays* 39(1):e201600159.

Lange, E. M. S., S. Rao, and P. Toledo. 2017. Racial and ethnic disparities in obstetric anesthesia. *Seminars in Perinatology* 41(5):293–298.

Lee, B., Y. Wang, S. A. Carlson, K. J. Greenlund, H. Lu, Y. Liu, J. B. Croft, P. I. Eke, M. Town, and C. W. Thomas. 2023. National, state-level, and county-level prevalence estimates of adults aged ≥18 years self-reporting a lifetime diagnosis of depression—United States, 2020. *MMWR* 72(24):644–650.

Lemaître, J.-F., V. Ronget, M. Tidière, D. Allainé, V. Berger, A. Cohas, F. Colchero, D. A. Conde, M. Garratt, A. Liker, G. A. B. Marais, A. Scheuerlein, T. Székely, and J.-M. Gaillard. 2020. Sex differences in adult lifespan and aging rates of mortality across wild mammals. *Proceedings of the National Academy of Sciences* 117(15):8546–8553.

Liese, K. L., M. Mogos, S. Abboud, K. Decocker, A. R. Koch, and S. E. Geller. 2019. Racial and ethnic disparities in severe maternal morbidity in the United States. *Journal of Racial and Ethnic Health Disparities* 6(4):790–798.

Liu, K. A., and N. A. Mager. 2016. Women's involvement in clinical trials: Historical perspective and future implications. *Pharmacy Practice* 14(1):708.

Long, M., B. Frederiksen, U. Ranji, A. Salganicoff, and K. Diep. 2022. *Experiences with Health Care Access, Cost, and Coverage: Findings from the 2022 KFF Women's Health Survey.* https://www.kff.org/womens-health-policy/report/experiences-with-health-care-access-cost-and-coverage-findings-from-the-2022-kff-womens-health-survey/ (accessed August 20, 2024).

Long, M., B. Frederiksen, U. Ranji, K. Diep, and A. Salganicoff. 2023. *Women's Experiences with Provider Communication and Interactions in Health Care Settings: Findings from the 2022 KFF Women's Health Survey.* https://www.kff.org/womens-health-policy/issue-brief/womens-experiences-with-provider-communication-interactions-health-care-settings-findings-from-2022-kff-womens-health-survey/ (accessed August 20, 2024).

Lopes, L., A. Montero, M. Presiado, and L. Hamel. 2024. *Americans' Challenges with Health Care Costs.* https://www.kff.org/health-costs/issue-brief/americans-challenges-with-health-care-costs/ (accessed August 8, 2024).

Lu, Z., J. K. Guo, Y. Wei, D. R. Dou, B. Zarnegar, Q. Ma, R. Li, Y. Zhao, F. Liu, H. Choudhry, P. A. Khavari, and H. Y. Chang. 2020. Structural modularity of the Xist ribonucleoprotein complex. *Nature Communications* 11(1):6163.

Magnan, S. 2021. Social determinants of health 201 for health care: Plan, do, study, act. *NAM Perspectives* 2021.

Marsh, E. E., G. Wegienka, and D. R. Williams. 2024. Uterine fibroids. *JAMA* 331(17):1492–1493.

Mauvais-Jarvis, F., D. J. Clegg, and A. L. Hevener. 2013. The role of estrogens in control of energy balance and glucose homeostasis. *Endocrine Reviews* 34(3):309–338.

McPhee, C., I. O. Aninye, and L. Horan. 2022. Recommendations for improving women's bone health throughout the lifespan. *Journal of Women's Health* 31(12):1671–1676.

MD Anderson Cancer Center. 2023. *ESMO: PARP Inhibitor Plus Immunotherapy Lowers Risk of Endometrial Cancer Progression Over Chemotherapy Alone.* https://www.mdanderson.org/newsroom/esmo-parp-inhibitor-plus-immunotherapy-lowers-risk-of-endometrial-cancer-progression-over-chemotherapy-alone.h00–159622590.html (accessed October 21, 2024).

Mishra, S., H.-F. Chung, M. Waller, and G. Mishra. 2021. Duration of estrogen exposure during reproductive years, age at menarche and age at menopause, and risk of cardiovascular disease events, all-cause and cardiovascular mortality: A systematic review and meta-analysis. *BJOG* 128(5):809–821.

Montalmant, K. E., and A. K. Ettinger. 2024. The racial disparities in maternal mortality and impact of structural racism and implicit racial bias on pregnant Black women: A review of the literature. *Journal of Racial and Ethnic Health Disparities* 11(6):3658–3677.

Muehlenbein, M. P., J. Gassen, E. C. Shattuck, and C. S. Sparks. 2022. Lower testosterone levels are associated with higher risk of death in men. *Evolution, Medicine, and Public Health* 11(1):30–41.

NAMS 2022 Hormone Therapy Position Statement Advisory Panel. 2022. The 2022 hormone therapy position statement of the North American Menopause Society. *Menopause* 29(7):767–794.

NASEM (National Academies of Sciences, Engineering, and Medicine). 2017. *Communities in action: Pathways to health equity.* Washington, DC: The National Academies Press.

NASEM. 2019. *Vibrant and healthy kids: Aligning science, practice, and policy to advance health equity.* Washington, DC: The National Academies Press.

NASEM. 2022. *Improving representation in clinical trials and research: Building research equity for women and underrepresented groups.* Washington, DC: The National Academies Press.

NASEM. 2023a. *Federal policy to advance racial, ethnic, and tribal health equity.* Washington, DC: The National Academies Press.

NASEM. 2023b. *Inclusion of pregnant and lactating persons in clinical trials: Proceedings of a workshop.* Washington, DC: The National Academies Press.

NASEM. 2024a. *Advancing research on chronic conditions in women.* Washington, DC: The National Academies Press.

NASEM. 2024b. *Ending unequal treatment: Strategies to achieve equitable health care and optimal health for all.* Washington, DC: The National Academies Press.

National Commission for the Protection of Human Subjects of Biomedical and Behavioral Research. 1979. *The Belmont Report.* Washington, DC: Department of Health, Education, and Welfare.

Nichols, T. R., A. Welborn, M. R. Gringle, and A. Lee. 2021. Social stigma and perinatal substance use services: Recognizing the power of the good mother ideal. *Contemporary Drug Problems* 48(1):19–37.

OASH (Office of the Assistant Secretary for Health). 2023. *Menopause Symptoms and Relief.* https://www.womenshealth.gov/menopause/menopause-symptoms-and-relief (accessed September 13, 2024).

Okoro, O. N., L. A. Hillman, and A. Cernasev. 2020. "We get double slammed!": Healthcare experiences of perceived discrimination among low-income African-American women. *Women's Health* 16:1745506520953348.

Opoku, A. A., M. Abushama, and J. C. Konje. 2023. Obesity and menopause. *Best Practice & Research Clinical Obstetrics & Gynaecology* 88:102348.

ORWH (Office of Research on Women's Health). n.d.-a. *Clinical Research and Trials.* https://orwh.od.nih.gov/womens-health-equity-inclusion/clinical-research-and-trials (accessed August 21, 2024).

ORWH. n.d.-b. *NIH Inclusion Outreach Toolkit: How to Engage, Recruit, and Retain Women in Clinical Research: History of Women's Participation in Clinical Research.* https://orwh.od.nih.gov/toolkit/recruitment/history (accessed August 8, 2024).

ORWH. 2021. *Historical Timeline—30 Years of Advancing Women's Health.* Bethesda, MD: National Institutes of Health.

Öztürk, R., T. L. Bloom, Y. Li, and L. F. C. Bullock. 2021. Stress, stigma, violence experiences and social support of U.S. infertile women. *Journal of Reproductive and Infant Psychology* 39(2):205–217.

Payne, J. L., and J. Maguire. 2019. Pathophysiological mechanisms implicated in postpartum depression. *Frontiers in Neuroendocrinology* 52:165–180.

Plevkova, J., M. Brozmanova, J. Harsanyiova, M. Sterusky, J. Honetschlager, and T. Buday. 2020. Various aspects of sex and gender bias in biomedical research. *Physiological Research* 69(Suppl 3):S367–S378.

Prather, C., T. R. Fuller, K. J. Marshall, and W. L. Jeffries. 2016. The impact of racism on the sexual and reproductive health of African American women. *Journal of Women's Health* 25(7):664–671.

Puhl, R. M., T. Andreyeva, and K. D. Brownell. 2008. Perceptions of weight discrimination: Prevalence and comparison to race and gender discrimination in America. *International Journal of Obesity* 32(6):992–1000.

Raman, S., and A. Cohen. 2023. *Ob-Gyn Workforce Shortages Could Worsen Maternal Health Crisis.* https://burgess.house.gov/news/documentsingle.aspx?DocumentID=403659 (accessed August 8, 2024).

Robson, M., S. A. Im, E. Senkus, B. Xu, S. M. Domchek, N. Masuda, S. Delaloge, W. Li, N. Tung, A. Armstrong, W. Wu, C. Goessl, S. Runswick, and P. Conte. 2017. Olaparib for metastatic breast cancer in patients with a germline BRCA mutation. *New England Journal of Medicine* 377(6):523–533.

Salsberg, E., C. Richwine, S. Westergaard, M. Portela Martinez, T. Oyeyemi, A. Vichare, and C. P. Chen. 2021. Estimation and comparison of current and future racial/ethnic representation in the U.S. health care workforce. *JAMA Network Open* 4(3):e213789.

Saylor, P. J., R. B. Rumble, and J. M. Michalski. 2020. Bone health and bone-targeted therapies for prostate cancer: American Society of Clinical Oncology endorsement summary of a Cancer Care Ontario guideline. *JCO Oncology Practice* 16(7):389–393.

Sayres Van Niel, M., and J. L. Payne. 2020. Perinatal depression: A review. *Cleveland Clinic Journal of Medicine* 87(5):273–277.

Schmidt, P. J., L. Nieman, M. A. Danaceau, M. B. Tobin, C. A. Roca, J. H. Murphy, and D. R. Rubinow. 2000. Estrogen replacement in perimenopause-related depression: A preliminary report. *American Journal of Obstetrics and Gynecology* 183(2):414–420.

Schofield, C. A., S. Brown, I. E. Siegel, and C. A. Moss-Racusin. 2024. What you don't expect when you're expecting: Demonstrating stigma against women with postpartum psychological disorders. *Stigma and Health* 9(3).

Schreier, H. M. C., M. Bosquet Enlow, T. Ritz, B. A. Coull, C. Gennings, R. O. Wright, and R. J. Wright. 2016. Lifetime exposure to traumatic and other stressful life events and hair cortisol in a multi-racial/ethnic sample of pregnant women. *Stress* 19(1):45–52.

Shamsi, H. A., A. G. Almutairi, S. A. Mashrafi, and T. A. Kalbani. 2020. Implications of language barriers for healthcare: A systematic review. *Oman Medical Journal* 35.

Soares, C. N., and B. Zitek. 2008. Reproductive hormone sensitivity and risk for depression across the female life cycle: A continuum of vulnerability? *Journal of Psychiatry and Neuroscience* 33(4):331–343.

Soldin, O. P., and D. R. Mattison. 2009. Sex differences in pharmacokinetics and pharmacodynamics. *Clinical Pharmacokinetics* 48(3):143–157.

Sosinsky, A. Z., J. W. Rich-Edwards, A. Wiley, K. Wright, P. A. Spagnolo, and H. Joffe. 2022. Enrollment of female participants in United States drug and device Phase 1–3 clinical trials between 2016 and 2019. *Contemporary Clinical Trials* 115:106718.

Srikanth, N., L. Xie, J. Francis, and S. E. Messiah. 2023. Association of social determinants of health, race and ethnicity, and age of menarche among U.S. women over 2 decades. *Journal of Pediatric and Adolescent Gynecology* 36(5):442–448.

Stall, N. M., N. R. Shah, and D. Bhushan. 2023. Unpaid family caregiving—the next frontier of gender equity in a postpandemic future. *JAMA Health Forum* 4(6):e231310.

Steele, L. S., A. Daley, D. Curling, M. F. Gibson, D. C. Green, C. C. Williams, and L. E. Ross. 2017. LGBT identity, untreated depression, and unmet need for mental health services by sexual minority women and trans-identified people. *Journal of Women's Health* 26(2):116–127.

Still, C. H., S. Tahir, H. N. Yarandi, M. Hassan, and F. A. Gary. 2020. Association of psychosocial symptoms, blood pressure, and menopausal status in African-American women. *Western Journal of Nursing Research* 42(10):784–794.

Superville, D. R. 2023. *Women in the K–12 Workforce, by the Numbers.* https://www.edweek.org/leadership/women-in-the-k-12-workforce-by-the-numbers/2023/03 (accessed October 3, 2024).

Taylor, A. M., D. L. H. Chan, M. Tio, S. M. Patil, T. A. Traina, M. E. Robson, and M. Khasraw. 2021. PARP (poly ADP-ribose polymerase) inhibitors for locally advanced or metastatic breast cancer. *Cochrane Database of Systematic Reviews* 4(4):Cd011395.

Temkin, S. M., S. Noursi, J. G. Regensteiner, P. Stratton, and J. A. Clayton. 2022. Perspectives from advancing National Institutes of Health research to inform and improve the health of women: A conference summary. *Obstetrics and Gynecology* 140(1):10–19.

Temkin, S. M., E. Barr, H. Moore, J. P. Caviston, J. G. Regensteiner, and J. A. Clayton. 2023. Chronic conditions in women: The development of a National Institutes of Health framework. *BMC Women's Health* 23(1):162.

Thase, M. E., R. Entsuah, M. Cantillon, and S. G. Kornstein. 2005. Relative antidepressant efficacy of venlafaxine and SSRIs: Sex-age interactions. *Journal of Women's Health* 14(7):609–616.

Trost, S., J. Beauregard, G. Chandra, F. Njie, J. Berry, A. Harvey, and D. A. Goodman. 2022. *Pregnancy-related deaths: Data from maternal mortality review committees in 36 U.S. states, 2017–2019.* Atlanta, GA: Centers for Disease Control and Prevention.

Valentine, J. A., L. F. Delgado, L. T. Haderxhanaj, and M. Hogben. 2022. Improving sexual health in U.S. rural communities: Reducing the impact of stigma. *AIDS and Behavior* 26(1):90–99.

van Oosterhout, R. E. M., A. R. de Boer, A. H. E. M. Maas, F. H. Rutten, M. L. Bots, and S. A. E. Peters. 2020. Sex differences in symptom presentation in acute coronary syndromes: A systematic review and meta-analysis. *Journal of the American Heart Association* 9(9):e014733.

Vohra-Gupta, S., L. Petruzzi, C. Jones, and C. Cubbin. 2023. An intersectional approach to understanding barriers to healthcare for women. *Journal of Community Health* 48(1):89–98.

Wang, S. S. Y., Y. E. Jie, S. W. Cheng, G. L. Ling, and H. V. Y. Ming. 2023. PARP inhibitors in breast and ovarian cancer. *Cancers* 15(8).

Weinberger, A. H., S. A. McKee, and C. M. Mazure. 2010. Inclusion of women and gender-specific analyses in randomized clinical trials of treatments for depression. *Journal of Women's Health* 19(9):1727–1732.

Whitman, A., N. De Lew, A. Chappel, V. Aysola, R. Zuckerman, and B. D. Sommers. 2022. *Addressing social determinants of health: Examples of successful evidence-based strategies and current federal efforts.* Washington, DC: Assistant Secretary for Planning and Evaluation.

WHO (World Health Organization). n.d. *Social Determinants of Health.* https://www.who.int/health-topics/social-determinants-of-health#tab=tab_1 (accessed October 21, 2024).

Williamson, L. 2024. *Families Often Have Chief Medical Officers—and They're Almost Always Women.* https://www.heart.org/en/news/2024/04/17/families-often-have-chief-medical-officers-and-theyre-almost-always-women (accessed October 3, 2024).

Yan, B. W., E. Arias, A. C. Geller, D. R. Miller, K. D. Kochanek, and H. K. Koh. 2024. Widening gender gap in life expectancy in the U.S., 2010–2021. *JAMA Internal Medicine* 184(1):108–110.

Yermachenko, A., and V. Dvornyk. 2014. Nongenetic determinants of age at menarche: A systematic review. *BioMed Research International* 2014(1):371583.

Zhao, H., M. DiMarco, K. Ichikawa, M. Boulicault, M. Perret, K. Jillson, A. Fair, K. DeJesus, and S. S. Richardson. 2023. Making a "sex-difference fact": Ambien dosing at the interface of policy, regulation, women's health, and biology. *Social Studies of Science* 53(4):475–494.

3

Review of National Institutes of Health Structure, Policies, and Programs

OVERVIEW OF THE NATIONAL INSTITUTES OF HEALTH'S STRUCTURE

To elucidate improvements that might be made to advance progress on women's health research (WHR) at the National Institutes of Health (NIH), it is critical to understand the policies, programs, and structures that shape how NIH supports this work. With an annual budget of approximately $48 billion, NIH is the largest and most influential and complex biomedical research sponsor in the world (NIH, n.d.-a). This chapter does not provide a comprehensive overview of NIH but rather focuses on major aspects of NIH's history, policies, programs, and structures relevant to WHR.

NIH Mission and Goals

NIH's mission is to "seek fundamental knowledge about the nature and behavior of living systems and the application of that knowledge to enhance health, lengthen life, and reduce illness and disability" (NIH, 2017b). NIH's goals, and therefore the research it conducts and supports, center around fostering scientific discovery and developing innovative research with high scientific integrity to expand medical and related knowledge to support health (see Box 3-1). To achieve this mission, NIH invests the majority of its budget on basic sciences and clinical research, with almost 83 percent awarded for extramural research. Most extramural research is funded through competitive grants to more than 300,000 researchers at more than 2,700 universities, medical schools, and other research institutions in every state.

BOX 3-1
NIH Goals

- To foster fundamental creative discoveries, innovative research strategies, and their applications as a basis for ultimately protecting and improving health;
- To develop, maintain, and renew scientific human and physical resources that will ensure the nation's capability to prevent disease;
- To expand the knowledge base in medical and associated sciences in order to enhance the nation's economic well-being and ensure a continued high return on the public investment in research; and
- To exemplify and promote the highest level of scientific integrity, public accountability, and social responsibility in the conduct of science.

In realizing these goals, NIH provides leadership and direction to programs designed to improve the health of the nation by conducting and supporting research in:

- the causes, diagnosis, prevention, and cure of human diseases;
- the processes of human growth and development;
- the biological effects of environmental contaminants;
- the understanding of mental, addictive and physical disorders; and
- directing programs for the collection, dissemination, and exchange of information in medicine and health, including the development and support of medical libraries and the training of medical librarians and other health information specialists.

SOURCE: Excerpt from NIH, 2017b.

Approximately 11 percent of the NIH budget supports projects conducted by the nearly 6,000 scientists in NIH laboratories. The remaining 6 percent covers research support, administrative, and facility construction, maintenance, or operational costs (Lauer, 2024; NIH, n.d.-a). The fiscal year (FY) 2023 program level was $47.683 billion, with an additional $1.5 billion going to the Advanced Research Projects Agency for Health. Each year, through its annual appropriations process, Congress approves the funding for all federal agencies, including NIH. Congress does not generally specify funding amounts for individual health conditions at NIH but instead sets an overall amount for each NIH Institute, Center, and Office (ICO). Each ICO determines how to allocate those funds, though some are earmarked by Congress for specific programs within each ICO (CRS, 2024; Rodgers, 2024).

NIH Organization

NIH funds research in every U.S. state and a small number of studies in other countries (NIH, 2024d, n.d.-a). Its core revolves around its 21 Institutes and six Centers (ICs) coordinated through its Office of the Director (OD) (NIH, 2023f, 2024g). All the Institutes award and administer grants, while most but not all Centers provide grant funding. For example, the Center for Scientific Review (CSR) coordinates peer review of grant applications but does not provide direct funding to investigators. The Center for Information Technology (CIT) mainly provides computer support services, and the Clinical Center provides clinical services, houses clinical research, and offers training. Other Centers, including the Fogarty International Center (FIC), National Center for Advancing Translational Sciences (NCATS), and National Center for Complementary and Integrative Health (NCCIH), function like Institutes. Although their budgets are small, these Centers fund research in their areas of interest (NIH, 2023f). The budgets of the ICs vary (see Figure 3-1).

In addition to ICs, the OD oversees about a dozen Offices and the Division of Program Coordination, Planning, and Strategic Initiatives (DPCPSI). Within the OD, DPCPSI oversees several offices, many of which are specifically tasked with broad responsibility for coordinating research across the 27 ICs, for example, the Office of Research on Women's Health (ORWH), Office of Behavioral and Social Sciences Research (OBSSR), Office of Disease Prevention (ODP), and Office of AIDS Research (OAR) (NIH, n.d.-c) (see Figure 3-2 for a listing of all offices). These coordinating Offices each have a director and work closely with the directors and staff of the ICs to identify areas of potential collaboration. For example, virtually all ICs fund research relevant to behavioral science, women's health, and prevention. The coordinating Offices explore the potential for pooling resources, reducing duplication, and stimulating new directions; each director also holds the title of NIH associate director (NIH, 2024f; OAR, n.d.; OBSSR, n.d.; ODP, n.d.-a; ORWH, n.d.-j).

In addition to the coordinating Offices, DPCPSI also oversees several other Offices (see Figure 3-2). A consequence of this structure is that both DPCPSI and the OD (see Figure 3-3) are tasked with the nearly impossible roles of fully supporting the missions of the dozens of Offices they oversee. The complexity of the NIH organization is shown in Figures 3-3 and 3-4.[1]

Office Budgets

Budgets for select programmatic Offices are shown in Table 3-1. In contrast to ICs, programmatic Offices do not have sufficient funds to support grants independently, nor is that their major role. Office budgets support their mission to initiate the development of collaborative funding that

---

[1] The section was changed after release of the report to clarify the offices in the NIH OD specifically tasked with research coordination.

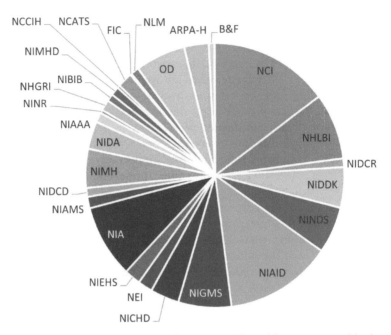

FIGURE 3-1 Distribution of National Institutes of Health 2023 enacted budget, by Institutes, Centers, and Offices.

NOTE: ARPA-H = Advanced Research Projects Agency for Health; B&F = Buildings and Facilities; FIC = Fogarty International Center; NCATS = National Center for Advancing Translational Sciences; NCCIH = National Center for Complementary and Integrative Health; NCI = National Cancer Institute; NEI = National Eye Institute; NHGRI = National Human Genome Research Institute; NHLBI = National Heart, Lung, and Blood Institute; NIA = National Institute on Aging; NIAAA = National Institute on Alcohol Abuse and Alcoholism; NIAID = National Institute of Allergy and Infectious Diseases; NIAMS = National Institute of Arthritis and Musculoskeletal and Skin Diseases; NIBIB = National Institute of Biomedical Imaging and Bioengineering; NICHD = *Eunice Kennedy Shriver* National Institute of Child Health and Human Development; NIDA = National Institute on Drug Abuse; NIDCD = National Institute on Deafness and Other Communication Disorders; NIDCR = National Institute of Dental and Craniofacial Research; NIDDK = National Institute of Diabetes and Digestive and Kidney Diseases; NIEHS = National Institute of Environmental Health Sciences; NIGMS = National Institute of General Medical Sciences; NIMH = National Institute of Mental Health; NIMHD = National Institute on Minority Health and Health Disparities; NINDS = National Institute of Neurological Disorders and Stroke; NINR = National Institute of Nursing Research; NLM = National Library of Medicine; OD = Office of the Director.

SOURCE: Data from NIH, 2023a,b.

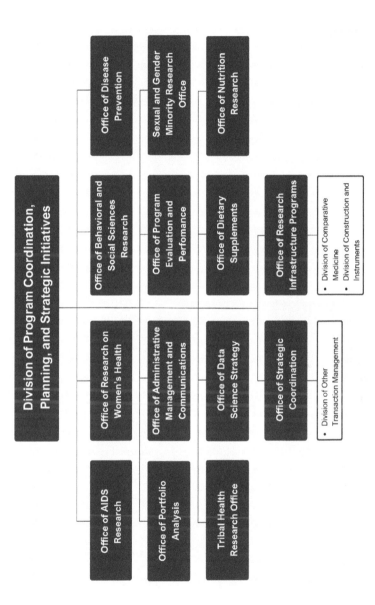

FIGURE 3-2 Organizational structure of Division of Program Coordination, Planning, and Strategic Initiatives (DPCPSI).
NOTE: This figure was changed after release of the report to clarify the offices in the NIH OD specifically tasked with research coordination.
SOURCE: Adapted from NIH, n.d.-c.

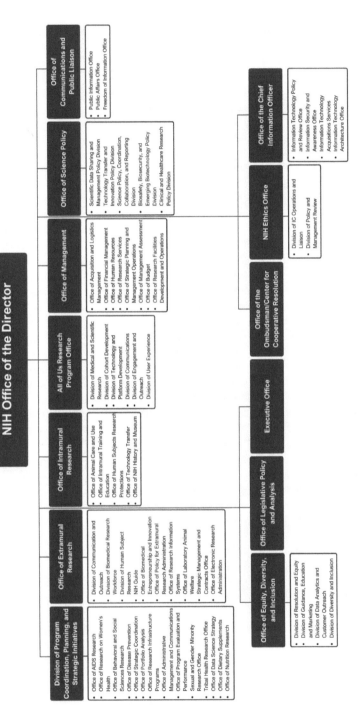

FIGURE 3-3 Organizational structure of National Institutes of Health Office of the Director.
SOURCE: Adapted from NIH, n.d.-c.

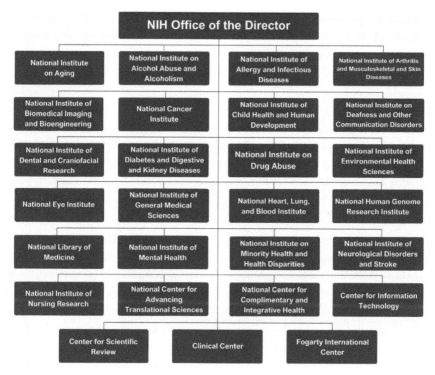

FIGURE 3-4 Complexity of National Institutes of Health (NIH) organizational structure.
SOURCE: Adapted from OMA, n.d.

TABLE 3-1 Budgets of Select National Institutes of Health Programmatic Offices in Dollars

Office	Fiscal Year 2023 Budget
Office of AIDS Research	$67,587,000
Office of Behavioral and Social Sciences Research	$40,047,000
Office of Dietary Supplements	$28,500,000
Office of Disease Prevention	$17,873,000
Office of Nutrition Research	$1,313,000
Office of Research Infrastructure Programs	$309,393,000
Office of Research on Women's Health	$76,648,000 *Includes:* $10 million for new OADR, $5 million in new funding for BIRCWH, and $2 million for NASEM study. Remainder: $59,648,000

NOTE: BIRCWH = Building Interdisciplinary Research Careers in Women's Health; NASEM = National Academies of Sciences, Engineering, and Medicine; OADR = Office of Autoimmune Disease Research.
SOURCE: Data from Clayton, 2023; NIH, n.d.-e.

aligns with the mutual interests and goals of the ICs (NIH, 2024f; OAR, n.d.; OBSSR, n.d.; ODP, n.d.-a; ORWH, n.d.-j).

WHR AT NIH

ORWH

No IC is charged with addressing women's health, but some women's health conditions fall within the purview and expertise of the 27 ICs (NIH, 2023f). The task of ORWH is to ensure that the research conducted and supported by the ICs adequately addresses women's health. As discussed in Chapter 1, NIH created ORWH in 1990 to coordinate and promote research on the health of women, both within and outside the NIH scientific community (ORWH, n.d.-k). Congressional action to address the lack of inclusion of women in NIH-sponsored research, via the NIH Revitalization Act of 1993, was the key impetus for the Office's creation (ORWH, n.d.-k) (see Box 3-2 for ORWH's key responsibilities as outlined by Congress). The 21st Century Cures Act,[2] signed in 2016, reaffirmed NIH's commitment to advancing WHR, including by advocating for the importance of considering sex as a biological variable (SABV) in research and ensuring that women, people of all ages, and underrepresented racial and ethnic groups are appropriately represented in clinical research (ORWH, n.d.-k).

ORWH Organization and Funding

ORWH became part of DPCPSI as a result of the NIH Reform Act of 2006.[3] DPCPSI coordinates agency-wide initiatives and works to identify emerging scientific opportunities. Thus, it is well suited to oversee the work of ORWH (ORWH, n.d.-k). See Figure 3-5 for a visual contextualizing ORWH's organizational position within NIH.

ORWH's budget increased steadily during its first decade but was stagnant between 2003 and 2020 (see Figure 3-6). The president's FY 2025 ORWH budget request includes $154 million, an increase of $76 million from FY 2023 and 2024, but as of September 2024, Congress has not yet approved it (OD, n.d.). The additional funds would support research on peri- and postmenopause and diabetes, opioid use disorder in pregnant women, and alcohol use during pregnancy. In addition, NIH plans to create a nationwide network of centers of excellence and innovation in women's health (OD, n.d.).

---

[2] Public Law No. 114–255.
[3] Public Law No. 109–482.

BOX 3-2
ORWH Mission

Congress assigned a far-reaching leadership role for ORWH by mandating that the ORWH director:

- Advise the NIH director and staff on matters relating to research on women's health
- Strengthen and enhance research related to diseases, disorders, and conditions that affect women
- Ensure that research conducted and supported by NIH adequately addresses issues regarding women's health
- Ensure that women are appropriately represented in biomedical and biobehavioral research studies supported by NIH
- Develop opportunities and support for recruitment, retention, reentry, and advancement of women in biomedical careers
- Support and advance rigorous research that is relevant to the health of women
- Ensure NIH-funded research accounts for SABV

ORWH crafts and implements the NIH Strategic Plan for Women's Health Research in partnership with NIH ICs and co-funds research on the role of sex and gender on health. ORWH also collaborates with NIH ICs, the NIH Office of Extramural Research, and the NIH Office of Intramural Research to monitor adherence to NIH's inclusion policies, which ensure that women and minorities are represented in NIH-supported clinical research.

ORWH's interdisciplinary research and career development initiatives stimulate research on sex and gender differences and provide career support to launch promising women's health researchers. These programs set the stage for improved health for women and their families and career opportunities and advancement for a diverse biomedical workforce.

SOURCE: Excerpt from ORWH, n.d.-j.

ORWH Advisory Groups

ORWH's work is guided by two advisory groups, both established by Congress as part of the NIH Revitalization Act of 1993: the Advisory Committee on Research on Women's Health (ACRWH) and the Coordinating Committee on Research on Women's Health (CCRWH). Both make recommendations on research priorities to ORWH based on their consideration of gaps in knowledge and emerging scientific opportunities (ORWH, n.d.-c,d,i).

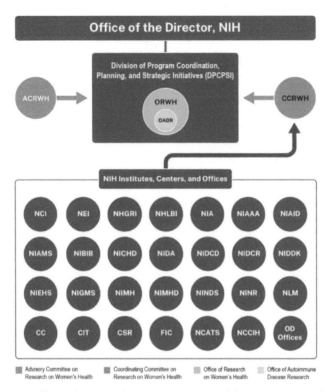

FIGURE 3-5 Office of Research on Women's Health's (ORWH's) place in the National Institutes of Health (NIH) Office of the Director and its relationship to other NIH entities.

NOTE: CC = Clinical Center; CIT = Center for Information Technology; CSR = Center for Scientific Review; FIC = Fogarty International Center; NCATS = National Center for Advancing Translational Sciences; NCCIH = National Center for Complementary and Integrative Health; NCI = National Cancer Institute; NEI = National Eye Institute; NHGRI = National Human Genome Research Institute; NHLBI = National Heart, Lung, and Blood Institute; NIA = National Institute on Aging; NIAAA = National Institute on Alcohol Abuse and Alcoholism; NIAID = National Institute of Allergy and Infectious Diseases; NIAMS = National Institute of Arthritis and Musculoskeletal and Skin Diseases; NIBIB = National Institute of Biomedical Imaging and Bioengineering; NICHD = *Eunice Kennedy Shriver* National Institute of Child Health and Human Development; NIDA = National Institute on Drug Abuse; NIDCD = National Institute on Deafness and Other Communication Disorders; NIDCR = National Institute of Dental and Craniofacial Research; NIDDK = National Institute of Diabetes and Digestive and Kidney Diseases; NIEHS = National Institute of Environmental Health Sciences; NIGMS = National Institute of General Medical Sciences; NIH = National Institutes of Health; NIMH = National Institute of Mental Health; NIMHD = National Institute on Minority Health and Health Disparities; NINDS = National Institute of Neurological Disorders and Stroke; NINR = National Institute of Nursing Research; NLM = National Library of Medicine; OD = Office of the Director.

SOURCE: ORWH, n.d.-k.

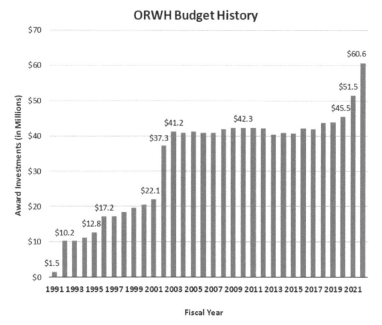

FIGURE 3-6 Office of Research on Women's Health (ORWH) budget history: 1991–2022.
SOURCE: Clayton, 2023.

ACRWH is a Federal Advisory Committee Act committee comprising nonfederal employees and provides advice and recommendations on priority issues affecting women's health and sex differences research. Its responsibilities include advising the ORWH director on appropriate research activities in women's health, reviewing the WHR portfolio, assessing scientific career development goals, and evaluating the inclusion of women and minoritized individuals in NIH clinical research. ACRWH meets at least once per fiscal year and produces biennial reports that discuss the NIH-wide programs conducted to fulfill ORWH's core mission and its accomplishments and highlight research on the health of women and the influence of sex and gender on health and disease (ORWH, n.d.-c,f).

CCRWH comprises IC directors or their designees who serve as liaisons between ORWH and the ICs. It provides guidance, collaboration, and support to ORWH program goals and is a resource for women's health activities across the agency, including assisting with data collection and the development and expansion of clinical trials to include women (ORWH, n.d.-i).

ORWH Research Areas and Activities

ORWH's work focuses on several key areas, all aligned with its mission. Only 8.9 percent of the ORWH budget in 2023 was used to support R01 grants in partnership with ICs (Clayton, 2023). Other ORWH investments include (ORWH, n.d.-m) the following:

- The Science of Sex & Gender: ORWH's activities in this area aim to advance knowledge of how sex and gender influence health and disease.
- Women's Health Equity and Inclusion: ORWH coordinates, promotes, and supports research to advance women's health equity and enhance understanding of intersectionality.
- Supporting Women in Biomedical Careers: ORWH funds programs that address the underrepresentation of women in biomedical careers.

Specific ORWH workforce-related programs include (see Chapter 8 for more information on these and other programs) the following:

- The Building Interdisciplinary Research Careers in Women's Health program was established in 2000 to connect scholars who are junior faculty to senior faculty with a shared interest in women's health and sex differences research (ORWH, n.d.-g).
- The Specialized Centers of Research Excellence on Sex Differences program funds pilot funding, training, and education at NIH-supported centers that serve as research hubs focusing on sex and gender (ORWH, n.d.-r).

Other examples of ORWH activities and initiatives include the following:

- The U3 Administrative Supplement Program provides funding for research focused on intersectionality and health among populations of women that are understudied, underrepresented, and underreported (U3).
- The sex and gender program, started in 2013, offers supplemental funding to NIH grantees to support research on influences of sex and gender (ORWH, n.d.-m). The administrative supplements provide 1-year awards of approximately $100,000, and ORWH has invested $38.87 million since inception, supporting 383 investigators in FY 2013–2021 across ICOs. For FY 2021, ORWH committed $1 million, enough to cover only approximately 10 supplements (Agarwal et al., 2021; ORWH, n.d.-b).

- The Pathways to Prevention program convenes federal agencies, researchers, and community members to identify research gaps in a scientific area of broad public health importance. It also works to develop an action plan to address these gaps (ODP, n.d.-c).

See Figure 3-7 for ORWH's extramural grant awards by program in 2022.

Office of Autoimmune Disease Research (OADR)

OADR sits within ORWH. Congress created OADR in the Consolidated Appropriations Act, 2023[4] in response to the 2022 National Academies of Sciences, Engineering, and Medicine report, *Enhancing NIH Research on Autoimmune Disease* (NASEM, 2022; ORWH, n.d.-a).[5] The Office is charged with evaluating NIH's autoimmune disease research portfolio and was directed to

- Coordinate development of a multi-IC strategic research plan;
- Identify emerging areas of innovation and research opportunity;

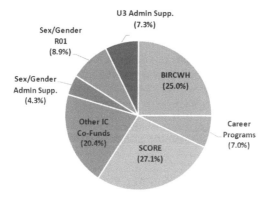

FIGURE 3-7 Distribution of Office of Research on Women's Health (ORWH) extramural grant awards by program, fiscal year 2022.
NOTES: ORWH total investments = $43,222,779. Funding portfolio excludes research and development contracts, interagency/intra-agency agreements., and loan repayment awards. BIRCWH = Building Interdisciplinary Research Careers in Women's Health; IC = Institutes and Centers; SCORE = Specialized Centers of Research Excellence on Sex Differences; U3 Admin Supp. = U3 (underrepresented, underserved, and underreported) Administrative Supplement Program.
SOURCE: Clayton, 2023 (based on frozen data from NIH IMPAC II, Fiscal Year 2022).

---

[4] Public Law 117–328.
[5] The report recommended that an office be created in the NIH Office of the Director, not within ORWH.

- Coordinate and foster collaborative research across ICs;
- Annually evaluate the NIH autoimmune disease research (ADR) portfolio;
- Provide resources to support planning, collaboration, and innovation; and
- Develop a publicly accessible central repository for ADR.

To start, the Office is collaborating with leading experts to review NIH-funded research from the past 5 years to create an initial overview of the research portfolio (ORWH, n.d.-a). OADR-ORWH has begun supporting research, such as two multi-year awards for the collaborative Accelerating Medicines Partnership® Autoimmune and Immune-Mediated Diseases (AMP® AIM) program in FY23 and FY24.[6] Launched in 2021, the program is managed by the Foundation for the NIH and supported by several ICOs, private partners, and not-for-profit organizations. Its goal is to advance the fields understanding of the cellular and molecular interactions that drive inflammation and autoimmune diseases.[7,8]

ORWH Policy Oversight

SABV

The SABV Policy, implemented in 2016, requires that "sex as a biological variable will be factored into research designs, analyses, and reporting in vertebrate animals and human studies" and "strong justification from the scientific literature, preliminary data, or other relevant considerations [if] proposing to study only one sex" (NOT-OD-15-103).[9] ORWH leads the Trans-NIH SABV Working Group in its efforts to inform policy development and implementation (ORWH, 2021). Greater detail on the policy is provided later in this chapter.

Clinical trial inclusion policies

In the 1993 NIH Revitalization Act, Congress turned an existing NIH inclusion policy into federal law and directed the NIH to establish guidelines for broader inclusion of women and minoritized individuals in clinical research, with requirements including:

- "NIH [should ensure] that women and minorities are included in all human subject research.

---

[6] For more information, see https://orwh.od.nih.gov/OADR-ORWH/Funding-Information#card-1797 (accessed January 25, 2025).

[7] For more information, see https://www.niams.nih.gov/grants-funding/niams-supported-research-programs/accelerating-medicines-partnership-amp (accessed January 25, 2025).

[8] This paragraph was updated after release of the report to add the AMP® AIM program as an example.

[9] See https://grants.nih.gov/grants/guide/notice-files/NOT-OD-15-103.html (accessed September 9, 2024).

- Phase III clinical trials [should] include women and minorities in numbers adequate to allow for valid analyses of differences in intervention effects.
- Cost is not allowed as an acceptable reason for excluding these groups.
- NIH [should initiate] programs and support for outreach efforts to recruit and retain women and minorities and their subpopulations as volunteers in clinical studies" (ORWH, n.d.-h).

A 2017 amendment to the NIH inclusion policy adds a "requirement that recipients conducting applicable NIH-defined Phase III clinical trials ensure results of valid analyses by sex/gender, race, and/or ethnicity are submitted to Clinicaltrials.gov" (NIH, 2017a). ORWH supports the NIH inclusion policy by collecting and analyzing data on clinical trial diversity (ORWH, n.d.-h).

NIH-Wide Strategic Plan for Research on the Health of Women

In May 2024, NIH released its NIH-Wide Strategic Plan for Research on the Health of Women 2024–2028, which ORWH led in collaboration with ACRWH, ICO representatives, and federal partners (ORWH, 2024, n.d.-k). The plan includes agency-wide strategic goals and objectives in the areas of "biological, behavioral, social, structural, and environmental factors; data science and data management practices; scientific workforce training and education; biology underlying sex influences; and community-engaged science across the research and practice continuum" (ORWH, n.d.-k, p. 4).

The NIH strategic plan places importance on both sex and gender in research. Guiding principles for the plan include "consider[ing] the complex intersection among multiple factors that affect the health of women, includ[ing] diverse populations of women in clinical research, and integrat[ing] perspectives from a diverse workforce of scientists with differing skills, knowledge and experience" (ORWH, n.d.-k, p. 9). Strategic goals outlined in the plan include the following:

- "Research: Advance research that examines the multiple biological, behavioral, social, structural, and environmental factors that influence the health of women, as well as the intersections of these factors" (ORWH, n.d.-k, p. 13).
- "Data science and management: Improve data science and data management practices with innovative research methods, measurements, and cutting-edge technologies to prevent and treat conditions affecting women" (ORWH, n.d.-k, p. 14).
- "Training and education: Foster women scientists' career development and promote scientific workforce training and education that advances the health of women and the science of sex and gender influences" (ORWH, n.d.-k, p. 15).

- "Basic and translational science: Support the basic and translational study of the biology underlying sex influences and its intersection with disease and health preservation in women across the life course" (ORWH, n.d.-k, p. 16).
- "Community engagement: Advance community-engaged science across the research and practice continuum and enhance the dissemination and implementation of evidence-based solutions to improve the health of women" (ORWH, n.d.-k, p. 17).

Role of ICOs in WHR

Most ICOs have an important role in advancing WHR. For example, reproductive health and pregnancy fall under the purview of the *Eunice Kennedy Shriver* National Institute of Child Health and Human Development (NICHD), while issues affecting lesbian and bisexual women, nonbinary and transgender individuals assigned female at birth, or transgender women are under the Sexual & Gender Minority Research Office (SGMRO) (NICHD, 2021; SGMRO, 2024). Issues specific to American Indian and Alaska Native (AIAN) women fall under the purview of the NIH Tribal Health Research Office (THRO), which serves as the hub for coordination of tribal health–related activities across NIH (THRO, 2023). Specific conditions, such as breast, uterine, endometrial and cervical cancers, are under the National Cancer Institute (NCI), and the menopause transition is under the National Institute on Aging (NIA) (NCI, n.d.-a; NIA, 2022). However, many women's health conditions, such as endometriosis, fibroids, pelvic floor disorders, polycystic ovary syndrome (PCOS), and vulvodynia, are not prioritized by ICs based on a review of IC strategic plans as well as low levels of funding for these conditions from 2013–2023 (see Chapter 4).[10] Collaboration across NIH ICOs is therefore critical to ensure that WHR is being addressed fully and comprehensively. While ORWH is tasked with coordinating women's health across NIH Institutes, coordinating across ICOs presents a significant strategic challenge (ORWH, n.d.-k). This section highlights the role of SGMRO, THRO, and two ICs—National Institute on Minority Health and Health Disparities (NIMHD) and NICHD—given their unique roles for advancing various aspects of women's health, followed by an overview of IC strategic planning for women's health and sex differences research.

SGMRO

Similarly to ORWH, SGMRO coordinates research across NIH related to sexual and gender minorities (SGM), including individuals who identify as lesbian, gay, bisexual, asexual, transgender, Two-Spirit, queer, or intersex

---

[10] This sentence was changed after release of the report to clarify the scope of NIH ICs.

(SGMRO, 2024). Therefore, issues specific to SGM women fall under its umbrella. While speaking at one of the committee's information-gathering meetings, its director highlighted the following as challenges for it and women's health: scant research focusing on SGM women; inadequate and inaccurate data collection on sexual orientation, gender identity, and sex characteristics; the SABV policy's treatment of sex as binary; the NIH inclusion policy's treatment of gender as binary; and the marginalization of SGM women in STEM fields and the health science workforce (NASEM, 2024b; Parker, 2024b).

NIMHD

NIMHD has been a leader in increasing the scientific community's focus on nonbiological factors, such as socioeconomics, politics, discrimination, culture, and environment, in relation to health disparities. NIMHD has added several populations to its purview since its creation, including those defined by disability, rurality, socioeconomic status, sexual orientation, and gender identity with a focus on gender minorities (NIH, 2023g; NIMHD, 2024a; Pérez-Stable, 2024). In addition to research on women and girls within racially and ethnically minoritized, disability, and lower socioeconomic status groups, the addition of SGM, in particular, demonstrate a focus on subpopulations included within WHR frameworks through research on cisgender lesbian and bisexual women, nonbinary and transgender people assigned female at birth, and transgender women. Though women and girls are not a minority group in the United States, they experience well-documented discrimination, bias, and subjugation that are root causes of health disparities and reduced health care access (see Chapter 6). Women's health concerns are minoritized in terms of treatment in society and corresponding allocation of research funds to understand and improve their health. Based on the committee's funding analysis, NIMHD spent 13 percent of its grant funding on WHR 2013–2023 (see Chapter 4).

NIMHD is the most likely IC to fund research on minoritized women and research centering these groups, but based on input from researchers who spoke at the committee's information-gathering meetings and submitted input in writing and the experience of committee members, grants examining women or pregnant women submitted to NIMHD will often be transferred to NICHD for peer review in study section. While it is unclear how often this is the case, based on the committee's funding analysis, NICHD funds the majority of maternal-child health grants. Studying women, pregnancy, and minoritized populations each pose different methodological challenges and considerations; increased capacity at both NIMHD and NICHD would improve the evaluation of studies at the intersection of these topics. Where reviewers with expertise in both areas cannot be recruited, recruiting more than one, each with the respective expertise, is critical.

NICHD

NICHD's mission is to lead research and training to "understand human development, improve reproductive health, enhance the lives of children and adolescents, and optimize abilities for all" (NICHD, 2019). Its priorities are reproduction, pregnancy, child health, and pregnant and lactating women, children, and people with disabilities (NICHD, 2021). The health of women before or after pregnancy and sex differences do not easily fall within the purview of these stated objectives. In 1993, the NIH Revitalization Act (Public Law 103–43) mandated the establishment of an intramural laboratory and clinical research program on obstetrics and gynecology at NICHD and, in 2000, gynecologic health was added to its description of purpose (Public Law 106–554). In 2012, NICHD added its Gynecologic Health and Disease Branch (GHDB), to support "basic, translational, and clinical research programs related to gynecologic health throughout the reproductive lifespan," including conditions such as menstrual disorders, uterine fibroids, endometriosis, adenomyosis, ovarian cysts, PCOS, and pelvic floor disorders, as well as gynecologic pain syndromes such as chronic pelvic pain, vulvodynia, and dysmenorrhea (NICHD, 2018). GHDB supports this work through its research programs on Menstruation and Menstrual Disorders, Uterine Fibroids, Endometriosis and Adenomyosis, Pelvic Floor Disorders, and Gynecological Pain Syndromes, and through additional programs such as the Pelvic Floor Disorders Network, established in 2001 to spur collaborative research and improve patient care (NICHD, 2023a, 2024c). Endometriosis research is stated as an NICHD "aspirational goal," though this is a multisystem disease that requires additional funding and scientific inquiry (NICHD, n.d.). One mechanism through which NICHD has made progress on this goal is Centers to Advance Research in Endometriosis, which support synergistic research programs on endometriosis that span basic, translational, and human subjects research (RFA-HD-21-002).

Based on its review, the committee found that NICHD focuses primarily on women's health as a mechanism to produce healthy offspring. However, not all women experience pregnancy, and even for those who do, it is a relatively brief phase in the context of an average woman's life-span. Many health conditions experienced during pregnancy have implications for health later in life (see Chapters 5 and 7). Based on the committee's funding analysis (see Chapter 4), NICHD allocated 37 percent of its grant funding on WHR at NIH from FY 2013 to 2023, with nearly 69 percent of that funding going to maternal-child health studies, where women were involved in the studies, but the study design tended to include at least some or more focus on fetal, infant, or child health outcomes.

Another mechanism through which NICHD supports women's health is the Implementing a Maternal Health and Pregnancy Outcomes Vision for Everyone (IMPROVE) initiative, which aims to address key causes of maternal morbidity and mortality, including cardiovascular disease, hypertension, hemorrhage, mental health disorders, substance use, and infectious disease. In FY23, IMPROVE awarded $43.4 million in funding, including $30 million in support from NICHD plus $13.4 million from other Institutes and Centers (NICHD, 2023b).[11]

Tribal Health Research Office (THRO)

NIH established THRO in 2015 to "ensure meaningful input from and collaboration with Tribal Nations on NIH policies, programs, and priorities." THRO serves as the hub for coordination of tribal health–related activities across NIH and as the main point of contact at NIH for federally recognized AIAN tribes (THRO, 2023). It provides a unique opportunity to meaningfully collaborate with and receive input from Tribal Nations on WHR, enabling tribal consultation, incorporation of Indigenous SDOH (see Chapter 6), and ethical conduct of research with Tribal Nations. One specific example of needed coordination is to address barriers to inclusion in grants and workforce development. Due to the rurality of many Tribal Nations, their public health workforce includes community health workers, doulas, early childhood home visitors, and other paraprofessionals. To effectively build the WHR workforce, it is essential to involve these experts in NIH-funded initiatives. In addition, tribal colleges and universities are an important career pathway for many (especially rural) AIAN youth in the trajectory to becoming a health researcher, and ICs could work with THRO to ensure outreach and inclusion.

Women's Health in IC Strategic Plans

Most ICs develop strategic plans that outline their goals and priorities. For the most part, these plans lack a strong emphasis on women's health. A possible reason is that individual ICs, which are mainly organized by body systems and diseases or conditions, tend to focus on their specific areas of research and may fail to integrate women's health as a crosscutting theme (NIH, 2023f). While ORWH collaborates with ICs to coordinate WHR across the organization, the committee's review of the integration of and attention to WHR into the strategic plans of these Institutes found it to be inconsistent and sparse, failing to comprehensively address the gaps in WHR (ORWH, n.d.-j).

---

[11] This section was changed after release of the report to make corrections and clarifications on the scope of NICHD's stated objectives, clarify information on statutes affecting NICHD research activities and changes in NICHD organizational structure, and update/add descriptions of example programs.

Positive Examples

Overall, the IC strategic plans do not demonstrate prioritization of women's health. However, some Institutes have set significant goals regarding women's health and sex differences research; this section highlights a few.

The National Institute on Drug Abuse (NIDA) 2022–2026 strategic plan notes that women become addicted to substances more quickly than men, have comorbid mental illness more often, and respond differently to treatments (NIDA, 2022). As one of its crosscutting priorities, it emphasizes the need to understand sex differences in addiction and translate these findings into treatments tailored to women and also consider the unique experiences of LGBTQ+ individuals who are marginalized because of their gender identity or sexual orientation and at greater risk of substance use because of discrimination and other stressors (NIDA, 2022).

One of the National Institute on Alcohol Abuse and Alcoholism (NIAAA) 2024–2028 strategic goals is to advance research related to women's health. Its strategic plan highlights the importance of understanding the effects of sex on the development of alcohol use disorder and co-occurring mental health conditions, including the mechanisms of these effects and the relationship between alcohol misuse and common comorbidities. The plan acknowledges that women face higher risk of developing certain alcohol-related diseases, such as alcohol-associated liver disease and alcohol-related heart disease and sets goals to evaluate and adapt screening and support services to understudied populations, including women. The plan specifies collaboration with ORWH and other partners across NIH to advance integrated WHR (NIAAA, n.d.-b).[12]

In its 2020–2025 strategic plan, NIA specifically aims to support research on women's health, including sex and gender differences in health and disease overall, cognitive decline and Alzheimer's disease and related dementias, and topics unique to women. The plan notes the Institute's support of a diverse portfolio of research on aging women, including studying sex differences in the basic biology of aging and hormonal influences on cognitive health and age-related diseases more common in women, such as osteoporosis, breast and ovarian cancer, and urinary tract dysfunction. The plan includes specific initiatives and goals focused on women's health, including a commitment to ensure women are fully represented in research and track, monitor, and report on adherence to the SABV policy. Surprisingly, however, the plan mentions menopause only three times, despite this being a significant aging-related concern for half the U.S. population (NIA, 2024).

---

[12] This paragraph was changed after release of the report to clarify the scope of the NIAAA strategic goals.

The National Heart, Lung, and Blood Institute (NHLBI) strategic plan includes a number of strategic goals related to women's health and sex and gender in research (the plan does not cover a specified period). These include improving the representation of women in clinical research, ensuring the applicability of findings to them, and elucidating and further investigating the various factors and environmental, genetic, epigenetic, molecular, cellular, and systemic mechanisms responsible for sex differences in heart, lung, blood, and sleep health and disease (NHLBI, n.d.-a,b).

NICHD is among those ICs that do emphasize women's health, though primarily reproductive health. Its 2020 strategic plan spells out the goal of advancing the understanding and treatment of health conditions and aspects of reproduction unique to women, such as pregnancy and menstruation. NICHD's approach includes supporting research on the health of women and girls, focusing on infertility for both men and women, pregnancy, childbirth, lactation, and the postpartum period (NICHD, n.d.).

Overall Lack of Prioritization of Women's Health

Surprisingly, of the 24 IC strategic plans (CIT does not have a published strategic plan, NCI has strategic priorities, and NIAID has strategic plans for 7 specific diseases/vaccines but not NIAID overall), only NIMH, National Eye Institute (NEI), National Institute of Arthritis and Musculoskeletal and Skin Diseases (NIAMS), NIMHD, and NIAAA explicitly mention collaboration with ORWH (NEI, n.d.; NIAAA, n.d.-b; NIAMS, n.d.; NIMH, 2024; NIMHD, 2024b). ORWH itself has an NIH-Wide Strategic Plan for Research on the Health of Women 2024–2028. This plan aims to, among other goals, integrate women's health across the biomedical research enterprise and develop a workforce that advances research on women's health and the science of sex and gender (ORWH, n.d.-k).

The SABV policy, which is meant to be applied to human and animal studies across NIH, is specifically mentioned by name in only 5 of the 24 strategic plans (NIA, NIMH, NEI, NIAMS, and NCCIH) (NCCIH, 2021; NEI, n.d.; NIA, 2024; NIAMS, n.d.; NIMH, 2024). The National Institute of Environmental Health Sciences' draft strategic plan for FY 2025–2029 also emphasizes the importance of research that benefits the health of all people across the life-span, including through consideration of SABV and collaboration with ORWH, though its previous 2018-2023 strategic plan did not (NIEHS, n.d.-a,b).

The National Institute of Neurological Disorders and Stroke (NINDS) strategic plan acknowledges the importance of health equity for all groups, including all sexes and genders, but women specifically are mentioned only once, in relation to migraines (NINDS, n.d.). Similarly, the National Library of Medicine emphasizes the significance of addressing health disparities, including those based on sex and gender, but otherwise makes no mention of women (NLM, n.d.). NCATS makes no mention of women, sex, or gender, except in relation to workforce in its 2016 strategic plan; its May 2024 plan generally mentions women, however women and sex differences are not specifically mentioned in its strategic objectives (NCATS, 2016, 2024a).[13]

Overall, the picture is inconsistent, with some ICs giving greater importance to the subject than others. Although many ICs support research aimed at understanding sex differences in the development and progression of various diseases, not all of them have strategic priorities related to women's health. As a result, integrating it into the broader NIH strategic plans remains limited. This can be attributed to a variety of factors, including historical research biases, funding priorities, and the specific missions of the different NIH ICs, which may not always align with the goals of ORWH. The committee's review of these strategic plans suggests the need for more comprehensive and coordinated efforts across NIH to address these issues uniformly.

NIH-Wide Strategic Plan

Per the 21st Century Cures Act, NIH updates its strategic plan every 5 years. The most recent iteration is for FY 2021–2025. "The Strategic Plan outlines NIH's vision for biomedical research direction, capacity, and stewardship, by articulating the highest priorities of NIH over the next 5 years" and is designed to complement and harmonize the IC strategic plans (NIH, 2021a). Although enhancing women's health is one of the five crosscutting themes in the framework of the plan, it does not offer much in terms of strategic priorities to address gaps in WHR. It discusses efforts around addressing institutional and environmental barriers that restrict women's potential to advance their careers, some specific ongoing programs and initiatives related to maternal health, including women in clinical trials, and mentions the SABV policy. It has four "bold predictions" or ambitious goals for its 5-year period related to women's health specifically:

- Research on new approaches to cervical cancer screening will lead to developing self-sampling,[14] with the potential to substantially reduce disease incidence and mortality.
- At least one novel, nonhormonal pharmacologic treatment for endometriosis will be identified and moved to clinical trials.
- U.S. maternal deaths per year will be significantly decreased,

---

[13] This sentence was changed after release of the report to include information from the NCATS strategic plan released in May 2024.

[14] Progress has been made on this—in May 2024, the Food and Drug Administration approved a primary human papillomavirus self-collection for cervical cancer screening in a health care setting (American Cancer Society, 2024).

particularly among Black and AIAN women, by implementing results of research studies focusing on links between social determinants and biological risk factors.

- Following findings of the Task Force on Research Specific to Pregnant Women and Lactating Women showing that almost no data exist on medications in these women, label changes will be facilitated by results of clinical trials for at least three therapeutics specific to pregnant and lactating women and children (NIH, 2021b).

While these predictions are important aspirations for women's health, no accompanying steps lay out how these goals will be accomplished.

Does the Current Structure of NIH Serve the Needs for WHR?

The committee considered whether the current organizational structure is adequate to address the pressing need for high-quality WHR. Today, no IC focuses exclusively on WHR. However, it is part of the portfolio of many different ICs. As noted, coordination of research across the 27 ICs is the responsibility of ORWH. As part of its charge, the committee needed to determine whether ORWH has the budget, staffing, and political clout to assure that NIH demonstrates global leadership in WHR.

The committee heard from a wide range of experts from the WHR community during its information-gathering meetings. It also heard testimony from a range of scientific, clinical, and community leaders. One particularly important session featured several NIH grantees.[15] One is studying scientific and clinical challenges associated with uterine fibroids. A second works on endometriosis, and a third focuses on pelvic floor disorders (NASEM, 2024c). Although each of these three problem areas is a central area of investigation in WHR, the grant applications are likely to be evaluated in different study sections in peer review, and the grants may be administered by different ICs. While studies on endometriosis and fibroids are likely to be funded by NICHD, studies on pelvic floor disorders are more likely to be funded through the National Institute of Diabetes and Digestive and Kidney Diseases (NIDDK) (NICHD, 2021; NIDDK, 2024b). In addition, these conditions all received low levels of grant funding from 2013–2023 (see Chapter 4) and have significant research gaps (see Chapter 7).[16]

Therefore, one concern is that these ICs, although committed to high-quality research involving women, do not necessarily have women's health as a core component of their strategic plans. The studies on pelvic floor disorders, for example, go to an Institute that manages priorities in not only kidney and urological diseases, but also endocrinology, metabolism, and

---

[15] See https://www.nationalacademies.org/event/41979_03–2024_assessment-of-nih-research-on-womens-health-meeting-3 for more information (accessed June 15, 2024).

[16] This sentence was changed after release of the report to clarify the scope of NIH ICs.

digestive diseases. Furthermore, urology is largely separate from urogyne-cology; while there are some overlapping conditions involving incontinence and other urinary symptoms, urology does not cover all urogynecological conditions (Rajan et al., 2007). Additionally, review of NIDDK's National Advisory Council revealed that none of its 12 health and science experts appears to focus on WHR (NIDDK, 2024a). Studies on pelvic floor disorders are not likely to be prioritized or reviewed adequately under a strategic plan with no specific mention of urogynecology and by an advisory council with no related expertise (NIDDK, 2021).

NICHD has the greatest proportion of funding for WHR among the NIH ICs (see Chapter 4). However, its emphasis does not include the entire range of issues in women's health. The NICHD Strategic Plan emphasizes "healthy pregnancies, healthy children, healthy and optimal lives" (NICHD, n.d.). The 18-person National Advisory Child Health and Human Development Council includes six members who appear to specialize in WHR, with a heavy focus on pregnancy (NICHD, 2024a).

Problems with NIH Programmatic Offices

DPCPSI houses 14 Offices, four of which have responsibility for coordinating programs across ICs; OBSSR, ODP, OAR, and ORWH coordinate and support research in behavioral and social sciences, prevention research, HIV/AIDS research, and women's health (DPCPSI, n.d.). Theoretically, the coordinating Offices can help avoid duplication, stimulate synergy, and encourage innovation. In practice, that potential may not have been realized. Through presentations from NIH and other experts at the committee's information-gathering meetings, several explanations for these shortcomings surfaced, including their low budgets, limited authority, and reporting structure.

Low budgets and limited authority

Table 3-1 shows the budgets for select programmatic Offices. Although these budgets have grown in recent years, they are insufficient for funding research relevant to their missions (NIH, n.d.-d,e). Rather, their role is more to coordinate and support research and policies in their given area across NIH. For example, although ORWH has the largest budget among the coordinating Offices, it still functions primarily to coordinate WHR across ICs, facilitate implementation of the SABV policy, and engage in other supportive work (see earlier in this chapter for more information). ORWH and OAR have external advisory councils, but OBSSR and ODP do not (OAR, 2024; ORWH, n.d.-d). Although ORWH cofunds women's health–related applications and research projects with ICs, its budget and infrastructure are insufficient to administer grants independently without an IC partner (Clayton, 2023). Actual funding of research on women's health therefore depends primarily on ICs with a range of other priorities, which may explain why only 8.8 percent (based on the committee's analysis, see Chapter 4) of NIH research expenditure is spent on WHR.

The committee considered these factors when assessing what is needed to confront the challenges of WHR under the NIH structure. ORWH's limited resources and inability to fund research independent of existing ICs or administer a women's health study section pose a barrier to addressing these challenges. The ORWH strategic plan, although laudable, has not been executed by NIH across its many ICs in a way that successfully addresses the pressing demand for more and better-coordinated research relevant to women and girls within its current structure.

Since the 2006 NIH reauthorization, the NIH structure has been relatively unchanged, in part because the number of ICs is fixed in statute.[17] This is in contrast to an organizational structure that had flexibly responded to new challenges for over a century. The following section briefly addresses the history of NIH as it is relevant to the committee's recommendations.

The Evolution of NIH

The roots of NIH date back to 1887, when a one-room laboratory was established as part of the Marine Hospital Service providing medical care to merchant seamen. Congress asked it to take responsibility for examining itinerant sailors who might be vectors for infectious diseases, such as cholera and yellow fever. By 1912, it became part of the Public Health Service. It had a relatively limited mission until the middle of the 20th century, when it evolved into NIH. In 1940, President Franklin D. Roosevelt dedicated a building in Bethesda, Maryland, to house it (Kaplan et al., 2017).

In the years leading up to World War II, an influential academic engineer, Vannaver Bush, made an impassioned plea for the United States to make major investments in original research. Following the war, Bush published a report entitled *Science: The Endless Frontier*. It argued that massive investments in basic and applied research were needed to establish the United States as the world leader in science and technology (Bush, 1945). The vision included transforming leading universities into research-intensive institutions that would reward faculty research productivity. To make this transformation attractive, universities would receive substantial overhead payments that they could use to build laboratories and support infrastructure services, including university libraries (Kaplan et al., 2017). This approach continues at NIH today (UMR, 2024).

NIH has evolved, regularly modifying its organizational structure to reflect changes in science and clinical practice. In 1948, it created Institutes for heart disease, dentistry, and microbiology. NIMH was founded in 1949,

---

[17] Public Law 109–482.

and new Institutes on diabetes and stroke were established in 1950 (Kaplan et al., 2017).

Between 1950 and about 2005, NIH was continually reorganizing in response to evolving scientific directions and societal demands. For example, in 1971, President Richard Nixon declared a war on cancer. The resulting National Cancer Act allowed a redistribution of NIH funds that shifted some resources away from other areas of investigation. To this day, NCI has greater power and resources in relation to the other Institutes (Kaplan et al., 2017).

The HIV epidemic led to considerable public pressure for an expansion of NIH funding. Influential groups of citizens and scientists persuaded Congress that greater NIH research was essential (IOM, 1991; Padamsee, 2018). Without this research, the United States would be at a strategic disadvantage in relation to rival nations. Between 1999 and 2002, the NIH budget nearly doubled (Kaplan et al., 2017). Overall, it has increased fourfold over the past 30 years (CRS, 2024).

NIMH has been in and out of NIH over the past 80 years. It separated from NIH in 1967 and became a component of the Health Services and Mental Health Administration. By the 1970s, a serious concern about an epidemic of recreational drug use caused Congress to authorize NIDA within NIMH. A year later, NIMH briefly rejoined NIH but exited again to become part of the new Alcohol, Drug Abuse, and Mental Health Administration (Kaplan et al., 2017). The Hughes Act of 1970 paved the way for NIAAA to be a component of NIMH (NIAAA, n.d.-a). In 1992, NIMH moved back to NIH, and NIDA and NIAAA were spun off as separate Institutes (Kaplan et al., 2017).

NIMHD evolved as well—it did not start as an Institute. In 1990, the Office of Minority Programs was established in the NIH OD, and in 1993, the Health Revitalization Act established the Office of Research on Minority Health.[18] In 2000, the National Center on Minority Health and Health Disparities was established; it was redesignated as an Institute in 2010, as part of the Patient Protection and Affordable Care Act,[19] due to decades of work to bring attention to the unequal burden of illness and death experienced by certain U.S. populations (NIH, 2010; NIMHD, 2024a).

This detour into history reveals that NIH has a long tradition of reorganizing in response to scientific and societal needs. However, the NIH Reform Act of 2006[20] set 27 as NIH's maximum number of national ICs; the Secretary of HHS has the authority to add or remove an IC as long as they stay within the limit. It was not clear to the committee that a fixed

---

[18] Public Law 103–143.
[19] Public Law 111–148.
[20] Public Law 109–482.

organizational structure is in the best interest of science and society. With this in mind, the committee reviewed NIH programs, structures, and funding to determine how to best to support WHR at NIH (see Chapter 9 for the committee's recommendations).

Summary of WHR at NIH

No clear comprehensive approach to strategic planning or evaluating progress in WHR exists across NIH and between individual ICs. Each IC has its own individual and unique approach to women's health and focus on specific disease processes relevant to that content area. Moreover, the IC strategic plans cover different time frames that often do not align with the NIH-Wide Strategic Plan for Research on the Health of Women. This decentralized approach poses a significant barrier to generating research that will improve the health of women throughout the life-span and tracking progress in any given scientific field of women's health. Furthermore, this structure decentralizes and effectively prevents central accountability from managing failures or progress in the field. Consistent with the findings in *Enhancing NIH Research on Autoimmune Diseases*, this committee finds that without a clear strategic plan for NIH as a whole, it is difficult to track progress or achievement of important milestones (NASEM, 2022).

ORWH has a large and important charge. It oversees essential programs and policies to support the advancement of WHR. It is also responsible for coordination of WHR across NIH—research that spans countless conditions and diseases and is relevant to almost every IC (ORWH, n.d.-j). However, its budget and level of authority are not commensurate with its mission or charge.

NIH SABV POLICY

History of the SABV Policy and Related Requirements

NIH implemented the SABV policy in 2016 to recognize the importance of sex in research and address the persistent exclusion or underrepresentation of females in preclinical and clinical research (Miller et al., 2017; ORWH, 2023). The policy expects that "sex as a biological variable will be factored into research designs, analyses, and reporting in vertebrate animals and human studies" and "strong justification from the scientific literature, preliminary data, or other relevant considerations [if] proposing to study only one sex" (NOT-OD-15–103) (NIH, 2015a).

The SABV policy requires researchers to consider biological sex in their research and describe in their proposals how they will consider it with respect to factors such as study design; the population of interest and study sample, such as sampling or recruitment procedures and power analyses; and statistical analysis plans. The policy language is broad and allows latitude to incorporate SABV in ways specific to the research questions (Miller and Reckelhoff, 2016; ORWH, n.d.-l). Despite some misconceptions of the policy early on, it does not require researchers to study mechanisms or contributors to sex differences (Clayton, 2018; Dalla et al., 2024; NIH, 2015a; White et al., 2021). What it does require is that investigators provide a justification for not factoring sex into the design (ORWH, n.d.-l). Considerable challenges and limitations remain in implementation of the SABV policy, described next.

Examples of SABV-Related Analyses and Resources for Applicants

Concrete examples of how investigators may incorporate biological sex into their analyses include reporting primary outcomes by sex, including sex as a covariate in models, and reporting sex-disaggregated data in

---

BOX 3-3
NIH Resources and Training Materials on Sex as a Biological Variable and Sex and Gender Research

SABV Primer:
    Developed by ORWH and the National Institute of General Medical Sciences and available free to the public, the primer includes four modules that provide an overview of the importance of the SABV policy for scientific rigor, transparency, and discovery across the spectrum of biomedical sciences and how to incorporate SABV in experimental design, analyses, and reporting: *SABV and the Health of Women and Men*, *SABV and Experimental Design*, *SABV and Analyses*, and *SABV and Research Reporting* (ORWH, n.d.-n,q). In FY 2022, 733 people accessed the primer training, and about three-quarters completed it (ORWH, 2023). There is opportunity to expand this primer by including more contemporary examples of appropriate and inappropriate applications of SABV (e.g., missed opportunities) in practice and in the context of currently used research methods across different fields.

SABV Primer: Train the Trainer:
    A six-module course developed by ORWH that guides training of the SABV policy in in-person, virtual, and one-on-one and group training environments and includes SABV best practices (ORWH, n.d.-o). This primer can be expanded to include more specific training modules for researchers who practice in certain fields, such as fundamental biology, population genetics, and interventional studies.

analytic models. The relative appropriateness and potential scientific yield of an approach will vary depending on the research question and context. ORWH has developed resources and training materials on the SABV policy and sex and gender research for the research community, including a Bench-to-Bedside series and core concepts training materials (NIH, n.d.-b; ORWH, n.d.-e). Still, room remains for additional improvement regarding training—particularly tailoring education for scientists who are conducting research in certain fields and using certain methodologies for which SABV considerations may not be intuitive (see Box 3-3).

Effect of SABV

The potential effect of SABV is broad. If it is implemented completely and successfully, effective ongoing training in it would lead to improved and optimal scientific methods and, in turn, scientific discoveries generating new knowledge that could benefit the health of all. Thus, policies such

---

Sex and Gender Research Modules:

The *Bench-to-Bedside: Integrating Sex and Gender to Improve Human Health* course includes six modules on sex and gender differences in disease areas, including immunology, cardiovascular and pulmonary diseases, neurology, endocrinology, and mental health (ORWH, n.d.-e). *Introduction to Sex and Gender: Core Concepts for Health-Related Research* includes a video and slide set on sex, gender, and intersectionality as health-related variables (NIH, n.d.-b). The modules could be expanded to tailor them toward researchers practicing in certain fields whose conventional forms of training do not typically include a primary consideration of SABV, such as experimental studies, population genetics, and artificial intelligence (Cirillo et al., 2020; Naqvi et al., 2019; Zhang et al., 2022).

In addition to augmenting education and training resources, an opportunity exists to make evaluating SABV in the peer-review process clearer so that reviewers are able to facilitate more consistent implementation (Arnegard et al., 2020; Woitowich and Woodruff, 2019). The review training slides from the CSR briefly mention SABV in the criterion scores (NIH, 2024h) and the NIH Reviewer Orientation guide does not include information about SABV beyond linking to the decision tree that guides reviewers through steps to evaluate applications for it (NIH, 2018); outcomes include acknowledging the lack of a strong justification for a single-sex study "as a weakness in the critique and discussion and score accordingly" (NIH, n.d.-f). The scoring systems and procedure guidance do not mention SABV (NIH, 2015b). When NIH solicited feedback on the peer-review process, it was unclear to respondents how SABV would be incorporated in the rubric (NIH, 2023h).

as SABV are needed not only to raise awareness of and help fill knowledge gaps in women's health but also for achieving precision medicine and equity in health care more broadly. Pertaining to health equity, establishing policies requiring investigators to conduct research in a way that produces knowledge that can be applied to both female and male patients is a needed step to ensure that patients are receiving evidenced-base care rather than care that has been investigated adequately only in narrow demographics. Furthermore, methods such as sex disaggregation that fall under the umbrella of SABV can lead to discoveries of sex-specific effects or associations and translate to precision medicine interventions that will ultimately improve outcomes for the entire population (Ji et al., 2020, 2021; Shapiro et al., 2021).

Understanding the successes, limitations, and barriers to implementing the SABV policy requires accepting that SABV and sex differences research are not equivalent. SABV requires all investigators submitting proposals to NIH to include females and males in their study samples unless they have a strong justification otherwise and consider how to best incorporate biological sex into study design and analysis strategies based on the specific research question (Miller and Reckelhoff, 2016; NIH, 2015a). In contrast, sex differences research describes projects in which identifying sex differences in a particular condition or intervention is a primary or at least a secondary objective (Miller and Reckelhoff, 2016). It may require increases in sample sizes and funding based on power analyses designed to detect such differences. Furthermore, though SABV is required for all NIH grant submissions, and incorporating biological sex into study design as more than a control variable can increase the frequency of generating research findings that can benefit the sexes in different ways, it does not mitigate the need for true sex differences research, which fully assesses whether findings apply to the sexes, whether differences exist, and the mechanisms underlying and driving such differences (Galea et al., 2020; Peters and Woodward, 2023). Such research can further advance knowledge of how to care for women as well as men and ultimately lead to better health for all (Galea et al., 2020; Peters and Woodward, 2023).

Limited Appreciation and Uptake of SABV

Several years have passed since NIH enacted the SABV policy (Arnegard et al., 2020; Clayton, 2018). Despite efforts by NIH and other sponsors to implement it across investigator-initiated scientific projects, along with efforts by journals to implement sex and gender in research guidelines in research reporting, uptake and application in practice have been suboptimal (Arnegard et al., 2020; Carmody et al., 2022; Waltz et al., 2021a,b; White et al., 2021). Limited incorporation persists in researchers using preclinical models (Waltz et al., 2021a,b), and similar issues abound among clinical and population scientists (Willingham, 2022). As a result, the potential generation of new knowledge that could help to address sex disparities and improve women's health has been stymied.

The problem of limited uptake and application stems from multiple sources, including limited appreciation for the potential scientific yield of applying SABV in research and limited understanding of how to apply it in practice to gain maximal new knowledge. The former has led to many investigators citing a perceived low estimated value-to-cost ratio when considering the resources needed to include animals of both sexes in an experiment or enroll enough women and men to ensure adequate statistical power for sex differences analyses in a clinical study (Waltz et al., 2021a,b) and also perpetuated the perception that SABV should be at most a secondary consideration in research and, in turn, is dispensable if resources are limited. It is coupled to limited understanding of the scientific yield that can arise from when SABV is treated as primary consideration. The scientific knowledge to be gained from treating SABV as a primary versus secondary consideration can be illustrated using examples with a review of relevant fundamental statistical concepts (see Box 3-4).

There are additional considerations regarding SABV as it could be applied in current and future research practice, including the conventional binary definitions of sex and gender (Clayton, 2018; ORWH, n.d.-p; Parker, 2024a). A binary conceptualization of sex excludes other categories, such as intersex, and technically misrepresents how sex frequently manifests as a bimodal distribution of continuous measures with respect to anatomy, physiology, biochemical, and even hormonal measures (Peters and Woodward, 2023; Yang and Rubin, 2024). A wealth of data is now available to clarify how genetic, transcriptomic, and phenotypic traits consistently demonstrate broadly overlapping diversity spanning the sexes. This consistent phenomenon of nature, which manifests, for example, as broad and overlapping bell-shaped curves representing the distributions of height measured across a population of female and male adults, is also seen across many other biological measures, including gene expression (Ahmed et al., 2023; Yang and Rubin, 2024).

Similarly, the SABV policy does not mention gender-related constructs, such as gender identity and gender roles. Advancing progress in women's health will require that gender be incorporated more systematically into research. This is unlikely without developing and implementing policies requiring researchers to, at a minimum, report the gender identity of their human participants. Accordingly, future SABV training and policy implementation may be developed to include the concepts of sex diversity rather than sex difference, in addition to gender diversity rather than gender difference, as considerations for research on a given topic and in a given context.

BOX 3-4
Examples of Primary versus Secondary Consideration of
Sex as a Biological Variable in Research

The examples in Figure 3-8 are extrapolated from real data collected and reported in published studies (Cheng et al., 2010; Llamosas-Falcón et al., 2022). Scenario A finds that sex is a confounder when examining the association between age and heart cavity size. The rate of reduction in heart cavity size with advancing age is similar by sex, indicating no significant sex interaction (i.e., similar slopes) (Cheng et al., 2010). In Scenario B, sex has a significant interaction, revealed by different slopes, on the association of age and heart wall thickness, also known as "left ventricular hypertrophy," an established significant risk factor for cardiovascular and all-cause mortality (Cheng et al., 2010; Levy, 1988, 1990). Similarly, in Scenario C, sex also has a significant interaction on the association of alcohol intake and liver cirrhosis, a well-known finding that has led to sex-specific recommendations for alcohol intake, yet understanding remains limited of underlying mechanisms (Llamosas-Falcón et al., 2022; USDA, 2020).

In statistical terms, sex is an effect modifier and not just a confounder in Scenarios B and C. When sex is only a confounder, as in Scenario A, a potential treatment implication may be as simple as a dose adjustment. When it is an effect modifier, as in Scenarios B and C, the potential treatment implication may be more complex and even require an alternate therapy altogether (Diao et al., 2024; Kavousi, 2016). In many biomedical research settings, researchers attempting to address SABV often consider Scenario A and stop there, with relatively few considering Scenarios B or C and following up with the requisite sex-stratified analyses needed to understand further implications of the observed sex difference. These examples illustrate why and how the need for comprehensive training and tailored and pragmatic education in how to apply SABV in research persists and how a small amount of additional analytical effort can lead to a large amount of potential scientific gain.

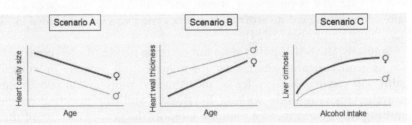

FIGURE 3-8 Illustration of the potential to discover new insights when fully considering SABV. In Scenario A, sex is a confounder. In Scenarios B and C, sex is an effect modifier, and the significant interaction on the association between the predictor (x axis) and the outcome (y axis) warrants follow-up with sex-specific analyses.

Limited Oversight of SABV Policy

Another major impediment to successful implementation of the SABV policy relates to oversight. There is a lack of systems or procedures to ensure that investigators follow through with their stated plans to incorporate and account for biologic sex into their projects. Grant reviewers are required to consider SABV as a criterion that can affect the overall grant score (NIH, n.d.-f). Unfortunately, it is not clear if attention to SABV during the NIH grant review process is consistent across reviewers and study sections. Based on committee expertise and input from NIH researchers at its public meetings, the merits of investigators' justifications for not factoring sex into study design are not routinely evaluated. Rewards or penalties in scoring based on implementing SABV in study design are not applied consistently despite NIH guidance to reviewers (NIH, n.d.-f), even where it would contribute to addressing significant knowledge gaps in the evidence base on women's health and health care.

Several factors may limit adherence to the SABV policy, including the level of reviewer expertise, experience of the NIH program official overseeing the grant, and content area. The lack of a mechanism to ensure that researchers complete and report planned analyses by sex also limits the policy's effectiveness. This lack of accountability substantially lessens the knowledge that federally funded proposals could generate. Furthermore, there are lessons to learn from policies of other research organizations that not only require grantees to describe sex- and gender-based analyses in their proposals but also hold applicants and reviewers accountable for them (CIHR, 2018; Haverfield and Tannenbaum, 2021; Johnson et al., 2009).

Technical Considerations for Implementing SABV

Certain technical issues merit discussion, given that they represent perceived barriers to incorporating SABV into research studies. For example, investigators have often incorrectly cited marked hormonal variability as a legitimate reason to exclude females from certain studies. It exists in both females and males according to certain time scales and at certain life stages,[21] and this variability is important to include and account for across all study types to enhance the potential gain in new knowledge that may be translated to benefit the health of women as well as men (Beery and Zucker, 2011; Bell, 2018; Dalla et al., 2024; Lew et al., 2022). For example, whereas female rats tend to exhibit rhythms occurring over the course of days in physiological trait variations associated with the estrous cycle, this is less robust in mice (Kopp et al., 2006). Accordingly, the aggregate evidence to date from basic models, such as mouse models, has mirrored evidence from human biology studies

---

[21] Hormonal variation in males occurs in the postnatal period and then at puberty. After that point, testosterone levels in males decline and level off (Bell, 2018).

in demonstrating both sex-specific and sex-similar variations in hormonal, neurohormonal, and other biochemical measures. Such accumulating data have led to a growing awareness and understanding that studying both sexes in a given experiment will increase its translational impact and help avoid inappropriate generalization of findings from males to females or vice versa.

There remains a commonly held perception that adhering to SABV in a proposal will incur greater costs because it would require researchers to increase the sample size of the proposed studies so that they are adequately powered to detect sex differences (Waltz et al., 2021a). However, incorporating SABV into a given study design does not require this in every experimental situation (see Costs and Implementation of SABV in Basic Science section). Applying SABV in many or most scenarios will maximize the opportunity to gain more information on sex-specific or sex-differential findings up front, potentially precluding the need for follow-up studies to investigate sex-divergent effects. For instance, in several examples, lack of prespecified study of sex-specific effects in a trial has required post-hoc, de novo studies of the same intervention (Sohani et al., 2023; Zhao et al., 2024). Thus, given the potential for incorporating SABV in studies to maximize their scientific yield and generalizability, doing so is likely to be more rather than less cost efficient over the long term.

Nonetheless, the SABV policy remains a complex issue, given the situations where it may be scientifically justifiable not to incorporate SABV. For example, in certain basic science models, background sex-based genetic differences and hormonal variation have not been shown to affect endpoints of interest. Assessing how to apply SABV in these situations is based on published studies demonstrating that variation in females in a given context is negligible. The SABV policy allows for and encourages describing all scientific justifications for any proposed study designs.

Costs and Implementation of SABV in Basic Science

Sometimes, addressing SABV adds no increased cost. In many cases, sample size does not have to change or requires a small increase to meet the SABV criteria (Dalla et al., 2024). For basic science, implementing SABV would include using females with intact ovaries, ovariectomized females with and without estrogen treatment, and aged females, depending on the study question (Allegra et al., 2023; Dalla et al., 2024; Miller et al., 2011). This does not address changes in postcoital, pregnant, or lactating and weaning animals. Depending upon the parameters being measured, the sample sizes for each cohort can vary from as low as 7 for physiological parameters to at least 10 for standard behavioral assays (Corrigan et al., 2020; Crawley, 1999). With at least six stages in the female life cycle, incorporating SABV can become expensive in these cases.

There is an opportunity to provide additional funding for basic science studies to include sex diversity in model organisms. This may be substantially cheaper than in many types of clinical studies, and scientists would be more likely to do so if NIH increased grant funding for this purpose. At approximately $1 per cage per 4–5 group-housed mice per day, including two sexes will double cage costs (Ohio State University, n.d.; UCSF, n.d.; University of Kentucky, n.d.; University of Michigan, n.d.). Researchers are disinclined to include sex diversity without adequate funding, and funding for this purpose is often limited in the standard R01 grant. NIH needs to consider whether cutting costs by excluding female or male animals would also produce less rigorous science and could therefore result in increased health care costs, since the resulting science may lead to inadequately treating women or men based on studies in only one sex.

Implementation of SABV Within NIH Institutes

The 2019–2020 Biennial Report of the ACRWH includes a report of the NIH ICOs, including information on their SABV implementation efforts. NIDA, for example, notes that its history of supporting research on sex differences in substance use disorders precedes SABV and that from 2019 to 2020, the success rate of grants analyzing sex differences was higher than the average, at 21 percent versus 16 percent, respectively (ORWH, 2021). NIDA uses its Extramural Project System to track inclusion of both sexes in animal studies and experiments that analyze sex differences. Similarly, the National Institute on Deafness and Other Communication Disorders uses its Science Tracking and Reporting System to track funded research in women's health. Others, such as NIAID, National Institute of Environmental Health Sciences, and NIDDK, note their use of funding opportunity announcements to emphasize their interest in applications that address women's health and sex differences (ORWH, 2021).

Many Institutes, however, simply report on their compliance with SABV during the peer-review process, with the National Human Genome Research Institute even noting "absent including information about NIH's SABV policy on the NIH checklists and [Funding Opportunity Announcement] templates, there is no way to ensure complete compliance" (ORWH, 2021, p. 162).

SABV Summary

Opportunities exist to improve the implementation of the 2016 SABV policy for NIH-funded research studies and concomitantly incentivize or require researchers to be accountable for proposing and carrying out the sex-specific analyses and research that was the policy's intent. For example, one way to improve accountability and reporting could be to require researchers to report how they plan to analyze their results to explore sex differences (when applicable) in yearly and final progress reports. In addition, expanding grantee reporting requirements to include both sex and gender categories in

NIH RePORTER annually in the tables submitted to NIH, including their postaward enrollment projections, would also improve accountability.

Although more journals are supporting changes in reporting by sex and gender, a significant gap remains in publishing findings that focus specifically on women or gender science (Arnegard et al., 2020; Clayton, 2018; Heidari et al., 2016; ORWH, 2021, 2023; Woitowich et al., 2020). Notwithstanding organizational efforts, journal editors could further require that NIH-funded studies published in peer-reviewed journals address SABV directly, along with a statement of reasoning if they did not use female animals, enroll women in human subjects research, or present analytic results by sex (Arnegard et al., 2020; Clayton, 2018). This approach could be implemented in the same way that many journals require specific statements regarding conflicts of interest or guidelines for accepted language for marginalized groups. Improving SABV policy implementation would normalize the concept that funding studies focused on conditions that affect women are rigorous and evidence based.

NIH RESEARCH STRUCTURE

NIH's extramural program funds the full spectrum of research, including basic, preclinical, clinical, population-based, and implementation science, all of which are critical to advancing knowledge of women's health (see Box 3-5). Across NIH, numerous mechanisms are used to solicit extramural applications, including parent announcements, program announcements, requests for applications, and notices of special interest (see Box 3-6), in addition to Requests for Proposals, Research Opportunity Announcements, and prize challenges.[22]

Peer Review

According to NIH, "the peer review process forms the cornerstone of the NIH extramural research mission and seeks to ensure that applications submitted to the NIH are evaluated by scientific experts in a manner free from inappropriate influences" (NIH, 2019). NIH highlights the following as core values of the peer-review process: expert assessment, transparency, impartiality, fairness, confidentiality, security, integrity, and efficiency.

Peer review is a two-step process comprising initial peer review, performed by a Scientific Review Group (SRG),[23] and council review, performed

---

[22] This sentence was updated after release of the report to add additional solicitation mechanisms.

[23] SRGs are groups of scientists who review grant applications made up of mostly nonfederal scientists and led by a Scientific Review Officer (SRO) at NIH who is responsible for overseeing the review. The term encompasses any review panel. There are two types of SRGs—standing study sections and Special Emphasis Panels (SEPs).

BOX 3-5
Research Types Funded by NIH

1. Basic science research, such as animal models that have examined sex differences to study mechanisms of chronic disease in females.
2. Preclinical research that connects basic science research with human medicine to understand the basis of a disease or disorder and find ways to treat it, including research on biomarkers.
3. Clinical research that includes testing new technologies or interventions, behavioral and observational studies, and outcomes and health services research.
4. Population-based research that focuses on health outcomes at the population level to determine the effects of diseases and efforts to prevent, diagnose, and treat them.
5. Implementation research on how evidence-based practices, interventions, and policies can be translated to use in settings like hospitals and schools.

SOURCES: Excerpts from NASEM, 2024a; ODP, n.d.-b.

---

by National Advisory Councils or Boards for ICs (NIH, 2019). CSR is centered entirely around peer review, ensuring that all applications "receive fair, independent, expert, and timely scientific reviews—free from inappropriate influence—so NIH can fund the most promising research" (NIH, 2023c). It oversees the peer-review process, "serving as the central receipt point for all research and training grant applications submitted to NIH" (NIH, 2023c). It assigns review of these applications to the appropriate review branches of funding ICs or to SRGs within CSR (NIH, 2023c). It is largely responsible for initial peer review, reviewing approximately 75 percent of grant applications submitted to NIH (CSR, 2022). CSR may administer peer review through either standing study sections or special emphasis panels (SEPs). SEPs are used for a range of reasons, such as when assigning an application to the appropriate standing study section would create a conflict of interest, or for particular types of grants, such as fellowships, Small Business Innovation Research grants, and Academic Research Enhancement Award grants. SEPs can be recurring or for one-time initiatives or conflicts (Rubinstein, 2022).

During initial peer review, external scientists with relevant expertise assess applications on technical and scientific merit. Members of standing SRGs serve for up to 6 years (the typical term length is 4 years), attend three meetings each year, and need to be approved by the NIH deputy director or, for NCI, the NCI director. The collective expertise of the SRG

BOX 3-6
Examples of Mechanisms Used Across NIH to Solicit
Extramural Applications*

Notice of Funding Opportunities:

- Parent Announcements: broad opportunities for unsolicited or investigator-initiated applications that allow applicants to submit an application for a specific activity code. They are open for up to 3 years and use standard due dates. Not all ICs participate on all parent announcements.
- Program Announcements: issued by one or more ICs that aim to highlight areas of scientific interest and solicit applications for a new or ongoing program and typically open for 3 years.
- Request for Applications (RFA): issued by one or more ICs and highlight a well-defined area of scientific interest to accomplish particular program goals. An RFA will indicate the amount of funds available and the anticipated number of awards. ICs typically convene a review panel for applications received.
- Notice of Special Interest: an invitation for grant applications on high-priority or high-opportunity topics that usually identifies one or more active notices of funding opportunity. With rare exceptions, these do not have set-aside funding. NIH ICs do not presuppose support levels ahead as is commonly done for several types of requests for applications and program announcements that have set-aside funds.

NOTE: *The title of Box 3-6 was updated after release of the report to clarify its content.
SOURCES: NIAID, 2023; NIH, 2023i.

---

has to suit the applications it will consider and is judged based on publication record, research and funding history, other scientific achievements, and recommendations from colleagues. While it is uncommon, CSR may recruit public representatives to provide a patient or advocacy perspective, and it pays close attention to balance in an SRG's membership. During initial peer review, research project grant (RPG) applications are evaluated based on five criteria: significance, investigators, innovation, approach, and environment (NIH, 2019). This process will be updated and simplified for most RPGs beginning in 2025 (see the Simplified Framework section for more information). The outcome of the initial peer review is relayed to the funding IC and the application's project director/principal investigator (PI) in an NIH

Summary Statement (NIH, 2019). IC advisory councils or boards are composed of individuals with demonstrated interests in the health program areas of the particular IC. They include not only biomedical, behavioral, social, and public health scientists but also leaders in such fields as law, economics, management, health policy, and public policy. Patients, relatives of patients, and advocates who represent the concerns of the community may also be asked to serve. Members typically serve for 4 years, or 6 years for NCI. They perform the second level of peer review for research grant applications and offer advice and recommendations on policy and program development, program implementation, evaluation, and other matters of significance to the mission and goals of the respective ICs and recommendations on research conducted by each Institute's or Center's intramural program.

With input from staff and the advisory council or board, the IC director makes final funding decisions within the constraints of the available budget (NIH, 2019). Most grants are issued for 3-, 4-, or 5-year periods. Investigators have to file progress reports (i.e., noncompeting continuation applications) each year. Investigators often can submit renewal applications for additional funding for a period after that provided by the current award. These applications have to compete for funding through the peer review system (NIH, 2019).[24]

Key Steps in the Review Process

Before submission, the grant cycle for extramural investigators usually begins with consulting with a program official (PO) at a specific IC to discuss the potential match with its mission and priorities. If the PO does not believe the proposal is a good fit, they may recommend another IC. In addition to the scientific proposal, typical grant applications for R01 mechanisms may require investigator biosketches, letters of support, budgets, facilities and environment descriptions, and other documentation, resulting in a total package often exceeding 100 pages (NIH, 2024c).

Investigators submitting applications to NIH may indicate their preferred Institute and study section. CSR assigns the submitted application to a funding IC for funding consideration and to either a review branch at the funding IC or a review branch or SRG within CSR for review (CSR, 2023a). The role of the Scientific Review Officer (SRO) is to oversee the study section review and ensure integrity in the process. The SRO reaches out to potential reviewers on the study section to confirm their availability, recruits ad hoc reviewers as needed for the round of applications, and, once the roster is complete, instructs reviewers to check for conflicts

---

[24] Email communication with Kristin Kramer, Center for Scientific Review, National Institutes of Health and Stephanie Constant, Office of Extramural Research, National Institutes of Health, on September 26, 2024, and September 27, 2024.

of interest, such as the possibility of a financial benefit from the applicant institution or a history of collaboration with personnel on the application. Reviewers are assigned based on their area of expertise, considering their workloads and avoiding identified conflicts of interest (NIH, 2024b,e).

Assignments are typically released about 6 weeks before the SRG convenes. Reviewers are to assess the scientific and technical merit of all assigned grant applications using the established NIH review criteria and assign scores to reflect their overall assessment of a project (overall impact score). Scores range from 1 to 9, with 1 being the highest impact score and 9 indicating low impact (NIH, 2024b). Scores ranging from 1 to 3 indicate an application with minor or no weaknesses and high impact, 4–6 indicate a good application but more than one major or several minor weaknesses, and 7–9 indicating a low-impact application with many weaknesses (NIH, 2024b; Rockey, 2011).

The study section then enters the "read" phase, where assigned reviewers read the critiques of the other reviewers and decide if they want to adjust their scores. The SRO reviews all the scores; typically, those applications with the top 50 percent of scores (based on the mean of the three reviewers' overall impact scores) are moved forward for discussion.

Within 6 weeks of the meeting, overall impact scores are assigned to applications that average the final scores submitted by the study section reviewers and multiplying by 10, yielding scores ranging from 10 (high impact) to 90 (low impact). Often, a percentile is calculated using the scores from the previous two and the scores from the current meeting, to provide a rank percentile relative to other applications, allowing for comparison across committees with potentially different scoring behaviors (NIH, 2024b; Rockey, 2011). The IC staff prepare a funding plan for the director. The top-scoring grants are then discussed with the Council of the IC, and the director decides which applications to fund based on scores and alignment with the funding priorities and mission of the IC. Directors have the discretion to fund out of order, even if the application was not in the top scoring percentiles.[25]

Effect of Institute Paylines

Institutes set paylines that determine which grant applications are likely to be considered for funding, though not all paylines are published. These paylines are set based on application impact scores or percentile rank (see Box 3-7 for definitions of these terms). For example, a grant ranked in the 10th percentile has a more favorable score than 90 percent of the applications reviewed by that study section. When an Institute sets a payline at the 10th percentile, it means that applications scoring from the first through

---

[25] Email communication with Kristin Kramer, Center for Scientific Review, National Institutes of Health and Stephanie Constant, Office of Extramural Research, National Institutes of Health, on September 26, 2024 and September 27, 2024.

BOX 3-7
Definitions for Payline and Related Terms

Impact Score/Overall Impact Score/Priority Score: Reviewers assign applications an impact score based on scientific and technical merit. Impact scores range between 1 and 9, where 1 is indicative of a very strong application, and 9 is indicative of an application with substantial weaknesses. The normalized average of all reviewer impact scores constitutes the final/overall impact/priority score—these range from 10 to 90, where 10 is best. Generally, scores of 10–30 are most likely to be funded.

Percentile Rank: The percentile rank is based on a ranking of the impact scores assigned by a peer-review committee. It is typically calculated by ordering the impact score of an application against that of all applications reviewed in the current and preceding two review rounds. An application ranked in the 5th percentile is considered more meritorious than 95 percent of the applications reviewed by that committee. This ranking allows for comparison across committees with potentially different scoring behaviors.

Payline: Many Institutes calculate a percentile rank up to which most applications can be funded. For grant applications that do not receive percentile ranks, the payline may be expressed as an impact score. Institutes that choose to publish paylines in advance calculate them based on expectations about the availability of funds, application loads, and the average cost of RPGs during the current fiscal year.

SOURCES: Edited excerpts from NIH, 2023e; Rockey, 2011.

10th percentiles are likely to be funded (NIH, 2023e; Rockey, 2011). Paylines vary from one Institute to another and within an Institute by type of grant (see Table 3-2). Applications that score under an IC's payline are then considered by the council and director for funding. Occasionally, an IC will fund applications that are scored above the payline.

For FY 2024, NICHD has set the payline for R15 grants at a Priority Score of 28. For R01, R21, and R03 grants, NICHD notes that it considers scientific merit, program priorities, portfolio balance, and the availability of funds in making funding decisions but does not have set paylines. In addition, NICHD states that new competing R01 applications will be reduced by an average of 14 percent below the level of support recommended by the study section (NICHD, 2024b).

TABLE 3-2 Paylines of Select Institutes, Fiscal Year 2024

	R Grants				K Grants					F Grants	
	R01	R21	R03	R15	K01	K08	K25	K99	F30	F31	F32
NCI	10th percentile (ESI* = 17th)	10th percentile	Scores up to and including 25	Scores up to and including 25	X	X	X	X	X	X	X
NICHD	X	X	X	Priority score 28	Priority score 28	Priority score 28	Priority score 28	Priority score 37	Priority score 26	28th percentile (34th for diversity F31)	35th percentile
NIAID	10th percentile (New PIs = 14th)	28 overall impact score	28 overall impact score	23 overall impact score	20 overall impact score	20 overall impact score	20 overall impact score	X	20 overall impact score	24 overall impact score	31 overall impact score
NHLBI	14th percentile (ESI* = 24th)	X	X	Priority score 30	Priority score 30	Priority score 30	Priority score 30	Priority score 30	Priority score 20	35th percentile	35th percentile
NIMHD	Priority score range 10-30	Priority score range 10-35	X	Priority score range 10-35	Priority score range 10-35	Priority score range 10-35	Priority score range 10-35	Priority score range 10-35	Priority score range 10-35	Priority score range 10-35	Priority score range 10-35
NIAAA	X	X	X	X	X	X	X	X	X	X	X
NEI	X	X	X	X	X	X	X	X	X	X	X
NCATS	X	X	X	X	X	X	X	X	X	X	X
NIAMS	8th percentile (ESI* = 15th)	8th percentile	Priority score 21	27th percentile	Priority score 30	Priority score 30	Priority score 30	Priority score 30	19th percentile	22nd percentile	22nd percentile

NOTES: * ESI = early-stage investigator. X indicates that an Institute does not set or does not publish its paylines for that grant. NIMHD information is based on fiscal year (FY) 2023; all other Institutes are based on FY 2024. NCATS = National Center for Advancing Translational Sciences; NCI = National Cancer Institute; NEI = National Eye Institute; NHLBI = National Heart, Lung, and Blood Institute; NIAAA = National Institute on Alcohol Abuse and Alcoholism; NIAID = National Institute of Allergy and Infectious Diseases; NIAMS = National Institute of Arthritis and Musculoskeletal and Skin Diseases; NICHD = *Eunice Kennedy Shriver* National Institute of Child Health and Human Development; NIMHD = National Institute on Minority Health and Health Disparities.
SOURCES: NCATS, 2024b; NCI, n.d.-b; NEI, 2024; NHLBI, 2024; NIAAA, 2024; NIAID, 2024; NIAMS, 2024; NICHD, 2024b; NIMHD, 2023.

NCI, on the other hand, has set FY 2024 R01 paylines at the 10th percentile for experienced investigators and 17th percentile for early-stage investigators. NCI notes that funding for new R01s with costs below or above $175,000 will be reduced by 6.5 and 8.5 percent below the recommended level of support, respectively. R21 grants have a payline set at the 10th percentile, and, for R03 and R15 grants, scores up to and including 25 are likely to be funded (NCI, n.d.-b).

This variation in paylines and budget cuts across IC illustrates the potential for inequity in funding across research topics. Based on the funding analysis commissioned by the committee, it is clear that the amount spent on women's health varies greatly between ICs. For example, from 2013 to 2023, NCI spent $9.2 billion and NICHD $5.3 billion (15.9 and 36.6 percent of their overall spending, respectively), while the National Eye Institute spent $80.6 million and NINDS $600 million (1.0 and 2.8 percent of their overall spending, respectively) (see Chapter 4). Budget differences between the ICs, and therefore payline variations, could result in inequitable funding for WHR.

Early Career Reviewer (ECR) Program

CSR's ECR program provides early-career scientists with peer-review experience while helping to diversify the reviewer pool at CSR. To be eligible, researchers need to have at least 1 year of experience as a full-time faculty member in an assistant professor or equivalent role (associate professors may participate if they have NIH early-stage investigator status),[26] evidence of an active and independent research program, one first-authored research publication in a peer-reviewed journal within the past 2 years, one additional senior-authored research publication since receiving a doctorate, and no prior experience serving on an NIH study section. ECR provides an opportunity to gain experience in peer review working alongside accomplished researchers in their area of study, understand how grant applications are evaluated, contribute to the scientific community, and develop skills in grant writing and research evaluation (CSR, 2024).

This program could provide an opportunity to recruit more reviewers with expertise in women's health and train reviewers on sex differences and how to properly apply and assess the SABV policy. This is important given NIH's need for more reviewers overall and more reviewers with expertise in women's health and sex differences in particular.

Simplified Framework

NIH will implement a simplified peer-review process for most RPGs beginning in 2025. This effort aims to address criticisms from reviewers

---

[26] Email communication with Kristin Kramer, Center for Scientific Review, National Institutes of Health on September 26, 2024.

regarding the complexity of the process and increasing responsibilities placed on them for policy compliance. NIH has also received feedback about applicant reputation biasing the outcomes of peer review, which these changes also aim to address. Simplified peer review will apply to many R and U grant mechanisms[27] (NIH, 2024a, 2024i). The Simplified Framework for NIH Peer Review consolidates the five regulatory criteria (significance, investigators, innovation, approach, and environment) into three factors (see Figure 3-9). Several additional review considerations have shifted to NIH staff to reduce the burden on reviewers (NIH, 2024i).

Peer Review and WHR: Barriers and Opportunities

In addition to the feedback on the peer-review process that led to creating the Simplified Framework, stakeholders, including those who spoke at the committee's open meetings (see Box 3-8 for examples), have raised a number of concerns about how the peer-review process at NIH presents obstacles to equitable funding for WHR.

One concern is the lack of study sections focusing specifically on women's health issues within CSR. Although some ICs carry out peer review for certain applications and have their own study sections, CSR oversees 75 percent of grant applications submitted to NIH (CSR, 2022). Therefore, although over 200 study sections review the majority of grants, none of these focuses on women's health issues outside of pregnancy and reproductive health (CSR, 2023b). Favorable peer-review evaluation by an NIH CSR study section is a prerequisite for extramural funding of an awarded NIH grant. When examining which CSR study sections have been the most likely to favorably evaluate WHR, the committee's analysis shows a large proportion of grants on women's health evaluated by SEPs that are organized and administered by an individual IC rather than by CSR, which oversees standing study sections (Figure 3-10).

Relatedly, stakeholders have also raised the possibility that reviewers' expertise is not sufficiently suited to grant applications on women's health or sex differences research, unfairly and negatively affecting the performance of these applications. Although difficult to measure, this merited consideration based on committee member experience and public input. This report is focused on WHR, but lack of study section expertise exists in other research areas as well. For example, concerns regarding inadequately experienced reviewers have also been raised in the field of cardiovascular research, with one recent manuscript asserting that "it is almost impossible for a single SRO to find proper reviewers for the diverse pool of

---

[27] R01, R03, R15, R16, R21, R33, R34, R36, R61, RC1, RC2, RC4, RF1, RL1, RL2, U01, U34, U3R, UA5, UC1, UC2, UC4, UF1, UG3, UH2, UH3, and UH5 (including phased awards: R21/R33, UH2/UH3, UG3/UH3, R61/R33).

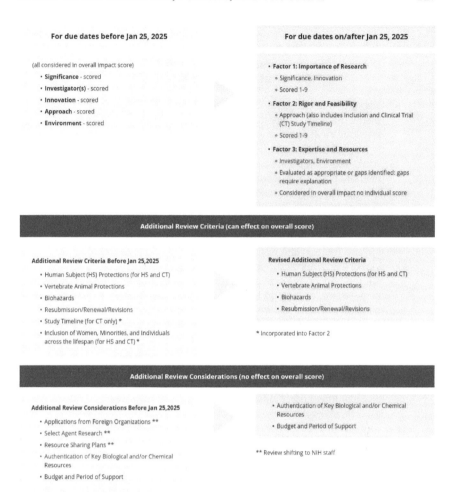

For due dates before Jan 25, 2025

(all considered in overall impact score)
- **Significance** - scored
- **Investigator(s)** - scored
- **Innovation** - scored
- **Approach** - scored
- **Environment** - scored

For due dates on/after Jan 25, 2025

- **Factor 1: Importance of Research**
  ○ Significance, Innovation
  ○ Scored 1-9
- **Factor 2: Rigor and Feasibility**
  ○ Approach (also includes Inclusion and Clinical Trial (CT) Study Timeline)
  ○ Scored 1-9
- **Factor 3: Expertise and Resources**
  ○ Investigators, Environment
  ○ Evaluated as appropriate or gaps identified: gaps require explanation
  ○ Considered in overall impact no individual score

Additional Review Criteria (can effect on overall score)

Additional Review Criteria Before Jan 25,2025
- Human Subject (HS) Protections (for HS and CT)
- Vertebrate Animal Protections
- Biohazards
- Resubmission/Renewal/Revisions
- Study Timeline (for CT only) *
- Inclusion of Women, Minorities, and Individuals across the lifespan (for HS and CT) *

Revised Additional Review Criteria
- Human Subject (HS) Protections (for HS and CT)
- Vertebrate Animal Protections
- Biohazards
- Resubmission/Renewal/Revisions

* Incorporated into Factor 2

Additional Review Considerations (no effect on overall score)

Additional Review Considerations Before Jan 25,2025
- Applications from Foreign Organizations **
- Select Agent Research **
- Resource Sharing Plans **
- Authentication of Key Biological and/or Chemical Resources
- Budget and Period of Support

- Authentication of Key Biological and/or Chemical Resources
- Budget and Period of Support

** Review shifting to NIH staff

FIGURE 3-9 Simplified Framework for National Institutes of Health peer review. SOURCE: NIH, 2024i.

applications that are assigned to each study section" and therefore "this flawed approach is reflected in the composition of the study sections, which include reviewers who are mismatched to the scientific contents of the applications they are assigned to review" (Marian, 2023). Concerns have also been raised regarding the lack of adequately experienced reviewers for research on race, racism, and equity (Headen, 2024).

A WHR-specific study section, while unlikely to solve the problem of insufficient funding for WHR on its own, could bring together experts with a broad perspective on women's health. Further employing SEPs to review

---

BOX 3-8
Excerpts from Researchers on the Peer-Review
Process at Committee Meetings

- Disparities still exist, and there are limitations of the current peer-review process. There is research showing that applications led by principal investigators who identify as African American or Black do not get funded as often as those led by White researchers. We would like to see NIH continue to explore efforts and strategies to diversify peer-review committees.
- This puts urology research in competition with other fields that have significantly more resources, and it means that our studies are reviewed by people who, for the most part, have limited or no expertise in pelvic floor disorders. This means reviewers may favor grants that are more in line with their own clinical and research interests.
- A lot of the gynecologic-specific conditions either go to study sections that may only have one or two individuals that have the expertise to review them, or they go to SEPs in which case many of these communities are so small that they still end up going to people who do not know the science. Primarily because everybody who does know the science has applied for that opportunity.
- The grant review process should be reviewed and evaluated to better support meritorious research on topics of women's health research. One recommendation is to ensure that every grant application in women's health has at least one reviewer with relevant specialized expertise.
- There is a lack of reviewer expertise in understanding the constructs of race and racism in equity-based work that I have actually found challenging in receiving effective peer review.
- Those who engage in research on women's health need and deserve a home where their applications are reviewed by peers with expertise on female physiology and women's lived experience, rather than scientists with no knowledge, or very little knowledge or interest, in these areas.
- Often, grant reviewers do not have adequate expertise, and there can even be bias among grant reviewers. A quotation from a recent review that I had was that biomarkers of risk in postpartum depression are not needed or interesting.

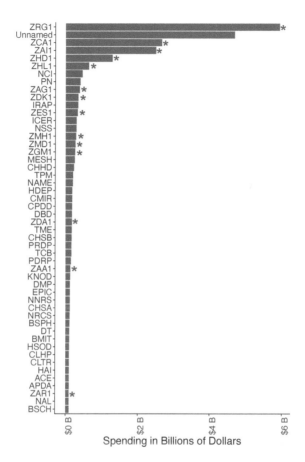

FIGURE 3-10 National Institutes of Health spending on women's health research by study section, 2013–2023.
NOTES: *ZRG1, ZCA1, ZAI1, ZHD1, ZHL1, ZAG1, ZDK1, ZES1, ZMH1, ZMD1, ZGM1, ZDA1, ZAA1, and ZAR1 represent a broad range of topics among special emphasis panels that have been the most likely to favorably evaluate WHR. ACE = AIDS Clinical Studies and Epidemiology Study Section; APDA = Adult Psychopathology and Disorders of Aging Study Section; BMIT = Biomedical Imaging Technology A Study Section; BSCH = Behavioral and Social Consequences of HIV/AIDS Study Section; BSPH = Behavioral and Social Science Approaches to Preventing HIV/AIDS Study Section; CHHD = Child Health and Human Development Study Section; CLHP = Community-Level Health Promotion Study Section; CHSA = Cancer, Heart, and Sleep Epidemiology A Study Section; CHSB = Cancer, Heart, and Sleep Epidemiology B Study Section; CLTR = Clinical Trials Review Committee; CMIR = Cellular, Molecular and Integrative Reproduction Study Section; CPDD = Child Psychopathology and Developmental Disabilities Study Section;

continued

FIGURE 3-10 Continued

DBD = Developmental Brain Disorders Study Section; DMP: Drug Discovery and Molecular Pharmacology Study Section; DT = Developmental Therapeutics Study Section; EPIC = Epidemiology of Cancer Study Section; HAI = Hypersensitivity, Autoimmune, and Immune-mediated Diseases Study Section; HDEP = Health Disparities and Equity Promotion Study Section; HSOD = Health Services Organization and Delivery Study Section; ICER = Integrative and Clinical Endocrinology and Reproduction Study Section; IRAP = Infectious Diseases, Reproductive Health, Asthma and Pulmonary Conditions Study Section; KNOD = Kidney, Nutrition, Obesity and Diabetes Study Section; MESH = Biobehavioral Mechanisms of Emotion, Stress and Health Study Section; NAL = Neurotoxicology and Alcohol Study Section; NAME = Neurological, Aging and Musculoskeletal Epidemiology; NCI = National Cancer Institute; NNRS = Neuroendocrinology, Neuroimmunology, Rhythms and Sleep Study Section; NRCS = Nursing and Related Clinical Sciences Study Section; PDRP = Psychosocial Development, Risk and Prevention Study Section; PN = Pregnancy and Neonatology Study Section; PRDP = Psychosocial Risk and Disease Prevention Study Section; TCB = Tumor Cell Biology Study Section; TME = Tumor Microenvironment Study Section; TPM = Tumor Progression and Metastasis Study Section.
SOURCE: Committee funding analysis, see Chapter 4.

applications related to women's health or sex differences is another potential short-term solution.

Another concern is the potential for bias in the NIH grant-making process. For example, an analysis of NIH grants to first-time awardees from 2006 to 2017 found sex differences in the size of awards in the N01, U01, and R01 categories, even at top research institutions, despite a lack of statistically significant sex differences in baseline performance measures. Women were awarded less in N01 and U01 but more in R01 (the most common award for first-time grantees). Women at Ivy League universities received statistically significantly smaller grants ($52,190 for women vs. $71,703 for men; median difference –$19,513). At the top 50 NIH-funded institutions, first-time female awardees received significantly smaller grants ($93,916 for women vs. $134,919 for men; median difference, –$41,003). While female awardees received lower funding on other measures, most were not statistically significant (Oliveira et al., 2019). One limitation of this study is that it does not report how much funding the investigator requested.

A recent analysis describing the representation of women on NIH study sections reported that men were more likely to be reviewers on study sections across ICs and chairs of study sections. Women were also more likely to serve on study sections with lower total funding and research grants awarded and to have temporary affiliations (Volerman et al., 2021). Though this was a cross-sectional study of one review cycle in 2019, the lack of representation on study sections and of influential power and positions on review panels has important implications for the review of grants focused on WHR. The SRO is often present during the funding discussion and may advocate for a particular proposal or communicate feedback directly to investigators.

Another analysis of data from 1991 to 2020 found sex, gender, racial, and ethnic inequities for super-PIs (SPIs)—PIs holding three or more research project grants—even after adjusting for career stage and degree. The analysis found that women and Black PIs were 34 and 40 percent less likely to be an SPI than their male and White counterparts, respectively, with Black women the least likely to be represented—they were 71 percent less likely to be SPIs than White men (Nguyen et al., 2023).

The results of these analyses are significant for WHR, since data also suggest women researchers are more likely to study women's health topics and enroll more women in clinical trials (Nielsen et al., 2017; Sugimoto et al., 2019; Yong et al., 2023). An analysis of NIH- and industry-funded cardiovascular studies from 2010 to 2019 found that women led just 18.4 percent of all trials and that women-led trials enrolled more female participants than trials led by men, at 44.9 percent and 37.9 percent female participation, respectively (Yong et al., 2023). These documented disparities signal the need for further work to understand the role of gender bias in research (Nguyen et al., 2023; Schmaling and Gallo, 2023).

CSR has already made commitments to address bias in peer review through various initiatives, including developing the simplified review process (Lauer and Byrnes, 2023). As of December 2022, 16,646 reviewers had completed the Bias Awareness and Mitigation Training for reviewers, chairs, and SROs, with 91 percent of reviewers finding the training helpful in improving their ability to identify peer-review bias to a large or moderate extent and 93 percent finding it helpful in improving their comfort intervening in review bias to a large or moderate extent (NIH, 2023d). CSR is also working to increase diversity among reviewers, including in their scientific background, demographics, geography, career stage, and level of experience with peer review. For example, in 2020, CSR expanded its ECR Program (discussed in this chapter) by requiring standing study sections to include two ECRs at each meeting. While underrepresented minoritized individuals were just 10.3 percent of all CSR reviewers in 2021, they were 16.8 percent of ECRs. CSR has also developed tools to allow SROs to track diversity on SEPs and assist them in identifying new reviewers among scientists who have not yet been involved at NIH (NIH, 2023d).

Another consideration is the impact pregnancy and parenting have on women's ability to take on additional professional service roles and how caregiving responsibilities of all researchers may impact their presence in NIH study sections, meetings, and critical networking opportunities. This includes issues related to on-site childcare for reviewers and related activities that require travel and financial support. Caregiving continues to be a hurdle for a women's ability to fully participate in the scientific community and requires additional organization, money, and reliance on informal support. See Chapter 8 and the 2024 report, *Supporting Family Caregivers in STEMM: A Call to Action*, for more information (NASEM, 2024d).

Summary of NIH Peer Review

The peer review process is complex, with CSR overseeing tens of thousands of grants each year through a rigorous and thorough review process on incredibly varied topics and areas. While progress has been made in many aspects of the peer review process, and concerted efforts by CSR continue, efforts to increase expertise on women's health in the peer review process will continue to be essential moving forward. The committee's public comment sessions and review of the literature raised numerous suggestions for improving the peer review process and to advance WHR. These include recommendations to continue increasing diversity in peer-review committees; report information on race, ethnicity, gender, and geography among committees; add experts in women's health and sex differences research to committees; create study sections in CSR specifically dedicated to women's health and sex differences research; create a review branch for multidisciplinary research in obstetrics, gynecology, and reproductive sciences; and undertake a review and evaluation of the peer-review process to determine how it could better support WHR. The committee's recommendations regarding improvements to the peer-review process to improve WHR can be found in Chapter 9.

Intramural Research Program (IRP)

NIH's IRP supports basic, translational, and clinical biomedical research throughout NIH (NIH, 2022a). It includes intramural programs embedded in 23 of the ICs located at one or more of the six NIH campuses and also conducts research in Detroit, Michigan, and Framingham, Massachusetts (NIH Intramural Research Program, 2022). It supports about 1,200 PIs who lead intramural research projects involving nearly 6,000 trainees (see Chapter 8 for more background) (NIH, 2022a,b). Intramural researchers are not eligible for extramural NIH grants and infrequently supported by competitive non-NIH grants, although this is permitted (NIH, 2017c).

IRP Review Process

Research support for intramural scientists is primarily determined by the scientific directors, clinical directors, and IC directors, based on past scientific achievements (Schor, 2024). This process differs from the evaluation of extramural competitive grants, which focuses on the proposed research's quality. Instead, the intramural review looks at the scientist's accomplishments since the previous review (NIH, 2017c). For new or less consistent investigators, future research plans are given more weight. The review assesses the overall quality, impact, and long-term goals of each research program. While the criteria are similar to those used for extramural grants, there is an added consideration of whether the investigator is leveraging the unique resources and features of the NIH intramural environment (NIH, 2017c).

The IRP's review process for its researchers varies by IC (NIH Intramural Research Program, 2022). In general, IRP researchers are reviewed on the entirety of their program every 4 years. Criteria used to conduct reviews include scientific significance, their approach, level of innovation, environment, level of support, use of training, productivity, and efforts related to mentoring. Intramural researchers are required to specify the sex(es) to be included in their proposed studies and report in the NIH Intramural Database[28] if their results have suggested differences between male and female subjects.

External reviewers appointed as boards of scientific counselors conduct these reviews. In-person site visits may also be conducted. After the review, the assessment of the board of scientific counselors is reviewed internally and the evaluation is presented to the NIH deputy director for intramural research, who discusses it with the relevant scientific director (NIH, 2022a). Once funding levels, core service provision, and staffing are determined, these decisions are provided to the relevant IC Council.[29]

CONCLUDING OBSERVATIONS

NIH is large and complex. NIH's structure, comprising numerous ICOs, each with its own specific focus and funding mechanisms, can create challenges in coordinating and prioritizing research efforts. This fragmentation has led to inefficiencies or gaps in addressing the unique aspects of women's health. As a result, critical issues have not received the needed attention or prioritization, hindering the development of targeted treatments and interventions.

REFERENCES

Agarwal, R. K., A. Apostoli, C . Hampp, and C. Hunter. 2021. *ORWH Sex/Gender Administrative Supplement Program: Evaluation and Concept Clearance.* https://orwh.od.nih.gov/sites/orwh/files/docs/13-Agarwal_508C.pdf (accessed October 23, 2024).

---

[28] See https://intramural.nih.gov/index.taf (accessed January 23, 2025).

[29] This section was changed after release of the report to clarify the IRP review process and to add information on reporting requirements.

Ahmed, A., S. Köhler, R. Klotz, N. Giese, T. Hackert, C. Springfeld, D. Jäger, and N. Halama. 2023. Sex differences in the systemic and local immune response of pancreatic cancer patients. *Cancers* 15(6).

Allegra, S., F. Chiara, D. Di Grazia, M. Gaspari, and S. De Francia. 2023. Evaluation of sex differences in preclinical pharmacology research: How far is left to go? *Pharmaceuticals* 16(6).

American Cancer Society. 2024. *American Cancer Society Statement: FDA Approval of HPV Self-Collection for Cervical Cancer Screening.* https://pressroom.cancer.org/releases?item=1325#. (accessed October 22, 2024).

Arnegard, M. E., L. A. Whitten, C. Hunter, and J. A. Clayton. 2020. Sex as a biological variable: A 5-year progress report and call to action. *Journal of Women's Health* 29(6):858–864.

Beery, A. K., and I. Zucker. 2011. Sex bias in neuroscience and biomedical research. *Neuroscience Biobehavioral Reviews* 35(3):565–572.

Bell, M. R. 2018. Comparing postnatal development of gonadal hormones and associated social behaviors in rats, mice, and humans. *Endocrinology* 159(7):2596–2613.

Bush, V. 1945. *Science the endless frontier: A report to the president by Vannevar Bush, director of the Office of Scientific Research and Development, July 1945.* Washington, DC: Office of Scientific Research and Development.

Carmody, C., C. G. Duesing, A. E. Kane, and S. J. Mitchell. 2022. Is sex as a biological variable still being ignored in preclinical aging research? *Journals of Gerontology* 77(11):2177–2180.

Cheng, S., V. Xanthakis, L. M. Sullivan, W. Lieb, J. Massaro, J. Aragam, E. J. Benjamin, and R. S. Vasan. 2010. Correlates of echocardiographic indices of cardiac remodeling over the adult life course: Longitudinal observations from the Framingham Heart Study. *Circulation* 122(6):570–578.

CIHR (Canadian Institutes of Health Research). 2018. *How CIHR Is Supporting the Integration of SGBA.* https://cihr-irsc.gc.ca/e/50837.html (accessed July 17, 2024).

Cirillo, D., S. Catuara-Solarz, C. Morey, E. Guney, L. Subirats, S. Mellino, A. Gigante, A. Valencia, M. J. Rementeria, A. S. Chadha, and N. Mavridis. 2020. Sex and gender differences and biases in artificial intelligence for biomedicine and healthcare. *NPJ Digital Medicine* 3(1):81.

Clayton, J. A. 2018. Applying the new SABV (sex as a biological variable) policy to research and clinical care. *Physiology & Behavior* 187:2–5.

Clayton, J. A. 2023. *NASEM Committee on the Assessment of NIH Research on Women's Health. Presentation to NASEM Committee on the Assessment of NIH Research on Women's Health, Meeting 1 (December 14, 2023).* https://www.nationalacademies.org/event/41452_12–2023_assessment-of-nih-research-on-womens-health-meeting-1-part-3 (accessed August 22, 2024).

Corrigan, J. K., D. Ramachandran, Y. He, C. J. Palmer, M. J. Jurczak, R. Chen, B. Li, R. H. Friedline, J. K. Kim, J. J. Ramsey, L. Lantier, O. P. McGuinness, and A. S. Banks. 2020. A big-data approach to understanding metabolic rate and response to obesity in laboratory mice. *eLife* 9.

Crawley, J. N. 1999. Behavioral phenotyping of transgenic and knockout mice: Experimental design and evaluation of general health, sensory functions, motor abilities, and specific behavioral tests. *Brain Research* 835(1):18–26.

CRS (Congressional Research Service). 2024. *National Institutes of Health (NIH) funding: FY1996–FY2025 (CRS Report R43341).* Washington, DC: Congressional Research Service.

CSR (Center for Scientific Review). 2022. *Center for Scientific Review NIH 2022–2027 strategic plan.* Bethesda, MD: National Institutes of Health.

CSR. 2023a. *The Assignment Process.* https://public.csr.nih.gov/ForApplicants/SubmissionAndAssignment/DRR/assignmentprocess (accessed October 22, 2024).

CSR. 2023b. *Regular Standing Study Sections and Continuing Special Emphasis Panels (SEPs).* https://public.csr.nih.gov/StudySections/StandingStudySections (accessed August 26, 2024).

CSR. 2024. *Early Career Reviewer (ECR) Program.* https://public.csr.nih.gov/ForReviewers/ BecomeAReviewer/ECR#ecr1 (accessed August 22, 2024).

Dalla, C., I. Jaric, P. Pavlidi, G. E. Hodes, N. Kokras, A. Bespalov, M. J. Kas, T. Steckler, M. Kabbaj, H. Würbel, J. Marrocco, J. Tollkuhn, R. Shansky, D. Bangasser, J. B. Becker, M. McCarthy, and C. Ferland-Beckham. 2024. Practical solutions for including sex as a biological variable (SABV) in preclinical neuropsychopharmacological research. *Journal of Neuroscience Methods* 401:110003.

Diao, K., X. Lei, W. He, R. Jagsi, S. H. Giordano, G. L. Smith, A. Caudle, Y. Shen, S. K. Peterson, and B. D. Smith. 2024. Racial and ethnic differences in long-term adverse radiation therapy effects among breast cancer survivors. *International Journal of Radiation Oncology, Biology, Physics* 118(3):626–631.

DPCPSI (Division of Program Coordination, Planning, and Strategic Initiatives). n.d. *DPCPSI Offices.* https://dpcpsi.nih.gov/offices (accessed October 22, 2024).

Galea, L. A. M., E. Choleris, A. Y. K. Albert, M. M. McCarthy, and F. Sohrabji. 2020. The promises and pitfalls of sex difference research. *Frontiers in Neuroendocrinology* 56:100817.

Haverfield, J., and C. Tannenbaum. 2021. A 10-year longitudinal evaluation of science policy interventions to promote sex and gender in health research. *Health Research Policy and Systems* 19(1):94.

Headen, I. 2024. *Structural Changes to Support Structural Determinants Research in Women's Health: Presentation to the NASEM Committee on the Assessment of NIH Research on Women's Health, Meeting 4 (April 11, 2024).* https://www.nationalacademies.org/ documents/embed/link/LF2255DA3DD1C41C0A42D3BEF0989ACAECE3053A6A9B/ file/DA81A7014AD0D94CBE0B576E4271A1563640B19949CF?noSaveAs=1 (accessed August 27, 2024).

Heidari, S., T. F. Babor, P. De Castro, S. Tort, and M. Curno. 2016. Sex and gender equity in research: Rationale for the Sager Guidelines and recommended use. *Research Integrity and Peer Review* 1:2.

IOM (Institute of Medicine). 1991. *The AIDS research program of the National Institutes of Health.* Washington, DC: The National Academy Press.

Ji, H., A. Kim, J. E. Ebinger, T. J. Niiranen, B. L. Claggett, C. N. Bairey Merz, and S. Cheng. 2020. Sex differences in blood pressure trajectories over the life course. *JAMA Cardiology* 5(3):19–26.

Ji, H., T. J. Niiranen, F. Rader, M. Henglin, A. Kim, J. E. Ebinger, B. Claggett, C. N. B. Merz, and S. Cheng. 2021. Sex differences in blood pressure associations with cardiovascular outcomes. *Circulation* 143(7):761–763.

Johnson, J. L., L. Greaves, and R. Repta. 2009. Better science with sex and gender: Facilitating the use of a sex and gender-based analysis in health research. *International Journal for Equity in Health* 8(1):14.

Kaplan, R. M., S. B. Johnson, and P. C. Kobor. 2017. NIH behavioral and social sciences research support: 1980–2016. *American Psychologist* 72(8):808–821.

Kavousi, M. 2016. Tools and techniques—statistical. Confounding and effect measure modification: Analysing sex in cardiovascular research. *EuroIntervention* 12(3):404–407.

Kopp, C., V. Ressel, E. Wigger, and I. Tobler. 2006. Influence of estrus cycle and ageing on activity patterns in two inbred mouse strains. *Behavioural Brain Research* 167(1):165–174.

Lauer, M. 2024. *FY 2023 by the Numbers: Extramural Grant Investments in Research.* https:// nexus.od.nih.gov/all/2024/02/21/fy-2023-by-the-numbers-extramural-grant-investments-in-research/ (accessed August 11, 2024).

Lauer, M., and N. Byrnes. 2023. *Announcing a Simplified Review Framework for NIH Research Project Grant Applications.* https://nexus.od.nih.gov/all/2023/10/19/announcing-a-simplified-review-framework-for-nih-research-project-grant-applications/ (accessed August 22, 2024).

Levy, D. 1988. Left ventricular hypertrophy. Epidemiological insights from the Framingham Heart Study. *Drugs* 35(Suppl 5):1–5.

Levy, D., R. J. Garrison, D. D. Savage, W. B. Kannel, and W. P. Castelli. 1990. Prognostic implications of echocardiographically determined left ventricular mass in the Framingham Heart Study. *New England Journal of Medicine* 322(22):1561–1566.

Lew, L. A., J. S. Williams, J. C. Stone, A. K. W. Au, K. E. Pyke, and M. J. MacDonald. 2022. Examination of sex-specific participant inclusion in exercise physiology endothelial function research: A systematic review. *Frontiers Sports and Active Living* 4:860356.

Llamosas-Falcón, L., C. Probst, C. Buckley, H. Jiang, A. M. Lasserre, K. Puka, A. Tran, and J. Rehm. 2022. Sex-specific association between alcohol consumption and liver cirrhosis: An updated systematic review and meta-analysis. *Frontiers in Gastroenterology* 1:1005729.

Marian, A. J. 2023. What ails the NIH peer review study sections and how to fix the review process of the grant applications. *Journal of Cardiovascular Aging* 3(1):11.

Miller, L. R., C. Marks, J. B. Becker, P. D. Hurn, W. J. Chen, T. Woodruff, M. M. McCarthy, F. Sohrabji, L. Schiebinger, C. L. Wetherington, S. Makris, A. P. Arnold, G. Einstein, V. M. Miller, K. Sandberg, S. Maier, T. L. Cornelison, and J. A. Clayton. 2017. Considering sex as a biological variable in preclinical research. *FASEB Journal* 31(1):29–34.

Miller, V. M., J. R. Kaplan, N. J. Schork, P. Ouyang, S. L. Berga, N. K. Wenger, L. J. Shaw, R. C. Webb, M. Mallampalli, M. Steiner, D. A. Taylor, C. N. Merz, and J. F. Reckelhoff. 2011. Strategies and methods to study sex differences in cardiovascular structure and function: A guide for basic scientists. *Biology of Sex Differences* 2:14.

Miller, V. M., and J. F. Reckelhoff. 2016. Sex as a biological variable: Now what?! *Physiology* 31(2):78–80.

Naqvi, S., A. K. Godfrey, J. F. Hughes, M. L. Goodheart, R. N. Mitchell, and D. C. Page. 2019. Conservation, acquisition, and functional impact of sex-biased gene expression in mammals. *Science* 365(6450).

NASEM (National Academies of Sciences, Engineering, and Medicine). 2022. *Enhancing NIH research on autoimmune disease.* Washington, DC: The National Academies Press.

NASEM. 2024a. *Advancing research on chronic conditions in women.* Washington, DC: The National Academies Press.

NASEM. 2024b. *Discussion of policies, systems, and structures for research on women's health at the National Institutes of Health: Proceedings of a workshop—in brief.* Washington, DC: The National Academies Press.

NASEM. 2024c. *Overview of research gaps for selected conditions in women's health research at the National Institutes of Health: Proceedings of a workshop—in brief.* Washington, DC: The National Academies Press.

NASEM. 2024d. *Supporting family caregivers in STEMM: A call to action.* Washington, DC: The National Academies Press.

NCATS (National Center for Advancing Translational Sciences). 2016. *NCATS Strategic Plan.* Bethesda, MD: National Institutes of Health.

NCATS. 2024a. *2025–2030 NCATS Strategic Plan.* https://ncats.nih.gov/sites/default/files/2024-09/NCATS-Strategic-Plan-2025-2030_508.pdf (accessed January 6, 2025).

NCATS. 2024b. *Funding Policy & Operating Guidelines.* https://ncats.nih.gov/funding/funding-policy-operating-guidelines (accessed October 23, 2024).

NCCIH (National Center for Complementary and Alternative Medicine). 2021. *NCCIH Strategic Plan FY 2021–2025: Mapping a pathway to research on whole person health.* Bethesda, MD: National Center for Complementary and Integrative Health.

NCI (National Cancer Institute). n.d.-a. *Comprehensive Cancer Information.* https://www.cancer.gov/ (accessed October 22, 2024).

NCI. n.d.-b. *NCI Full Year Funding Policy for RPG Awards FY 2024.* https://deainfo.nci.nih.gov/funding/rpg-awards/index.htm (accessed August 15, 2024).

NEI (National Eye Institute). n.d. *NEI strategic plan vision for the future 2021–2025.* Bethesda, MD: National Insitutes of Health.

NEI. 2024. *Fiscal Operations Plan.* https://www.nei.nih.gov/grants-and-training/policies-and-procedures/fiscal-operations-plan (accessed October 23, 2024).

Nguyen, M., S. I. Chaudhry, M. M. Desai, K. Dzirasa, J. E. Cavazos, and D. Boatright. 2023. Gender, racial, and ethnic inequities in receipt of multiple National Institutes of Health research project grants. *JAMA Network Open* 6(2):e230855–e230855.

NHLBI (National Heart, Lung, and Blood Institute). n.d.-a. *Charting the future together: the NHLBI strategic vision.* Bethesda, MD: National Institutes of Health.

NHLBI. n.d.-b. *Strategic Vision.* https://www.nhlbi.nih.gov/about/strategic-vision (accessed October 22, 2024).

NHLBI. 2024. *Available Funding and Operating Guidelines.* https://www.nhlbi.nih.gov/current-operating-guidelines (accessed October 23, 2024).

NIA (National Institute on Aging). 2022. *Research Explores the Impact of Menopause on Women's Health and Aging.* https://www.nia.nih.gov/news/research-explores-impact-menopause-womens-health-and-aging (accessed July 30, 2024).

NIA. 2024. *The National Institute on Aging: Strategic directions for research, 2020–2025.* Bethesda, MD: National Insitutes of Health.

NIAAA (National Institute on Alcohol Abuse and Alcoholism). n.d.-a. *History of NIAAA.* https://www.niaaa.nih.gov/about-niaaa/our-work/history-niaaa (accessed October 7, 2024).

NIAAA. n.d.-b. *National Institute on Alcohol Abuse and Alcoholism strategic plan: Fiscal years 2024–2028 advancing alcohol research to promote health and well-being.* Bethesda, MD: National Insitutes of Health.

NIAAA. 2024. *FY 2024 Financial Management Plan.* https://www.niaaa.nih.gov/management-reporting/fy-2024-financial-management-plan (accessed October 23, 2024).

NIAID (National Institute of Allergy and Infectious Diseases). 2023. *Notice of Special Interest (NOSI) SOP.* https://www.niaid.nih.gov/research/notice-special-interest-nosi-sop (accessed August 21, 2024).

NIAID. 2024. *Archive of Final NIAID Paylines by Fiscal Year.* https://www.niaid.nih.gov/grants-contracts/archive-paylines-fiscal-year (accessed October 23, 2024).

NIAMS (National Institute of Arthritis and Musculoskeletal and Skin Diseases). n.d. *Strategic plan fiscal years 2020–2024: Turning discovery into health.* Bethesda, MD: National Institutes of Health.

NIAMS. 2024. *FY 2024 Funding Plan.* https://www.niams.nih.gov/fy-2024-funding-plan (accessed October 23, 2024).

NICHD (*Eunice Kennedy Shriver* National Institute of Child Health and Human Development). n.d. *NICHD: Strategic plan 2020.* Bethesda, MD: National Insitutes of Health.

NICHD. 2018. Gynecologic health and disease research at NICHD. Bethesda, MD: National Institutes of Health.

NICHD. 2019. *About NICHD.* https://www.nichd.nih.gov/about (accessed October 22, 2024).

NICHD. 2021. *Scientific Research Themes and Objectives.* https://www.nichd.nih.gov/about/org/strategicplan/researchthemes (accessed August 20, 2024).

NICHD. 2023a. *GHDB Research Programs.* https://www.nichd.nih.gov/about/org/der/branches/ghdb/programs (accessed January 23, 2025).

NICHD. 2023b. *Implementing a Maternal Health and Pregnancy Outcomes Vision for Everyone (IMPROVE) initiative fact sheet.* https://www.nichd.nih.gov/sites/default/files/inline-files/IMPROVE-Fact-Sheet-2023-Final.pdf (accessed December 13, 2024).

NICHD. 2024a. *National Advisory Child Health and Human Development Council Roster.* https://www.nichd.nih.gov/about/advisory/council/public-roster (accessed August 20, 2024).

NICHD. 2024b. *NICHD Funding Strategies For Fiscal Year 2024.* https://www.nichd.nih.gov/grants-contracts/process-strategies/strategies/2024 (accessed August 22, 2024).

NICHD. 2024c. *Pelvic Floor Disorders Network.* https://www.nichd.nih.gov/research/supported/pelvicfloor (accessed January 23, 2025).

NIDA (National Institute on Drug Abuse). 2022. *Cross-Cutting Priorities.* https://nida.nih.gov/about-nida/2022–2026-strategic-plan/cross-cutting-themes (accessed August 20, 2024).

NIDDK (National Institute of Diabetes and Digestive and Kidney Diseases). 2021. *Strategic plan for research: Pathways to health for all.* Bethesda, MD: National Institutes of Health.

NIDDK. 2024a. *NIDDK Advisory Council: Members.* https://www.niddk.nih.gov/about-niddk/advisory-coordinating-committees/national-diabetes-digestive-kidney-diseases-advisory-council/members (accessed August 15, 2024).

NIDDK. 2024b. *Research Areas.* https://www.niddk.nih.gov/about-niddk/research-areas (accessed October 22, 2024).

NIEHS (National Institute of Environmental Health Sciences). n.d.-a. *2025–2029 strategic plan: Health at the intersection of people and their environments.* Bethesda, MD: National Institutes of Health.

NIEHS. n.d.-b. *National Institute of Environmental Health Sciences 2018–2023 Strategic Plan: Advancing environmental health sciences improving health.* Bethesda, MD: National Institutes of Health.

Nielsen, M. W., J. P. Andersen, L. Schiebinger, and J. W. Schneider. 2017. One and a half million medical papers reveal a link between author gender and attention to gender and sex analysis. *Nature Human Behaviour* 1(11):791–796.

NIH (National Institutes of Health). n.d.-a. *Budget.* https://www.nih.gov/about-nih/what-we-do/budget (accessed August 20, 2024).

NIH. n.d.-b. *Introduction to Sex and Gender: Core Concepts For Health-Related Research.* https://orwh.od.nih.gov/e-learning/introduction-to-sex-and-gender-core-concepts-for-health-related-research (accessed August 2, 2024).

NIH. n.d.-c. *OD Organizational Chart.* https://oma.od.nih.gov/IC_Organization_Chart/OD%20Organizational%20Chart.pdf (accessed August 21, 2024).

NIH. n.d.-d. *Office of the Director: Congressional justification FY 2021.* Bethesda, MD: National Institutes of Health.

NIH. n.d.-e. *Office of the Director: Congressional justification FY 2024.* Bethesda, MD: National Institutes of Health.

NIH. n.d.-f. *Reviewer Guidance to Evaluate Sex as a Biological Variable (SABV).* https://grants.nih.gov/grants/peer/guidelines_general/sabv_decision_tree_for_reviewers.pdf (accessed August 2, 2024).

NIH. 2010. *NIH record: "We have unfinished business": Minority Health Center now an Institute.* Bethesda, MD: National Institutes of Health.

NIH. 2015a. *Enhancing Reproducibility Through Rigor and Transparency: Notice Number: NOT-OD-15-103.* https://grants.nih.gov/grants/guide/notice-files/NOT-OD-15-103.html (accessed October 9, 2024).

NIH. 2015b. *Scoring system and procedure.* Bethesda, MD: National Institutes of Health.

NIH. 2017a. *Amendment: NIH Policy and Guidelines on the Inclusion of Women and Minorities as Subjects in Clinical Research.* https://grants.nih.gov/grants/guide/notice-files/NOT-OD-18-014.html (accessed August 21, 2024).

NIH. 2017b. *Mission and Goals.* https://www.nih.gov/about-nih/what-we-do/mission-goals (accessed August 20, 2024).

NIH. 2017c. *Policies and Procedures to Guide: Boards of Scientific Counselors: In Reviewing Intramural Research at the NIH.* https://oir.nih.gov/system/files/media/file/2021-08/policy-guide_bsc_reviewing_intramural_research.pdf (accessed August 22, 2024).

NIH. 2018. *NIH reviewer orientation.* Bethesda, MD: National Institutes of Health.

NIH. 2019. *NIH Peer Review: Grants and Cooperative Agreements.* https://grants.nih.gov/grants/peerreview22713webv2.pdf (accessed August 21, 2024).

NIH. 2021a. *NIH-Wide Strategic Plan.* https://www.nih.gov/about-nih/nih-wide-strategic-plan (accessed August 20, 2024).

NIH. 2021b. *NIH-wide strategic plan for fiscal years 2021–2025.* Bethesda, MD: National Institutes of Health.

NIH. 2022a. *IRP Review Process.* https://irp.nih.gov/our-research/irp-review-process (accessed August 22, 2024).

NIH. 2022b. *Report of the director, National Institutes of Health: Fiscal Years 2019–2021.* Bethesda, MD: National Institutes of Health.

NIH. 2023a. *Appropriations (Section 1)*. https://www.nih.gov/about-nih/what-we-do/nih-almanac/appropriations-section-1 (accessed August 23, 2024).

NIH. 2023b. *Appropriations (Section 2)*. https://www.nih.gov/about-nih/what-we-do/nih-almanac/appropriations-section-2 (accessed August 23, 2024).

NIH. 2023c. *Center for Scientific Review (CSR)*. https://www.nih.gov/about-nih/what-we-do/nih-almanac/center-scientific-review-csr (accessed August 21, 2024).

NIH. 2023d. *CSR Initiatives to Address Bias in Peer Review*. https://public.csr.nih.gov/AboutCSR/Address-Bias-in-Peer-Review (accessed August 22, 2024).

NIH. 2023e. *Frequently Asked Questions (FAQ)*. https://www.nlm.nih.gov/ep/FAQScores.html (accessed August 22, 2024).

NIH. 2023f. *Lists of Institutes and Centers*. https://www.nih.gov/institutes-nih/list-institutes-centers (accessed September 4, 2024).

NIH. 2023g. *NIH Designates People with Disabilities as a Population with Health Disparities*. https://www.nih.gov/news-events/news-releases/nih-designates-people-disabilities-population-health-disparities (accessed August 20, 2024).

NIH. 2023h. *Simplifying review framework: Feedback from the request for information*. Bethesda, MD: National Institutes of Health.

NIH. 2023i. *Understand Funding Opportunities*. https://grants.nih.gov/grants/how-to-apply-application-guide/prepare-to-apply-and-register/understand-funding-opportunities.htm (accessed August 21, 2024).

NIH. 2024a. *Background—NIH Peer Review Process*. https://grants.nih.gov/policy/peer/simplifying-review/background.htm (accessed August 22, 2024).

NIH. 2024b. *First Level: Peer Review*. https://grants.nih.gov/grants-process/review/first-level#scoring (accessed October 22, 2024).

NIH. 2024c. *Grants and Funding: Sample Applications and Documents*. https://grants.nih.gov/grants-process/write-application/samples-applications-and-documents (accessed October 23, 2024).

NIH. 2024d. *Information for Foreign Grants*. https://grants.nih.gov/new-to-nih/information-for/foreign-grants (accessed October 22, 2024).

NIH. 2024e. *Managing Conflicts of Interest in NIH Peer Review of Grants and Contracts*. https://grants.nih.gov/policy-and-compliance/policy-topics/peer-review/coi (accessed October 23, 2024).

NIH. 2024f. *NIH Associate Directors*. https://www.nih.gov/about-nih/what-we-do/nih-almanac/associate-directors (accessed October 22, 2024).

NIH. 2024g. *Office of the Director, NIH*. https://www.nih.gov/about-nih/what-we-do/nih-almanac/office-director-nih (accessed October 22, 2024).

NIH. 2024h. *Reviewer Training: For Research Project Grants*. https://public.csr.nih.gov/sites/default/files/2024-04/Core_Reviewer_Training_Slides_3_24.pptx (accessed August 2, 2024).

NIH. 2024i. *Simplified Peer Review Framework*. https://grants.nih.gov/policy/peer/simplifying-review/framework.htm (accessed August 22, 2024).

NIH Intramural Research Program. 2022. *Our Programs*. https://irp.nih.gov/about-us/our-programs (accessed October 23, 2024).

NIMH (National Institute of Mental Health). 2024. *National Institute of Mental Health: Strategic plan for research*. Bethesda, MD: National Institutes of Health.

NIMHD (National Institute on Minority Health and Health Disparities). 2023. *NIMHD Financial Management Plan for Grant Awards*. https://www.nimhd.nih.gov/funding/nimhd-funding/funding-strategy.html (accessed October 23, 2024).

NIMHD. 2024a. *About NIMHD*. https://www.nimhd.nih.gov/about/ (accessed September 10, 2024).

NIMHD. 2024b. *NIH minority health and health disparities strategic plan 2021–2025: Taking the next steps*. Bethesda, MD: National Institutes of Health.

NINDS (National Institute of Neurological Disorders and Stroke). n.d. *National Institute of Neurological Disorders and Stroke (NINDS) strategic plan: 2021–2026 investing in the future of neuroscience*. Bethesda, MD: National Institutes of Health.

NLM (National Library of Medicine). n.d. *Synopsis of a platform for biomedical discovery and data-powered health: Strategic plan 2017–2027.* Bethesda, MD: National Institutes of Health.

OAR (Office of AIDS Research). n.d. *About the Office of AIDS Research.* https://www.oar.nih.gov/about (accessed October 22, 2024).

OAR. 2024. *Office of AIDS Research Advisory Council.* https://www.oar.nih.gov/about/oarac (accessed October 23, 2024).

OBSSR (Office of Behavioral and Social Sciences Research). n.d. *About OBSSR.* https://obssr.od.nih.gov/about (accessed October 22, 2024).

OD (Office of the Director). n.d. *Office of the Director: Congressional justification FY 2025.* Bethesda, MD: National Institutes of Health.

ODP (Office of Disease Prevention). n.d.-a. *About ODP.* https://prevention.nih.gov/about-odp (accessed October 22, 2024).

ODP. n.d.-b. *Dissemination & Implementation (D&I) Research.* https://prevention.nih.gov/research-priorities/dissemination-implementation (accessed August 20, 2024).

ODP. n.d.-c. *Pathways to Prevention (P2P) Program.* https://prevention.nih.gov/research-priorities/research-needs-and-gaps/pathways-prevention (accessed July 30, 2024).

Ohio State University. n.d. *Research Responsibilities and Compliance: Per Diem Rates and Fees.* https://research.osu.edu/research-responsibilities-and-compliance/animal-care-and-use/diem-rates-and-fees (accessed October 24, 2024).

Oliveira, D. F. M., Y. Ma, T. K. Woodruff, and B. Uzzi. 2019. Comparison of National Institutes of Health grant amounts to first-time male and female principal investigators. *JAMA* 321(9):898–900.

OMA (Office of Management Assessment). n.d. *NIH Organizational Chart.* https://oma.od.nih.gov/IC_Organization_Chart/NIH%20Organizational%20Chart.pdf (accessed October 22, 2024).

ORWH (Office of Research on Women's Health). n.d.-a. *About the Office of Autoimmune Disease Research (OADR-ORWH).* https://orwh.od.nih.gov/OADR-ORWH (accessed August 21, 2024).

ORWH. n.d.-b. *Administrative Supplements for Research on Sex & Gender Differences.* https://orwh.od.nih.gov/sex-gender/orwh-mission-area-sex-gender-in-research/administrative-supplements-for-research-on-sex-gender-differences (accessed October 22, 2024).

ORWH. n.d.-c. *Advisory Committee on Research on Women's Health.* https://orwh.od.nih.gov/about/advisory-committee-on-research-on-womens-health (accessed August 20, 2024).

ORWH. n.d.-d. *Advisory Committees.* https://orwh.od.nih.gov/about/advisory-committees (accessed August 20, 2024).

ORWH. n.d.-e. *Bench to Bedside: Integrating Sex and Gender to Improve Human Health Course.* https://orwh.od.nih.gov/e-learning/bench-to-bedside-integrating-sex-and-gender-to-improve-human-health-course (accessed August 2, 2024).

ORWH. n.d.-f. *Biennial Reports.* https://orwh.od.nih.gov/our-work/biennial-reports (accessed August 20, 2024).

ORWH. n.d.-g. *Career Development Programs & Projects.* https://orwh.od.nih.gov/career-development-education#card-1154 (accessed August 21, 2024).

ORWH. n.d.-h. *Clinical Research and Trials.* https://orwh.od.nih.gov/womens-health-equity-inclusion/clinical-research-and-trials (accessed August 21, 2024).

ORWH. n.d.-i. *Coordinating Committee on Research on Women's Health.* https://orwh.od.nih.gov/about/coordinating-committee-on-research-on-womens-health (accessed August 20, 2024).

ORWH. n.d.-j. *Mission and History.* https://orwh.od.nih.gov/about/mission-history (accessed August 20, 2024).

ORWH. n.d.-k. *NIH-wide strategic plan for research on the health of women.* Bethesda, MD: National Institutes of Health.

ORWH. n.d.-l. *NIH Policy on Sex as a Biological Variable.* https://orwh.od.nih.gov/sex-gender/orwh-mission-area-sex-gender-in-research/nih-policy-on-sex-as-biological-variable (accessed February 9, 2024).

ORWH. n.d.-m. *ORWH Research Programs & Initiatives.* https://orwh.od.nih.gov/our-work (accessed July 30, 2024).

ORWH. n.d.-n. *SABV Primer Supplement.* https://orwh.od.nih.gov/e-learning/sabv-primer-supplement (accessed August 2, 2024).

ORWH. n.d.-o. *SABV Primer: Train the Trainer.* https://orwh.od.nih.gov/e-learning/sabv-primer-train-trainer (accessed August 2, 2024).

ORWH. n.d.-p. *Sex as a biological variable (SABV) primer course instructor guide.* Bethesda, MD: National Institutes of Health.

ORWH. n.d.-q. *Sex as a Biological Variable: A Primer.* https://orwh.od.nih.gov/e-learning/sex-as-biological-variable-primer (accessed August 2, 2024).

ORWH. n.d.-r. *Specialized Centers of Research Excellence on Sex Differences (U54 Clinical Trial Optional).* https://orwh.od.nih.gov/sex-gender/orwh-mission-area-sex-gender-in-research/specialized-centers-of-research-excellence-on-sex-differences-u54-clinical-trial (accessed August 11, 2024).

ORWH. 2021. *Report of the Advisory Committee on Research on Women's Health, fiscal years 2019–2020: Office of Research on Women's Health and NIH support for research on women's health.* Bethesda, MD: National Institutes of Health.

ORWH. 2023. *Report of the Advisory Committee on Research on Women's Health, fiscal years 2021–2022: Office of Research on Women's Health and NIH support for research on women's health.* Bethesda, MD: National Institutes of Health.

ORWH. 2024. *Introducing the NIH-Wide Strategic Plan for Research on the Health of Women 2024–2028.* https://orwh.od.nih.gov/in-the-spotlight/all-articles/introducing-nih-wide-strategic-plan-for-research-on-health-of-women-2024-2028-0 (accessed October 22, 2024).

Padamsee, T. J. 2018. Fighting an epidemic in political context: Thirty-five years of HIV/AIDS policy making in the United States. *Social History of Medicine* 33(3):1001–1028.

Parker, K. 2024a. *Advancing Sexual & Gender Minority Health Research at NIH & Beyond.* https://dpcpsi.nih.gov/sites/default/files/2024-05/KLP-Regional-Workshop-2024-v-FINAL_508.pdf (accessed August 2, 2024).

Parker, K. 2024b. *Overview of the Sexual & Gender Minority Research Office. Presentation to the NASEM Committee on the Assessment of NIH Research on Women's Health, Meeting 2 (January 25, 2024).* https://www.nationalacademies.org/documents/embed/link/LF2255DA3DD1C41C0A42D3BEF0989ACAECE3053A6A9B/file/D25E955998B9271BEA8D547B0AE0ADF31DE0620DC05C?noSaveAs=1 (accessed February 16th, 2024).

Pérez-Stable, E. J. 2024. *Overview of NIMHD Research on Women's Health. Presentation to the NASEM Committee on the Assessment of NIH Research on Women's Health, Meeting 2 (January 25, 2024).* https://acrobat.adobe.com/id/urn:aaid:sc:va6c2:12690ec1-5b6c-4048-bf77-104189517bb3 (accessed February 16th, 2024).

Peters, S. A. E., and M. Woodward. 2023. A roadmap for sex- and gender-disaggregated health research. *BMC Medicine* 21(1):354.

Rajan, S. S., N. Kohli, R. M. Rogers, R. P. Goldberg, P. Tulikangas, P. L. Rosenblatt, E. Elkadry, J.-J. R. Miller, P. K. Sand, P. J. Culligan, C. R. Rardin, M. Murphy, V. R. Lucente, L. A. C. Berman, K. A. Grow McLean, C. A. LaSala, D. L. Myers, and M. C. Shaw. 2007. *Urogynecology in primary care.* London, U.K.: Springer-Verlag London Limited.

Rockey, S. 2011. *Paylines, Percentiles and Success Rates.* https://nexus.od.nih.gov/all/2011/02/15/paylines-percentiles-success-rates/ (accessed August 22, 2024).

Rodgers, C. M. 2024. *Reforming the National Institutes of Health: Framework for discussion.* Washington, DC: House Committee on Energy and Commerce.

Rubinstein, A. 2022. *Peer Review at NIH. Presentation at NCI Division of Cancer Biology January 12–13, 2022 21st Annual New Grantee Workshop.* https://www.cancer.gov/about-nci/organization/dcb/funding/resources/rubinsteinngw2022 (accessed August 21, 2024).

Schmaling, K. B., and S. A. Gallo. 2023. Gender differences in peer reviewed grant applications, awards, and amounts: A systematic review and meta-analysis. *Research Integrity and Peer Review* 8(1):2.

Schor, N. F. 2024. Developing the next-generation cancer research workforce in the National Institutes of Health Intramural Research Program. *Journal of the National Cancer Institute* 116(5):637–641.

SGMRO (Sexual & Gender Minority Research Office). 2024. *About SGMRO.* https://dpcpsi. nih.gov/sgmro (accessed August 20, 2024).

Shapiro, J. R., S. L. Klein, and R. Morgan. 2021. Stop "controlling" for sex and gender in global health research. *BMJ Global Health* 6(4):e005714.

Sohani, Z. N., H. Behlouli, C. S. de Moura, M. Abrahamowicz, and L. Pilote. 2023. Sex differences in the effectiveness of angiotensin-converting enzyme inhibitors, angiotensin II receptor blockers, and sacubitril–valsartan for the treatment of heart failure. *Journal of the American Heart Association* 12(14):e028865.

Sugimoto, C. R., Y.-Y. Ahn, E. Smith, B. Macaluso, and V. Larivière. 2019. Factors affecting sex-related reporting in medical research: A cross-disciplinary bibliometric analysis. *Lancet* 393(10171):550–559.

THRO (Tribal Health Research Office). 2023. *About Us.* https://dpcpsi.nih.gov/thro/about (accessed October 22, 2024).

UCSF (University of California, San Francisco). n.d. *Preclinical Therapeutics Recharge Rates.* https://cancer.ucsf.edu/research/cores/preclinical/preclinical-rates (accessed October 24, 2024).

UMR (United for Medical Research). 2024. *NIH's role in sustaining the U.S. Economy: Every state benefits.* Washington, DC: United for Medical Research.

University of Kentucky. n.d. *Division of Laboratory Animal Resources: Services and Rates.* https://www.research.uky.edu/division-laboratory-animal-resources/services-and-rates (accessed October 24, 2024).

University of Michigan. n.d. *Animal Care and Use Program: Rates.* https://animalcare.umich. edu/business-services/rates/ (accessed October 24, 2024).

USDA (U.S. Department of Agriculture). 2020. *Dietary guidelines for Americans: 2020–2025, 9th edition.* Washington, DC: U.S. Department of Agriculture.

Volerman, A., V. M. Arora, J. F. Cursio, H. Wei, and V. G. Press. 2021. Representation of women on National Institutes of Health study sections. *JAMA Network Open* 4(2):e2037346.

Waltz, M., J. A. Fisher, A. D. Lyerly, and R. L. Walker. 2021a. Evaluating the National Institutes of Health's sex as a biological variable policy: Conflicting accounts from the front lines of animal research. *Jounal of Womens Health* 30(3):348–354.

Waltz, M., K. W. Saylor, J. A. Fisher, and R. L. Walker. 2021b. Biomedical researchers' perceptions of the NIH'S Sex as a Biological Variable policy for animal research: Results from a U.S. national survey. *Journal of Women's Health* 30(10):1395–1405.

White, J., C. Tannenbaum, I. Klinge, L. Schiebinger, and J. Clayton. 2021. The integration of sex and gender considerations into biomedical research: Lessons from international funding agencies. *Journal of Clinical Endocrinology and Metabolism* 106(10):3034–3048.

Willingham, E. 2022. The fraught quest to account for sex in biology research. *Nature* 609:456–459.

Woitowich, N. C., and T. K. Woodruff. 2019. Implementation of the NIH sex-inclusion policy: Attitudes and opinions of study section members. *Journal of Women's Health* 28(1):9–16.

Woitowich, N. C., A. Beery, and T. Woodruff. 2020. A 10-year follow-up study of sex inclusion in the biological sciences. *eLife* 9:e56344.

Yang, W., and J. B. Rubin. 2024. Treating sex and gender differences as a continuous variable can improve precision cancer treatments. *Biology of Sex Differences* 15(1):35.

Yong, C., A. Suvarna, R. Harrington, S. Gummidipundi, H. M. Krumholz, R. Mehran, and P. Heidenreich. 2023. Temporal trends in gender of principal investigators and patients in cardiovascular clinical trials. *Journal of the American College of Cardiology*81(4):428–430.

Zhang, C., Y. Ye, and H. Zhao. 2022. Comparison of methods utilizing sex-specific PRSS derived from GWAS summary statistics. *Frontiers in Genetics* 13:892950.

Zhao, G., Y. Wang, S. Wang, and N. Li. 2024. Reporting outcome comparisons by sex in oncology clinical trials. *Nature Communications* 15(1):3051.

4

Overview of the National Institutes of Health Investment in Women's Health Research

INTRODUCTION

This chapter describes how the National Institutes of Health (NIH) tracks funding and undertakes portfolio analysis; it then presents the committee's assessment of NIH funding for women's health research (WHR). Because women's health includes diseases and conditions that are sex specific or affect women and men differently or disproportionally, the task of measuring the state of NIH funding for research on the health of women, the nature of the gaps, and establishing a standard for allocation each present challenges.

The easiest of these challenges may be assessing the funding for female-specific diseases and conditions. However, the domain also includes studying female development, including the effect of sex hormones over the life course, which have also been understudied and lack an institutional home within NIH (see Chapter 5). Adding to the complexity are decisions regarding how to account for research on pregnancy, which often focuses primarily or exclusively on fetal or infant outcomes rather than the health of the pregnant person. Such work may be of interest and importance to women, and presumably men, without being directly tied to their health.

Gaps in sex-specific research on women's health include areas discussed in prior chapters, such as in the funding of research on endometriosis and reproductive cancers specific to women. This also raises the issue of how to count research on diseases and conditions experienced predominantly but not exclusively by women, such as rheumatoid arthritis and osteoporosis; the disease burden and research have focused largely on female patients, but the evidence base and funding fall far below that of diseases experienced by male patients, either predominantly or exclusively (Mirin, 2021; Salari et al., 2021).

The more challenging category to assess is diseases that affect women and girls differently from men and boys. This depends on not just the funding that went to research on such diseases but also the extent to which that research examined whether there are sex or gender differences and the underlying mechanisms or drivers of those differences. Moreover, there is an additional question of what proportion of the study's funding should be categorized as examining women's health. At one extreme, that could include all the funding on a study that reported whether and how findings differed for women compared to men and the implications for treatment and future research. At the other extreme, it might only include the marginal costs of the additional analyses required. That proportion also might be seen as a function of both their representation in the research and the analyses proposed or conducted that contribute to evidence-based care for them. With perfect information, such a gold standard would be informative.

This chapter focuses on the proportion of NIH funding going to research on women's health, not on what the gold standard could be. That would ideally reflect objective measures, including the relative and absolute burden of diseases and conditions. However, since the gaps in the evidence base also include a lack of research on the range of female development, it would be difficult, if not impossible, to hold all assessments to that standard. In addition, individual rare diseases, also known as "orphan diseases,"[1] have a small effect relative to those experienced by a larger share of the population. The study of them not only is humane and needed but also can create opportunities for breakthrough science, as they almost by definition fall outside the existing evidence base and are often undercounted as a result.

A question frequently arises as to what portion of the NIH budget funds research on the health of men. Until the 1993 NIH Revitalization Act,[2] that answer was simpler, as the vast majority of funding was for not only sex-specific diseases and conditions but also those that affect men and women. Unfortunately, including women as research participants and female animals and tissues in studies has had a limited effect on informing women's health by having been built primarily on theories and evidence from a focus on men. For example, work ranging from heart disease to autism has been limited in part by diagnostic tools, criteria, and interventions based on studying male participants as normal and including female participants who either fit that model or were labeled "atypical presentation." These limitations have been confounded by a lack of work

---

[1] According to the Orphan Drug Act, orphan diseases or conditions are defined as those affecting fewer than 200,000 in the United States (Public Law 97–414). [*This footnote was changed after release of the report to clarify the source of the definition.*]

[2] Public Law 103–143, 107 Stat. 122 (June 10, 1993).

systematically assessing whether and to what extent findings from studies conducted in mixed-sex samples hold for female patients. Assessing the extent to which studies propose to and do carry out such analyses is unfortunately beyond the resources and time frame of this report. However, the goal of clearly establishing to whom findings of a given study applies warrants considerable attention as part of the effort to build an evidence base on the health of women (IOM, 2001; Liu and Mager, 2016).

What is the ideal or optimal balance between spending on sex-specific diseases and conditions depends in large part on how much a given sex experiences and is burdened by them. For example, to the extent that women experience more diseases and disease burden from cancer in or related to reproductive organs or hormones, a higher allocation to funding of research on diseases specific to them is warranted. The size of the existing evidence base is also relevant; the issue is how well the sex-specific diseases and conditions have been studied and are understood. The gap is a function of the disease burden and the extent of the evidence base to date.

The long-standing emphasis of NIH funding on diseases and conditions affecting men has reinforced the idea that male bodies are the standard and treated female bodies as an exception. For example, most urologic conditions in men fall under the general practice of urology, whereas many in women are addressed almost exclusively in the subspecialty of urogynecology. Thus, the relative need for research specific to females versus males is in part a function of the long-standing and erroneous assumption that the latter could routinely be generalized to women's health and health care.

ASSESSING DISEASE AND CONDITION FUNDING LEVELS AT NIH

The committee faced a fundamental challenge in evaluating NIH investment in WHR. It sought to examine current spending and the trajectory of spending on WHR over the past 10 years. On the surface, this should be a straightforward exercise. NIH expenditures are matter of public record, and the agency has a strong commitment to transparency. However, NIH uses multiple systems to account for its research expenditures, and the data needed for such an evaluation can be difficult to interpret. Some of the evaluation systems, such as the Research Portfolio Online Reporting Tools (RePORT) website and associated RePORT Expenditures and Results (RePORTER) tool, are public facing, meaning anyone can access them. Other tools, such as the Research, Condition, and Disease Categorization (RCDC) system and Search and Visualize intersect tool, are for internal use and people outside the government cannot access them. These tools can help NIH Institutes and Centers (ICs) analyze their portfolios in more depth and recognize trends and gaps in their research funding (Cebotari and Praskievicz, 2024; ORWH, 2023).

Reporting Categorical Funding: Process and Challenges

Tracking NIH research expenditures is a monumental task. Each year, more than 58,000 NIH grants support more than 300,000 investigators at more than 2,700 different institutions (Lauer, 2024; NIH, 2023a). Since fiscal year (FY) 2008, the primary system used to account for NIH categorical expenditures is RCDC (NIH, n.d.-a). Congress mandated creating it in the NIH Reform Act of 2006[3] to uniformly categorize NIH-funded research projects at all ICs and better understand how research dollars are used (NASEM, 2024a; NIH, 2024a). The Division of Scientific Categorization and Analysis (DSCA) within the Office of Extramural Research in the NIH Office of the Director (OD) maintains and curates RCDC categories with the assistance of IC subject matter experts. Data and scientific information analysts and computational linguists staff DSCA (Cebotari and Praskievicz, 2024).

NIH is required to use RCDC to publicly report how much is spent for research through grants and other funding mechanisms annually in NIH-wide defined categories. The number of RCDC categories has increased over time, and each year, new ones are introduced (Cebotari and Praskievicz, 2024). For FY 2023 reporting, there were 324 public categories;[4] NIH also uses nonpublic categories internally (Cebotari and Praskievicz, 2024). Requests from Congress, the White House, NIH leadership, and advocacy groups, as well as evolving research (Cebotari and Praskievicz, 2024; NIH, n.d.-c,d), drive the development of new RCDC categories. An internal NIH working group decides if a newly proposed category should be added, with approvals prioritized by research urgency and the number of requests (Cebotari and Praskievicz, 2024). For example, because of the obvious omission, Congress requested a category for menopause, which was reported via RCDC in 2024 (Cebotari and Praskievicz, 2024; NIH, 2024b). Subject matter experts from across NIH define the scientific parameters for RCDC categories and also validate individual projects to ensure category accuracy (Cebotari and Praskievicz, 2024). The RePORT website offers public access to a downloadable spreadsheet that summarizes NIH expenditures for each category; many advocacy groups have used these data to educate their constituents, lobby for additional funding, and highlight inequities in NIH funding (Baird et al., 2021; NASEM, 2024a,b; NIH, 2024a). New RCDC categories are not retroactively applied to past fiscal years, but NIH internally examines past research trends (Cebotari and Praskievicz, 2024; NASEM, 2024a; NIH, n.d.-b). This limits public understanding of the trajectory of NIH funding. For example, the category for cervical cancer

---

[3] Public Law 109–482, 120 Stat. 3675 (January 15, 2007).

[4] See https://report.nih.gov/funding/categorical-spending#/ for a listing of all RCDC categories (accessed July 25, 2024).

was created in 2008, vaginal cancer in 2015, and polycystic ovary syndrome (PCOS) in 2022 (NIH, 2024a). Research on these women's health topics was occurring before their RCDC categories were established, limiting the accuracy of funding totals for diseases by NIH over time.

The RCDC system's fundamental methodology has not changed, though improvements in natural language processing have been integrated to increase specificity and accuracy (Cebotari and Praskievicz, 2024). A category is made up of a list of weighted biomedical concepts, known as a "category fingerprint," sourced from the RCDC Thesaurus that are relevant to it and may have many synonyms. For example, the ALS category comprises concepts such as "ALS pathology," "ALS patients," and "amyotrophic lateral sclerosis" (Cebotari and Praskievicz, 2024; NIH, n.d.-c). The Thesaurus is foundational to the RCDC system and amended as science and language advance.

To index a project, the automated system mines the title, abstract, public health relevance, and specific aims sections of each project application using natural language processing techniques. Thesaurus concepts in project text are compared to category fingerprints, and if enough overlap[5] appears between these and the text, the project is reported in that category (Cebotari and Praskievicz, 2024; NIH, n.d.-b,c). Nearly all RCDC categories are reported in this automated way, and dollars are reported at the full project amount for each category in which the project is listed (Cebotari and Praskievicz, 2024; NIH, n.d.-b). According to NIH, the Women's Health RCDC category is reported manually[6]—subject matter experts determine if projects need to be reported in a category. Dollars can be prorated (1–100 percent) based on the portion of the project that meets the category definition (Cebotari and Praskievicz, 2024; Lauer, 2018; NIH, n.d.-b).

As the official source of categorical reporting for NIH-funded research projects, the system is consistent in its budgetary allocation methodology and offers standardized project-level reporting (Cebotari and Praskievicz, 2024). However, interpreting RCDC data has some important caveats. While new research areas continue to be added based on official requests, the RCDC categories do not encompass all types of biomedical research or all health conditions (Lauer, 2018). RCDC categories are not a sum of the total NIH expenditure, and NIH does not budget by RCDC categories (Cebotari and Praskievicz, 2024; NIH, n.d.-a).

---

[5] NIH has an empirical threshold value for each RCDC category that it has determined minimizes false positives and false negatives; "enough overlap" means a project has crossed that threshold (Cebotari and Praskievicz, 2024; NIH, n.d.-b).

[6] Email communication with Nancy Praskievicz, Division of Scientific Categorization and Analysis, National Institutes of Health on October 7, 2024.

In addition, categories overlap and are not mutually exclusive, so individual projects may be reported in multiple categories (Cebotari and Praskievicz, 2024; NIH, n.d.-a). For example, a grant for a clinical trial to treat cachexia in breast cancer might meet the threshold for five different categories: Clinical Trials and Supportive Activities, Cachexia, Breast Cancer, Cancer, and Women's Health (Cebotari and Praskievicz, 2024). As described, the entire budget of the grant is attributed to each RCDC category that it falls into, or, for manually reported categories, prorated to account for the percentage of the project meeting the category definition. The automated system cannot parse project funding by category, such as deciding that 50 percent went to one category, 30 percent to a second, and 20 percent to a third. According to NIH, this would require a burdensome manual process that could introduce data discrepancies (Cebotari and Praskievicz, 2024; Lauer, 2018; NASEM, 2024a). As a result, the overall total research spending reported via the RCDC system will be higher than the NIH budget (Lauer, 2018). Since the grants cannot be prorated across multiple categories, this approach results in an overestimate in spending for many categories, given that the full amount of a grant is included even if it focuses on more than one disease or condition. As a result, if members of the public were to use RCDC categories to sum the funding allocated for various women's health–related categories, such as all female-specific cancers, this would overestimate the total funding because many grants study more than one female-specific cancer, so they would be counted across multiple categories.

NIH Reporting of Funding for WHR

Of particular interest to the committee is the RCDC category and reporting algorithm for Women's Health.[7] The specific definition used by RCDC to categorize Women's Health grants is not publicly available, though it includes conditions that exclusively affect women, while other conditions that affect women either predominantly or differently are reviewed

---

[7] NIH notes, "Reporting for this category now more closely follows the standard RCDC process compared with the project identification, cost pro-ration, and validation procedures used for FY 2018 and prior fiscal years. Individual Institutes, Centers, and Offices (ICOs) previously classified reportable awards using subjectively-defined criteria and assigned funding based on percentages of female subjects included in the studies. In FY 2019, subject matter experts across ICOs achieved consensus that the allocation of women's health-related spending should be grounded on scientific relevance and developed new prorating guidance, accordingly. To ensure a robust reporting transition, starting FY 2019, ICOs applied the new definitions only to the competing projects and retained the previous prorating schemes for the non-competing awards and will gradually roll-out from the inclusion-based approach in the subsequent fiscal years. In conjunction with the described efforts, NIH also instituted the use of an automated Manual Categorization System (MCS) to enhance workflow efficiency and standardize the NIH-wide cost allocation practices" (NIH, 2024a).

by IC subject matter experts for relevance to Women's Health; because it is a manual effort, approaches are unique to each IC, and reporting is at each IC's discretion.[8] As of 2023, NIH IC experts can include projects that (1) recruit female participants and (2) focus on female-specific diseases or conditions, such as breast or cervical cancers, endometriosis, PCOS, and maternal health.

NIH IC experts, at their discretion, can also include conditions that predominately affect women.[9] Projects centering on child health outcomes are not included unless they focus mainly on girls. Funding for studies that involve both women and men or partially address women's health can be manually prorated (1–100 percent of the obligated dollar amount) based on, for example, disease burden or the proportion of study aims related to women's health, depending on each IC's approach to coding and proration.[10] Basic science studies can be prorated by the proportion of women's health-related study aims or percentage of female research subjects; if that information is unknown, funding can be reported at 50 percent. DSCA has also confirmed that the category includes topics that do not have their own categories. For example, projects on menstruation could appear in the Women's Health RCDC category even though no menstruation category exists.[11] The Women's Health category also includes relevant grants for women's health career development and conferences. The RePORT website includes individual projects listed in the Women's Health RCDC category since FY 2020 (NIH, 2024a).

However, based on its review of abstracts from RePORTER when preparing for its funding analysis (see Appendix A), the committee identified a large number of grants coded as Women's Health that did not appear to be related, in that the grant did not focus on a female-specific condition or a condition more common in women and was not assessing sex differences for a condition present in both sexes. The committee did not have access to the full grant and so could only base this assessment on the title, abstract, and public health relevance statement. However, the committee found a smaller proportion of grants on WHR than what is reported in the Women's Health category (see funding analysis), further indicating that some of the grants in that category could be miscategorized, leading to an overestimate of funding for WHR.

---

[8] Email communication with Nancy Praskievicz, Division of Scientific Categorization and Analysis, National Institutes of Health on October 7, 2024.

[9] Email communication with Nancy Praskievicz, Division of Scientific Categorization and Analysis, National Institutes of Health on October 7, 2024.

[10] Email communication with Nancy Praskievicz, Division of Scientific Categorization and Analysis, National Institutes of Health on October 7, 2024.

[11] Email communication with Nancy Praskievicz, Division of Scientific Categorization and Analysis, National Institutes of Health on January 26, 2024.

Based on current RCDC methods, NIH is estimated to spend $4.6 billion on Women's Health in FY 2024 (approximately 10 percent of the NIH Congressional appropriation) and $5 billion in FY 2025 (NIH, 2024a). Recent evaluations by NIH of its spending for Women's Health are documented in the biennial *Report of the Advisory Committee on Research on Women's Health: Fiscal Years 2021–2022* (ORWH, 2023). It defined women's health using language from Section 141 of the NIH Revitalization Act of 1993,[12] which also established the Office of Research on Women's Health (ORWH). Specifically, the advisory committee defined women's health as "all diseases, disorders, and conditions: (1) that are unique to, more serious in, or more prevalent in women, (2) for which the factors of medical risk or types of medical intervention are different for women or for which it is unknown whether such factors or types are different for women, and (3) with respect to which there has been insufficient clinical research involving women as subjects or insufficient clinical data on women." This definition also includes research on prevention of such conditions (ORWH, 2023).

ORWH summarized funding data for three broad areas in the report: (1) female-specific diseases and conditions, (2) diseases and conditions that occur predominantly among women, and (3) other ORWH-selected diseases and conditions that have particularly important implications for women even though they may affect both men and women.

Before FY 2020, NIH (and all Department of Health and Human Services agencies) used the Moyer Women's Health Crosscutting Category report (Moyer Report) to classify research funding by disease and condition categories annually using mandated specific categories and budget allocation definitions. Since then, the best available data come from the RCDC system and some of its internal tools. Among the 315 RCDC categories in FY 2022, about 40 were regarded as highly relevant to women's health and analyzed in the biennial report from the advisory committee (ORWH, 2023). Unfortunately, the change in policy for reporting created a discontinuity, and categories used after FY 2022 may not be directly comparable to those used in prior years (ORWH, 2023).

ORWH reports NIH's spending for WHR was $4.59 billion in FY 2022, a 2.8 percent increase from FY 2020 (ORWH, 2023). For many RCDC categories, exclusive focus on women—Fibroid Tumors (Uterine), Endometriosis, and Uterine Cancer, for example—can be identified clearly, so all expenditures are justifiably attributable to Women's Health. For conditions that affect both women and men, however, it is necessary to estimate the proportion of expenditures that apply to Women's Health. To make these estimates, ORWH used the internal Search and Visualize intersect tool (ORWH, 2023). As expected, variability in expenditure was wide across

---

[12] Public Law 103–143, 107 Stat. 122 (June 10, 1993).

RCDC categories. Categories with the greatest total expenditure in FY 2022 include Breast Cancer; Maternal Health, including Maternal Morbidity and Mortality as a subcategory; Pregnancy; and Contraception/Reproduction. However, Aging, Autoimmune Disease, Cardiovascular, Diabetes, Mental Health, and Substance Misuse RCDC categories had the largest expenditures overall, in the billions of dollars. The proportion attributed to women's health within these categories was estimated to be 16–28 percent of the total. Except for breast cancer, total investments for female-specific diseases tend to be more modest (ORWH, 2023).

ORWH also reports significant increases in expenditure from FY 2020 to FY 2022 for several conditions within each of the three broad categories analyzed. For example, among female-specific diseases and conditions, ORWH reported increases in the research budget for Cervical and Uterine Cancers (29.5 percent and 13.5 percent increases, respectively), Endometriosis (89.7 percent), and Maternal Health (37.2 percent) (ORWH, 2023). Cervical cancer and maternal health funding have benefited in part from efforts that focused more attention on these issues, including the Congressionally mandated 2021 ORWH conference on Advancing NIH Research on the Health of Women, which included static cervical cancer survival rates and maternal morbidity and mortality as two of three major priority areas (ORWH, n.d.), and NIH-wide Implementing a Maternal Health and Pregnancy Outcomes Vision for Everyone Initiative and its associated national network of Maternal Health Research Centers of Excellence launched in FY 2022 (NICHD, n.d.; NIH, 2023b). Ovarian Cancer, Fibroid Tumors (Uterine), and Vulvodynia were among the categories with decreased research expenditures from FY 2020 to FY 2022 (5.5, 15.1, and 37.9 percent decreases, respectively) (ORWH, 2023).

PORTFOLIO ANALYSIS

NIH established the Office of Portfolio Analysis (OPA) in 2011 within the Division of Program Coordination, Planning, and Strategic Initiatives under the OD, in response to the NIH Reform Act of 2006.[13] OPA's goal is "to accelerate biomedical research by providing access to improved methods of data-driven decision making" (OPA, 2021). This goal guides OPA's objectives of improving data and tools to help NIH policy makers optimize decisions and investments and creating and distributing high-quality metrics and standards for portfolio analysis at NIH (OPA, 2021). OPA's strategic plan emphasizes enhancing decision-making processes through refined analytics and tools, supporting NIH's strategic goals. OPA supports NIH leadership and ICs and Offices (ICOs) through data cleaning and analysis

---

[13] Public Law 109–482, 120 Stat. 3675 (January 15, 2007).

and developing new analytics and computational tools to answer critical questions about the NIH portfolio, including potential gaps (OPA, 2021). OPA also maps research topics and can measure productivity and effect of NIH-funded research. It disseminates best practices for portfolio analysis through trainings and symposiums. OPA collaborates across NIH, such as with the National Library of Medicine and Offices within the OD, such as the Offices of Extramural and Intramural Research and the Office of Science Policy. These actions help NIH in strategic planning and portfolio management and in assessing resource allocation to ensure a comprehensive distribution of biomedical research investment (OPA, 2021).

OPA uses a variety of internal- and external-facing methods and tools to evaluate current and emerging research areas and the progress of the scientific enterprise. For example, OPA uses artificial intelligence and machine learning algorithms to create metrics to quantify research investment productivity and effect, characterize the scientific workforce, and predict breakthroughs in key research areas likely to yield significant advances within 2–12 years (NASEM, 2024a; OPA, 2021). Data sources for these metrics include grant applications and awards, publications, clinical trials, patents, and associated metadata, such as authorship, affiliations, and citations (OPA, 2021). Specific tools include iSearch, an internal, next-generation analysis suite, and iCite, a public dashboard of bibliometrics for published papers associated with a research portfolio, such as endometriosis or osteoporosis. Tools within iCite quantify scientific influence of published papers and predict the likelihood of citation by clinical trials and clinical guidelines (iCite, n.d.; OPA, 2021).

However, focusing on publications as a measure of effect, even via a sophisticated metric, does not necessarily capture whether research grants are leading to improved health outcomes (see Chapter 8 for a discussion of publication bias, which also affects the usefulness of this measure). It would be beneficial to track and publish information on the WHR workforce, including how many NIH-funded early-career investigators continue to publish, continue to be awarded NIH grants, remain in academia, or remain in science, for example (see Chapter 9 for a discussion of metrics).

OPA's approach to analyzing topics such as NIH-funded WHR starts with the women's health RCDC category and then extends beyond that using machine learning, input from subject matter experts, and artificial intelligence and language modeling to examine the whole NIH portfolio. OPA trains its artificial intelligence model on scientific data from the whole research landscape of 40 million publications and 4 million grant documents categorized based on computational model–based assessments and then checked by subject matter experts (NASEM, 2024a).

SUMMARY OF NIH ASSESSMENTS OF FUNDING FOR WHR

In summary, the approach used to assess funding for WHR at NIH has limitations. The major limitations include inaccurate grant content curation, lack of transparency, and the potential for overestimation of spending in RCDC categories. First, the system does not always accurately identify grants as related or unrelated to women's health, and the full definition of women's health NIH uses for research expenditures is not public, limiting transparency and reproducibility. This issue is intrinsic to research topics or areas that are broad or crosscutting, given that conventional search tools are unable to easily distinguish, for example, if a grant is actually focused on women's health or mentions that women are in the study but is not focused on measuring outcomes directly or indirectly related to their health. When grants are manually categorized by NIH, it is not clear what process (i.e., for coding and proration of dollars) is used because it is implemented differently by each IC and not done systematically across NIH. Second, the publicly available data (i.e., NIH RePORTER) overestimate the total expenditure on WHR (and other research areas) because it allows for each relevant grant to be counted multiple times. Because of these limitations, in addition to other limitations discussed (e.g., some RCDC codes were only recently created, so cannot be used to assess trends over time, and many diseases and conditions do not have a code), the committee undertook a different approach, described in Appendix A and the following section.

The committee suggests implementing alternative accounting systems and methods to improve accuracy. First, more advanced systems and tools are needed to curate grant content to more accurately discern relevance to a given topic or area, such as women's health. This may involve asking grantees to assist with classifying and categorizing their topic area and focus. It may also involve using more advanced tools, such as large language models, to curate grant content to more accurately identify any grant relevance and then discern the degree of relevance to a given topic area such as women's health. An ideal solution might use both approaches.

Second, more systematic approaches are needed when reporting spending categories in RePORTER to avoid multiple counting of grants with potential relevance to a given topic. This could involve categorizing grants by main funding priorities for NIH first, such as women's, children's, or men's health, and then subcategorizing by disease or condition. This could also involve applying a weighting system to assign proportions of the expenditure for each grant relevant to multiple spending categories in a consistent manner so that the full amount is not simultaneously assigned to multiple diseases and condition spending categories. For example, the full budget of a cancer center grant should not be counted multiple times for each of the many different types of cancers being studied, as this would not accurately reflect the resources devoted to study each cancer. Ultimately, the sum of expenditures across categories would equal the actual research budget.

The committee heard from DSCA staff, in addition to leaders from OPA and the Office of Evaluation, Performance, and Reporting, at its second committee meeting (see Appendix C for public meeting agendas), and these groups acknowledged the limitations of the RCDC system.

THE COMMITTEE'S ANALYSIS OF NIH FUNDING FOR WHR

As noted in Chapter 1, the committee defines WHR as the scientific study of the range of and variability in women's health and the mechanisms and outcomes in disease and non-disease states across the life course. It considers both sex and gender and how these affect women's health and well-being, disease risk, pathophysiology, symptoms, diagnosis, and treatment. This work also addresses interacting concerns related to women's bodies, roles, and social and structural determinants and systems[14] (see Key Terms at the beginning of this report).

As described in Chapter 3, NIH funds several types of research, including basic science, preclinical, clinical, population-based, and implementation research, all of which have a role in broadening understanding of women's health (e.g., exploring risk and protective factors; see Recommendation 8 for more examples). Funding for research on women's health is provided through both extramural and intramural grants awarded by various ICOs at NIH, including the OD. Of the total 27 ICs, two do not provide funding, the Center for Scientific Review and NIH Clinical Center. The remaining 25, in addition to the OD, receive funding each FY for awarding grants across various domains of biomedical research. Using publicly available data from NIH RePORTER[15] and the methodology in Appendix A,[16] the committee conducted an analysis to determine trends over time in the allocation of NIH grants to fund WHR. It involved a comprehensive review of the abstract text extracted for all NIH grants funded during FY 2013–FY 2023. The grants related to WHR were identified from systematic abstract text curation coupled with human adjudication. Funding data on WHR was examined for

---

[14] Adapted from Canada's National Women's Health Research Initiative.

[15] RePORTER is an electronic database that "allows users to search a repository of NIH-funded projects and access publications and patents resulting from NIH funding" (NIH, n.d.-d). It draws data from several databases, including eRA databases, Medline, PubMed Central, the NIH Intramural Database, and iEdison. It is updated weekly to reflect both new projects and revisions to existing projects (such as if a grantee's institution has changed or the award amount has changed) (NASEM, 2022; NIH, n.d.-d).

[16] See Appendix A for a description of the methods for this analysis, limitations, and supplemental data tables and figures. Additional data tables are available in the project's Public Access File and upon request from PARO@nas.edu.

NIH as a whole and each of the 25 funding ICs plus the OD, henceforth referred to as the "ICs" for the purposes of this analysis.

Overall Funding Trends

During FY 2013–FY 2023, the total grant funding for WHR amounted to 8.8 percent of all NIH spending on research grants awarded for these years, while NIH has reported 10 percent of its budget is spent on WHR[17] (Clayton, 2023; ORWH, 2023). The proportion of total NIH grant funding for WHR was 7.9 percent in FY 2023 (see Figure 4-1). A low proportion

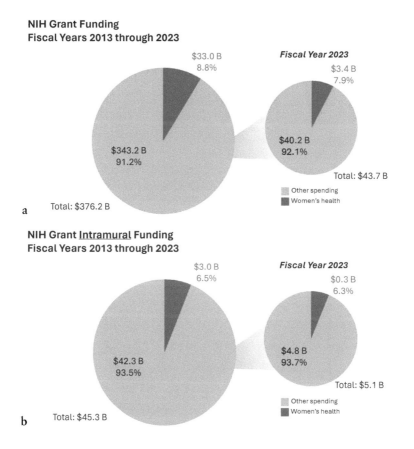

FIGURE 4-1 Total National Institutes of Health (NIH) grant funding on women's health research for the study period fiscal years (FY) 2013–2023 and for FY 2023 (inset) (Panel A) and intramural funding (Panel B).

---

[17] See the Concluding Observations section for a discussion about this discrepancy.

of funding for WHR was seen for NIH intramural grants (6.5 percent) and the aggregate of extramural and internal grants (see Figure 4-1). Overall, NIH grant funding has steadily increased FY 2013–FY 2023 in both dollars spent and the number of projects funded. However, the proportion of funding for research related to women's health remained low and decreased during the same period (Figure 4-2 and Appendix Table A-1). Of the $33 billion NIH spent on WHR grants in the analysis period, the National Cancer Institute (NCI) accounted for approximately $9.2 billion,

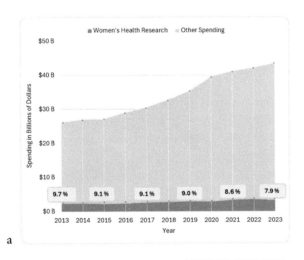

a

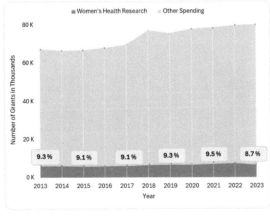

b

FIGURE 4-2 Overall National Institutes of Health (NIH) grant funding and the proportion of NIH funding on women's health research, fiscal years 2013–2023, including amount spent (Panel A) and number of research grants awarded (Panel B). NOTE: Percentages in both panels indicate the specific proportion of spending (Panel A) or grants (Panel B) designated as women's health research.

Eunice Kennedy Shriver National Institute of Child Health and Human Development (NICHD) $5.3 billion, National Institute of Allergy and Infectious Diseases (NIAID) $4.1 billion, and the other ICs about $2 billion or less (see Figure 4-3).

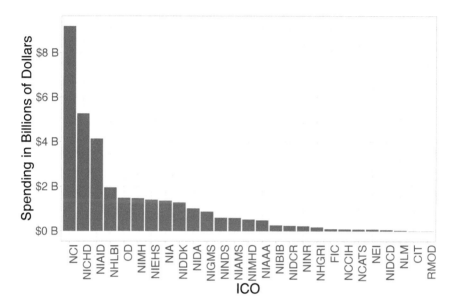

FIGURE 4-3 Portion of total National Institutes of Health (NIH) women's health research grant spending, by Institutes, Centers, or Offices, for fiscal years 2013–2023. NOTE: CIT = Center for Information Technology; FIC = Fogarty International Center; ICO = Institute, Center, or Office; NCATS = National Center for Advancing Translational Sciences; NCCIH = National Center for Complementary and Integrative Health; NCI = National Cancer Institute; NEI = National Eye Institute; NHGRI = National Human Genome Research Institute; NHLBI = National Heart, Lung, and Blood Institute; NIAAA = National Institute on Alcohol Abuse and Alcoholism; NIA = National Institute on Aging; NIAID = National Institute of Allergy and Infectious Diseases; NIAMS = National Institute of Arthritis and Musculoskeletal and Skin Diseases; NIBIB = National Institute of Biomedical Imaging and Bioengineering; NICHD = *Eunice Kennedy Shriver* National Institute of Child Health and Human Development; NIDA = National Institute on Drug Abuse; NIDCD = National Institute on Deafness and Other Communication Disorders; NIDCR = National Institute of Dental and Craniofacial Research; NIDDK = National Institute of Diabetes and Digestive and Kidney Diseases; NIEHS = National Institute of Environmental Health Sciences; NIGMS = National Institute of General Medical Sciences; NIMH = National Institute of Mental Health; NIMHD = National Institute on Minority Health and Health Disparities; NINDS = National Institute of Neurological Disorders and Stroke; NINR = National Institute of Nursing Research; NLM = National Library of Medicine; OD = Office of the Director; RMOD = Road Map/Common Fund.

Grant Funding for WHR by NIH Institute or Center

The low proportion of funding for WHR was seen across all ICs (see Figure 4-4 and Appendix Table A-2). The temporal trend of a flat or decreasing proportion of funding for WHR was seen in each IC, including those with the largest portfolio of spending on it (see Appendix Figure A-2). The IC with the largest proportion of its funding allocated to WHR was the NICHD (37 percent of its spending); all other ICs spent less than 20 percent, and many less than 10 percent, on WHR (see Figure 4-4 and Appendix Table A-2).

Grant Mechanisms for Funding WHR

All NIH grant funding is awarded through a selection of established mechanisms, each designated to fund a certain type of research project or program. These include extramural research (R and P grants); cooperative agreements (U grants); fellowship, training, and training center activities (F, K, and T grants); and intramural research activities (Z grants) (Table 4-1). WHR funding is provided across ICs through a variety of grant mechanisms, though it is predominantly through research project grants (R series) (Figure 4-5).

Distribution of NIH Grant Funding for Women's Health Conditions

To understand how NIH grant funding for WHR has been spent over time, the committee selected funding patterns for a list of 67 conditions (and a category for other diseases and conditions) it prespecified as relevant (see Appendix Table A-3). Given the committee's time frame, resources, and lack of access to full grant content, it was not able to prorate spending on each grant by topic, a limitation noted in the current spending category reporting by NIH. This will be an essential step to include in future assessments to gain a clearer picture of spending on each condition (see Appendix A for additional limitations of the committee's analysis).

NIH grants funded to study conditions relevant to women's health favored certain conditions; among the studied conditions, the 10 highest funded included breast cancer and some female-specific cancers, pregnancy and infertility, and perimenopause and menopause, as well as conditions that also affect men, such as HIV/AIDS, diabetes, and depressive disorders (see Figure 4-6). For FY 2013–FY 2023, the women's health condition that received the most grant funding was breast cancer, with most granted by NCI. Relatively disparate rates of funding were seen for other female-specific cancers, with uterine, vaginal, and vulvar cancer receiving far less research investment (see Figure 4-7). The second most funded area among

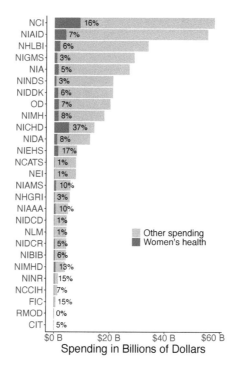

FIGURE 4-4 National Institutes of Health (NIH) grant funding for women's health research for fiscal years 2013 through 2023. Percentage spent on women's health research is shown across each of the funding ICs.

NOTE: CIT = Center for Information Technology; FIC = Fogarty International Center; NCATS = National Center for Advancing Translational Sciences; NCCIH = National Center for Complementary and Integrative Health; NCI = National Cancer Institute; NEI = National Eye Institute; NHGRI = National Human Genome Research Institute; NHLBI = National Heart, Lung, and Blood Institute; NIAAA = National Institute on Alcohol Abuse and Alcoholism; NIA = National Institute on Aging; NIAID = National Institute of Allergy and Infectious Diseases; NIAMS = National Institute of Arthritis and Musculoskeletal and Skin Diseases; NIBIB = National Institute of Biomedical Imaging and Bioengineering; NICHD = *Eunice Kennedy Shriver* National Institute of Child Health and Human Development; NIDA = National Institute on Drug Abuse; NIDCD = National Institute on Deafness and Other Communication Disorders; NIDCR = National Institute of Dental and Craniofacial Research; NIDDK = National Institute of Diabetes and Digestive and Kidney Diseases; NIEHS = National Institute of Environmental Health Sciences; NIGMS = National Institute of General Medical Sciences; NIMH = National Institute of Mental Health; NIMHD = National Institute on Minority Health and Health Disparities; NINDS = National Institute of Neurological Disorders and Stroke; NINR = National Institute of Nursing Research; NLM = National Library of Medicine; OD = Office of the Director; RMOD = Road Map/Common Fund.

TABLE 4-1 Types of NIH Grants

Activity Code		Purpose
Extramural Research		
R	Research Projects	Research project grants may be awarded for discrete, specific research projects to individuals at universities, medical and other health professional schools, colleges, hospitals, research institutes, for-profit organizations, and government institutions. Typically, these grants are awarded for 3–5 years. The most common award is R01.
P	Program Project/ Center Grants	"Program project/center grants are large, multi-project efforts that generally include a diverse array of research activities."
Cooperative Agreements		
U	Cooperative Agreements	Cooperative agreements are "a support mechanism frequently used for high-priority research areas that require substantial involvement from NIH program or scientific staff."
Fellowships, Training, Training Centers		
F	Fellowships	Fellowships "provide individual research training opportunities (including international) for trainees at the undergraduate, graduate, and postdoctoral levels."
K	Career Development Awards	Career Development awards "provide individual and institutional research training opportunities (including international) to trainees at the undergraduate, graduate, and postdoctoral levels."
T	Institutional Training Grants	Institutional Training awards enable institutions "to provide individual research training opportunities (including international) to trainees at the undergraduate, graduate, and postdoctoral levels."
Intramural Research		
Z	Intramural Research	Z grants support research activities of NIH intramural researchers.

SOURCES: Excerpts from NIAID, 2023; NIH, 2017a,b,c, 2023c.

selected conditions related to women's health was HIV/AIDS research, with most granted by NIAID and NICHD. Relatively low rates of funding were seen for many other conditions that affect women differently than men, such as coronary heart disease, and female-specific conditions, such as endometriosis, PCOS, and fibroids.

In analyses of funding trends over time, the relative predominance of funding for the 10 highest women's health conditions was fairly consistent for FY 2013–FY 2023, except for an increase for pregnancy-related conditions

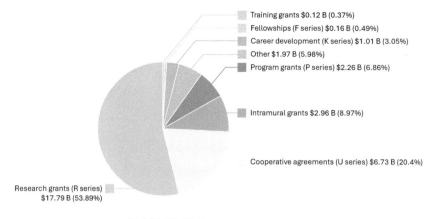

Training grants $0.12 B (0.37%)
Fellowships (F series) $0.16 B (0.49%)
Career development (K series) $1.01 B (3.05%)
Other $1.97 B (5.98%)
Program grants (P series) $2.26 B (6.86%)
Intramural grants $2.96 B (8.97%)
Cooperative agreements (U series) $6.73 B (20.4%)
Research grants (R series) $17.79 B (53.89%)
Total: $33.02 B (100%)

FIGURE 4-5 National Institutes of Health (NIH) grant funding, fiscal years 2013–2023, on women's health research is provided across Institutes and Centers through a variety of grant mechanisms.

NOTES: Dollars are presented in billions. Percentages represent the portions of women's health research funded by different grant mechanisms. FY = fiscal year.

(see Figure 4-8). Trends in funding for cancers specific to and more common in women were relatively flat for FY 2013–FY 2023 (see Figure 4-9). For prevalent chronic conditions that affect both sexes, funding oriented toward women's health increased over time for some but not all (see Figure 4-10). Substantial increases were seen for Alzheimer's disease and related dementias, coronary heart disease, and diabetes, with relatively little or no change for osteoporosis, osteoarthritis, and pulmonary hypertension. Among other select female-specific conditions, funding increased for perimenopause and menopause and endometriosis but was static for conditions such as fibroids, pelvic inflammatory disease, PCOS, premature ovarian failure, and menstrual disorders (see Figure 4-11). Among select autoimmune diseases relevant to women's health, systemic lupus erythematosus was the highest funded, though it experienced a recent decrease, and funding for the others was relatively constant (see Figure 4-12).

Overall, when compared to the steady and significant rise in total NIH grant funding for FY 2013–FY 2023 (see Figure 4-1), the proportionate funding for women's health in general, and for funding that is specific to many morbid and fatal conditions, has not kept pace. These trends have contributed to the persistently low and even decreasing rate of funding for WHR that is most recently estimated at 7.9 percent of total NIH funding (see Figure 4-1). Notably, the funding for several conditions, such as diabetes, pregnancy-related conditions, and menopause and perimenopause, appeared

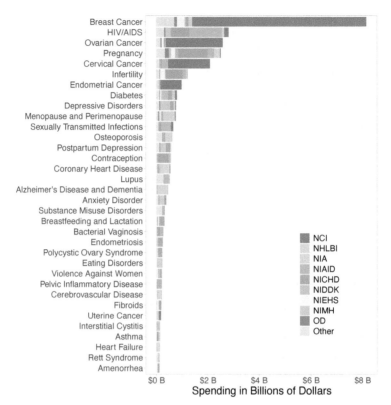

FIGURE 4-6 National Institutes of Health (NIH) grant funding for select conditions relevant to women's health, fiscal years 2013–2023.

NOTE: NCI = National Cancer Institute; NHLBI = National Heart, Lung, and Blood Institute; NIA = National Institute on Aging; NIAID = National Institute of Allergy and Infectious Diseases; NICHD = *Eunice Kennedy Shriver* National Institute of Child Health and Human Development; NIDDK = National Institute of Diabetes and Digestive and Kidney Diseases; NIEHS = National Institute of Environmental Health Sciences; NIH = National Institutes of Health; NIMH = National Institute of Mental Health; OD = Office of the Director.

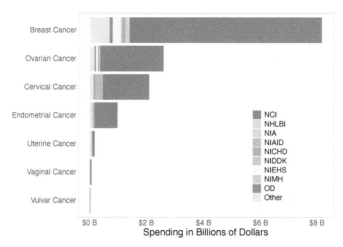

FIGURE 4-7 National Institutes of Health (NIH) grant funding for select cancers relevant to women's health, fiscal years 2013–2023.

NOTE: NCI = National Cancer Institute; NHLBI = National Heart, Lung, and Blood Institute; NIA = National Institute on Aging; NIAID = National Institute of Allergy and Infectious Diseases; NICHD = *Eunice Kennedy Shriver* National Institute of Child Health and Human Development; NIDDK = National Institute of Diabetes and Digestive and Kidney Diseases; NIEHS = National Institute of Environmental Health Sciences; NIMH = National Institute of Mental Health; OD = Office of the Director.

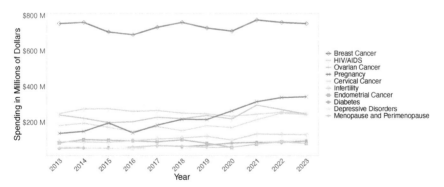

FIGURE 4-8 National Institutes of Health (NIH) grant funding over time for women's health research, fiscal years 2013–2023, for the top 10 highest funded among select conditions relevant to women's health.

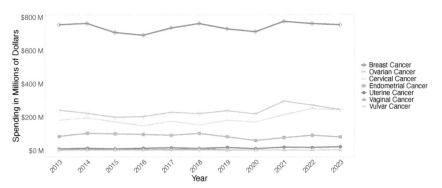

FIGURE 4-9 National Institutes of Health (NIH) grant funding over time for women's health research, fiscal years 2013–2023, for select cancers.

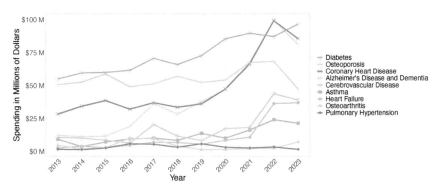

FIGURE 4-10 National Institutes of Health (NIH) grant funding over time for women's health research, fiscal years 2013–2023, for prevalent chronic diseases.

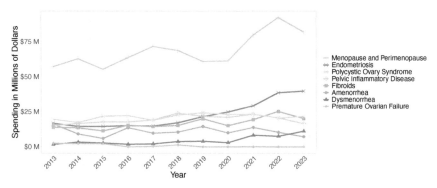

FIGURE 4-11 National Institutes of Health (NIH) grant funding over time for select female-specific health conditions, fiscal years 2013–2023.

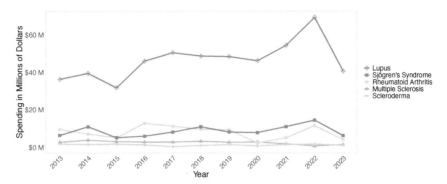

FIGURE 4-12 National Institutes of Health (NIH) grant funding over time for women's health research, fiscal years 2013–2023, for select autoimmune diseases relevant to women's health.

to derive from multiple IC sources (see Figure 4-6), indicating that these have not been consistently identified as within the purview of any single IC. The relatively scant funding for the majority of the 67 conditions determined to be relevant to women's health suggests that they have also lacked a consistent IC source of funding or, in some cases, any IC funding at all.

CONCLUDING OBSERVATIONS

In summary, the committee's analysis of NIH funding for WHR found that despite steady increases in total grant funding over the past 11 years, the proportion for WHR has remained low, at an overall average of 8.8 percent, and decreased over time, from 9.7 percent in FY 2013 to 7.9 percent in FY 2023. This analysis produced consistently lower estimates than those NIH reported for two main reasons: the analysis employed recently available advanced tools that allowed for more reliably identifying grants related to women's health and used an approach that avoids duplicate or multiplicative counting of grants when tabulating total funding amounts. Differences could have also occurred due to the definitions used. Since the committee did not have access to NIH's full definition for the women's health RCDC category, it is difficult to determine if some of the variance resulted from definitional differences of what constitutes WHR. Another limitation of the analysis is the inability to determine an ideal funding level or percent allocation for WHR. The nature and scope of conditions and diseases that exclusively or predominantly affect women are recognized to change over time, and highly prevalent conditions and diseases affecting both women and men can involve varying degrees of sex-divergent presentations and outcomes in ways that have yet to be fully understood, thus warranting more research (Pattisapu et al., 2021; Taqueti, 2018). Additionally, conditions and diseases with sex-differential effects can emerge from year to year—and involve a prevalence and burden in women that require time and effort to estimate (Bai et al., 2022; Cantrell et al., 2024). For all of these reasons, the ideal research funding level or allocation could not be reliably predicted. Notwithstanding these limitations, the analysis produced reproducible results regarding observable trends in NIH funding for WHR over time.

In addition to the overall low and declining funding rates for WHR, the analysis revealed several additional key findings. Although many research areas pertinent to women's health could fall under the purview of the existing ICs, the rate of funding was low across all ICs. The limited funds granted for WHR have had markedly uneven distribution across the major conditions affecting women's health. Furthermore, the analysis showed that many conditions that predominantly or exclusively affect women's health have received relatively little to no funding. Taken together, these findings indicate the need for substantially augmented funding for WHR across the existing ICs and a well-defined and stable funding home to enable research on underfunded or unfunded conditions affecting up to half the U.S. adult population.

REFERENCES

Bai, F., D. Tomasoni, C. Falcinella, D. Barbanotti, R. Castoldi, G. Mulè, M. Augello, D. Mondatore, M. Allegrini, A. Cona, D. Tesoro, G. Tagliaferri, O. Viganò, E. Suardi, C. Tincati, T. Beringheli, B. Varisco, C. L. Battistini, K. Piscopo, E. Vegni, A. Tavelli, S. Terzoni, G. Marchetti, and A. D. Monforte. 2022. Female gender is associated with long COVID syndrome: A prospective cohort study. *Clinical Microbiology and Infection* 28(4):611.e619–611.e616.

Baird, M. D., M. A. Zaber, A. Chen, A. W. Dick, C. E. Bird, M. Waymouth, G. Gahlon, D. D. Quigley, H. Al-Ibrahim, and L. Frank. 2021. *The WHAM report: The case to fund women's health research: An economic and societal impact analysis.* Santa Monica, CA: RAND Corporation.

Cantrell, C., C. Reid, C. S. Walker, S. J. Stallkamp Tidd, R. Zhang, and R. Wilson. 2024. Post-COVID postural orthostatic tachycardia syndrome (POTS): A new phenomenon. *Frontiers in Neurology* 15.

Cebotari, E., and N. Praskievicz. 2024. *NIH's research, condition, and disease categorization (RCDC) system. Presentation to the NASEM Committee on the Assessment of NIH Research on Women's Health, Meeting 2 (January 25, 2024).* https://www.nationalacademies.org/event/docs/D0195AEF81CCEAE1E0BEA79C3AA37C7D6EE52D5DFAF3?noSaveAs=1 (accessed February 26, 2024).

Clayton, J. A. 2023. *NASEM Committee on the Assessment of NIH Research on Women's Health. Presentation to NASEM Committee on the Assessment of NIH Research on Women's Health, Meeting 1 (December 14, 2023).* https://www.nationalacademies.org/event/41452_12-2023_assessment-of-nih-research-on-womens-health-meeting-1-part-3 (accessed August 22, 2024).

iCite. n.d. *iCite.* https://icite.od.nih.gov/ (accessed August 15, 2024).

IOM (Institute of Medicine). 2001. *Exploring the biological contributions to human health: Does sex matter?* Washington, DC: National Academy Press.

Lauer, M. 2018. *RCDeCade: 10 Years and Still Counting.* https://nexus.od.nih.gov/all/2018/06/12/rcdecade-10-years-and-still-counting/ (accessed August 7, 2024).

Lauer, M. 2024. *FY 2023 by the Numbers: Extramural Grant Investments in Research.* https://nexus.od.nih.gov/all/2024/02/21/fy-2023-by-the-numbers-extramural-grant-investments-in-research/ (accessed August 11, 2024).

Liu, K. A., and N. A. Mager. 2016. Women's involvement in clinical trials: Historical perspective and future implications. *Pharmacy Practice* 14(1):708.

Mirin, A. A. 2021. Gender disparity in the funding of diseases by the U.S. National Institutes of Health. *Journal of Women's Health* 30(7):956–963.

NASEM (National Academies of Sciences, Engineering, and Medicine). 2022. *Enhancing NIH research on autoimmune disease.* Washington, DC: The National Academies Press.

NASEM. 2024a. *Discussion of policies, systems, and structures for research on women's health at the National Institutes of Health: Proceedings of a workshop—in brief.* Washington, DC: The National Academies Press.

NASEM. 2024b. *Overview of research gaps for selected conditions in women's health research at the National Institutes of Health: Proceedings of a workshop—in brief.* Washington, DC: The National Academies Press.

NIAID (National Institute of Allergy and Infectious Diseases). 2023. *Cooperative agreements (U).* https://www.niaid.nih.gov/grants-contracts/cooperative-agreements (accessed August 22, 2024).

NICHD (*Eunice Kennedy Shriver* National Institute of Child Health and Human Development). n.d. *Implementing a Maternal Health and pregnancy Outcomes Vision for Everyone (IMPROVE) initiative.* https://www.nichd.nih.gov/research/supported/IMPROVE (accessed August 7, 2024).

NIH (National Institutes of Health). n.d.-a. *About RCDC.* https://report.nih.gov/funding/categorical-spending/rcdc (accessed August 7, 2024).

NIH. n.d.-b. *Frequently Asked Questions About Research, Condition, Disease Categorization (RCDC) System and the NIH Categorical Spending Reports.* https://report.nih.gov/funding/categorical-spending/rcdc-faqs (accessed August 7, 2024).

NIH. n.d.-c. *RCDC: Categorization Process.* https://report.nih.gov/funding/categorical-spending/rcdc-process (accessed August 7, 2024).

NIH. n.d.-d. *Report: Frequently Asked Questions.* https://report.nih.gov/faqs (accessed October 2, 2024).

NIH. 2017a. *Individual Fellowships (F) Kiosk.* https://researchtraining.nih.gov/programs/fellowships (accessed August 22, 2024).

NIH. 2017b. *Institutional Training Grants (T) Kiosk.* https://researchtraining.nih.gov/programs/training-grants (accessed August 22, 2024).

NIH. 2017c. *Research Career Development Awards (K) Kiosk.* https://researchtraining.nih.gov/programs/career-development (accessed August 22, 2024).

NIH. 2023a. *Impact of NIH Research: Direct Economic Contributions.* https://www.nih.gov/about-nih/what-we-do/impact-nih-research/serving-society/direct-economic-contributions (accessed August 7, 2024).

NIH. 2023b. *News Release: NIH Establishes Maternal Health Research Centers of Excellence.* https://www.nih.gov/news-events/news-releases/nih-establishes-maternal-health-research-centers-excellence (accessed September 8, 2023).

NIH. 2023c. *Type of Grant Programs.* https://grants.nih.gov/grants/funding/funding_program.htm (accessed August 22, 2024).

NIH. 2024a. *Estimates of Funding for Various Research, Condition, and Disease Categories (RCDC).* https://report.nih.gov/funding/categorical-spending#/ (accessed August 7, 2024).

NIH. 2024b. *New FY 2023 Categorical Spending Data Are Now Available.* https://nexus.od.nih.gov/all/2024/05/14/new-fy-2023-categorical-spending-data-are-now-available/ (accessed August 7, 2024).

OPA (Office of Portfolio Analysis). 2021. *Office of Portfolio Analysis strategic plan: Fiscal years 2021–2025.* Bethesda, MD: National Institutes of Health.

ORWH (Office of Research on Women's Health). n.d. *Advancing NIH Research on the Health of Women: A 2021 Conference.* https://orwh.od.nih.gov/research/2021-womens-health-research-conference (accessed August 7, 2024).

ORWH. 2023. *Report of the Advisory Committee on Research on Women's Health, fiscal years 2021–2022: Office of Research on Women's Health and NIH support for research on women's health.* Bethesda, MD: National Institutes of Health.

Pattisapu, V. K., H. Hao, Y. Liu, T. T. Nguyen, A. Hoang, C. N. Bairey Merz, and S. Cheng. 2021. Sex- and age-based temporal trends in Takotsubo Syndrome incidence in the United States. *Journal of the American Heart Association* 10(20):e019583.

Salari, N., H. Ghasemi, L. Mohammadi, M. H. Behzadi, E. Rabieenia, S. Shohaimi, and M. Mohammadi. 2021. The global prevalence of osteoporosis in the world: A comprehensive systematic review and meta-analysis. *Journal of Orthopaedic Surgery and Research* 16(1):609.

Taqueti, V. R. 2018. Sex differences in the coronary system. *Advances in Experimental Medicine and Biology* 1065:257–278.

5

The Biological Basis for Women's Health Through the Lens of Chromosomes and Hormones

As Chapter 2 outlines, women's health is uniquely affected by a number of biological and societal factors. This chapter details the need for sex differences research, including supporting examples; how understanding chromosomal and hormonal contributors to female health helps to advance male health; the complexity and current understanding of female hormonal physiology; and the need to advance our knowledge of how the unique female hormonal physiology contributes to mental and physical health. Understanding female physiology is essential to advance our understanding of how to address female-specific conditions and conditions that affect women differently than men.

NEED FOR SEX DIFFERENCES RESEARCH

The first step to improving women's health in the United States is to understand sex differences in diseases across the life-span and invest in discovery and implementation science that will improve the lifelong health of both women and men (see later in this chapter for a discussion on the effect of hormones and sex chromosomes across the life course). The following provides a brief background on sex chromosomes and examples from both preclinical and clinical studies demonstrating the importance of studying sex and sex chromosomes to understanding pathophysiology, disease progression, and the effects of treatment in both sexes.

The Role of Sex Chromosomes

Although the majority of this chapter focuses on hormonal changes during the female life course and their effects on health and disease, the role of sex chromosomes also warrants consideration. Sex differences begin with the sex chromosomes, most commonly with females having two X chromosomes and males having only one along with a smaller Y chromosome. To prevent a double dose of X gene expression, one of the X chromosomes in every cell of the female body is randomly inactivated by several cellular mechanisms, one of which is mediated by a long piece of functional RNA (Xist) and the more than 80 proteins associated with it—together called the "Xist ribonucleoprotein (RNP) complex" (Dou et al., 2024; Lu et al., 2020).

The initial information gained on the contributions of sex chromosomes came primarily from preclinical models. The discovery of *Sry*, a gene found on the Y chromosome, as the main testis-determining gene in the early 1990s provided the framework to begin thinking about how the presence or absence of the Y chromosome would set in motion the production of sex steroids in males and females (Sinclair et al., 1990). The absence of *Sry* and the activity of autosomal genes coordinate development of the female reproductive tract and postnatal steroid production (Rey et al., 2020). Decoding the genetic information of sex chromosomes has lagged far behind that of the autosomal chromosomes, with the human X and Y sequenced fully in 2020 (Miga et al., 2020) and 2023 (Rhie et al., 2023), respectively, nearly 20 years after researchers sequenced the first human genome.

Despite the much smaller size of the Y chromosome, genetic and mechanistic high-impact studies have focused almost exclusively on its role and its contribution to male fitness. While the Y chromosome has shrunk during evolution, its genetic information is critical for ensuring proper testis determination and spermatogenesis and also may account for large phenotypic sex differences in health and disease (Bellott et al., 2014). However, studies focused on sex chromosomes, especially those that include the sex chromosomes in genome-wide association studies (GWAS), are underrepresented in the literature.

Only a small fraction of GWAS have captured any data from the X or Y chromosome (Wise et al., 2013). One recent study concluded that the density of detected single nucleotide polymorphisms (SNPs) for the X chromosome was sixfold lower than for frequencies reported for autosomal chromosomes (Gorlov and Amos, 2023), arguing that the lack of SNPs is not a result of a methodological bias (e.g., differences in coverage or call rates) but rather has an underlying biological reason (a lower density of functional SNPs on the X-chromosome vs. autosomes). As a consequence, within the published GWAS catalog, only 25 percent provided results for the X chromosome, and this value dropped even lower, to 3 percent, for the Y chromosome (Sun et al., 2023).

To capture the full potential of the human genome and the role of sex chromosomes in predicting health outcomes for both women and men, it will be essential to include sex chromosomes in GWAS for annotating how genetic variations track with disease. The majority of the research implicating sex chromosomes in disease etiology originates from preclinical models in mice, which is why the lack of X and Y inclusion in most GWAS, whether it be technical or other, created a gap in our ability to investigate and translate those findings to human studies. The lack of information suggests that the GWAS catalog is limited, although increased awareness and newer technology should help overcome this knowledge gap even as each sex chromosome comes with its own unique challenges (Sun et al., 2023).

In addition to the limited efforts in human studies linking sex chromosomes with female-specific or -relevant diseases, their role in disease-relevant phenotypic outcomes in preclinical models has largely been addressed by chance observation or systematically assessing the four core genotypes (FCG) mouse models (Arnold and Chen, 2009). These models take advantage of the phenotypic female-to-male transition after stably expressing *Sry* in XX mice after reproductive maturity. Conversely, a male-to-female transition is observed when *Sry* is genetically ablated in XY mice. Comparison with control XX or XY mice enables uncoupling the role of sex chromosomes from hormonal output from the ovary or testes (Arnold, 2020a; De Vries et al., 2002). This system may also inform physiological changes that occur in individuals with differences in or disorders of sex development or the interplay of chromosomes and hormonal treatment in the gender-affirming care of trans individuals. One issue with these models is that for investigators funded by the National Institutes of Health (NIH), the financial burden to successfully breed and maintain FCG mouse cohorts and achieve sufficient statistical power is significant, greatly exceeding a simple comparison between males and females. NIH (and Center for Scientific Review panels) need to recognize and address this large financial obstacle to accelerate question-driven, curiosity-based science.

From preclinical models, researchers are learning that the long, non-coding RNA, Xist, a key player in regulating X-inactivation or silencing, interacts with a myriad of other proteins to drive female-specific autoimmunity (Dou et al., 2024) (see the section on autoimmune diseases later in this chapter for more detail). Less well-documented roles for sex chromosomes involve their developmental programming of neurons (Arnold, 2020b).

Female Sex Chromosome Affects Adverse Effects of an FDA-Approved Medication: Cardiometabolic Disease and Statins

Researchers often evaluate the efficacy of medications to treat common diseases, such as hypercholesterolemia, in large clinical trials that enroll both men and women. The trials use a sample size sufficient to detect a significant difference between those treated with the active medication or the placebo. However, they often do not include enough people to also look for sex differences in the effects (Galea et al., 2020). Medications may behave differently in women and men, resulting in variations in efficacy or the rate and type of adverse effects; analyzing these data together obscures any heterogeneity in response (Soldin and Mattison, 2009; Zucker and Prendergast, 2020). This oversight has implications for clinical practice, given that medications that have been shown to be effective for men and women together may be less so or cause more adverse effects for women.

A clear example is sex differences in cardiometabolic diseases and their treatment. Serum metabolite concentrations in healthy men and women differ significantly (Mittelstrass et al., 2011; Reue, 2024). In addition, the risk of several metabolic parameters and diseases differs in prevalence, including adipose distribution, plasma lipid profiles, insulin resistance, hypertension, fatty liver, myocardial infarct risk, and ischemic stroke risk (Chella Krishnan et al., 2018). These differences most likely result from sex chromosomes active in every cell throughout the lifetime. Sex chromosomes, especially XX, are known to influence several cardiometabolic traits, including body fat, fatty liver, insulin resistance, and atherosclerosis, and X escape genes appear to modulate fat mass and energy expenditure (Link et al., 2013).

Individuals with two X chromosomes experience a nearly 50 percent increased risk of adverse events with statin therapy compared to those with one X chromosome, including myopathy and new-onset Type 2 diabetes (Bytyçi et al., 2022; Goodarzi et al., 2013; Nguyen et al., 2018; Reue, 2024). To determine the source of this increased risk, investigators performed a preclinical study in mice; they added statin to the chow of male and female mice and found that fasting blood glucose increased in the female but not male mice, and female mice developed significant glucose intolerance after 4 weeks of statin treatment (Zhang et al., 2024). The researchers also found a reduction in grip strength and number of mitochondria in muscle only in the female mice treated with statin on the diet, which they could prevent by reducing the dosage of the X chromosome or *Kdm5c* gene (a sex chromosome gene), which is normally expressed at higher levels in females (Zhang et al., 2024). Given that statins reduced omega-3 free fatty acids in the female mice, the investigators tested fish oil as a therapy to prevent the side effects in female mice and found that glucose intolerance decreased and grip strength increased. The research team conducted a clinical study where they confirmed that statin treatment reduced omega-3 fatty acid levels and mitochondrial respiration more in women than men (Zhang et al., 2024). While this research was primarily in mice, the findings could have sizable implications for the approximately 92 million U.S. individuals, particularly the women, who are prescribed statins to treat high cholesterol and reduce the risk of primary and secondary cardiac events (Matyori et al., 2023).

Though more than 35 years have elapsed since the Food and Drug Administration (FDA) first approved statins, research has not examined the cardiometabolic differences influenced by the XX chromosome dosage and sex differences in fatty acid metabolism that induce more side effects in women than men, leaving gaps in implementing preventive strategies that could have reduced the rate of adverse events and side effects for many women prescribed statins (Endo, 2010). Given the simple solution of adding omega-3 fatty acids to prevent blood sugar and muscle-related adverse effects, this finding should motivate further studies on women and men separately to understand the biology of the disease state and how much the adverse effects of medications are influenced by sex. See Box 5-1 for additional examples of research needs in this area that affect treatment of women.

BOX 5-1
Effect of Sex on Cardiometabolic Health and
Disease—Research Needs

- Define values for cardiometabolic parameters in health and disease states in men and women separately.
- Determine changes in cardiometabolic parameters in women throughout the life-span, including effects of puberty, pregnancy, and the menopause transition.
- Assess the effects of the intersection of sex with genetic background, environment (including the mediating and moderating effects of weight bias), and gender on cardiometabolic traits.
- Identify molecular differences between sexes in metabolic tissues at the level of chromatin organization, DNA methylation, and gene expression using state-of-the-art techniques, such as single cell-omics, multi-omics, and spatial-omics, in experimental models and human tissues.
- Characterize drug action and adverse effects in both sexes and disaggregate data by sex. Use experimental models to identify mechanisms, particularly for studies of widely used and newer drugs aimed at reducing cardiometabolic disease risk, including statins, Glucagon-like peptide-1 receptor agonists, and sodium-glucose cotransporter-2 inhibitors.

Female Sex Chromosomes Affect the Pathogenesis of a Common Disease Class: Autoimmune Diseases

Autoimmune diseases, which result from the immune system mistakenly attacking the body's own healthy cells, affect up to 50 million U.S. individuals, and at least 80 percent of them are female (Angum et al., 2020; Ngo et al., 2014; NIEHS, 2024). Autoimmune diseases include lupus, multiple sclerosis, rheumatoid arthritis, and over 70 other disorders (NASEM, 2022, 2024). It is thought that a combination of genetic risk factors and exposures to one or more stressors on the body give rise to the majority of autoimmune diseases (NASEM, 2022, 2024), but researchers have not yet identified differences in genes and hormones that may explain this sex difference in incidence and prevalence (NIH, 2024). In recent years, an exciting breakthrough has occurred in understanding a pathophysiology of autoimmune diseases in women that appears to be mediated by female sex chromosomes (Dou et al., 2024; Jiwrajka and Anguera, 2022; Pyfrom et al., 2021; Syrett et al., 2019, 2020; Wang et al., 2016).

Research examined the relationship between the Xist RNP complex and autoimmunity (Dou et al., 2024). Considering that this complex is only expressed in females, the investigators sought to determine if Xist expression in males alters the immune response and produces features of autoimmune disease typically observed in females. The researchers used two strains of mice—one resistant and the other susceptible to autoimmune challenges—and genetically engineered them to express Xist. Only male mice from the autoimmune-susceptible genetic background with the transplanted Xist gene developed severe autoimmune disease after exposure to a known chemical inducer of lupus. The extent of disease pathology was similar to that observed in female mice from the same background after trigger exposure. However, susceptible male mice that did not make Xist also did not develop features of autoimmunity in response to the trigger. The investigators also observed that autoantibodies—the immune system proteins that attack normal cells in autoimmune diseases—recognized some of the proteins associated with the Xist RNP complex in this mouse model (Dou et al., 2024). Together, these findings suggest that the Xist RNP complex may be a key mediator of mechanisms that predispose females to an increased vulnerability to autoimmune disease.

The researchers next looked at autoantibodies to XIST—the human version of Xist—and related proteins in human blood (Dou et al., 2024). They found autoantibodies to dozens of proteins associated with the XIST RNP complex in people with autoimmune diseases—including many that they found in mice that developed autoimmune disease—but not in those without the conditions. Previous studies had identified some of the autoantibodies as being associated with autoimmune disease, but others were novel (Arbuckle et al., 2003; Rosen and Casciola-Rosen, 2016). While the XIST RNP complex alone does not cause an autoimmune response, these findings suggest that it may help trigger it in people who are vulnerable. More work is needed to understand exactly which proteins in the complex may be responsible, which could lead to more sensitive tests that could catch autoimmune diseases earlier and lead to the development of new prevention approaches.

Although it was known that every cell in the female body produces XIST, researchers have continued to rely on male animals and cell lines for their studies (Kim et al., 2021), and when they have included both male and female animals and cell lines, they are usually not analyzed separately. Thus, the standard practice in cell physiology research made it highly unlikely these anti-XIST-complex antibodies would ever have been discovered. This recent breakthrough underscores the role of basic science in helping to explain the disproportionately high number of women who suffer from autoimmune disorders, which are only one of many conditions that disproportionally and differentially affect women, so discovering the role of X-linked proteins here may lead to discoveries in other conditions as well.

Importance of Sex-Stratified Analyses in Clinical Research

Exercise physiology offers an example of the utility and benefits of sex-stratified analyses in research. Women have statistically lagged men in engaging in meaningful exercise. In addition, it was assumed that men and women needed the same amount of exercise to derive cardiovascular benefits. However, when a study analyzed National Health Interview Survey data from 412,413 U.S. adults (55 percent female) for gender-specific outcomes related to leisure-time physical activity, researchers found that men achieved maximal survival benefit from moderate to vigorous aerobic activity (e.g., cycling) for about 5 hours per week (Ji et al., 2024). In contrast, women achieved similar benefits from approximately 2.5 hours of exercise per week. In addition, engaging in regular physical activity resulted in 24 percent lower mortality risk in women compared to only 15 percent in men (Ji et al., 2024). Therefore, by studying women and men together but analyzing their data separately, the investigators found that women can get more out of each minute of moderate to vigorous activity than men do. This study, if replicated, could lead to sex-specific exercise recommendations to improve the health of both men and women.

Studying Women Leads to Findings That Improve All People's Health

Studying women independently can also inform men's health research. This section highlights examples in two disease areas—bone health and cancer treatment.

Bone Health

As described in Chapter 2, osteoporosis is a disease in which there is a loss of both bone mass and structure such that the bone can fracture with very little force. Both men and women achieve peak bone mass in their early twenties, but women lose bone earlier and more rapidly than men because of hormone changes in the menopause transition (Karlamangla et al., 2021; Lu et al., 2016).

A class of medications that decrease bone resorption, bisphosphonates, were approved more than 2 decades ago as the first nonhormonal treatment for osteoporosis in women (Russell, 2011). Subsequent research found that after the rapid loss of bone during the menopause transition, the slower loss of trabecular bone resulted from reduced activity of osteoblasts, the cells responsible for new bone formation (Ji and Yu, 2015; Thapa et al., 2022). This led to the development and approval of two medications—a truncated form of human parathyroid hormone (hPTH (1–34)) and romosozumab—that stimulate osteoblasts to form new bone (Bandeira and Lewiecki, 2022). In addition, developing medications that could both prevent and treat osteoporosis in women led to creating and adopting guidelines for when to evaluate them. Today, women without significant risk factors are recommended to obtain a bone mineral density scan by age 65 years and be treated with bone-active medications if their bone mass is found to be low, putting them at increased risk of fractures (Kling et al., 2014; McPhee et al., 2022). The knowledge gained about bone loss in women and the medications to prevent and treat osteoporosis have also been applied to men. Based on the observation that men did not have the rapid loss seen in women, the guidelines recommend waiting until age 70 to screen men for osteoporosis, if no risk factors are present (Adler, 2000; Bello et al., 2024). In addition, all the medications approved for treating osteoporosis in women are also effective for maintaining bone mass in men (Tu et al., 2018). Therefore, the extensive knowledge base built on understanding and treating osteoporosis in women led to additional research in men that identified new surveillance and treatment recommendations, with implications for health coverage and costs.

Cancer Treatment and Care

Another example of how studying a condition in women can lead to breakthroughs for men's health comes from the contributions of breast and ovarian cancer research to prostate cancer treatment, such as groundbreaking research regarding aromatase inhibitors, which deplete estrogen levels, and poly(adenosine diphosphate-ribose) polymerase (PARP) inhibitors. Adverse events related to aromatase inhibitors, used as adjunct therapies for breast cancer in women, informed researchers and laid a pathway to approach androgen depletion in men treated for prostate cancer (Clinical Education at JAX, 2024; Michmerhuizen et al., 2020; Ulm et al., 2019).

Breast cancer treatment in women has evolved such that adjunctive therapies, especially aromatase inhibitors, have become standard of care. However, early in their clinical adoption, it became clear the treatments that reduce serum estrogen levels could cause rapid reduction in bone mass and increase the risk of incident fractures. This led to recommendations for bone mineral density screening of women with breast cancer before initiating these treatments; if the bone mass was low and osteoporosis fracture risk high, nonhormonal treatments to maintain bone density and prevent fractures were instituted with bisphosphonates or denosumab. These recommendations for assessment and preservation of bone mass were drafted and published in 2003 by the American Society of Clinical Oncology. This is another example of how studying women's health and disease advanced men's health, especially in the use of bone-active agents to prevent bone loss when hormone-depleting agents are instituted to prevent cancer recurrence (Brown et al., 2020; Diana et al., 2021; Johnson et al., 2021; Pineda-Moncusí et al., 2020; Shapiro, 2020; Suarez-Almazor et al., 2022). However, it took another 17 years to translate recommendations regarding screening and treatment to men when androgen-depleting treatments of prostate cancer were adopted (Bruning et al., 1990; Chen et al., 2005; Ramin et al., 2018).

PARP inhibitors, which block DNA repair in tumor cells by inhibiting the PARP enzyme, are FDA-approved treatments for women with breast and ovarian hereditary cancer syndromes with *BRCA* mutations (Menezes et al., 2022). Cancers characterized by *BRCA1* and/or *BRCA2* mutations have deficient DNA-damage repair. The overlying hypothesis that *BRCA1/2* mutated cancers and other cancers with defective DNA repair are more sensitive to PARP inhibitors compared to normal cells has been demonstrated in preclinical models and clinical trials. In 2014, FDA approved olaparib, the first PARP inhibitor, for patients with advanced ovarian cancers harboring *BRCA* mutations (Drugs.com, 2023; FDA, 2017). A randomized double-blind Phase III study of maintenance olaparib compared to placebo in patients with a *BRCA* mutation found a 70 percent reduction in risk of disease progression or death and higher progressive-free survival in those receiving olaparib compared to placebo (Moore et al., 2018). All subsequent studies of other PARP inhibitors demonstrated significant improvements in progression-free survival compared to placebo, leading to additional FDA approvals for olaparib in 2018, niraparib in 2020, and olaparib in combination with bevacizumab, which blocks tumor-triggered blood vessel formation, in select patients in 2020 (FDA, 2018, 2020a, 2020b). This exemplifies the need for sex-difference and sex-specific research to apply findings accurately to the care of women.

Two PARP inhibitors are also approved to treat breast cancer with *BRCA* mutations. These discoveries have also benefited men with *BRCA*-mutated prostate cancer. FDA then approved PARP inhibitors, either alone or in combination with other agents, for specific indications, such as prostate cancers that are castration resistant or have *BRCA* mutations. Overall, the successful evaluation of PARP inhibitors for metastatic cancer is the culmination of over 60 years of work since the first PARP enzyme was identified (Drew, 2015). The research and clinical opportunities, which were first recognized in women with breast and ovarian hereditary cancer syndromes, ultimately led to clinical trials in men with *BRCA*-mutated prostate cancer, improving cancer outcomes for both men and women (Drew, 2015).

Summary of the Need for Sex Differences Research

This section provided examples highlighting the importance of studying sex and sex chromosomes at the levels of cells and organisms in preclinical, observational, and clinical trials research. Sex chromosomes influence the cardiometabolic traits that underly some of the most chronic, burdensome, and costly health conditions, including cardiovascular disease (CVD), Type 2 diabetes, and osteoporosis. Moreover, sex and sex chromosomes influence the effects of interventions—medication and behavioral—on health outcomes. Research on the effects of sex chromosomes on health and disease, however, is only in its infancy. The dominance of male cell lines and male animals in basic physiologic research persists, and therefore, many gaps persist in knowledge related to conditions that differentially affect women (Kim et al., 2021).

Because this research is relatively new, researchers are not yet able to accurately identify all the research gaps or quantify their effect on the health of women and men. Sex and sex chromosomes have been viewed as playing a role only in fetal development. However, evidence is growing of the sizable impact that sex chromosomes have on health throughout the lifespan, dictating the development of the fetus, child, adolescent, and adult, and interacting both independently of and synergistically with sex steroids, which vary over the life course. This research urgently warrants attention to improve health outcomes for all people. The next section describes sex steroid variation over the life course in women, provides examples of how such changes affect women's health, and identifies gaps in knowledge on sex steroids and health.

THE FEMALE HORMONAL LIFE COURSE— IMPLICATIONS FOR UNDERSTANDING MENTAL AND PHYSICAL HEALTH MANIFESTATIONS

Understanding female physiology is necessary to accelerate progress and fully elucidate underlying mechanisms of conditions that affect women's health. Female physiology is more dynamic because of hormonal fluctuations throughout the life cycle. Understanding this complexity of normal physiology in females can help inform how natural changes and fluctuations in hormone signaling contribute to physical and mental health in women. It is important to summarize the current understanding of normal female hormonal physiology. In this section, the committee provides a comprehensive overview of basic knowledge of female hormonal physiology and, where applicable, questions that have yet to be answered or investigated. See Box 5-2 for key findings from this section.

BOX 5-2
Key Findings

- Much of women's health research has focused primarily on the associations of estrogens and progestins with various female disease states; however, other known, less-well-characterized hormones are sure to play a role in basic female physiology and health over the life-span. Without well-funded, sustained efforts that focus on women and female model systems, the hormonal and chromosomal contributions to disease pathophysiology and potential therapeutic targets in improving human health represent a missed opportunity.
- While much is known about female hormonal physiology with respect to the reproductive cycle, researchers still do not understand why hormonal fluctuations across the female life course are tightly coupled to diseases of the brain and peripheral tissues.
- Data on sex hormones, including sex hormone–binding globulin, a sex steroid transporter, androgens, and follicle-stimulating hormone, and cardiometabolic disease suggest important associations with cardiometabolic disease, but more data and analysis are needed to understand the underlying mechanisms and potential therapeutic implications.

CURRENT UNDERSTANDING OF FEMALE
HORMONAL PHYSIOLOGY

Puberty

Two discrete physiological processes—the growth and maturation of the gonads, or gonadarche, and increased production of adrenal hormones, or adrenarche (Bangalore Krishna and Witchel, 2024)—characterize puberty. The pubertal transition and gonadarche begins with activation of the hypothalamic-pituitary-gonadal (HPG) axis and pulsatile secretion of gonadotropin releasing hormone (GnRH) from the hypothalamus, which stimulates the pituitary to release follicle-stimulating hormone (FSH) and luteinizing hormone (LH) (Wolf and Long, 2016). In girls, FSH promotes growth of ovarian follicles, skeletal maturation, and growth plate fusion, leading to cessation of growth (Wolf and Long, 2016). FSH and LH together stimulate the ovarian follicles to synthesize estradiol, which promotes cornification of the vaginal mucosa and uterine growth, in addition to breast development. This process culminates in ovulation and menses (Bangalore Krishna and Witchel, 2024) (see next section).

Even before the physical signs of puberty are visible, pulsatile secretion of GnRH and resultant pulsatile release of FSH and LH occurs, primarily at night initially. As puberty progresses, this pattern transitions to the adult pulsatile pattern throughout the day (Wolf and Long, 2016). It is unclear what prompts initiation of pulsatile GnRH release and what factors keep the "pulse generator" quiescent throughout childhood (Wolf and Long, 2016). Proposed signals stimulating GnRH neurons include kisspeptins, neurokinin B, leptin, and gonadal steroids, but additional research is needed in this area (Bangalore Krishna and Witchel, 2024; Wolf and Long, 2016).

Adrenarche is defined by increased release of adrenal hormones: dehydroepiandrosterone (DHEA) sulfate, androstenedione, testosterone, and 11-oxyandrogens. These hormones lead to development of pubic and axillary hair, increased apocrine body odor, and acne (changes known as "pubarche") (Bangalore Krishna and Witchel, 2024). While knowledge about adrenal physiology continues to grow, the trigger for adrenarche remains unknown (Bangalore Krishna and Witchel, 2024).

For girls, in general, breast development occurs before pubic hair development, although both processes become more synchronized as puberty proceeds (Bangalore Krishna and Witchel, 2024). The growth spurt occurs simultaneously with breast budding, peaking in mid-puberty. Menarche generally occurs 2–3 years following onset of breast development with only a small amount of linear growth thereafter (Bangalore Krishna and Witchel, 2024). Longitudinal studies suggest that puberty is starting at younger ages, which may be the result of rising rates of obesity, environmental factors, stress and perinatal growth, and epigenetic factors (Bangalore Krishna and

Witchel, 2024). This warrants ongoing research to understand the implications of these exposures on not only puberty but also health in adulthood.

Menstruation

The unique reproductive demands placed on females result in dynamic hormonal fluctuations marked by significant and cyclical changes in multiple hormonal systems. The HPG axis largely regulates these hormonal fluctuations in female physiology. It is these three tissues that primarily coordinate hormonal changes during the female reproductive life course, which is marked by the onset of puberty and menarche (the first menstrual period). Throughout the reproductive years, this female-specific physiology is initiated in the brain, mainly through the hypothalamic release of GnRH. Within the pituitary, FSH and LH act on ovaries to elicit monthly cyclical secretions of the sex steroids estradiol (E2) and progesterone (P4) from the ovaries. Hormonal secretions controlled by the HPG axis coordinate ovulation and prepare the uterine lining for implantation and support of a fertilized ovum (Bulun, 2016).

Other endocrine systems, including the adrenal and thyroid axes, also participate in ovulation. Aside from their role in the central control of GnRH pulsatility, neurotransmitters and neuropeptides, including dopamine, norepinephrine, serotonin, and opioids have profound effects on the HPG axis (Bulun, 2016). Similarly, ovarian sex steroids and polypeptide hormones, inhibin, activin, and follistatin (Bulun, 2016), influence gonadotropin production (see Figure 5-1). For reproductive success, a preovulatory surge of LH is required during the mid-cycle to trigger ovulation; the empty shell transforms into the corpus luteum, which secretes steroids for sustaining an implanted fertilized gamete. Specifically, E2 stimulates the proliferation of the endometrium, whereas P4 promotes endometrial differentiation (Bulun, 2016). Without fertilization, the corpus luteum involutes, E2 and P4 subside, and uterus sheds its lining, resulting in a monthly menstrual cycle (Bulun, 2016).

Pregnancy

Pregnancy results when an ovum is fertilized and implants successfully into the uterine lining. Throughout gestation, multiple hormones ensure the uterine environment will support fetal growth and development and prepare the pregnant person for delivery and nursing. An important aspect of pregnancy in humans is the luteal-placental shift that involves reliance on placental human chorionic gonadotropin instead of the corpus luteum. However, because trophoblasts—the cells that provide nutrients to the embryo and develop into a large part of the placenta—lack the enzymes necessary to convert progesterone to estrogen (17α-hydroxylase

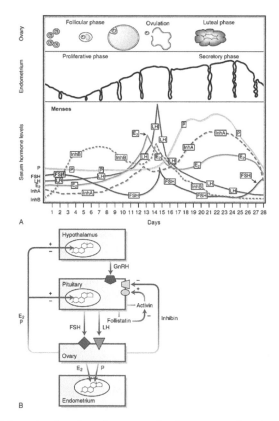

FIGURE 5-1 The role of various hormones in the menstrual cycle.
NOTES: **A,** Changes in the ovarian follicle, endometrial thickness, and serum hormone levels during a 28-day menstrual cycle. Menses occur during the first few days of the cycle. **B,** Endocrine interactions in the female reproductive axis, including some of the well-characterized endocrine interactions among the hypothalamus, pituitary, ovary, and endometrium for regulation of the menstrual cycle. E2 = estradiol; FSH = follicle-stimulating hormone; GnRH = gonadotropin-releasing hormone; InhA = Inhibin A; InhB = Inhibin B; LH = luteinizing hormone.
SOURCE: Bulun, 2016; Used with permission of Elsevier, permission conveyed through Copyright Clearance Center, Inc.

and 17,20-lyase), estrogens are synthesized through a combination of fetal adrenal and liver precursors that are metabolized in placental trophoblasts to generate estriol (E3), the major estrogen in the maternal circulation (Tal and Taylor, 2021). Other estrogens synthesized by the maternal-fetal-placental unit include E2, estrone (E1), and estetrol (E4). During pregnancy, estrogens have multiple roles, including enhancing receptor-mediated uptake of low-density lipoprotein-bound cholesterol for steroid production, increasing uteroplacental blood flow, increasing endometrial prostaglandin synthesis, and preparing the breasts for lactation (Tal and Taylor, 2021). Before birth, estrogens help to stimulate pituitary prolactin synthesis and secretion in anticipation of future lactation or breastfeeding (Al-Chalabi et al., 2023). Aside from these hormonal changes, pregnancy induces a suite of physiological responses involving metabolic responses with respect to how fuel is absorbed, stored, or allocated. Other major changes include the increased demands on the cardiovascular system and hemodynamic properties, which are discussed later in this chapter.

Perimenopause and Menopause

Menopause marks the end of cyclical menstrual periods resulting from the loss of ovarian function and the end of the reproductive phase of the female life course; the final menstrual period can only be determined retrospectively after 1 year without menses (El Khoudary et al., 2019; Harlow et al., 2012). The menopause transition may occur naturally, as ovaries stop producing eggs and ovarian synthesis and secretion of E2 gradually declines and then stabilizes postmenopause (El Khoudary et al., 2019; Harlow et al., 2012). Early menopause can occur by surgical removal of the ovaries, resulting in an abrupt decline in E2, or by anti-hormone therapies commonly used in breast cancer survivors that eliminate E2 biosynthesis (Bulun, 2016; Okeke et al., 2013; Rosenberg and Partridge, 2013). Perimenopause occurs in the years preceding menopause, characterized by anovulatory cycles and irregular menses, through one year after the final menstrual period (Bulun, 2016; Santoro, 2016).[1] Hormonal changes in perimenopause include elevation of FSH, decreased inhibin levels, normal LH, and slightly elevated and variable estradiol (Bulun, 2016; El Khoudary et al., 2019; Harlow et al., 2012). As the ovary ages and follicular reserves begin to decline after age 30, inhibin and anti-Mullerian hormone (AMH) levels begin to drop; these drop even further after age 40, allowing FSH to rise (Bulun, 2016; de Kat et al., 2016). One of the best biomarkers for the ovarian reserve is AMH, which has become a useful tool in assisted reproductive technology for humans (Bedenk et al., 2020).

Following menopause, a host of disorders and diseases increase, including vasomotor instability, urogenital atrophy, adiposity and Type 2 diabetes, osteoporosis, musculoskeletal symptoms, and CVD (Bulun, 2016; Jiang et al., 2019; OASH, 2023; Opoku et al., 2023). Post-menopause, androgens increase from both the ovaries and the adrenal glands, which produce a suite of androgens, including DHEA and DHEA-S. The lower amounts of postmenopausal estrogen are derived from the conversion of androstenedione to estrone in adrenal glands and further modification of estrone to estradiol via aromatase in adipose tissue. These hormonal changes cause

---

[1] This sentence was changed after release of the report to clarify the definition of perimenopause.

a precipitous drop in estradiol that effectively increases the androgen-to-estrogen ratio in postmenopausal women, potentially contributing to the many changes reported in the postmenopausal state (Bulun, 2016).

Menopause hormone therapy, or hormone replacement therapy, is used to ease symptoms of the menopause transition and can improve quality of life (Santoro, 2016). In 2002, the Women's Health Initiative, evaluating the effect of hormone replacement therapy on CVD among other trial aims and outcomes, found increased risk of coronary heart disease, stroke, and breast cancer among participants taking estrogen plus progestin (though estrogen-only therapy reduced the risk of those same outcomes) and recommended that postmenopausal women not be treated with hormone replacement therapy to prevent CVD or other chronic conditions (Chlebowski et al., 2015; Madsen et al., 2023; Manson et al., 2013, 2024; Manson and Kaunitz, 2016; Rossouw et al., 2002). Use of hormone therapy among peri- and postmenopausal women decreased precipitously after publication of the initial findings (Crawford et al., 2018; Madsen et al., 2023; Manson et al., 2024; Sprague et al., 2012). Since that time, however, additional analyses of Women's Health Initiative data and other studies have led women's health experts to further elucidate the role of hormone replacement therapy for peri- and postmenopausal women. Specifically, subgroup data from the Women's Health Initiative, along with data from other trials and cohorts, support the use of short-term hormone therapy for vasomotor symptoms in subgroups of women for whom benefits outweigh the risks (i.e., women younger than 60 and in early perimenopause without other significant comorbidities) (Madsen et al., 2023; Manson et al., 2024; Manson and Kaunitz, 2016).

Understanding the effect of female hormone physiology on physical and mental health across the life course is important in providing insight into how fluctuations in the normal hormonal profile, particularly the changes in estrogen noted in Figure 5-2, may increase the risk for mental and physical health disorders throughout life.

The next sections summarize the current understanding of the association of changes and perturbations in female hormonal physiology with mental and physical health conditions across the life-span and gaps in current knowledge (see Figure 5-3).

HORMONAL ASSOCIATIONS WITH MENTAL HEALTH DISORDERS ACROSS THE LIFE COURSE

Given the chemical nature of estrogen as a lipophilic steroid, its uptake and subsequent regulation of genetic pathways can occur in any cell within central and peripheral tissues that also express one of the three cognate receptors (Chen et al., 2022). Thus, in addition to reproductive organs, estrogen signaling can occur in nearly all organs, including the brain

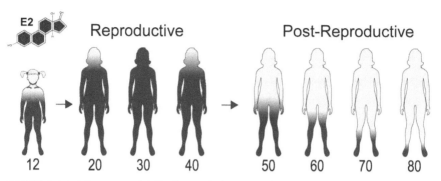

FIGURE 5-2 The rise and fall of estradiol (e2) levels over the female lifespan.
SOURCE: Adapted from ID 142070810, Estrogen Testosterone ©Designua,
Dreamstime.com.

(Chen et al., 2022). However, a molecular understanding of the key cellular
E2 targets in tissues other than the breast or uterus has been understudied
over the past 2 decades and remains elusive. This is especially true of the
brain, where both neuronal and nonneuronal cell types, such as microglia, astrocytes, and ependymal cells, are replete with the nuclear estrogen
receptor-alpha (Elzer et al., 2010; Osterlund et al., 2000). Although it has
been well documented in rodent models that ovarian steroids modulate

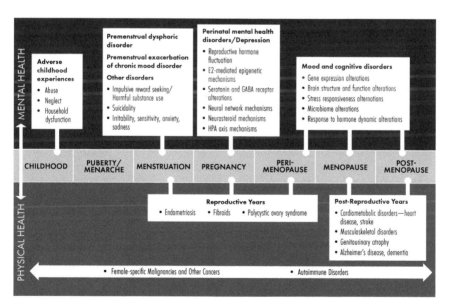

FIGURE 5-3 Female hormonal life course and physical and mental disorders.
NOTE: E2 = estradiol; GABA = gamma-aminobutyric acid; HPA = hypothalamic-
pituitary-adrenal axis.

brain activity and behaviors that maximize reproductive success in females, including feeding, mating, defensive, and maternal behaviors, researchers still do not understand why female-related affective disorders are linked to hormonal fluctuations across the life course (Etgen et al., 1999; McCarthy and Pfaus, 1996).

Despite the centrality of ovarian steroids, research also suggests that normative changes in sex steroids during sensitive windows, including puberty, the menstrual cycle, pregnancy and postpartum, and the menopause transition, trigger psychiatric symptoms in some women (Kundakovic and Rocks, 2022; Schweizer-Schubert et al., 2020). Decades of research focused on understanding the role of ovarian steroids in mood disorders in women have led to limited breakthroughs in the past decade. The bench-to-bedside application of extant knowledge of sex steroids and preclinical models of perinatal depression (PND) has helped researchers to identify novel treatments and resulted in two new FDA-approved medications for postpartum depression in the past 5 years (FDA, 2019, 2023). Sleep also plays an important role in mental health, with sex differences in sleep patterns and sleep disorders (e.g., women are more likely than men to report insomnia, and a bidirectional relationship exists between sleep disturbance and mental health conditions, such as depression and anxiety) (Perger et al., 2024; Rumble et al., 2023). Changing hormone levels throughout female life stages may affect sleep, and sleep is an important factor in the conditions described in the following section. For example, premenstrual dysphoric disorder (PMDD) is associated with poor-quality sleep, insomnia, and fatigue in the premenstrual phase, affecting mood and emotional processing (Lin et al., 2021; Meers and Nowakowski, 2020). Poor-quality sleep during pregnancy is also associated with PND, and increased maternal and gestational ages worsen sleep quality (Fu et al., 2023; Poeira and Zangão, 2022). Finally, sleep disturbances are common during perimenopause, and vasomotor symptoms coupled with chronic sleep disturbance increase the risk of depression during the menopause transition (Brown et al., 2024; Joffe et al., 2010).

Researchers have begun mapping the effects of ovarian steroids on the brain during puberty, the menstrual cycle, pregnancy, and the menopause transition. This work, however, has taken substantial time—80 years from identifying allopregnanolone to the FDA approval of brexanolone as an efficacious treatment for postpartum depression—and the majority of studies of hormone effects on the brain have been underpowered (Pinna, 2020; Reddy et al., 2023). The lack of statistical significance, rather than being interpreted as needing larger, adequately powered studies, has sometimes led researchers to assume an absence of an effect of hormones on the brain (Bachmann et al., 2024; Leeners et al., 2017; Petersen et al., 2021; Smart et al., 2019; Smith et al., 2019).

Although depression affects 57 percent of adolescent girls and 24 percent of women each year, human imaging studies examining sex differences, women's health, or female endocrinology remain relatively scant (CDC, 2023; Lee et al., 2023; Taylor et al., 2021). A recent analysis showed that only 2 percent of human brain imaging studies published in the top five neuroscience journals mentioned women's health, and of those, 83 percent included the women's health variable to justify *excluding* women, characterize the sample without further analysis, such as reporting the number taking oral contraceptives, or control for sex steroids in statistical models (Taylor et al., 2021). While private philanthropy has begun to support such research (Jacobs, 2023; Stevens, 2019), publicly funded efforts at a national level have yet to be prioritized or implemented.

Other than laying out the basic framework of hormonal changes during puberty, the menstrual cycle, pregnancy, and the menopause transition, there is relatively little understanding of how the female endocrine system affects nonreproductive target organs in nondisease and disease states, such as the heart. This is particularly apparent in mental health, where preclinical studies have identified the neuromodulatory effects of ovarian steroids, but the precise neuronal circuits affected or molecular targets in the brain have yet to be elucidated. Other major initiatives on the brain, such as Brain Research Through Advancing Innovative Neurotechnologies, do not adequately address this lack of information because they have not prioritized research on the female brain or sex differences (NIH, n.d.; BRAIN Initiative Alliance, n.d.). For the human brain, the effects of ovarian steroids are only beginning to receive attention, as evidenced by smaller university- or foundation-led research initiatives that specifically prioritize women's brain health (BWH, n.d.; Weill Cornell Medicine Neurology, n.d.). In the following sections, the committee describes the clinical state of knowledge on how hormonal fluctuations during the female life course correlate with and might contribute to mental health disorders and the remaining gaps in knowledge.

Pubertal Depression

The increased risk of depression in women, compared with men, begins at mid-puberty and persists through the female reproductive lifespan. Before puberty, depression rates are similar in boys and girls. After menarche, girls are twice as likely to experience depression and suicidal thoughts and behaviors, leading some to hypothesize a role for ovarian steroids in triggering depression in girls. The first year following menarche is characterized by irregular and anovulatory menstrual cycles, which increase ovarian steroid instability and may, in turn, trigger depression. Recent research suggests the confluence of increased ovarian steroid fluctuations and interpersonal stress during puberty triggers depression in girls. One recent study demonstrated that 57 percent of girls reported depressed mood during periods of ovarian steroid change (Andersen et al., 2022). A subsequent study showed that recent stressful life events interacted with estrogen to predict depressed mood in pubertal girls (Andersen et al., 2024).

Despite these advances, research has been correlational, and few pre-clinical models identifying neuroendocrine mechanisms of pubertal depression exist. The neurobiological mechanisms that explain how stress and ovarian steroid fluctuation interact to trigger depression remain unknown, and research has only just begun to focus on how the hypothalamic-pituitary-adrenal (HPA) axis, HPG axis, and central nervous system interact to determine affective states in humans (Ludwig et al., 2019; Zhu et al., 2021). Research in this area, particularly in puberty, is sorely needed given the alarming increases in child and adolescent stress during the COVID-19 pandemic, rates of self-reported loneliness and suicidality, and prevalence of depression in girls (Chavira et al., 2022; Madigan et al., 2023).

PMDD and Other Menstrual-Related Mood Disorders

Hormonal changes during the menstrual cycle trigger emotional and behavioral changes in some people (see Figure 5-4). Symptoms include impulsive reward seeking and harmful substance use during the follicular phase of the cycle and irritability, sensitivity, anxiety, and sadness during the luteal phase. The latter set of symptoms generally remit after the onset of

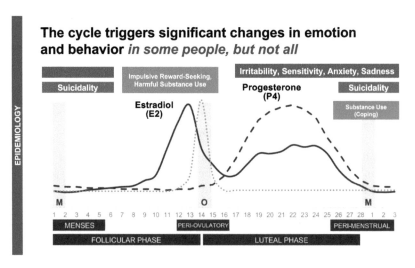

FIGURE 5-4 Timing of mental health symptoms observed during the menstrual cycle.
SOURCE: Eisenlohr-Moul, 2024.

menses. Suicidality and substance use as a coping mechanism occurs in some during the perimenstrual and menstrual phase (Eisenlohr-Moul, 2024).

PMDD is the sole diagnostic entity for mood symptoms that occur in predictable patterns during the menstrual cycle. It describes a pattern of at least five symptoms, at least one emotional, in the week before menses that resolve in the week after. Emotional symptoms include affective lability, irritability, anger, interpersonal conflicts, depressed mood, and anxiety. Individuals with PMDD may also experience an inability to experience joy or pleasure, poor concentration, lethargy, change in appetite, hypersomnia or insomnia, feeling overwhelmed or out of control, or physical symptoms, such as bloating and pain (Eisenlohr-Moul, 2024).

Prospective daily ratings are required during two or more menstrual cycles to make a diagnosis of PMDD, given the essential peak before menses and remission of symptoms postmenses. In those with prospectively confirmed PMDD, research has demonstrated that ovarian steroid stabilization with the GnRH agonist leuprolide acetate diminishes PMDD symptoms, and the administration of E2 and P4 provokes PMDD symptoms (Schmidt et al., 1998), suggesting that E2 and P4 play a central role in triggering symptoms in susceptible individuals. Although the source of this susceptibility has not been fully identified, research has shown that women with PMDD are sensitive to changing hormones at the cellular level. Cells from women with PMDD exposed to E2 and P4 experienced changes in gene expression in a gene complex known to regulate epigenetic responses to sex steroids and the environment (Dubey et al., 2017; Marrocco et al., 2020). In those with PMDD, changes in gene expression were associated with changes in regional cerebral blood flow during P4 administration (Wei et al., 2021). Exposure to sex steroids alters gene transcription in those with PMDD and changes patterns of blood flow to the brain, which helps explain the emergence of symptoms during the luteal phase of the menstrual cycle. The reason some women experience epigenetic changes in response to E2 and P4, however, remains unclear.

Despite these scientific advances, significant difficulty remains in diagnosis and clinical management of PMDD. Prospective daily ratings are only used by 12 percent of clinicians who routinely diagnose PMDD, and research shows that diagnosing based on retrospective symptom recall results in a 60 percent false positive rate (Eisenlohr-Moul, 2024). Aside from the difficulty in diagnosis, many women with symptoms tied to their menstrual cycle are missed by the diagnostic system. Significant heterogeneity between individuals exists in the timing of symptom onset relative to ovulation and menses and the specific symptoms that occur (Eisenlohr-Moul, 2024). For example, PMDD excludes those with premenstrual exacerbation of chronic depressive disorder, even if the degree of symptom change is the same as in those with PMDD (Epperson et al., 2012).

In addition, PMDD does not capture the periovulatory changes in impulsive reward seeking or substance use seen in many individuals (Eisenlohr-Moul, 2024; Epperson et al., 2012). As a result, the classification system misses the majority of individuals with mood symptoms provoked or exacerbated by the menstrual cycle, leading to an underrepresentation of women with such mood changes in psychiatric research and an underestimation of the associated prevalence and costs. Basic, epidemiologic, and clinical research is therefore needed to advance the understanding of how much ovarian hormones modulate mood in women across the population, not just those who are identified as having PMDD. It is critical to expand the research base to more specifically determine the source of differential sensitivity to hormonal changes, identify more efficient and user-friendly methods of clinical assessment and diagnosis, identify treatments for not only PMDD but also the premenstrual exacerbation of other psychiatric illness, and, critically, develop and make evidence-based treatments accessible to the potentially millions of women affected.

PND

The causes of PND, a major depressive disorder that occurs during pregnancy or the 3 months following childbirth, have been difficult to disentangle because it is determined by multiple etiologic pathways (see Chapter 7 for information on its high burden). Both neuroendocrine and psychosocial factors contribute to the expression of illness, which implicate the complex interplay between HPG and HPA axes. Changes in the levels of E2 and P4 during pregnancy and postpartum trigger affective dysregulation in those susceptible to PND (Bloch et al., 2000) and regulate key nodes of a brain network responsible for motivation and reward responsiveness (Schiller et al., 2022).

The rapid antidepressant effects of allopregnanolone, a progesterone metabolite that modulates that gamma-aminobutyric acid (GABA) A receptor, suggests dysfunctional GABA signaling in PND. Multiple trauma exposure, common to 65 percent of those with PND according to one study (Guintivano et al., 2018), and psychosocial stress, a known trigger of PND, alter GABA signaling (Meltzer-Brody and Kanes, 2020; Schalla and Stengel, 2024). Preclinical models have identified precise mechanisms by which changes in perinatal allopregnanolone levels trigger dysregulation of GABA signaling and provoke depression-like behavior in mice. Mice that lack the GABA-A receptor delta subunit are phenotypically indistinguishable from wild-type mice until the postpartum period, when they show deficits in maternal care that depend on corticotropin-releasing hormone (CRH) neurons and specifically the ability to suppress stress-induced activation of the HPA axis during the peripartum period, which is mediated by CRH neuron activity (Maguire and Mody, 2008; Melón et al., 2018). Treatment with allopregnanolone modulates neural oscillations in the basolateral amygdala and motivated behavior, which are mediated by GABA-A receptor delta subunit (Antonoudiou et al., 2022).

Recent scientific advances in the neuroendocrine mechanisms of PND and its treatment may be seen as a success of NIH investment, but the path from basic discovery to clinical intervention has been slow (Patterson et al., 2024; Payne and Maguire, 2019). Two new pharmacologic agents—both GABA-A receptor modulators—have been FDA approved in the past 7 years, allowing for more rapid, targeted treatment of PND than ever before (FDA, 2019, 2023; Patterson et al., 2024). These advances also come with important caveats. Allopregnanolone has been a focus of scientific inquiry since the 1940s. Its calming effects and the mediating role of GABA receptors were discovered in the 1980s (Majewska et al., 1986). By the 1990s, researchers had identified its role in modulating stress and effect on HPA axis function in pregnancy (Morrow et al., 1995), yet despite these critical advances and interest from talented scientists around the world, discovery might have proceeded more quickly if funding research on the neuroendocrinology of PND had been a priority (Paul et al., 2020).

The Menopause Transition and the Brain

Mood Disorders

Research has demonstrated the role of ovarian steroids in perimenopausal depression. Depression onset occurs during the reproductive stage when E2 levels decline, and some studies suggest that rapid fluctuations in ovarian steroids trigger depression in susceptible women (Schweizer-Schubert et al., 2020). E2 administration—either by stabilizing sex steroid levels or by increasing levels—rapidly reduces perimenopausal depression symptoms (Schmidt et al., 2000), whereas blinded E2 withdrawal provokes depression symptoms in women who had experienced perimenopausal depression (Schmidt et al., 2015).

Work using induced pluripotent stem cells developed from women with perimenopausal depression show dysregulated gene networks, including those responsible for inflammatory response and estradiol response, and these differences in cellular gene expression may account for individual differences in mood response to depression in the context of perimenopausal hormone withdrawal and treatment (Rudzinskas et al., 2021). As with mood symptoms experienced during the other reproductive windows, recent scientific advances in the understanding of how hormones may regulate mood during perimenopause have not yet translated into novel treatments or improved access to clinical care. In addition, few preclinical models of perimenopausal depression and anxiety exist, which has hampered the understanding of the triggering, neural pathways, and drug discovery. The standard of care relies on selective serotonin reuptake inhibitors, medications effective in fewer than 50 percent of women that were introduced to the market nearly 40 years ago (Hillhouse and Porter, 2015; Maki et al., 2019; Stute et al., 2020). Menopausal hormone therapy (MHT) is also a standard recommendation for those with comorbid hot flashes (Maki et al., 2019). The most common form of MHT, conjugated equine estrogen (CEE), was approved by FDA in 1942 (Stefanick, 2005). Identification of neural targets for new, targeted pharmacologic agents is urgently needed, as are more information and educational resources for physicians and women about mental well-being during this important life transition.

Cognition and Dementia

Early menopause, either spontaneous or resulting from bilateral removal of the ovaries, especially before the age of 40–45, is associated with an increased risk of mild cognitive impairment, Alzheimer's disease (AD) and dementia, and medial temporal lobe neurodegeneration (Bove et al., 2014; Gervais et al., 2020; Rocca et al., 2007, 2021; Zeydan et al., 2019). This risk is most pronounced among women who do not use MHT up until the age of 50. In addition, longitudinal declines in cerebral metabolism and hippocampal atrophy and increased brain amyloid-beta deposition are greater over the menopause transition compared with men of the same age, independent of the apolipoprotein E gene and cardiovascular risk factors (Mosconi et al., 2018). The underlying biological mechanisms that may explain these findings suggest that hormonal fluctuations and levels are critical to the development of this clinical syndrome and corresponding brain pathology. For example, compared with age-matched controls, reduced levels of 17-Beta-estradiol and testosterone are observed in female and male patients with AD (Barron and Pike, 2012)

There are three physiological estrogens in females, E1, E2, and E3, with E2 being the major product in the premenopausal period (Spencer et al., 2008). In addition to promoting dendritic growth, estrogen also has a protective effect on the brain through brain metabolism. Shifts in estrogens during the menopause transition could lead to the deficits seen in brain metabolism in AD, such as mitochondrial impairment, or disruption of neurogenesis and hippocampal atrophy in women with mild cognitive impairment (Fleisher et al., 2005; Long et al., 2012; Turek and Gąsior, 2023).

The protective effects of estrogen against amyloid-beta accumulation— the pathological hallmark of AD—are attributed to its influence on amyloid precursor processing, on clearance of amyloid-beta, and on the degradation of amyloid-beta, in addition to reducing levels of hyperphosphorylated tau, a component of the neurofilament tangles seen in AD (Gandy and Petanceska, 2000; Li et al., 2000; Muñoz-Mayorga et al., 2018; Zhao et al., 2011).

Despite these observations, data from clinical trials and translation approaches have been mixed. The Women's Health Initiative Memory Study remains the only randomized, placebo-controlled trial on MHT for primary prevention of dementia. It enrolled postmenopausal females with a uterus over 65 and randomized them to receive oral CEE plus medroxyprogesterone acetate (MPA) or a placebo; and females without a uterus received oral CEE or a placebo. The primary outcome was incident dementia and mild cognitive impairment. The results suggested that the risk of all-cause dementia was twice as high in the CEE/MPA group, translating to an additional 23 cases of dementia per 10,000 women per year. The group without a uterus did not reveal a significant effect on incidence of dementia or mild cognitive impairment. When data were pooled together from both arms, there was an increased risk of dementia for the active drug compared to placebo groups in late life (Shumaker et al., 2003, 2004).

Further analyses noted that cardiovascular risk factors did not modify the effects of hormone therapy on cognitive function, and brain magnetic resonance imaging studies found that ischemic brain volume did not differ between the hormone therapy and placebo groups. However, the rates of accumulation of white matter lesions and total brain lesion volumes were higher among females with a history of CVD treated with hormone therapy versus placebo (Coker et al., 2014; Volgman et al., 2019).

Results from more recently conducted randomized clinical trials suggest that the timing and type of MHT are important for cognitive decline—with data suggesting that initiating MHT shortly after the final menstrual period does not have either long-term detrimental effects on cognition or beneficial cognitive effects (Espeland et al., 2013; Gleason et al., 2015; Henderson et al., 2016; Jett et al., 2022). The use of MHT remains controversial, with difficulty interpreting the data from studies due to differences in the timing of hormone therapy initiation in relation to menopause, the type of hormone treatment, characterization of comorbidities, such as CVD and AD risk of the participants, study design (clinical trial vs. observational study), outcome metrics (measure of cognition or neuroimaging modality), and sample size.

These findings collectively highlight the need to conduct further randomized clinical trials and studies that examine the effect of perimenopause or early postmenopause hormone replacement therapy administration on cognitive function, neuroimaging markers, and *APOE4* carrier status to examine potential differences in the mechanistic basis of cognitive function and decline in women.

Summary of Hormonal Associations with Mental Health Disorders

Half the U.S. population will experience menopause should they live long enough, and the majority of women will have clinically significant symptoms (Peacock et al., 2023). Given the large number of affected people who will require clinical intervention, research is needed to guide the understanding of the pathophysiology such that illness expression can be prevented or treated effectively. Simultaneously, research focused on the clinical management of symptoms with existing treatments is sorely needed. Although risk of depression is elevated during and after the menopause transition, no randomized controlled trials have ever examined the comparative effectiveness of existing treatments for perimenopause-onset depression (Badawy et al., 2024; Bromberger et al., 2011). Moreover, since women comprise the majority of both the workforce and unpaid caregiving roles in the United States, preserving cognition and preventing dementia as they age is of high importance (Stall et al., 2023). The largest and most comprehensive large-scale, randomized, placebo-controlled trial for primary prevention, however, was completed over 20 years ago and conducted only in postmenopausal women, once illness progression may have already started (BLS, 2023; Hays et al., 2003).

The lack of well-powered clinical trials has left a large gap in knowledge essential for guiding the clinical care of midlife women in the menopause transition. Given that more recent research has demonstrated that hormone therapy may be safe when initiated earlier, with certain hormone formulations, and in subgroups of women with differential risk factors—accounting for those with AD risk and CVD, for example—additional large-scale, randomized, controlled trials are needed to disentangle the effects of hormonal treatments on cognition from the effects of aging and other risk factors and examine their synergistic effects on both risk and resilience (Cho et al., 2023; Faubion et al., 2022).

HORMONAL ASSOCIATIONS WITH PHYSICAL HEALTH DISORDERS ACROSS THE LIFE COURSE

Cancers Across the Life Course

Hormone-dependent cancers include breast, endometrial, and ovarian cancers (Hoadley et al., 2018). Risk factors for estrogen-dependent cancers include high natural endogenous levels, hormone replacement therapy, obesity, and polycystic ovary syndrome (PCOS). Oral contraceptive pills (OCPs) appear to reduce the risk of epithelial ovarian and endometrial cancer (American Cancer Society, 2024). OCP use is also associated with a decreased risk of colorectal cancer (Murphy et al., 2017). In contrast, oral contraception appears to increase the risk of breast cancer, and long-term use is associated with increased cervical cancer risk (American Cancer Society, 2024; Asthana et al., 2020; Barańska et al., 2021; NCI, 2018). Prenatal exposure to diethylstilbestrol, an artificial estrogen no longer in use, is a risk factor for clear cell cervical and vaginal cancers in females exposed in utero (White et al., 2022). Tamoxifen, a selective estrogen receptor modulator commonly used to treat breast cancer, is associated with a higher risk of uterine malignancies, including endometrial cancers and uterine sarcomas (American Cancer Society, 2024).

Excess body weight or gaining weight during adulthood and physical inactivity are associated with numerous cancers, including female-specific cancers (American Cancer Society, 2024). The link between obesity and hormone-dependent cancers may be related to hormonal synthesis in adipose tissue, leading to heightened circulating estrogen levels. Hormonal signaling pathways have been implicated in modulating cell growth, proliferation, invasion, angiogenesis, and metastasis (Ranhotra, 2022). Thanks to a large and sustained investment in breast cancer research, the relationship between estrogen and breast and endometrial cancers is much better understood compared to cancers such as ovarian and cervical, indicating an important knowledge gap.

Breast, endometrial, and ovarian cancers are more prevalent after menopause (Barry et al., 2014). The role of exogenous hormones and female-specific cancers is variable. For instance, high levels of estrogen, testosterone, and P4 increase breast cancer risk. In contrast, high levels of estrogen increase endometrial cancer risk, while progestins are protective. As described, after the initial Women's Health Initiative study, the use of combination estrogen and progesterone declined significantly, and some authors have speculated that the increasing incidence in endometrial cancer may be the result of decreased use of combination hormone replacement therapy, prolonged use of vaginal estrogens, or use of compounded bioidentical hormone therapy (Constantine et al., 2019).

Hormonal therapy is used to treat select patients with breast, endometrial, and ovarian cancer. For breast cancer, endocrine therapy with or without ovarian suppression/ablation is considered for patients with hormone receptor–positive cancers and based on risk of recurrence (Burstein et al., 2016). Endometrial cancers can be treated with several hormonal strategies, including megestrol acetate, medroxyprogesterone acetate, alternating tamoxifen with megestrol acetate, and an aromatase inhibitor (NCCN, 2023). Levonorgestrel intrauterine devices and oral progestins are used to treat patients with endometrial cancer who desire fertility or are not surgical candidates (NCCN, 2023). Hormonal therapy is used to treat patients with low-grade serous ovarian cancers and sex-cord stromal tumors (NCCN, 2024).

Breast and hormone-dependent gynecologic cancers share many similarities. Their development is in part driven by hormonal factors, and treatment options include hormonal therapies, aromatase inhibitors, and ovarian suppression/ablation. A better understanding of steroid sex hormone pathophysiology, role of signaling pathways, and mechanisms of carcinogenesis is needed to identify additional preventive and treatment strategies.

Reproductive and Postreproductive Years

Endometriosis is the presence of endometrium-like tissue outside of the uterine cavity—most often in the pelvic peritoneum and ovaries—leading to inflammation and scarring. Endometriosis and intrauterine endometrial tissue both respond to estrogen and P4 similarly, resulting in endometriosis proliferation and inhibition of endometrial growth, respectively. Ectopic endometrial tissue, however, does not respond as predictably to progestin and native progesterone, as it has a different secretory pattern of cytokines and prostaglandins, steroid biosynthesis and metabolism, and steroid receptor content (Bulun, 2016). This may explain why hormonal treatments are not effective in curing the disease and recurrence is common. Further research on its pathogenesis is needed in human and nonhuman primate models to identify nonsurgical diagnostic and treatment approaches that would significantly improve health and quality of life for millions of women. Similarly, additional research is needed to understand the role of estrogen, P4, and other hormones in the development of uterine fibroids and pelvic floor disorders, conditions that significantly affect quality of life for women during their reproductive and nonreproductive years (see Chapter 7).

Menopause, Hormones, and Cardiometabolic Disorders

Menopause as a Critical Transition for Cardiometabolic Health

During and after the menopausal transition, key changes in cardiometabolic health occur, notably the accumulation of risk factors resulting from changing hormonal profiles. These changes, including alterations in blood pressure trajectory and lipid profiles and increased visceral adiposity, contribute to increased risk of postmenopausal heart disease and stroke (Madsen et al., 2023; Samargandy et al., 2022). For example, in a longitudinal analyses of participants from the Women's Health Initiative, increases in FSH over a 5-year period were associated with increasing total body fat, total body fat mass, and subcutaneous adipose tissue (Mattick et al., 2022). Developing central obesity after menopause is of particular concern, as it confers a higher risk of cardiovascular and all-cause mortality, independent of body mass index (Sun et al., 2019).

Lipid profiles also change in peri- and postmenopause, and this may include increases in low-density lipoprotein, total cholesterol, apolipoproteins, and triglycerides and a decrease in the protection from high-density lipoprotein (Holven and Roeters van Lennep, 2023; Torosyan et al., 2022). Vascular aging and changes in endovascular function in peri- and postmenopause further contribute to changes in risk of CVD (Moreau and Hildreth, 2014), and data suggest sex-specific associations between endogenous sex hormones and measures of arterial stiffness, a key contributor to hypertension (Subramanya et al., 2018). Finally, though increasing blood pressure is known to occur with chronological age, data suggest an additional contribution from reproductive aging and changes in hormones occurring during the perimenopause transition (Samargandy et al., 2022).

Endogenous Hormones and Risk of Cardiometabolic Disease

Directly related to changes in cardiometabolic profiles during peri- and postmenopause, overall, data indicate key associations between endogenous sex hormones levels and cardiovascular endpoints and risk factors among postmenopausal women. Estrogen-level changes measured in postmenopausal women, however, do not seem to fully explain the increasing risk of CVD (Hu et al., 2020; Zhao et al., 2018). Despite some conflicting data on the association between endogenous estrogen and cardiovascular endpoints (Hu et al., 2020), data on sex hormone–binding globulin, a sex steroid transporter that helps to regulate circulating testosterone and estrogen and can act independently of sex steroids, is inversely associated with clinical diabetes, coronary heart disease, and stroke with some evidence for causality (Ding et al., 2006, 2009; Kalyani et al., 2009; Li et al., 2023; Madsen et al., 2020; Sun et al., 2024). Furthermore, despite data indicating a role for androgens in the etiology of CVD in men (Zhang et al., 2022), an adequate understanding of that role and the change in androgen-to-estrogen ratio in the cardiovascular health of older women is lacking (Rexrode et al., 2003), which is an area where research is needed (Sohrabji et al., 2019).

Osteoporosis

Menarche is associated with increased circulating levels of estrogen, and this results in a rapid gain in bone mass from ages 12 to 20, with women achieving their peak bone mass by approximately age 20 (Clarke and Khosla, 2010). Bone remains strong through the childbearing years as a result of the steady levels of estrogen and progestins through normal menstrual cycles (Clarke and Khosla, 2010; Seifert-Klauss and

Prior, 2010). Women maintain most of their bone mass until they enter perimenopause, when the sustained reduction in estrogen levels results in uncoupled bone remodeling, yielding increased resorption relative to formation (Clarke and Khosla, 2010). There is a rapid turnover of bone and a rapid loss of trabecular, or spongy, bone which is the porous component of bone that is highly enriched in the spine and, along with the cortical shell, gives bone its strength (Ott, 2018; Walker and Shane, 2023). Studies of women's bone mass through their life course found rapid bone loss within 10 years of the menopause transition, especially estrogen-sensitive trabecular bone in the lumbar spine, pelvis, and hips (Finkelstein et al., 2008; Nilas and Christiansen, 1988). This is followed by slow, steady loss that disproportionately affects trabecular/spongy bone (Finkelstein et al., 2008; Ji and Yu, 2015; Seeman, 2013; Walker and Shane, 2023). Over time, this bone loss leads to low bone mass and strength, culminating in osteoporosis, frailty, and increased risk of fractures, especially in the vertebra (Clarke and Khosla, 2010). However, women do generate estrogen from fat stores, which can slow some of the bone loss (Frisch et al., 1980; Gimble et al., 1996; Hetemäki et al., 2021). The natural onset of menopause is not the only condition that triggers significant bone loss. For example, millions of female breast cancer survivors use anti-estrogen therapies (aromatase inhibitors) for up to 10 years (Diana et al., 2021; Pineda-Moncusí et al., 2020; Shapiro, 2020). While these can reduce the risk of breast cancer reoccurrence, they can have a significant toll on bone quality and ultimately lead to unhealthy aging. Another group experiencing premature bone loss are those who undergo surgery to remove the ovaries, and while they are often prescribed hormone replacement therapy, it does not fully counteract that bone loss (Hibler et al., 2016). The risk of osteoporosis is higher in White and Asian compared to Black women, but the role of estrogens in this is not well understood (Office of the Surgeon General, 2004).

Despite medications that have been approved and are effective in preventing fractures of the lumbar spine and hip in elderly women and men, the best way to prevent osteoporosis is to achieve a high peak bone mass (IOF, n.d.; Rosen, 2000). No approved pharmacological treatments augment peak bone mass, which is affected by a combination of genetics, dietary choices that affect the intake of calcium and vitamin D, physical activity, and regular menstrual cycles (Rosen, 2000; Zumwalt and Dowling, 2014). Estrogen, however, remains a major prevention therapy for osteoporosis, and the timing and duration of use relative to the menopause transition to maximize bone and joint health is an area of continued investigation (Adler et al., 2016; Grigoryan and Clines, 2024; Rosen, 2000; Silverwood et al., 2015).

Hormonal Considerations Across the Life
Course for Transgender Individuals

Transgender individuals (XY women/girls and XX men/boys) have unique hormonal considerations across the life course, as outlined in the 2023 Endocrine Society Scientific Statement on Endocrine Health and Healthcare Disparities in Pediatric and Sexual and Gender Minority Populations (see Box 5-3) (Diaz-Thomas et al., 2023). Gender-affirming hormone therapy in transgender youth includes sex hormones and pubertal suppression with GnRH agonists. The long-term effect of these interventions on statural growth, CVD risk, bone mineral density, and reproductive health in both transgender women and men need further study. Tall stature in transgender girls may contribute to psychological distress, which may require rapid escalation of estrogen to facilitate closure of the epiphyses (Shumer and Araya, 2019). Similarly, for transgender boys, escalating testosterone therapy more slowly can provide a longer period of statural growth and greater height attainment to address short stature (Shumer and Araya, 2019). The effect of GnRH agonist therapy on final adult height and further manipulation of growth with additional therapies, such as aromatase inhibitors and growth hormone, require further investigation in transgender girls and boys (Diaz-Thomas et al., 2023; Roberts and Carswell, 2021).

Transgender individuals also have a higher rate of overweight, and one study noted a higher incidence and prevalence of Type 2 diabetes in transgender compared to cisgender women, despite no association with gender-affirming hormone therapy. In contrast, in another study, transgender women receiving gender-affirming hormone therapy (i.e., estrogen) had worse insulin resistance and adverse body composition alteration (Islam et al., 2022). Gender-affirming hormone therapy also significantly affects bone health due to the effects of testosterone-lowering therapy in transgender women and GnRH agonists in youth (Stevenson and Tangpricha, 2019). Because both testosterone and estrogen play major roles in bone formation in puberty and bone turnover in adulthood, the effect on long-term bone health may be significant; however, no long-term data exist on the association of GnRH agonists in adolescence with risk of osteopenia, osteoporosis, and/or bone fractures in transgender adult women (Diaz-Thomas et al., 2023).

Finally, it is important to recognize that transgender men who have not undergone total hysterectomy and oophorectomy are at risk and need to be screened for gynecologic malignancies (Diaz-Thomas et al., 2023). They may also experience pregnancy, even with gender-affirming hormone therapy (Diaz-Thomas et al., 2023). Little data exist on the long-term health impact of testosterone therapy in transgender men. All of these areas warrant further research to support the generation of evidence-based guidelines, as summarized in Box 5-3.

BOX 5-3
Future Research Needs for Transgender Individuals from
Endocrine Society Scientific Statement

- Design studies to quantify and elucidate endocrine health and health care disparities in non-White LGBTQIA youth.
- Design health care demographic data collection systems to allow patients to report self-identified sexual orientation and gender identity data.
- Determine the optimal timing and duration of gonadotropin hormone agonist therapy in transgender youth related to bone health.
- Design longitudinal studies to determine the prevalence of osteoporosis, osteopenia, and fractures among transgender youth and adults.
- Generate the evidence base to determine best practices in fertility preservation options and reproductive care of sexual and gender minority patients.
- Design studies to examine how sexual and gender identity may be impacted by chronic disease and how chronic disease management may be impacted by sexual and/or gender identity minority status.
- Develop policy changes to ensure broadening of insurance coverage for sexual and gender minorities and to de-pathologize sexual orientation and gender identity to remove further barriers to care.

SOURCE: Diaz-Thomas et al., 2023.

CONCLUDING OBSERVATIONS

Scientific research has predominantly used male participants as the norm, leading to a significant gap in understanding female-specific physiological and biological differences. This bias has resulted in a lack of comprehensive data on how female physiology uniquely contributes to and is affected by mental and physical health disorders and their treatments (Merone et al., 2022). The complex interplay between sex chromosomes, hormones, and physiology is not fully understood, creating a significant knowledge gap. While rodent models have provided some insights, translating these findings to humans remains challenging, given the additional influence of social and environmental factors that affect human development and behavior. There is a need for more diverse and sophisticated models to study the effects of sex chromosomes and hormones in a manner that is more representative of human biology.

Research is insufficient on the roles and effects of key sex hormones, such as estrogen, progesterone, and testosterone, in women, particularly how they influence nonreproductive systems and influence cardiovascular health, bone density, and mental health. Despite a growing recognition of the importance of considering sex as a biological variable in all areas of investigation, more focused attention by researchers and funders is needed. This includes understanding how sex hormones and chromosomes affect brain anatomy and neural regulation, immune system, vascular, and reproductive system function, and other systems. In addition, new fields of research, such as the role of epigenetics in sexual differentiation and disease development, are beginning to emerge. These areas hold promise for enriching the understanding of how sex differences are regulated at a molecular level, but they are still in their infancy and require more systematic investigation and research investment.

Advancing knowledge of the biological contributors to sex differences in the normal function of and dysregulation of multiple organ systems is crucial for developing more effective, personalized, and sex-specific treatments. The lack of research on female chromosomes and hormones, and even on understanding basic female physiology, has resulted in significant knowledge gaps that need to be addressed. Closing them is essential for advancing the understanding of sex differences and improving women's health outcomes across the life course.

REFERENCES

Adler, R. A. 2000. Osteoporosis in men. In *Endotext*, edited by K. R. Feingold, B. Anawalt, M. R. Blackman, A. Boyce, G. Chrousos, E. Corpas, W. W. de Herder, K. Dhatariya, K. Dungan, J. Hofland, S. Kalra, G. Kaltsas, N. Kapoor, C. Koch, P. Kopp, M. Korbonits, C. S. Kovacs, W. Kuohung, B. Laferrère, M. Levy, E. A. McGee, R. McLachlan, M. New, J. Purnell, R. Sahay, A. S. Shah, F. Singer, M. A. Sperling, C. A. Stratakis, D. L. Trence, and D. P. Wilson. South Dartmouth, MA: MDText.com, Inc.

Adler, R. A., G. El-Hajj Fuleihan, D. C. Bauer, P. M. Camacho, B. L. Clarke, G. A. Clines, J. E. Compston, M. T. Drake, B. J. Edwards, M. J. Favus, S. L. Greenspan, R. McKinney, Jr., R. J. Pignolo, and D. E. Sellmeyer. 2016. Managing osteoporosis in patients on long-term bisphosphonate treatment: Report of a Task Force of the American Society for Bone and Mineral Research. *Journal of Bone and Mineral Research* 31(1):16–35.

Al-Chalabi, M., A. Bass, and I. Alsalman. 2023. Physiology, prolactin. In *Statpearls*. Treasure Island, FL: StatPearls Publishing.

American Cancer Society. 2024. *Cancer facts & figures 2024*. Atlanta, GA: American Cancer Society.

Andersen, E., S. Fiacco, J. Gordon, R. Kozik, K. Baresich, D. Rubinow, and S. Girdler. 2022. Methods for characterizing ovarian and adrenal hormone variability and mood relationships in peripubertal females. *Psychoneuroendocrinology* 141:105747.

Andersen, E., H. Klusmann, T. Eisenlohr-Moul, K. Baresich, and S. Girdler. 2024. Life stress influences the relationship between sex hormone fluctuation and affective symptoms in peripubertal female adolescents. *Development and Psychopathology* 36(2):821–833.

Angum, F., T. Khan, J. Kaler, L. Siddiqui, and A. Hussain. 2020. The prevalence of autoimmune disorders in women: A narrative review. *Cureus* 12(5):e8094.

Antonoudiou, P., P. L. W. Colmers, N. L. Walton, G. L. Weiss, A. C. Smith, D. P. Nguyen, M. Lewis, M. C. Quirk, L. Barros, L. C. Melon, and J. L. Maguire. 2022. Allopregnanolone mediates affective switching through modulation of oscillatory states in the basolateral amygdala. *Biological Psychiatry* 91(3):283–293.

Arbuckle, M. R., M. T. McClain, M. V. Rubertone, R. H. Scofield, G. J. Dennis, J. A. James, and J. B. Harley. 2003. Development of autoantibodies before the clinical onset of systemic lupus erythematosus. *New England Journal of Medicine* 349(16):1526–1533.

Arnold, A. P. 2020a. Four Core Genotypes and XY* mouse models: Update on impact on SABV research. *Neuroscience and Biobehavioral Reviews* 119:1–8.

Arnold, A. P. 2020b. Sexual differentiation of brain and other tissues: Five questions for the next 50 years. *Hormones and Behavior* 120:104691.

Arnold, A. P., and X. Chen. 2009. What does the "Four Core Genotypes" mouse model tell us about sex differences in the brain and other tissues? *Frontiers in Neuroendocrinology* 30(1):1–9.

Asthana, S., V. Busa, and S. Labani. 2020. Oral contraceptives use and risk of cervical cancer—a systematic review & meta-analysis. *European Journal of Obstetrics, Gynecology, and Reproductive Biology* 247:163–175.

Bachmann, D., A. Buchmann, S. Studer, A. Saake, K. Rauen, E. Gruber, R. M. Nitsch, C. Hock, A. Gietl, and V. Treyer. 2024. Explaining variability in early stages of [18f]-flortaucipir tau-PET binding: Focus on sex differences. *Alzheimer's & Dementia: Diagnosis, Assessment & Disease Monitoring* 16(1):e12565.

Badawy, Y., A. Spector, Z. Li, and R. Desai. 2024. The risk of depression in the menopausal stages: A systematic review and meta-analysis. *Journal of Affective Disorders* 357:126–133.

Bandeira, L., and E. M. Lewiecki. 2022. Anabolic therapy for osteoporosis: Update on efficacy and safety. *Archives of Endocrinology and Metabolism* 66(5):707–716.

Bangalore Krishna, K., and S. F. Witchel. 2024. Normal puberty. *Endocrinology and Metabolism Clinics of North America* 53(2):183–194.

Barańska, A., A. Błaszczuk, W. Kanadys, M. Malm, K. Drop, and M. Polz-Dacewicz. 2021. Oral contraceptive use and breast cancer risk assessment: A systematic review and meta-analysis of case-control studies, 2009–2020. *Cancers* 13(22).

Barron, A. M., and C. J. Pike. 2012. Sex hormones, aging, and Alzheimer's disease. *Frontiers in Bioscience* 4(3):976–997.

Barry, J. A., M. M. Azizia, and P. J. Hardiman. 2014. Risk of endometrial, ovarian and breast cancer in women with polycystic ovary syndrome: A systematic review and meta-analysis. *Human Reproductive Update* 20(5):748–758.

Bedenk, J., E. Vrtačnik-Bokal, and I. Virant-Klun. 2020. The role of anti-Müllerian hormone (AMH) in ovarian disease and infertility. *Journal of Assisted Reproduction and Genetics* 37(1):89–100.

Bello, M. O., L. Rodrigues Silva Sombra, C. Anastasopoulou, and V. V. Garla. 2024. Osteoporosis in males. In *Statpearls*. Treasure Island, FL: StatPearls Publishing.

Bellott, D. W., J. F. Hughes, H. Skaletsky, L. G. Brown, T. Pyntikova, T. J. Cho, N. Koutseva, S. Zaghlul, T. Graves, S. Rock, C. Kremitzki, R. S. Fulton, S. Dugan, Y. Ding, D. Morton, Z. Khan, L. Lewis, C. Buhay, Q. Wang, J. Watt, M. Holder, S. Lee, L. Nazareth, J. Alföldi, S. Rozen, D. M. Muzny, W. C. Warren, R. A. Gibbs, R. K. Wilson, and D. C. Page. 2014. Mammalian Y chromosomes retain widely expressed dosage-sensitive regulators. *Nature* 508(7497):494–499.

BLS (Bureau of Labor Statistics), Department of Labor. 2023. *Labor Force Participation Rate for People Ages 25 to 54 in May 2023 Highest Since January 2007.* https://www.bls.gov/opub/ted/2023/labor-force-participation-rate-for-people-ages-25-to-54-in-may-2023-highest-since-january-2007.htm (accessed October 17, 2024).

Bloch, M., P. J. Schmidt, M. Danaceau, J. Murphy, L. Nieman, and D. R. Rubinow. 2000. Effects of gonadal steroids in women with a history of postpartum depression. *American Journal of Psychiatry* 157(6):924–930.

Bove, R., E. Secor, L. B. Chibnik, L. L. Barnes, J. A. Schneider, D. A. Bennett, and P. L. De Jager. 2014. Age at surgical menopause influences cognitive decline and Alzheimer pathology in older women. *Neurology* 82(3):222–229.

BRAIN Initiative Alliance. n.d. *The Brain Initiative Mission*. https://www.braininitiative.org/mission/ (accessed August 7, 2024).

BWH (Brigham and Women's Hospital). n.d. *Women's Brain Initiative: Tackling the Gap in Knowledge About Sex Differences and Brain Health*. https://www.bwhneurosciences.org/womens-brain-initiative/ (accessed August 7, 2024).

Bromberger, J. T., H. M. Kravitz, Y. F. Chang, J. M. Cyranowski, C. Brown, and K. A. Matthews. 2011. Major depression during and after the menopausal transition: Study of Women's Health Across the Nation (SWAN). *Psychological Medicine* 41(9):1879–1888.

Brown, J. E., C. Handforth, J. E. Compston, W. Cross, N. Parr, P. Selby, S. Wood, L. Drudge-Coates, J. S. Walsh, C. Mitchell, F. J. Collinson, R. E. Coleman, N. James, R. Francis, D. M. Reid, and E. McCloskey. 2020. Guidance for the assessment and management of prostate cancer treatment-induced bone loss. A consensus position statement from an expert group. *Journal of Bone Oncology* 25:100311.

Brown, L., M. S. Hunter, R. Chen, C. J. Crandall, J. L. Gordon, G. D. Mishra, V. Rother, H. Joffe, and M. Hickey. 2024. Promoting good mental health over the menopause transition. *Lancet* 403(10430):969–983.

Bruning, P. F., M. J. Pit, M. de Jong-Bakker, A. van den Ende, A. Hart, and A. van Enk. 1990. Bone mineral density after adjuvant chemotherapy for premenopausal breast cancer. *British Journal of Cancer* 61(2):308–310.

Bulun, S. 2016. Physiology and pathology of the female reproductive axis. In *Williams Textbook of Endocrinology* 13th ed., edited by S. Melmed, K. S. Polonsky, P. R. Larsen, and H. M. Kronenberg. Philadelphia, PA: Elsevier Health Sciences. Pp. 589–663.

Burstein, H. J., C. Lacchetti, H. Anderson, T. A. Buchholz, N. E. Davidson, K. E. Gelmon, S. H. Giordano, C. A. Hudis, A. J. Solky, V. Stearns, E. P. Winer, and J. J. Griggs. 2016. Adjuvant endocrine therapy for women with hormone receptor-positive breast cancer: American Society of Clinical Oncology clinical practice guideline update on ovarian suppression. *Journal of Clinical Oncology* 34(14):1689–1701.

Bytyçi, I., P. E. Penson, D. P. Mikhailidis, N. D. Wong, A. V. Hernandez, A. Sahebkar, P. D. Thompson, M. Mazidi, J. Rysz, D. Pella, Ž. Reiner, P. P. Toth, and M. Banach. 2022. Prevalence of statin intolerance: A meta-analysis. *European Heart Journal* 43(34):3213–3223.

CDC (Centers for Disease Control and Prevention). 2023. *U.S. Teen Girls Experiencing Increased Sadness and Violence*. https://www.cdc.gov/media/releases/2023/p0213-yrbs.html (accessed September 4, 2024).

Chavira, D. A., C. Ponting, and G. Ramos. 2022. The impact of COVID-19 on child and adolescent mental health and treatment considerations. *Behaviour Research and Therapy* 157:104169.

Chella Krishnan, K., M. Mehrabian, and A. J. Lusis. 2018. Sex differences in metabolism and cardiometabolic disorders. *Current Opinions in Lipidology* 29(5):404–410.

Chen, P., B. Li, and L. Ou-Yang. 2022. Role of estrogen receptors in health and disease. *Frontiers in Endocrinology* 13:839005.

Chen, Z., M. Maricic, M. Pettinger, C. Ritenbaugh, A. M. Lopez, D. H. Barad, M. Gass, M. S. LeBoff, and T. L. Bassford. 2005. Osteoporosis and rate of bone loss among postmenopausal survivors of breast cancer. *Cancer* 104(7):1520–1530.

Chlebowski, R. T., T. E. Rohan, J. E. Manson, A. K. Aragaki, A. Kaunitz, M. L. Stefanick, M. S. Simon, K. C. Johnson, J. Wactawski-Wende, M. J. O'Sullivan, L. L. Adams-Campbell, R. Nassir, L. S. Lessin, and R. L. Prentice. 2015. Breast cancer after use of estrogen plus progestin and estrogen alone: Analyses of data from 2 Women's Health Initiative randomized clinical trials. *JAMA Oncology* 1(3):296–305.

Cho, L., A. M. Kaunitz, S. S. Faubion, S. N. Hayes, E. S. Lau, N. Pristera, N. Scott, J. L. Shifren, C. L. Shufelt, C. A. Stuenkel, and K. J. Lindley. 2023. Rethinking menopausal hormone therapy: For whom, what, when, and how long? *Circulation* 147(7):597–610.

Clarke, B. L., and S. Khosla. 2010. Female reproductive system and bone. *Archives of Biochemistry and Biophysics* 503(1):118–128.

Clinical Education at JAX. 2024. *PARP Inhibitors: Overview and Indications*. https://www.jax.org/education-and-learning/clinical-and-continuing-education/clinical-topics/tumor-testing/parpi-detail# (accessed July 10, 2024).

Coker, L. H., M. A. Espeland, P. E. Hogan, S. M. Resnick, R. N. Bryan, J. G. Robinson, J. S. Goveas, C. Davatzikos, L. H. Kuller, J. D. Williamson, C. D. Bushnell, and S. A. Shumaker. 2014. Change in brain and lesion volumes after CEE therapies: The WHIMS-MRI studies. *Neurology* 82(5):427–434.

Constantine, G. D., G. Kessler, S. Graham, and S. R. Goldstein. 2019. Increased incidence of endometrial cancer following the Women's Health Initiative: An assessment of risk factors. *Journal of Women's Health* 28(2):237–243.

Crawford, S. L., C. J. Crandall, C. A. Derby, S. R. El Khoudary, L. E. Waetjen, M. Fischer, and H. Joffe. 2018. Menopausal hormone therapy trends before versus after 2002: Impact of the Women's Health Initiative study results. *Menopause* 26(6):588–597.

de Kat, A. C., Y. T. van der Schouw, M. J. Eijkemans, G. C. Herber-Gast, J. A. Visser, W. M. Verschuren, and F. J. Broekmans. 2016. Back to the basics of ovarian aging: A population-based study on longitudinal anti-Müllerian hormone decline. *BMC Medicine* 14(1):151.

De Vries, G. J., E. F. Rissman, R. B. Simerly, L. Y. Yang, E. M. Scordalakes, C. J. Auger, A. Swain, R. Lovell-Badge, P. S. Burgoyne, and A. P. Arnold. 2002. A model system for study of sex chromosome effects on sexually dimorphic neural and behavioral traits. *Journal of Neuroscience* 22(20):9005–9014.

Diana, A., F. Carlino, E. F. Giunta, E. Franzese, L. P. Guerrera, V. Di Lauro, F. Ciardiello, B. Daniele, and M. Orditura. 2021. Cancer treatment-induced bone loss (CTIBL): State of the art and proper management in breast cancer patients on endocrine therapy. *Current Treatment Options in Oncology* 22(5):45.

Diaz-Thomas, A. M., S. H. Golden, D. M. Dabelea, A. Grimberg, S. N. Magge, J. D. Safer, D. E. Shumer, and F. C. Stanford. 2023. Endocrine health and health care disparities in the pediatric and sexual and gender minority populations: An Endocrine Society scientific statement. *Journal of Clinical Endocrinology and Metabolism* 108(7):1533–1584.

Ding, E. L., Y. Song, V. S. Malik, and S. Liu. 2006. Sex differences of endogenous sex hormones and risk of Type 2 diabetes: A systematic review and meta-analysis. *JAMA* 295(11):1288–1299.

Ding, E. L., Y. Song, J. E. Manson, D. J. Hunter, C. C. Lee, N. Rifai, J. E. Buring, J. M. Gaziano, and S. Liu. 2009. Sex hormone-binding globulin and risk of Type 2 diabetes in women and men. *New England Journal of Medicine* 361(12):1152–1163.

Dou, D. R., Y. Zhao, J. A. Belk, Y. Zhao, K. M. Casey, D. C. Chen, R. Li, B. Yu, S. Srinivasan, B. T. Abe, K. Kraft, C. Hellström, R. Sjöberg, S. Chang, A. Feng, D. W. Goldman, A. A. Shah, M. Petri, L. S. Chung, D. F. Fiorentino, E. K. Lundberg, A. Wutz, P. J. Utz, and H. Y. Chang. 2024. Xist ribonucleoproteins promote female sex-biased autoimmunity. *Cell* 187(3):733–749.e716.

Drew, Y. 2015. The development of PARP inhibitors in ovarian cancer: From bench to bedside. *British Journal of Cancer* 113 (Suppl 1):S3–S9.

Drugs.com. 2023. *Olaparib.* https://www.drugs.com/olaparib.html (accessed August 5, 2024).

Dubey, N., J. F. Hoffman, K. Schuebel, Q. Yuan, P. E. Martinez, L. K. Nieman, D. R. Rubinow, P. J. Schmidt, and D. Goldman. 2017. The ESC/E(Z) complex, an effector of response to ovarian steroids, manifests an intrinsic difference in cells from women with premenstrual dysphoric disorder. *Molecular Psychiatry* 22(8):1172–1184.

Eisenlohr-Moul, T. 2024. *The Menstrual Cycle and Mental Health: Progress, Gaps, and Barriers. Presentation to the NASEM Committee on the Assessment of NIH Research on Women's Health, Meeting 3 (March 7, 2024).* https://www.nationalacademies.org/documents/embed/link/LF2255DA3DD1C41C0A42D3BEF0989ACAECE3053A6A9B/file/D200E053FE7DB EC81160D764F44F8C5682FD9C162A7A?noSaveAs=1 (accessed August 7, 2024).

El Khoudary, S. R., G. Greendale, S. L. Crawford, N. E. Avis, M. M. Brooks, R. C. Thurston, C. Karvonen-Gutierrez, L. E. Waetjen, and K. Matthews. 2019. The menopause transition and women's health at midlife: A progress report from the Study of Women's Health Across the Nation (SWAN). *Menopause* 26(10):1213–1227.

Elzer, J. G., S. Muhammad, T. M. Wintermantel, A. Regnier-Vigouroux, J. Ludwig, G. Schütz, and M. Schwaninger. 2010. Neuronal estrogen receptor-alpha mediates neuroprotection by 17beta-estradiol. *Journal of Cerebral Blood Flow and Metabolism* 30(5):935–942.

Endo, A. 2010. A historical perspective on the discovery of statins. *Proceedings of the Japan Academy, Series B* 86(5):484–493.

Epperson, C. N., M. Steiner, S. A. Hartlage, E. Eriksson, P. J. Schmidt, I. Jones, and K. A. Yonkers. 2012. Premenstrual dysphoric disorder: Evidence for a new category for DSM-5. *American Journal of Psychiatry* 169(5):465–475.

Espeland, M. A., S. A. Shumaker, I. Leng, J. E. Manson, C. M. Brown, E. S. LeBlanc, L. Vaughan, J. Robinson, S. R. Rapp, J. S. Goveas, D. Lane, J. Wactawski-Wende, M. L. Stefanick, W. Li, S. M. Resnick, and W. S. Group. 2013. Long-term effects on cognitive function of postmenopausal hormone therapy prescribed to women aged 50 to 55 years. *JAMA Internal Medicine* 173(15):1429–1436.

Etgen, A. M., H. P. Chu, J. M. Fiber, G. B. Karkanias, and J. M. Morales. 1999. Hormonal integration of neurochemical and sensory signals governing female reproductive behavior. *Behavioural Brain Research* 105(1):93–103.

Faubion, S. S., C. Crandall, L. C. Davis, S. R. E. Khoudaqry, H. N. Hodis, R. A. Lobo, P. M. Maki, J. E. Manson, Pinkerton. J. V., N. Santoro, J. L. Shifren, C. Shufelt, R. C. Thurston, and W. Wolfman. 2022. The 2022 hormone therapy position statement of the North American Menopause Society. *Menopause* 29(7):767–794.

FDA (Food and Drug Administration). 2017. *FDA Approves Olaparib Tablets for Maintenance Treatment in Ovarian Cancer.* https://www.fda.gov/drugs/resources-information-approved-drugs/fda-approves-olaparib-tablets-maintenance-treatment-ovarian-cancer (accessed September 17, 2024).

FDA. 2018. *FDA Approved Olaparib (Lynparza, Astrazeneca Pharmaceuticals LP) for the Maintenance Treatment of Adult Patients with Deleterious or Suspected Deleterious Germline or Somatic BRCA-Mutated (GBRCAM or SBRCAM) Advanced Epithelial Ovarian, Fallopian Tube or Primary Peritoneal Cancer Who Are in Complete or Partial Response to First-Line Platinum-Based.* https://www.fda.gov/drugs/fda-approved-olaparib-lynparza-astrazeneca-pharmaceuticals-lp-maintenance-treatment-adult-patients (accessed September 3, 2024).

FDA. 2019. *FDA Approves First Treatment for Post-Partum Depression.* https://www.fda.gov/news-events/press-announcements/fda-approves-first-treatment-post-partum-depression (accessed October 17, 2024).

FDA. 2020a. *FDA Approves Niraparib for First-Line Maintenance of Advanced Ovarian Cancer.* https://www.fda.gov/drugs/resources-information-approved-drugs/fda-approves-niraparib-first-line-maintenance-advanced-ovarian-cancer (accessed September 3, 2024).

FDA. 2020b. *FDA Approves Olaparib Plus Bevacizumab as Maintenance Treatment for Ovarian, Fallopian Tube, or Primary Peritoneal Cancers.* https://www.fda.gov/drugs/resources-information-approved-drugs/fda-approves-olaparib-plus-bevacizumab-maintenance-treatment-ovarian-fallopian-tube-or-primary (accessed September 3, 2024).

FDA. 2023. *FDA Approves First Oral Treatment for Postpartum Depression.* https://www.fda.gov/news-events/press-announcements/fda-approves-first-oral-treatment-postpartum-depression (accessed October 17, 2024).

Finkelstein, J. S., S. E. Brockwell, V. Mehta, G. A. Greendale, M. R. Sowers, B. Ettinger, J. C. Lo, J. M. Johnston, J. A. Cauley, M. E. Danielson, and R. M. Neer. 2008. Bone mineral density changes during the menopause transition in a multiethnic cohort of women. *Journal of Clinical Endocrinology and Metabolism* 93(3):861–868.

Fleisher, A., M. Grundman, C. R. Jack, Jr., R. C. Petersen, C. Taylor, H. T. Kim, D. H. Schiller, V. Bagwell, D. Sencakova, M. F. Weiner, C. DeCarli, S. T. DeKosky, C. H. van Dyck, and L. J. Thal. 2005. Sex, apolipoprotein E Epsilon 4 status, and hippocampal volume in mild cognitive impairment. *Archives of Neurology* 62(6):953–957.

Frisch, R. E., J. A. Canick, and D. Tulchinsky. 1980. Human fatty marrow aromatizes androgen to estrogen. *Journal of Clinical Endocrinology and Metabolism* 51(2):394–396.

Fu, T., C. Wang, J. Yan, Q. Zeng, and C. Ma. 2023. Relationship between antenatal sleep quality and depression in perinatal women: A comprehensive meta-analysis of observational studies. *Journal of Affective Disorders* 327:38–45.

Galea, L. A. M., E. Choleris, A. Y. K. Albert, M. M. McCarthy, and F. Sohrabji. 2020. The promises and pitfalls of sex difference research. *Frontiers in Neuroendocrinology* 56:100817.

Gandy, S., and S. Petanceska. 2000. Regulation of Alzheimer β-amyloid precursor trafficking and metabolism. *Biochimica et Biophysica Acta—Molecular Basis of Disease* 1502(1):44–52.

Gervais, N. J., A. Au, A. Almey, A. Duchesne, L. Gravelsins, A. Brown, R. Reuben, E. Baker-Sullivan, D. H. Schwartz, K. Evans, M. Q. Bernardini, A. Eisen, W. S. Meschino, W. D. Foulkes, E. Hampson, and G. Einstein. 2020. Cognitive markers of dementia risk in middle-aged women with bilateral salpingo-oophorectomy prior to menopause. *Neurobiology of Aging* 94:1–6.

Gimble, J. M., C. E. Robinson, X. Wu, and K. A. Kelly. 1996. The function of adipocytes in the bone marrow stroma: An update. *Bone* 19(5):421–428.

Gleason, C. E., N. M. Dowling, W. Wharton, J. E. Manson, V. M. Miller, C. S. Atwood, E. A. Brinton, M. I. Cedars, R. A. Lobo, G. R. Merriam, G. Neal-Perry, N. F. Santoro, H. S. Taylor, D. M. Black, M. J. Budoff, H. N. Hodis, F. Naftolin, S. M. Harman, and S. Asthana. 2015. Effects of hormone therapy on cognition and mood in recently postmenopausal women: Findings from the randomized, controlled KEEPS-cognitive and affective study. *PLoS Medicine* 12(6):e1001833; discussion e1001833.

Goodarzi, M. O., X. Li, R. M. Krauss, J. I. Rotter, and Y. D. Chen. 2013. Relationship of sex to diabetes risk in statin trials. *Diabetes Care* 36(7):e100–101.

Gorlov, I. P., and C. I. Amos. 2023. Why does the X chromosome lag behind autosomes in GWAS findings? *PLOS Genetics* 19(2):e1010472.

Grigoryan, S., and G. A. Clines. 2024. Hormonal control of bone architecture throughout the lifespan: Implications for fracture prediction and prevention. *Endocrine Practice* 30(7):687–694.

Guintivano, J., P. F. Sullivan, A. M. Stuebe, T. Penders, J. Thorp, D. R. Rubinow, and S. Meltzer-Brody. 2018. Adverse life events, psychiatric history, and biological predictors of postpartum depression in an ethnically diverse sample of postpartum women. *Psychological Medicine* 48(7):1190–1200.

Harlow, S. D., M. Gass, J. E. Hall, R. Lobo, P. Maki, R. W. Rebar, S. Sherman, P. M. Sluss, and T. J. de Villiers. 2012. Executive summary of the Stages of Reproductive Aging workshop + 10: Addressing the unfinished agenda of staging reproductive aging. *Menopause* 19(4):387–395.

Hays, J., J. K. Ockene, R. L. Brunner, J. M. Kotchen, J. E. Manson, R. E. Patterson, A. K. Aragaki, S. A. Shumaker, R. G. Brzyski, A. Z. LaCroix, I. A. Granek, and B. G. Valanis. 2003. Effects of estrogen plus progestin on health-related quality of life. *New England Journal of Medicine* 348(19):1839–1854.

Henderson, V. W., J. A. St John, H. N. Hodis, C. A. McCleary, F. Z. Stanczyk, D. Shoupe, N. Kono, L. Dustin, H. Allayee, and W. J. Mack. 2016. Cognitive effects of estradiol after menopause: A randomized trial of the timing hypothesis. *Neurology* 87(7):699–708.

Hetemäki, N., T. S. Mikkola, M. J. Tikkanen, F. Wang, E. Hämäläinen, U. Turpeinen, M. Haanpää, V. Vihma, and H. Savolainen-Peltonen. 2021. Adipose tissue estrogen production and metabolism in premenopausal women. *Journal of Steroid Biochemistry and Molecular Biology* 209:105849.

Hibler, E. A., J. Kauderer, M. H. Greene, G. C. Rodriguez, and D. S. Alberts. 2016. Bone loss after oophorectomy among high-risk women: An NRG Oncology/Gynecologic Oncology Group study. *Menopause* 23(11):1228–1232.

Hillhouse, T. M., and J. H. Porter. 2015. A brief history of the development of antidepressant drugs: From monoamines to glutamate. *Experimental and Clinical Psychopharmacology* 23(1):1–21.

Hoadley, K. A., C. Yau, T. Hinoue, D. M. Wolf, A. J. Lazar, E. Drill, R. Shen, A. M. Taylor, A. D. Cherniack, V. Thorsson, R. Akbani, R. Bowlby, C. K. Wong, M. Wiznerowicz, F. Sanchez-Vega, A. G. Robertson, B. G. Schneider, M. S. Lawrence, H. Noushmehr, T. M. Malta, J. M. Stuart, C. C. Benz, and P. W. Laird. 2018. Cell-of-origin patterns dominate the molecular classification of 10,000 tumors from 33 types of cancer. *Cell* 173(2):291–304.e296.

Holven, K. B., and J. Roeters van Lennep. 2023. Sex differences in lipids: A life course approach. *Atherosclerosis* 384:117270.

Hu, J., J. H. Lin, M. C. Jiménez, J. E. Manson, S. E. Hankinson, and K. M. Rexrode. 2020. Plasma estradiol and testosterone levels and ischemic stroke in postmenopausal women. *Stroke* 51(4):1297–1300.

IOF (International Osteoporosis Foundation). n.d. *Prevention*. https://www.osteoporosis.foundation/patients/prevention (accessed October 21, 2024).

Islam, N., R. Nash, Q. Zhang, L. Panagiotakopoulos, T. Daley, S. Bhasin, D. Getahun, J. Sonya Haw, C. McCracken, M. J. Silverberg, V. Tangpricha, S. Vupputuri, and M. Goodman. 2022. Is there a link between hormone use and diabetes incidence in transgender people? Data from the STRONG cohort. *Journal of Clinical Endocrinology and Metabolism* 107(4):e1549-e1557.

Jacobs, E. G. 2023. Bridging the neuroscience gender divide. *Nature* 623(667).

Jett, S., E. Schelbaum, G. Jang, C. Boneu Yepez, J. P. Dyke, S. Pahlajani, R. Diaz Brinton, and L. Mosconi. 2022. Ovarian steroid hormones: A long overlooked but critical contributor to brain aging and Alzheimer's disease. *Frontiers in Aging Neuroscience* 14.

Ji, H., M. Gulati, T. Y. Huang, A. C. Kwan, D. Ouyang, J. E. Ebinger, K. Casaletto, K. L. Moreau, H. Skali, and S. Cheng. 2024. Sex differences in association of physical activity with all-cause and cardiovascular mortality. *Journal of the American College of Cardiology* 83(8):783–793.

Ji, M. X., and Q. Yu. 2015. Primary osteoporosis in postmenopausal women. *Chronic Diseases and Translational Medicine* 1(1):9–13.

Jiang, J., J. Cui, A. Wang, Y. Mu, Y. Yan, F. Liu, Y. Pan, D. Li, W. Li, G. Liu, H. Y. Gaisano, J. Dou, and Y. He. 2019. Association between age at natural menopause and risk of Type 2 diabetes in postmenopausal women with and without obesity. *Journal of Clinical Endocrinology & Metabolism* 104(7):3039–3048.

Jiwrajka, N., and M. C. Anguera. 2022. The X in sex-biased immunity and autoimmune rheumatic disease. *Journal of Experimental Medicine* 219(6).

Joffe, H., A. Massler, and K. M. Sharkey. 2010. Evaluation and management of sleep disturbance during the menopause transition. *Seminars in Reproductive Medicine* 28(5):404–421.

Johnson, E. D., K. Butler, and S. Gupta. 2021. Bone health in patients with prostate cancer: An evidence-based algorithm. *Federal Practitioner* 38(Suppl 3):S20–S26.

Kalyani, R. R., M. Franco, A. S. Dobs, P. Ouyang, D. Vaidya, A. Bertoni, S. M. Gapstur, and S. H. Golden. 2009. The association of endogenous sex hormones, adiposity, and insulin resistance with incident diabetes in postmenopausal women. *Journal of Clinical Endocrinology and Metabolism* 94(11):4127–4135.

Karlamangla, A. S., A. Shieh, and G. A. Greendale. 2021. Hormones and bone loss across the menopause transition. *Vitamins and Hormones* 115:401–417.

Kim, J. Y., K. Min, H. Y. Paik, and S. K. Lee. 2021. Sex omission and male bias are still widespread in cell experiments. *American Journal of Physiology—Cell Physiology* 320(5):C742–C749.

Kling, J. M., B. L. Clarke, and N. P. Sandhu. 2014. Osteoporosis prevention, screening, and treatment: A review. *Journal of Women's Health* 23(7):563–572.

Kundakovic, M., and D. Rocks. 2022. Sex hormone fluctuation and increased female risk for depression and anxiety disorders: From clinical evidence to molecular mechanisms. *Frontiers in Neuroendocrinology* 66:101010.

Lee, B., Y. Wang, S. A. Carlson, K. J. Greenlund, H. Lu, Y. Liu, J. B. Croft, P. I. Eke, M. Town, and C. W. Thomas. 2023. National, state-level, and county-level prevalence estimates of adults aged ≥18 years self-reporting a lifetime diagnosis of depression—United States, 2020. *MMWR* 72(24):644–650.

Leeners, B., T. H. C. Kruger, K. Geraedts, E. Tronci, T. Mancini, F. Ille, M. Egli, S. Röblitz, L. Saleh, S. K., C. Schippert, Y. Zhang, and M. P. Hengartner. 2017. Lack of associations between female hormone levels and visuospatial working memory, divided attention and cognitive bias across two consecutive menstrual cycles. *Frontiers in Behavioral Neuroscience* 11(120).

Li, J., L. Zheng, K. H. K. Chan, X. Zou, J. Zhang, J. Liu, Q. Zhong, T. E. Madsen, W. C. Wu, J. E. Manson, X. Yu, and S. Liu. 2023. Sex hormone-binding globulin and risk of coronary heart disease in men and women. *Clinical Chemistry* 69(4):374–385.

Li, R., Y. Shen, L.-B. Yang, L.-F. Lue, C. Finch, and J. Rogers. 2000. Estrogen enhances uptake of amyloid β-protein by microglia derived from the human cortex. *Journal of Neurochemistry* 75(4):1447–1454.

Lin, P. C., C. H. Ko, Y. J. Lin, and J. Y. Yen. 2021. Insomnia, inattention and fatigue symptoms of women with premenstrual dysphoric disorder. *International Journal of Environmental Research and Public Health* 18(12).

Link, J. C., X. Chen, A. P. Arnold, and K. Reue. 2013. Metabolic impact of sex chromosomes. *Adipocyte* 2(2):74–79.

Long, J., P. He, Y. Shen, and R. Li. 2012. New evidence of mitochondria dysfunction in the female Alzheimer's disease brain: Deficiency of estrogen receptor-β. *Journal of Alzheimer's Disease* 30(3):545–558.

Lu, J., Y. Shin, M. S. Yen, and S. S. Sun. 2016. Peak bone mass and patterns of change in total bone mineral density and bone mineral contents from childhood into young adulthood. *Journal of Clinical Densitometry* 19(2):180–191.

Lu, Z., J. K. Guo, Y. Wei, D. R. Dou, B. Zarnegar, Q. Ma, R. Li, Y. Zhao, F. Liu, H. Choudhry, P. A. Khavari, and H. Y. Chang. 2020. Structural modularity of the Xist ribonucleoprotein complex. *Nature Communications* 11(1):6163.

Ludwig, B., B. Roy, and Y. Dwivedi. 2019. Role of HPA and the HPG axis interaction in testosterone-mediated learned helpless behavior. *Molecular Neurobiology* 56(1):394–405.

Madigan, S., N. Racine, T. Vaillancourt, D. J. Korczak, J. M. A. Hewitt, P. Pador, J. L. Park, B. A. McArthur, C. Holy, and R. D. Neville. 2023. Changes in depression and anxiety among children and adolescents from before to during the COVID-19 pandemic: A systematic review and meta-analysis. *JAMA Pediatrics* 177(6):567–581.

Madsen, T. E., X. Luo, M. Huang, K. E. Park, M. L. Stefanick, J. E. Manson, and S. Liu. 2020. Circulating SHBG (sex hormone-binding globulin) and risk of ischemic stroke: Findings from the WHI. *Stroke* 51(4):1257–1264.

Madsen, T. E., T. Sobel, S. Negash, T. Shrout Allen, M. L. Stefanick, J. E. Manson, and A. M.A. 2023. A review of hormone and non-hormonal therapy options for the treatment of menopause. *International Journal of Women's Health* 15:825–836.

Maguire, J., and I. Mody. 2008. GABA(A)R plasticity during pregnancy: Relevance to postpartum depression. *Neuron* 59(2):207–213.

Majewska, M. D., N. L. Harrison, R. D. Schwartz, J. L. Barker, and S. M. Paul. 1986. Steroid hormone metabolites are barbiturate-like modulators of the gaba receptor. *Science* 232(4753):1004–1007.

Maki, P. M., S. G. Kornstein, H. Joffe, J. T. Bromberger, E. W. Freeman, G. Athappilly, W. V. Bobo, L. H. Rubin, H. K. Koleva, L. S. Cohen, and C. N. Soares. 2019. Guidelines for the evaluation and treatment of perimenopausal depression: Summary and recommendations. *Journal of Women's Health* 28(2):117–134.

Manson, J. E., R. T. Chlebowski, M. L. Stefanick, A. K. Aragaki, J. E. Rossouw, R. L. Prentice, G. Anderson, B. V. Howard, C. A. Thomson, A. Z. LaCroix, J. Wactawski-Wende, R. D. Jackson, M. Limacher, K. L. Margolis, S. Wassertheil-Smoller, S. A. Beresford, J. A. Cauley, C. B. Eaton, M. Gass, J. Hsia, K. C. Johnson, C. Kooperberg, L. H. Kuller, C. E. Lewis, S. Liu, L. W. Martin, J. K. Ockene, M. J. O'Sullivan, L. H. Powell, M. S. Simon, L. Van Horn, M. Z. Vitolins, and R. B. Wallace. 2013. Menopausal hormone therapy and health outcomes during the intervention and extended poststopping phases of the Women's Health Initiative randomized trials. *JAMA* 310(13):1353–1368.

Manson, J. E., and A. M. Kaunitz. 2016. Menopause management—getting clinical care back on track. *New England Journal of Medicine* 374(9):803–806.

Manson, J. E., C. J. Crandall, J. E. Rossouw, R. T. Chlebowski, G. L. Anderson, M. L. Stefanick, A. K. Aragaki, J. A. Cauley, G. L. Wells, A. Z. LaCroix, C. A. Thomson, M. L. Neuhouser, L. Van Horn, C. Kooperberg, B. V. Howard, L. F. Tinker, J. Wactawski-Wende, S. A. Shumaker, and R. L. Prentice. 2024. The Women's Health Initiative randomized trials and clinical practice: A review. *JAMA* 331(20):1748–1760.

Marrocco, J., N. R. Einhorn, G. H. Petty, H. Li, N. Dubey, J. Hoffman, K. F. Berman, D. Goldman, F. S. Lee, P. J. Schmidt, and B. S. McEwen. 2020. Epigenetic intersection of BDNF Val66Met genotype with premenstrual dysphoric disorder transcriptome in a cross-species model of estradiol add-back. *Molecular Psychiatry* 25(3):572–583.

Mattick, L. J., J. W. Bea, L. Singh, K. M. Hovey, H. R. Banack, J. Wactawski-Wende, J. E. Manson, J. L. Funk, and H. M. Ochs-Balcom. 2022. Serum follicle-stimulating hormone and 5-year change in adiposity in healthy postmenopausal women. *Journal of Clinical Endocrinology and Metabolism* 107(8):e3455–e3462.

Matyori, A., C. P. Brown, A. Ali, and F. Sherbeny. 2023. Statins utilization trends and expenditures in the U.S. before and after the implementation of the 2013 ACC/AHA guidelines. *Saudi Pharmaceutical Journal* 31(6):795–800.

McCarthy, M. M., and J. G. Pfaus. 1996. Steroid modulation of neurotransmitter function to alter female reproductive behavior. *Trends in Endocrinology and Metabolism* 7(9):327–333.

McPhee, C., I. O. Aninye, and L. Horan. 2022. Recommendations for improving women's bone health throughout the lifespan. *Journal of Women's Health* 31(12):1671–1676.

Meers, J. M., and S. Nowakowski. 2020. Sleep, premenstrual mood disorder, and women's health. *Current Opinion in Psychology* 34:43–49.

Melón, L. C., A. Hooper, X. Yang, S. J. Moss, and J. Maguire. 2018. Inability to suppress the stress-induced activation of the HPA axis during the peripartum period engenders deficits in postpartum behaviors in mice. *Psychoneuroendocrinology* 90:182–193.

Meltzer-Brody, S., and S. J. Kanes. 2020. Allopregnanolone in postpartum depression: Role in pathophysiology and treatment. *Neurobiology of Stress* 12:100212.

Menezes, M. C. S., F. Raheem, L. Mina, B. Ernst, and F. Batalini. 2022. PARP inhibitors for breast cancer: Germline BRCA1/2 and beyond. *Cancers* 14(17).

Merone, L., K. Tsey, D. Russell, and C. Nagle. 2022. Sex inequalities in medical research: A systematic scoping review of the literature. *Women's Health Reports* (3(1):49–59.

Michmerhuizen, A. R., D. E. Spratt, L. J. Pierce, and C. W. Speers. 2020. Are we there yet? Understanding androgen receptor signaling in breast cancer. *NPJ Breast Cancer* 6:47.

Miga, K. H., S. Koren, A. Rhie, M. R. Vollger, A. Gershman, A. Bzikadze, S. Brooks, E. Howe, D. Porubsky, G. A. Logsdon, V. A. Schneider, T. Potapova, J. Wood, W. Chow, J. Armstrong, J. Fredrickson, E. Pak, K. Tigyi, M. Kremitzki, C. Markovic, V. Maduro, A. Dutra, G. G. Bouffard, A. M. Chang, N. F. Hansen, A. B. Wilfert, F. Thibaud-Nissen, A. D. Schmitt, J. M. Belton, S. Selvaraj, M. Y. Dennis, D. C. Soto, R. Sahasrabudhe, G. Kaya, J. Quick, N. J. Loman, N. Holmes, M. Loose, U. Surti, R. A. Risques, T. A. Graves Lindsay, R. Fulton, I. Hall, B. Paten, K. Howe, W. Timp, A. Young, J. C. Mullikin, P. A. Pevzner, J. L. Gerton, B. A. Sullivan, E. E. Eichler, and A. M. Phillippy. 2020. Telomere-to-telomere assembly of a complete human X chromosome. *Nature* 585(7823):79–84.

Mittelstrass, K., J. S. Ried, Z. Yu, J. Krumsiek, C. Gieger, C. Prehn, W. Roemisch-Margl, A. Polonikov, A. Peters, F. J. Theis, T. Meitinger, F. Kronenberg, S. Weidinger, H. E. Wichmann, K. Suhre, R. Wang-Sattler, J. Adamski, and T. Illig. 2011. Discovery of sexual dimorphisms in metabolic and genetic biomarkers. *PLOS Genetics* 7(8):e1002215.

Moore, K., N. Colombo, G. Scambia, B.-G. Kim, A. Oaknin, M. Friedlander, A. Lisyanskaya, A. Floquet, A. Leary, G. S. Sonke, C. Gourley, S. Banerjee, A. Oza, A. González-Martín, C. Aghajanian, W. Bradley, C. Mathews, J. Liu, E. S. Lowe, R. Bloomfield, and P. DiSilvestro. 2018. Maintenance olaparib in patients with newly diagnosed advanced ovarian cancer. *New England Journal of Medicine* 379(26):2495–2505.

Moreau, K. L., and K. L. Hildreth. 2014. Vascular aging across the menopause transition in healthy women. *Advances in Vascular Medicine* 2014.

Morrow, A. L., L. L. Devaud, R. H. Purdy, and S. M. Paul. 1995. Neuroactive steroid modulators of the stress response. *Annals of the New York Academy of Sciences* 771(1):257–272.

Mosconi, L., A. Rahman, I. Diaz, X. Wu, O. Scheyer, H. W. Hristov, S. Vallabhajosula, R. S. Isaacson, M. J. de Leon, and R. D. Brinton. 2018. Increased Alzheimer's risk during the menopause transition: A 3-year longitudinal brain imaging study. *PLoS One* 13(12):e0207885.

Muñoz-Mayorga, D., C. Guerra-Araiza, L. Torner, and T. Morales. 2018. Tau phosphorylation in female neurodegeneration: Role of estrogens, progesterone, and prolactin. *Frontiers in Endocrinology* 9:133.

Murphy, N., L. Xu, A. Zervoudakis, X. Xue, G. Kabat, T. E. Rohan, T. E. Wassertheil-Smoller, M. J. O'Sullivan, C. Thomson, C. Messina, H. D. Strickler, and M. J. Gunter. 2017. Reproductive and menstrual factors and colorectal cancer incidence in the Women's Health Initiative observational study. *British Journal of Cancer* 116(1):117–125.

NASEM (National Academies of Sciences, Engineering, and Medicine). 2022. *Enhancing NIH research on autoimmune disease.* Washington, DC: The National Academies Press.

NASEM. 2024. *Advancing research on chronic conditions in women.* Washington, DC: The National Academies Press.

NCCN (National Comprehensive Cancer Network). 2023. *NCCN guidelines for patients: Uterine neoplasms.* Plymouth Meeting, PA: National Comprehensive Cancer Network.

NCCN. 2024. *NCCN guidelines for patients: Ovarian cancer.* Plymouth Meeting, PA: National Comprehensive Cancer Network.

NCI (National Cancer Institute). 2018. *Oral Contraceptives and Cancer Risk.* https://www.cancer.gov/about-cancer/causes-prevention/risk/hormones/oral-contraceptives-fact-sheet#:~:text=The%20risk%20of%20breast%20cancer%20also%20increased%20the%20longer%20oral,have%20never%20used%20oral%20contraceptives. (accessed August 7, 2024).

Ngo, S. T., F. J. Steyn, and P. A. McCombe. 2014. Gender differences in autoimmune disease. *Frontiers in Neuroendocrinology* 35(3):347–369.

Nguyen, K. A., L. Li, D. Lu, A. Yazdanparast, L. Wang, R. P. Kreutz, E. C. Whipple, and T. K. Schleyer. 2018. A comprehensive review and meta-analysis of risk factors for statin-induced myopathy. *European Journal of Clinical Pharmacology* 74(9):1099–1109.

NIEHS (National Institute of Environmental Health Sciences). 2024. *Autoimmune Diseases.* https://www.niehs.nih.gov/health/topics/conditions/autoimmune (accessed August 5, 2024).

NIH (National Institutes of Health). n.d. *Research Overview.* https://braininitiative.nih.gov/research/research-overview (accessed August 7, 2024).

NIH. 2024. *Understanding Sex Differences in Autoimmune Disease.* https://www.nih.gov/news-events/nih-research-matters/understanding-sex-differences-autoimmune-disease (accessed August 6, 2024).

Nilas, L., and C. Christiansen. 1988. Rates of bone loss in normal women: Evidence of accelerated trabecular bone loss after the menopause. *European Journal of Clinical Investigation* 18(5):529–534.

OASH (Office of the Assistant Secretary for Health). 2023. *Menopause Symptoms and Relief.* https://www.womenshealth.gov/menopause/menopause-symptoms-and-relief (accessed September 13, 2024).

Office of the Surgeon General. 2004. *Bone health and osteoporosis: A report of the surgeon general.* Rockville, MD: Office of the Surgeon General, Department of Health and Human Services.

Okeke, T., U. Anyaehie, and C. Ezenyeaku. 2013. Premature menopause. *Annals of Medicine and Health Sciences Research* 3(1):90–95.

Opoku, A. A., M. Abushama, and J. C. Konje. 2023. Obesity and menopause. *Best Practice & Research Clinical Obstetrics & Gynaecology* 88:102348.

Osterlund, M. K., J. A. Gustafsson, E. Keller, and Y. L. Hurd. 2000. Estrogen receptor beta (ERbeta) messenger ribonucleic acid (mRNA) expression within the human forebrain: Distinct distribution pattern to ERalpha mRNA. *Journal of Clinical Endocrinology and Metabolism* 85(10):3840–3846.

Ott, S. M. 2018. Cortical or trabecular bone: What's the difference? *American Journal of Nephrology* 47(6):373–375.

Patterson, R., I. Balan, A. L. Morrow, and S. Meltzer-Brody. 2024. Novel neurosteroid therapeutics for post-partum depression: Perspectives on clinical trials, program development, active research, and future directions. *Neuropsychopharmacology* 49(1):67–72.

Paul, S. M., G. Pinna, and A. Guidotti. 2020. Allopregnanolone: From molecular pathophysiology to therapeutics. A historical perspective. *Neurobiology of Stress* 12:100215.

Payne, J. L., and J. Maguire. 2019. Pathophysiological mechanisms implicated in postpartum depression. *Frontiers in Neuroendocrinology* 52:165–180.

Peacock, K., K. Carlson, and K. M. Ketvertis. 2023. Menopause. In *Statpearls.* Treasure Island, FL: StatPearls Publishing.

Perger, E., R. Silvestri, E. Bonanni, M. C. Di Perri, M. Fernandes, F. Provini, G. Zoccoli, and C. Lombardi. 2024. Gender medicine and sleep disorders: From basic science to clinical research. *Frontiers in Neurology* 15:1392489.

Petersen, N., A. J. Rapkin, K. Okita, K. R. Kinney, T. Mizuno, M. A. Mandelkern, and E. D. London. 2021. Striatal dopamine D2-type receptor availability and peripheral 17β-estradiol. *Molecular Psychiatry* 26(6):2038–2047.

Pineda-Moncusí, M., N. Garcia-Giralt, A. Diez-Perez, S. Servitja, I. Tusquets, D. Prieto-Alhambra, and X. Nogués. 2020. Increased fracture risk in women treated with aromatase inhibitors versus tamoxifen: Beneficial effect of bisphosphonates. *Journal of Bone and Mineral Research* 35(2):291–297.

Pinna, G. 2020. Allopregnanolone, the neuromodulator turned therapeutic agent: Thank you, next? *Frontiers in Endocrinology* 11:236.

Poeira, A. F., and M. O. Zangão. 2022. Construct of the association between sleep quality and perinatal depression: A literature review. *Healthcare* 10(7).

Pyfrom, S., B. Paneru, J. J. Knox, M. P. Cancro, S. Posso, J. H. Buckner, and M. C. Anguera. 2021. The dynamic epigenetic regulation of the inactive X chromosome in healthy human B cells is dysregulated in lupus patients. *Proceedings of the National Academy of Sciences* 118(24).

Ramin, C., B. J. May, R. B. S. Roden, M. M. Orellana, B. C. Hogan, M. S. McCullough, D. Petry, D. K. Armstrong, and K. Visvanathan. 2018. Evaluation of osteopenia and osteoporosis in younger breast cancer survivors compared with cancer-free women: A prospective cohort study. *Breast Cancer Research* 20(1):134.

Ranhotra, H. S. 2022. Estrogen-related receptor alpha in select host functions and cancer: New frontiers. *Molecular and Cellular Biochemistry* 477(5):1349–1359.

Reddy, D. S., R. H. Mbilinyi, and E. Estes. 2023. Preclinical and clinical pharmacology of brexanolone (allopregnanolone) for postpartum depression: A landmark journey from concept to clinic in neurosteroid replacement therapy. *Psychopharmacology* 240(9):1841–1863.

Reue, K. 2024. *Mechanisms Underlying Sex Differences in Cardiometabolic Disease. Presentation to the NASEM Committee on the Assessment of NIH Research on Women's Health, Meeting 3.* https://www.nationalacademies.org/documents/embed/link/LF2255DA3D-D1C41C0A42D3BEF0989ACAECE3053A6A9B/file/D6CD67C8F77A41DD29AD85A BA5F56A4A95B87EC8C535?noSaveAs=1 (accessed July 30, 2024).

Rexrode, K. M., J. E. Manson, I. M. Lee, P. M. Ridker, P. M. Sluss, N. R. Cook, and J. E. Buring. 2003. Sex hormone levels and risk of cardiovascular events in postmenopausal women. *Circulation* 108(14):1688–1693.

Rey, R., N. Josso, and C. Racine. 2020. Sexual differentiation. In *Endotext*, edited by K. R. Feingold, B. Anawalt, M. R. Blackman, A. Boyce, G. Chrousos, E. Corpas, W. W. de Herder, K. Dhatariya, K. Dungan, J. Hofland, S. Kalra, G. Kaltsas, N. Kapoor, C. Koch, P. Kopp, M. Korbonits, C. S. Kovacs, W. Kuohung, B. Laferrère, M. Levy, E. A. McGee, R. McLachlan, M. New, J. Purnell, R. Sahay, A. S. Shah, F. Singer, M. A. Sperling, C. A. Stratakis, D. L. Trence, and D. P. Wilson. South Dartmouth, MA: MDText.com, Inc.

Rhie, A., S. Nurk, M. Cechova, S. J. Hoyt, D. J. Taylor, N. Altemose, P. W. Hook, S. Koren, M. Rautiainen, I. A. Alexandrov, J. Allen, M. Asri, A. V. Bzikadze, N.-C. Chen, C.-S. Chin, M. Diekhans, P. Flicek, G. Formenti, A. Fungtammasan, C. Garcia Giron, E. Garrison, A. Gershman, J. L. Gerton, P. G. S. Grady, A. Guarracino, L. Haggerty, R. Halabian, N. F. Hansen, R. Harris, G. A. Hartley, W. T. Harvey, M. Haukness, J. Heinz, T. Hourlier, R. M. Hubley, S. E. Hunt, S. Hwang, M. Jain, R. K. Kesharwani, A. P. Lewis, H. Li, G. A. Logsdon, J. K. Lucas, W. Makalowski, C. Markovic, F. J. Martin, A. M. Mc Cartney, R. C. McCoy, J. McDaniel, B. M. McNulty, P. Medvedev, A. Mikheenko, K. M. Munson, T. D. Murphy, H. E. Olsen, N. D. Olson, L. F. Paulin, D. Porubsky, T. Potapova, F. Ryabov, S. L. Salzberg, M. E. G. Sauria, F. J. Sedlazeck, K. Shafin, V. A. Shepelev, A. Shumate, J. M. Storer, L. Surapaneni, A. M. Taravella Oill, F. Thibaud-Nissen, W. Timp, M. Tomaszkiewicz, M. R. Vollger, B. P. Walenz, A. C. Watwood, M. H. Weissensteiner, A. M. Wenger, M. A. Wilson, S. Zarate, Y. Zhu, J. M. Zook, E. E. Eichler, R. J. O'Neill, M. C. Schatz, K. H. Miga, K. D. Makova, and A. M. Phillippy. 2023. The complete sequence of a human Y chromosome. *Nature* 621(7978):344–354.

Roberts, S. A., and J. M. Carswell. 2021. Growth, growth potential, and influences on adult height in the transgender and gender-diverse population. *Andrology* 9(6):1679–1688.

Rocca, W. A., J. H. Bower, D. M. Maraganore, J. E. Ahlskog, B. R. Grossardt, M. de Andrade, and L. J. Melton, 3rd. 2007. Increased risk of cognitive impairment or dementia in women who underwent oophorectomy before menopause. *Neurology* 69(11):1074–1083.

Rocca, W. A., C. M. Lohse, C. Y. Smith, J. A. Fields, M. M. Machulda, and M. M. Mielke. 2021. Association of premenopausal bilateral oophorectomy with cognitive performance and risk of mild cognitive impairment. *JAMA Network Open* 4(11):e2131448.

Rosen, A., and L. Casciola-Rosen. 2016. Autoantigens as partners in initiation and propagation of autoimmune rheumatic diseases. *Annual Review of Immunology* 34:395–420.

Rosen, C. J. 2000. The epidemiology and pathogenesis of osteoporosis. In *Endotext*, edited by K. R. Feingold, B. Anawalt, M. R. Blackman, A. Boyce, G. Chrousos, E. Corpas, W. W. de Herder, K. Dhatariya, K. Dungan, J. Hofland, S. Kalra, G. Kaltsas, N. Kapoor, C. Koch, P. Kopp, M. Korbonits, C. S. Kovacs, W. Kuohung, B. Laferrère, M. Levy, E. A. McGee, R. McLachlan, M. New, J. Purnell, R. Sahay, A. S. Shah, F. Singer, M. A. Sperling, C. A. Stratakis, D. L. Trence, and D. P. Wilson. South Dartmouth, MA: MDText.com, Inc.

Rosenberg, S. M., and A. H. Partridge. 2013. Premature menopause in young breast cancer: Effects on quality of life and treatment interventions. *Journal of Thoracic Disease* 5 (Suppl 1):S55–S61.

Rossouw, J. E., G. L. Anderson, R. L. Prentice, A. Z. LaCroix, C. Kooperberg, M. L. Stefanick, R. D. Jackson, S. A. Beresford, B. V. Howard, K. C. Johnson, J. M. Kotchen, and J. Ockene. 2002. Risks and benefits of estrogen plus progestin in healthy postmenopausal women: Principal results from the Women's Health Initiative randomized controlled trial. *JAMA* 288(3):321–333.

Rudzinskas, S., J. F. Hoffman, P. Martinez, D. R. Rubinow, P. J. Schmidt, and D. Goldman. 2021. In vitro model of perimenopausal depression implicates steroid metabolic and proinflammatory genes. *Molecular Psychiatry* 26(7):3266–3276.

Rumble, M. E., P. Okoyeh, and R. M. Benca. 2023. Sleep and women's mental health. *Psychiatric Clinics of North America* 46(3):527–537.

Russell, R. G. G. 2011. Bisphosphonates: The first 40 years. *Bone* 49(1):2–19.

Samargandy, S., K. A. Matthews, M. M. Brooks, E. Barinas-Mitchell, J. W. Magnani, R. C. Thurston, and S. R. El Khoudary. 2022. Trajectories of blood pressure in midlife women: Does menopause matter? *Circulation Research* 130(3):312–322.

Santoro, N. 2016. Perimenopause: From research to practice. *Journal of Women's Health* 25(4):332–339.

Schalla, M. A., and A. Stengel. 2024. The role of stress in perinatal depression and anxiety—a systematic review. *Frontiers in Neuroendocrinology* 72:101117.

Schiller, C. E., E. Walsh, T. A. Eisenlohr-Moul, J. Prim, G. S. Dichter, L. Schiff, J. Bizzell, S. L. Slightom, E. C. Richardson, A. Belger, P. Schmidt, and D. R. Rubinow. 2022. Effects of gonadal steroids on reward circuitry function and anhedonia in women with a history of postpartum depression. *Journal of Affective Disorders* 314:176–184.

Schmidt, P. J., L. K. Nieman, M. A. Danaceau, L. F. Adams, and D. R. Rubinow. 1998. Differential behavioral effects of gonadal steroids in women with and in those without premenstrual syndrome. *New England Journal of Medicine* 338(4):209–216.

Schmidt, P. J., L. Nieman, M. A. Danaceau, M. B. Tobin, C. A. Roca, J. H. Murphy, and D. R. Rubinow. 2000. Estrogen replacement in perimenopause-related depression: A preliminary report. *American Journal of Obstetrics and Gynecology* 183(2):414–420.

Schmidt, P. J., R. Ben Dor, P. E. Martinez, G. M. Guerrieri, V. L. Harsh, K. Thompson, D. E. Koziol, L. K. Nieman, and D. R. Rubinow. 2015. Effects of estradiol withdrawal on mood in women with past perimenopausal depression: A randomized clinical trial. *JAMA Psychiatry* 72(7):714–726.

Schweizer-Schubert, S., J. L. Gordon, T. A. Eisenlohr-Moul, S. Meltzer-Brody, K. M. Schmalenberger, R. Slopien, A. L. Zietlow, U. Ehlert, and B. Ditzen. 2020. Steroid hormone sensitivity in reproductive mood disorders: On the role of the GABA(A) receptor complex and stress during hormonal transitions. *Frontiers in Medicine* 7:479646.

Seeman, E. 2013. Age- and menopause-related bone loss compromise cortical and trabecular microstructure. *Journals of Gerontology* 68(10):1218–1225.

Seifert-Klauss, V., and J. C. Prior. 2010. Progesterone and bone: Actions promoting bone health in women. *Journal of Osteoporosis* 2010:845180.

Shapiro, C. L. 2020. Osteoporosis: A long-term and late-effect of breast cancer treatments. *Cancers* 12(11).

Shumaker, S. A., C. Legault, S. R. Rapp, L. Thal, R. B. Wallace, J. K. Ockene, S. L. Hendrix, B. N. Jones, III, A. R. Assaf, R. D. Jackson, J. Morley Kotchen, S. Wassertheil-Smoller, J. Wactawski-Wende, and WHIMS Investigators. 2003. Estrogen plus progestin and the incidence of dementia and mild cognitive impairment in postmenopausal women— the Women's Health Initiative memory study: A randomized controlled trial. *JAMA* 289(20):2651–2662.

Shumaker, S. A., C. Legault, L. Kuller, S. R. Rapp, L. Thal, D. S. Lane, H. Fillit, M. L. Stefanick, S. L. Hendrix, C. E. Lewis, K. Masaki, and L. H. Coker. 2004. Conjugated equine estrogens and incidence of probable dementia and mild cognitive impairment in postmenopausal women: Women's Health Initiative memory study. *JAMA* 291(24):2947–2958.

Shumer, D., and A. Araya. 2019. Endocrine care of transgender children and adolescents. In *Transgender Medicine: A Multidisciplinary Approach.* Pp. 165–181. Heidelberg, Germany: Springer International Publishing.

Silverwood, V., M. Blagojevic-Bucknall, C. Jinks, J. L. Jordan, J. Protheroe, and K. P. Jordan. 2015. Current evidence on risk factors for knee osteoarthritis in older adults: A systematic review and meta-analysis. *Osteoarthritis and Cartilage* 23(4):507–515.

Sinclair, A. H., P. Berta, M. S. Palmer, J. R. Hawkins, B. L. Griffiths, M. J. Smith, J. W. Foster, A.-M. Frischauf, R. Lovell-Badge, and P. N. Goodfellow. 1990. A gene from the human sex-determining region encodes a protein with homology to a conserved DNA-binding motif. *Nature* 346(6281):240–244.

Smart, K., S. M. L. Cox, S. G. Scala, M. Tippler, N. Jaworska, M. Boivin, J. R. Séguin, C. Benkelfat, and M. Leyton. 2019. Sex differences in [(11)C]ABP688 binding: A positron emission tomography study of mGlu5 receptors. *European Journal of Nuclear Medicine and Molecular Imaging* 46(5):1179–1183.

Smith, C. T., L. C. Dang, L. L. Burgess, S. F. Perkins, M. D. San Juan, D. K. Smith, R. L. Cowan, N. T. Le, R. M. Kessler, G. R. Samanez-Larkin, and D. H. Zald. 2019. Lack of consistent sex differences in D-amphetamine-induced dopamine release measured with [18F]fallypride PET. *Psychopharmacology* 236(2):581–590.

Sohrabji, F., A. Okoreeh, and A. Panta. 2019. Sex hormones and stroke: Beyond estrogens. *Hormones and Behavior* 111:87–95.

Soldin, O. P., and D. R. Mattison. 2009. Sex differences in pharmacokinetics and pharmacodynamics. *Clinical Pharmacokinetics* 48(3):143–157.

Spencer, J. L., E. M. Waters, R. D. Romeo, G. E. Wood, T. A. Milner, and B. S. McEwen. 2008. Uncovering the mechanisms of estrogen effects on hippocampal function. *Frontiers in Neuroendocrinology* 29(2):219–237.

Sprague, B. L., A. Trentham-Dietz, and K. A. Cronin. 2012. A sustained decline in postmenopausal hormone use: Results from the National Health and Nutrition Examination Survey, 1999–2010. *Obstetrics & Gynecology* 120(3):595–603.

Stall, N. M., N. R. Shah, and D. Bhushan. 2023. Unpaid family caregiving—the next frontier of gender equity in a postpandemic future. *JAMA Health Forum* 4(6):e231310-e231310.

Stefanick, M. L. 2005. Estrogens and progestins: Background and history, trends in use, and guidelines and regimens approved by the U.S. Food and Drug Administration. *American Journal of Medicine* 118(Suppl 12B):64–73.

Stevens, M. L. 2019. Medical philanthropy pays dividends: The impact of philanthropic funding of basic and clinical research goes beyond mere finances by reshaping the whole research enterprise. *EMBO Reports* 20(5):e48173.

Stevenson, M. O., and V. Tangpricha. 2019. Osteoporosis and bone health in transgender persons. *Endocrinology and Metabolism Clinics of North America* 48(2):421–427.

Stute, P., A. Spyropoulou, V. Karageorgiou, A. Cano, J. Bitzer, I. Ceausu, P. Chedraui, F. Durmusoglu, R. Erkkola, D. G. Goulis, A. Lindén Hirschberg, L. Kiesel, P. Lopes, A. Pines,

M. Rees, M. van Trotsenburg, I. Zervas, and I. Lambrinoudaki. 2020. Management of depressive symptoms in peri- and postmenopausal women: EMAS position statement. *Maturitas* 131:91–101.

Suarez-Almazor, M. E., X. Pundole, G. Cabanillas, X. Lei, H. Zhao, L. S. Elting, M. A. Lopez-Olivo, and S. H. Giordano. 2022. Association of bone mineral density testing with risk of major osteoporotic fractures among older men receiving androgen deprivation therapy to treat localized or regional prostate cancer. *JAMA Network Open* 5(4):e225432.

Subramanya, V., B. Ambale-Venkatesh, Y. Ohyama, D. Zhao, C. C. Nwabuo, W. S. Post, E. Guallar, P. Ouyang, S. J. Shah, M. A. Allison, C. E. Ndumele, D. Vaidya, D. A. Bluemke, J. A. Lima, and E. D. Michos. 2018. Relation of sex hormone levels with prevalent and 10-year change in aortic distensibility assessed by MRI: The Multi-Ethnic Study of Atherosclerosis. *American Journal of Hypertension* 31(7):774–783.

Sun, L., Z. Wang, T. Lu, T. A. Manolio, and A. D. Paterson. 2023. Exclusionary: 10 years later, where are the sex chromosomes in GWASs? *American Journal of Human Genetics* 110(6):903–912.

Sun, W., Y. Wang, C. Li, X. Yao, X. Wu, A. He, B. Zhao, X. Huang, and H. Song. 2024. Genetically predicted high serum sex hormone-binding globulin levels are associated with lower ischemic stroke risk: A sex-stratified mendelian randomization study. *Journal of Stroke and Cerebrovascular Diseases* 33(6):107686.

Sun, Y., B. Liu, L. G. Snetselaar, R. B. Wallace, B. J. Caan, T. E. Rohan, M. L. Neuhouser, A. H. Shadyab, R. T. Chlebowski, J. E. Manson, and W. Bao. 2019. Association of normal-weight central obesity with all-cause and cause-specific mortality among postmenopausal women. *JAMA Network Open* 2(7):e197337.

Syrett, C. M., B. Paneru, D. Sandoval-Heglund, J. Wang, S. Banerjee, V. Sindhava, E. M. Behrens, M. Atchison, and M. C. Anguera. 2019. Altered X-chromosome inactivation in T cells may promote sex-biased autoimmune diseases. *JCI Insight* 4(7).

Syrett, C. M., I. Sierra, Z. T. Beethem, A. H. Dubin, and M. C. Anguera. 2020. Loss of epigenetic modifications on the inactive X chromosome and sex-biased gene expression profiles in B cells from NZB/W F1 mice with lupus-like disease. *Journal of Autoimmunity* 107:102357.

Tal, R., and H. Taylor. 2021. Endocrinology of pregnancy. In *Endotext*, edited by K. R. Feingold, B. Anawalt, M. R. Blackman, A. Boyce, G. Chrousos, E. Corpas, W. W. de Herder, K. Dhatariya, K. Dungan, J. Hofland, S. Kalra, G. Kaltsas, N. Kapoor, C. Koch, P. Kopp, M. Korbonits, C. S. Kovacs, W. Kuohung, B. Laferrère, M. Levy, E. A. McGee, R. McLachlan, M. New, J. Purnell, R. Sahay, A. S. Shah, F. Singer, M. A. Sperling, C. A. Stratakis, D. L. Trence, and D. P. Wilson. South Dartmouth, MA: MDText.com, Inc.

Taylor, C. M., L. Pritschet, and E. G. Jacobs. 2021. The scientific body of knowledge—whose body does it serve? A spotlight on oral contraceptives and women's health factors in neuroimaging. *Frontiers in Neuroendocrinology* 60:100874.

Thapa, S., A. Nandy, and E. Rendina-Ruedy. 2022. Endocrinal metabolic regulation on the skeletal system in post menopausal women. *Frontiers in Physiology* 13.1052429.

Torosyan, N., P. Visrodia, T. Torbati, M. B. Minissian, and C. L. Shufelt. 2022. Dyslipidemia in midlife women: Approach and considerations during the menopausal transition. *Maturitas* 166:14–20.

Tu, K. N., J. D. Lie, C. K. V. Wan, M. Cameron, A. G. Austel, J. K. Nguyen, K. Van, and D. Hyun. 2018. Osteoporosis: A review of treatment options. *P & T* 43(2):92–104.

Turek, J., and Ł. Gąsior. 2023. Estrogen fluctuations during the menopausal transition are a risk factor for depressive disorders. *Pharmacology Reports* 75(1):32–43.

Ulm, M., A. V. Ramesh, K. M. McNamara, S. Ponnusamy, H. Sasano, and R. Narayanan. 2019. Therapeutic advances in hormone-dependent cancers: Focus on prostate, breast and ovarian cancers. *Endocrine Connections* 8(2):R10–R26.

Volgman, A. S., C. N. Bairey Merz, N. T. Aggarwal, V. Bittner, T. J. Bunch, P. B. Gorelick, P. Maki, H. N. Patel, A. Poppas, J. Ruskin, A. M. Russo, S. R. Waldstein, N. K. Wenger, K. Yaffe, and C. J. Pepine. 2019. Sex differences in cardiovascular disease and cognitive impairment: Another health disparity for women? *Journal of the American Heart Association* 8(19):e013154.

Walker, M. D., and E. Shane. 2023. Postmenopausal osteoporosis. *New England Journal of Medicine* 389(21):1979–1991.

Wang, J., C. M. Syrett, M. C. Kramer, A. Basu, M. L. Atchison, and M. C. Anguera. 2016. Unusual maintenance of X chromosome inactivation predisposes female lymphocytes for increased expression from the inactive X. *Proceedings of the National Academy of Sciences of the United States of America* 113(14):E2029–E2038.

Wei, S. M., E. B. Baller, P. E. Martinez, A. C. Goff, H. J. Li, P. D. Kohn, J. S. Kippenhan, S. J. Soldin, D. R. Rubinow, D. Goldman, P. J. Schmidt, and K. F. Berman. 2021. Subgenual cingulate resting regional cerebral blood flow in premenstrual dysphoric disorder: Differential regulation by ovarian steroids and preliminary evidence for an association with expression of ESC/E(Z) complex genes. *Translational Psychiatry* 11(1):206.

Weill Cornell Medicine Neurology. n.d. *Women's Brain Initiative.* https://neurology.weill. cornell.edu/research/womens-brain-initiative (accessed August 7, 2024).

White, M. C., H. K. Weir, A. V. Soman, L. A. Peipins, and T. D. Thompson. 2022. Risk of clear-cell adenocarcinoma of the vagina and cervix among U.S. women with potential exposure to diethylstilbestrol in utero. *Cancer Causes & Control* 33(8):1121–1124.

Wise, Anastasia L., L. Gyi, and Teri A. Manolio. 2013. Exclusion: Toward integrating the X chromosome in genome-wide association analyses. *American Journal of Human Genetics* 92(5):643–647.

Wolf, R. M., and D. Long. 2016. Pubertal development. *Pediatrics in Review* 37(7):292–300.

Zeydan, B., N. Tosakulwong, C. G. Schwarz, M. L. Senjem, J. L. Gunter, R. I. Reid, L. Gazzuola Rocca, T. G. Lesnick, C. Y. Smith, K. R. Bailey, V. J. Lowe, R. O. Roberts, C. R. Jack, Jr., R. C. Petersen, V. M. Miller, M. M. Mielke, W. A. Rocca, and K. Kantarci. 2019. Association of bilateral salpingo-oophorectomy before menopause onset with medial temporal lobe neurodegeneration. *JAMA Neurology* 76(1):95–100.

Zhang, P., J. J. Munier, C. B. Wiese, L. Vergnes, J. C. Link, F. Abbasi, E. Ronquillo, K. Scheker, A. Muñoz, Y. L. Kuang, E. Theusch, M. Lu, G. Sanchez, A. Oni-Orisan, C. Iribarren, M. J. McPhaul, D. K. Nomura, J. W. Knowles, R. M. Krauss, M. W. Medina, and K. Reue. 2024. X chromosome dosage drives statin-induced dysglycemia and mitochondrial dysfunction. *Nature Communications* 15(1):5571.

Zhang, X., J. Xiao, T. Liu, Q. He, J. Cui, S. Tang, X. Li, and M. Liu. 2022. Low serum dehydroepiandrosterone and dehydroepiandrosterone sulfate are associated with coronary heart disease in men with Type 2 diabetes mellitus. *Frontiers in Endocrinology* 13:890029.

Zhao, D., E. Guallar, P. Ouyang, V. Subramanya, D. Vaidya, C. E. Ndumele, J. A. Lima, M. A. Allison, S. J. Shah, A. G. Bertoni, M. J. Budoff, W. S. Post, and E. D. Michos. 2018. Endogenous sex hormones and incident cardiovascular disease in post-menopausal women. *Journal of the American College of Cardiology* 71(22):2555–2566.

Zhao, L., J. Yao, Z. Mao, S. Chen, Y. Wang, and R. D. Brinton. 2011. 17β-estradiol regulates insulin-degrading enzyme expression via an erβ/pi3-k pathway in hippocampus: Relevance to Alzheimer's prevention. *Neurobiology and Aging* 32(11):1949–1963.

Zhu, Y., X. Wu, R. Zhou, O. Sie, Z. Niu, F. Wang, and Y. Fang. 2021. Hypothalamic-pituitary-end-organ axes: Hormone function in female patients with major depressive disorder. *Neuroscience Bulletin* 37(8):1176–1187.

Zucker, I., and B. J. Prendergast. 2020. Sex differences in pharmacokinetics predict adverse drug reactions in women. *Biology of Sex Differences* 11(1):32.

Zumwalt, M., and B. Dowling. 2014. Effects of the menstrual cycle on the acquisition of peak bone mass. In *The Active Female: Health Issues Throughout the Lifespan*, edited by J. J. Robert-McComb, R. L. Norman, and M. Zumwalt. New York: Springer New York. Pp. 81–90.

6

Women, Health, and Society

INTRODUCTION

The previous chapter illustrates the role that biological factors, such as chromosomes and hormones, have on women's health. Biological sex shapes health in many ways, potentially offering vulnerability or resilience to various health conditions (NASEM, 2024a). However, women's health is also strongly shaped by the social and structural context of their lives, including their income and wealth, education, employment, location, family structure, and larger structural and policy forces. The social factors that contribute to gendered differences in men's and women's lives can also interact with each other and with biological differences, confounding or exacerbating the latter. Consequently, the health differences seen between women and among women compared to men are products of social and biological factors. Moreover, other identities, including gender identity, race, ethnicity,[1] and sexual orientation, shape women's health. These biological and social and structural factors intersect and can be bidirectional.

This chapter provides a high-level overview of how structural and social determinants of health can influence women's health, illustrating why the national research agenda needs to specifically focus research investments to

---

[1] As discussed in Chapter 1, this report strives to be consistent in its use of the following terms to describe specific racially and ethnically minoritized populations: "American Indian or Alaska Native," "Asian," "Black," "Hispanic or Latino/a/x/e," "Native Hawaiian or Pacific Islander," and "White." However, when describing data from cited studies, the terminology from source papers is used, introducing differences in language. This is also the case with the report's use of LGBTQIA+ and similar variations, such as LGBT, LGBTQ, and LGBTQ+. This is especially common in this chapter.

better understand how these factors shape the health of girls and women as it seeks to develop solutions to improve their health and well-being. While the structural and social determinants cover a large range of domains, this chapter offers an overview of select examples.

STRUCTURAL AND SOCIAL DETERMINANTS OF HEALTH

Healthy People 2030 organizes the social determinants of health (SDOH) into five domains: health care access and quality, economic stability, neighborhood and built environment, social and community context, and education access and quality (OASH, n.d.-a). The structural determinants of health are the

> macrolevel factors, such as laws, policies, institutional practices, governance processes, and social norms that shape the distribution (or maldistribution) of the SDOH (e.g., housing, income, employment, exposure to environmental toxins, interpersonal discrimination) across and within social groups. Structural determinants of health, also referred to as the 'determinants of the determinants of health,' include structural racism and other structural inequities and thus influence not only population health but also health equity. (NASEM, 2023b)

The 2024 National Academies of Sciences, Engineering, and Medicine (National Academies) report *Advancing Research on Chronic Conditions in Women* provides an overview as well as research gaps on the structural and SDOH as they specifically affect women, including structural sexism and health policy (NASEM, 2024a). See Figure 6-1 for a visualization from that report showing how biological, social, and structural determinants can affect women's health. As that report highlighted, gender-related social and cultural factors can lead to diverse exposures and experiences within the framework of structural and social determinants of health. These factors, through a range of mechanisms, affect not only preventive behaviors but also the onset, characteristics, and progression of various health conditions (NASEM, 2024a). In addition, women often face unique challenges in the health care system, including differences in clinical practices and patient-centered care, which can further influence their health outcomes. For example, weathering (see Figure 6-1) refers to the cumulative negative effect of chronic stress from social and economic adversity on the physical health of marginalized groups and results in premature biological aging and increased health vulnerability. It can yield adverse health outcomes (Geronimus et al., 2006; Simons et al., 2021).

Women navigate the world in ways distinct from men, and women who are additionally marginalized because of other facets of their identity face unique and additional challenges, making health equity a crucial

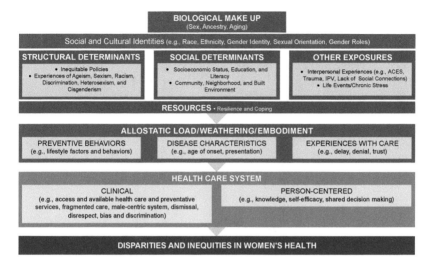

FIGURE 6-1 A bio-socio-cultural model for understanding women's health.
SOURCE: Adapted from NASEM, 2024a.

consideration within women's health. If equality is defined as treating all individuals in the same manner, it is important to emphasize that equity is not interchangeable. Equality assumes a level playing field for everyone without accounting for historical and current inequities. According to the World Health Organization, "equity is the absence of avoidable or remediable differences among groups of people, whether those groups are defined socially, economically, demographically, [or] geographically" (WHO, n.d.). In other words, equity is the process, and equality is the outcome. Equity focuses on justice (NASEM, 2023b).

In many areas, women experience not only differences in health outcomes compared to men but also inequities in health and health care. Health and health care inequities are driven by structural and social determinants, meaning they are more than just "differences." For example, the 2020 National Academies report *Birth Settings in America: Outcomes, Quality, Access and Choice* describes structural inequities and biases, including racism, on the systemic, institutional, and interpersonal levels that underlie SDOH for racially and ethnically minoritized women (NASEM, 2020a). Systematic oppression related to race, sexual orientation, gender identity, age, weight, ability, and more are especially harmful to women, who also experience sexism and misogyny. In addition, laws and policies are important macrolevel factors for consideration (Everett and Agénor, 2023; Jahn et al., 2023; Zubizarreta et al., 2024). These factors combined have contributed to deprioritizing and undervaluing women's health research (WHR). The remainder of this chapter outlines how social and structural determinants drive inequities in women's health and WHR, including consideration and examples of how the intersectional identities of women who are racially and ethnically minoritized, disabled, lesbian, bisexual, transgender, or otherwise marginalized further shape outcomes, and illustrates why these need to be considered in the development of the nation's research agenda on women's health.

STRUCTURAL DETERMINANTS OF HEALTH

Discrimination

Sexism

Structural sexism is "systematic gender inequalities between men and women in power and resources, as manifest in institutions, interactions, and individuals" (Homan, 2021). It is reflected in policies and institutions, such as how many women participate in the labor force, the ratio of men's to women's median weekly earnings, poverty rates, and percent of state legislative seats occupied by men versus women (Homan, 2019). Researchers have begun to explore how structural and systemic forms of gender-based discrimination affect women's health (Homan, 2019; Krieger, 2001, 2014; Philbin et al., 2024). For example, data suggest that bias against women in the workplace negatively affects women's health and, furthermore, that women living in states with high levels of structural sexism have approximately twice as many chronic health conditions compared to women in states with lower levels (Cunningham and Wicker, 2024; Homan, 2019). The health effects are substantial—women exposed to high structural sexism appear to have a health profile about 7 years older than women in low-sexism states (Homan, 2019). Additionally, structural sexism amplifies other forms of discrimination, such as structural racism, ableism, heterosexism, and classism, compounding negative health effects for women with multiple marginalized identities (Homan, 2019, 2021; Perry et al., 2013). For example, Everett et al. (2022a, 2024b) have linked structural heteropatriarchy (i.e., the combined impact of structural sexism and discrimination against lesbian, gay, and bisexual populations) to increased risk of preterm birth, decreased birthweight, and maternal cardiovascular morbidities. Moreover, the effects from such discrimination accumulate over time to affect women's health (Kelley and Gilbert, 2023).

Studies have also shown that structural sexism affects women's access to health care. For example, researchers examined state-level sexism using state-level indicators of administrative data, such as the ratio of men-to-women earnings, employment, poverty rate, and paid family leave policy, and their effect on access to health care. Higher state-level sexism was associated with greater barriers to accessing health care and affordability for Black and Hispanic but not White women, illustrating the effect of intersectional structural discrimination that racially and ethnically minoritized women face (Rapp et al., 2021).

Beyond access to health care, studies have examined the effect of structural sexism on the use of preventive health care, cesarean-section rates, breastfeeding, and disordered eating (Balistreri, 2024; Beccia et al., 2022; Dore et al., 2024; Nagle and Samari, 2021; NASEM, 2024a). Gender discrimination is also a major source of stress that directly affects mental health. Women who report experiencing discrimination are more likely to suffer from depression and anxiety (Vigod and Rochon, 2020). Moreover, research suggests there are fewer gender differences in mental illness rates in more gender-equal societies, suggesting discrimination may play a major role in these disparities (Yu, 2018). Future research on measuring structural sexism needs to consider the longitudinal nature of its effects, as most studies are cross-sectional; capture dynamic and complex ways in which systems of oppression affect women's health; and identify strategies to intervene (Beccia et al., 2024; Homan, 2019).

Racism, Colonialism, and Health Outcomes

A long history of colonialism and racism, reflected in policies, systems, and communities, drive U.S. health inequities (KFF, n.d.; NASEM, 2017, 2023b). The 2023 National Academies report *Federal Policy to Advance Racial, Ethnic, and Tribal Health Equity* details this history of racism, discrimination, and colonialism; its effect on health outcomes; and the need to address these root causes (NASEM, 2023b); to do so, research needs to account for these underlying structural causes to understand how they affect human biology and the ability to access needed services to prevent, diagnose, and treat health conditions.

Colonialism

Colonialism involves control of "people [and] the context of their lives—control of the economy through land appropriation, labor exploitation, and extraction of natural resources; control of authority through government, normative social institutions, and the military; control of gender and sexuality through oversight of the family and education; and control of subjectivity and knowledge through imposition of an epistemology and the formation of subjectivity" (IOM, 2013, p.13). The American Indian and Alaska Native (AIAN) population is a salient example in which colonialism affects health. To advance health for AIAN women, it is essential to understand the history of colonialism and how it continues to reverberate through all aspects of health at systems, community, and individual levels.[2]

The effects of colonialism have created modern health inequities through violence, targeted eradication of AIAN people, erasure of culture, dispossession of land, removal from tribal homelands, forced urbanization, and more (Brown-Rice, 2013; Carroll et al., 2022; Moss, 2019; NASEM, 2023b). AIAN women have been threatened with forcible removal of their children and endured forced sterilization (Newland, 2022; Stern, 2020). The forcible placement of AIAN children in boarding schools and non-AIAN homes has also resulted in cultural eradication (Newland, 2022). These historical events have negatively affected AIAN women's health, creating inequities in cancer, heart health, mental health, maternal mortality, violence, and more (American Heart Association, 2023; CDC, 2023a; KFF, 2022a; Kwon et al., 2024; Moss, 2019; NASEM, 2017, 2023b; Petrosky et al., 2021; Statista, n.d.; Urban Indian Health Institute, n.d.).

For example, the pregnancy-related death rate among AIAN women is nearly double that in White women (26.2 per 100,000 vs. 13.7) (KFF, 2022a). A review of pregnancy-related deaths among AIAN populations finds that about one in three is attributable to mental health conditions (Trost et al., 2022). Moreover, 2020 data suggest that approximately 92 percent of AIAN maternal mortality is preventable (CDC, 2024).

Like other health disparities affecting AIAN people, mental health outcomes need to be considered in the context of historical trauma resulting from colonialism. Suicide is one of the leading causes of mortality among AIAN people (Statista, n.d.). Although negative mental health outcomes are of great concern for AIAN women, the literature on AIAN mental health research is scant (Kwon et al., 2024). These health inequities exist, but it is important that solutions be framed to include community assets and viewed in terms of attaining balance among the components necessary for health and well-being in alignment with an Indigenous model of health, a concept based on the Medicine Wheel[3] (Greer and Lemacks, 2024; National Library of Medicine, n.d.).

When studying SDOH, it is also important to understand the Indigenous SDOH—that is, the factors that impact the health and well-being of Indigenous peoples uniquely. Seven Directions, the first national public health institute in the United States to focus solely on health and wellness for Indigenous people, asserts "[Indigenous SDOH] could include our

---

[2] The report *Federal Policy to Advance Racial, Ethnic, and Tribal Health Equity* provides a detailed history of tribal health and how it has led to significant health inequities (NASEM, 2023b).

[3] "The Medicine Wheel, sometimes known as the Sacred Hoop, has been used by generations of various Native American tribes for health and healing. It embodies the Four Directions, as well as Father Sky, Mother Earth, and Spirit Tree—all of which symbolize dimensions of health and the cycles of life" (National Library of Medicine, n.d.)

connection to our traditional lands, tribal sovereignty, tribal governance, our unique tribal or urban Indian health care system, the access we have to our traditional lifeways, native languages, traditional foods, ceremonies, relationships, and many more factors. The process of mapping social determinants of health with and for AIAN communities can and should include the factors or conditions that are only found in our tribal or urban Indian settings" (Seven Directions: A Center for Indigenous Public Health, 2023). These are all essential factors to consider not only for research (e.g., including tribal consultation) but also when developing programs, policies, and laws impacting AIAN communities.

Racism

Racism is a structural system resulting from the intersection of social and institutional power and racial prejudice. Policies, practices, and attitudes within this system operate to constrain or enhance access to resources, privileges, and advantages based on race. These privileges disproportionately accrue to some groups and are withheld from others according to social constructions of race and ethnicity (NASEM, 2023b). The psychological toll of racism can directly harm physical and mental health; it increases cortisol levels and weakens the immune system (Berger and Sarnyai, 2015; Chen and Mallory, 2021). In addition, chronic stress from racism is linked to increased risk of hypertension and poorer health at earlier ages (Dolezsar et al., 2014; Geronimus et al., 2006; Hicken et al., 2014).

As discussed in Chapter 2, Black women in the United States experience significant negative health outcomes relative to White women, such as early menopause transition with more severe symptoms, higher fibroid incidence, higher rates of pregnancy-related adverse events, and higher incidence of chronic conditions, such as heart disease and diabetes (Chinn et al., 2021; Harlow et al., 2022; Howell, 2018; Katon et al., 2023). Pregnancy-related mortality is highest among Black women, at 41.4 per 100,000 compared to 13.7, 11.2, 14.1, and 26.2 for White, Hispanic, Asian and Pacific Islander, and AIAN women, respectively (KFF, 2022a). Black, AIAN, Asian, and Pacific Islander women are more likely to experience preterm births, low-birthweight babies, or births after late or no prenatal care compared to White women (KFF, 2022a). Black women are almost two times more likely to experience infertility than White women, and Black, Latina, and Asian women are less likely to receive infertility and fertility preservation treatments (Dongarwar et al., 2022; Weiss and Marsh, 2023). The continuing effects of structural racism, rooted in a history of slavery and colonialism, impede advancing the health of Black women (Bleich et al., 2024), who constantly need to negotiate their identities based on a past entrenched in oppression, which influences their social interactions, mental health, and access to opportunities (Presumey-Leblanc and Sandel, 2024).

Hispanic and Latina women are more likely to be diagnosed with breast cancer at a more advanced stage, experience higher mortality rates from it, and, as breast cancer survivors, face a higher risk of cardiovascular disease (CVD) and related mortality compared to non-Hispanic White women (Gonzalo-Encabo et al., 2023; Paz and Massey, 2016). Black and Hispanic patients are significantly less likely than White patients to have minimally invasive surgery for uterine fibroids and more likely to undergo hysterectomies (Eltoukhi et al., 2014; Katon et al., 2023). These disparities reflect broader issues of racism and discrimination, which contribute to unequal access to health care and SDOH, exacerbating the health inequities faced by these communities.

Furthermore, research on structural determinants of health, including racism, is hampered by shortcomings in data collection and measurement of structural racism and other forms of discrimination (Hing et al., 2024; NASEM, 2023b). In addition, what the research enterprise considers "science" impacts the role of race and ethnicity and the types of studies conducted. For example, community-engaged research—representing a spectrum of approaches where community members and organizations and/or researchers collaborate—can be used to better identify mechanisms to prevent and address complex health issues impacted by bias, racism, and the structural and social determinants of health. These tools are underused and will be important to apply in future WHR (NASEM, 2024a; Wallerstein and Duran, 2006).

Lesbian, Gay, Bisexual, Transgender, Queer or Questioning, Intersex, and Asexual (LGBTQIA+) Discrimination

Sexual and gender minorities (SGM), including lesbian, bisexual, Two-Spirit, queer, and transgender and nonbinary (TNB) individuals, also experience unique challenges and barriers to health and health care compared to heterosexual cisgender women and men. While the term "TNB" is used throughout this chapter, the focus is on the ways social and structural determinants of health affect transgender women as well as transgender men and nonbinary individuals assigned female sex at birth. SGM are subject to marginalization and stigma that can have a number of downstream effects, such as poorer economic outcomes and increased vulnerability to interpersonal violence (Badgett et al., 2019; Coston, 2023; Flores et al., 2021; Movement Advancement Project and Center for American Progress, 2024; National Coalition of Anti-Violence Programs, 2018; Peitzmeier et al., 2020). On medical and biological dimensions, for example, when seeking gender-affirming care, TNB individuals sometimes need to navigate discrimination from health care providers and barriers to such care. Figure 6-2 shows a framework for multilevel social and structural determinants of health outcomes in SGM populations (Diaz-Thomas et al., 2023). The later sections

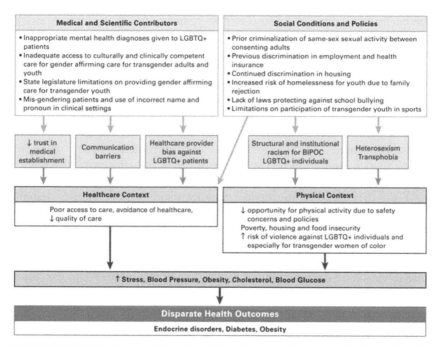

FIGURE 6-2 Medical, scientific and social policy contributors to health and health care disparities in sexual and gender minorities in the United States.
NOTES: LGBTQ+ = lesbian, gay, bisexual, transgender, queer, intersex, and asexual. Although not defined in the figure source, the acronym BIPOC can be used to refer to individuals who are Black, Indigenous, and people of color.
SOURCE: Diaz-Thomas et al., 2023. © Published by Oxford University Press on behalf of the Endocrine Society. All rights reserved.

of this chapter elaborate on several of these challenges and how they can affect health and well-being.

LGBT youth and young adults experience increased stress, labeled "minority stress," particularly during the pubertal transition (Mason et al., 2023). The minority stress model was introduced by Dr. Virginia R. Brooks (later known as Winn Kelly Brooks) in her 1981 book *Minority Stress and Lesbian Women* (Brooks, 1981). It proposes that members of minoritized communities experience specific and additional stressors compared to the everyday stress majority populations experience over the life-span (Meyer, 2003). Over time, this can lead to activation of the hypothalamic-pituitary-adrenal axis, one of the body's stress response systems, affecting physical and mental health (Diaz-Thomas et al., 2023; Hatzenbuehler and McLaughlin, 2014).

Although limited and underfunded, research points to unique sexual and reproductive health barriers among sexual minority women (SMW).

For example, compared to heterosexual women, SMW, including lesbian and bisexual women, may be more likely to experience pregnancy loss, stillbirth, low birthweight, and preterm birth (Charlton et al., 2020) and be at higher risk of developing cervical cancer (American Cancer Society, 2024). Data from Everett et al. suggest that these outcomes may be attenuated by policies that confer protections for SMW (Everett and Agénor, 2023; Everett et al., 2022b, 2024a). Contraceptive access is another area of concern; unintended pregnancy is higher among SMW compared to their heterosexual peers. Research on sexual and reproductive health inequities among racially and ethnically minoritized SMW remains especially limited (Agénor et al., 2021; Higgins et al., 2019).

For AIAN populations, gender is not a dichotomy of male or female. Precolonialism views on gender varied by tribe, with traditional languages including more than two genders. One modern term that applies only to Indigenous people is "Two-Spirit" (NASEM, 2020b; RRC Polytech, 2024). Two-Spirit people often face discrimination and marginalization from multiple directions. For example, they may experience racism and exclusion from non-Native LGBTQ communities, and within Native communities, they may encounter homophobia, transphobia, and rejection of their Two-Spirit identity (Tribal Information Exchange, n.d.). In broader society, Two-Spirit people face intersecting discrimination based on their racial, ethnic, gender, and sexual identities. The National Institutes of Health (NIH) funds little research on health outcomes for this population, with only three current NIH-funded studies with "Two-Spirit" in the title, abstract, or keywords based on a keyword search of RePORTER in October 2024 (NIH, n.d.). However, the limited evidence shows the discrimination Two-Spirit people face may contribute to health disparities, such as high rates of physical and sexual assault victimization, increased risk of mental health issues, such as depression and anxiety, greater likelihood of substance abuse, and elevated suicide risk (Robinson, 2022; Tribal Information Exchange, n.d.).

Weight Bias

Weight bias, also known as weight stigma, "refers to the negative attitudes, beliefs, stereotypes and discriminatory behaviors directed toward individuals based on their body weight or size" (Edwards-Gayfield, n.d.). This can manifest in various forms, including social exclusion and unfair treatment in both personal and professional settings. In health care, weight bias may lead to patients with higher weights receiving inadequate care, being blamed for their health conditions, or facing barriers to accessing necessary services. Weight bias often results in people seeking care later, avoiding it altogether, or receiving suboptimal treatment, which can exacerbate existing health issues and further marginalize this population (Lawrence et al., 2021). Furthermore, the lack of investment in developing medical technology and resources to care for people along the weight spectrum, such as too few magnetic resonance imaging devices sized for large bodies, creates problems with care and likely affects overall health (Brydon, 2022; Kukielka, 2020; Ordway, 2023).

Some research indicates that weight bias is more prominent for women than men, and women report more internalization of it than men, meaning they are more likely to have self-disparaging thoughts and feelings because of their weight (Sattler et al., 2018). Women, particularly those with higher weights, often face greater societal pressure regarding body image and are more likely to experience weight-related stigma in various aspects of life, including health care (Puhl and Heuer, 2010; Voges et al., 2022). Furthermore, Black and Hispanic women are, on average, heavier than White women, indicating a likely intersectional component to the experience of racialized weight stigma in society and health care (OMH, 2024a, 2024b; Strings, 2019).

Despite growing awareness of weight bias and its impact, a significant gap remains in research on how it mediates and moderates adverse health outcomes, particularly for individuals with higher weights. This gap is particularly critical given that weight bias can exacerbate disparities in health care access and treatment, compounding the challenges faced by those with higher weights and potentially leading to worse health outcomes. Addressing this gap is essential to comprehensively understanding and mitigating the effects of weight bias on overall health.

Disability

Disability[4] is an important consideration when undertaking research on women's health—across all ages, women have slightly higher rates of disability compared to men, and this gap widens with age (Office of Disability Employment Policy, 2021). Women with disabilities experience significant employment barriers compared to both nondisabled women and men with disabilities. Their employment rate (20.5 percent in 2023) is lower than both disabled men (24.8 percent) and nondisabled women (60.3 percent). Women with disabilities also earn less than men with disabilities (Ives-Rublee and Neal, 2024). This economic disparity leads to limited access to the positive SDOH (Friedman, 2024).

In general, women with disabilities have difficulty affording health care, medications, and other health-related needs (CDC, 2023b); those who face poverty, unemployment, and unmet health care needs because of financial

---

[4] Disability can be defined differently across the relevant literature, with some relying on individuals with disabilities to self-report and others relying on questions about diagnosed conditions or functional capacity.

constraints are also more likely to suffer from heightened mental distress (Cree et al., 2020). Women with physical, intellectual, or sensory disabilities face a wide range of sociocultural and structural factors that negatively affect their access to health care services, including reproductive health services, such as sexual education, contraceptive care, and pregnancy-related care, but this research is limited (Biggs et al., 2023; CDC, 2023b; Matin et al., 2021; Ransohoff et al., 2022).

Laws and Policies

Laws and policies are critical structural determinants of women's health. The following discussion provides a few examples focused on reproductive rights and rights for SGM.

Reproductive Rights and Justice

Reproductive justice, which encompasses the right to access reproductive health care and the socioeconomic and racial factors that influence health outcomes, is an important example for understanding the effect of structural determinants on women's health (SisterSong, n.d.). Addressing reproductive rights and health through this lens provides a comprehensive approach to improving women's overall health and well-being.

Regarding laws and policies, reproductive health and rights frameworks tend to focus on rights to abortion and contraception access. For example, the Supreme Court's ruling in *Dobbs v. Jackson Women's Health Organization*,[5] which struck down decisions guaranteeing abortion care access at the federal level, has resulted in abortion bans and early gestational restrictions with direct effects on those seeking abortion care in nearly half the country (KFF, 2024; NASEM, 2023b). This case is a defining moment regarding women's health and rights to bodily autonomy, and research has already identified numerous negative effects on women's health care access and health outcomes (Ahmed et al., 2023; Thornburg et al., 2024; Zhao et al., 2024; Zhu et al., 2024). These laws also interact with broader structural determinants to shape women's and girls' sexual and reproductive health outcomes. For example, restrictive abortion laws are linked to higher levels of preterm birth and low birthweight among Black people compared to non-Black people (Redd et al., 2021).

However, a reproductive justice framework extends the work of reproductive rights and health by identifying and addressing a set of gendered, racialized, and economically determined structural determinants of health. The term "reproductive justice" was coined in the 1990s as a Black feminist

---

[5] Dobbs v. Jackson Women's Health Organization, No. 19–1392, 597 U.S. 215 (2022).

response to White feminist movement approaches to reproductive health and rights (SisterSong, n.d.). It was intentionally intersectional, meaning that the goal was to include the myriad ways Black, Latina, AIAN, and other racially and ethnically minoritized women, as well low-income White women, in particular experienced threats to bodily autonomy and reproductive dignity, something largely excluded from early feminist movements that centered on middle class and wealthy White women. Reproductive justice as a movement and conceptual framework made more explicit that true reproductive freedom had to include rights to have a child under the condition of one's choosing (SisterSong, n.d.). This was responsive to injustices faced by Black, Latina, AIAN, and other racially and ethnically minoritized women, as well as women in poverty, including forced sterilization and medical experimentation with the first birth control pill on Puerto Rican women (Larson, 2021; NASEM, 2023b; Novak et al., 2018; Pendergrass and Raji, 2017; Stern, 2020; Washington, 2006). It is important to consider the evolution of NIH within this broader context and the effect this may have had on WHR.

Reproductive justice also includes as a central tenet that parents have a right to raise and care for their children in safe and healthy environments (SisterSong, n.d.). This final component focused on safe and healthy birthing and parental rights and has helped expand what it meant to advocate for reproductive justice and not just simply rights to reproductive control (Daniel, 2021). In this way, reproductive justice as a framework indicates that laws and policies that have allowed for forced sterilization of racially and ethnically minoritized women, unethical experimentation with the birth control pill on women, and other policies, such as the Indian Adoption Project, that have taken away parenting rights, fall under the rubric of gendered policies affecting women's health (Adoption History Project, n.d.; Larson, 2021; Lawrence, 2000; Lopez, 2008; Pendergrass and Raji, 2017; Price and Darity, 2010; Stern, 2005).

The reproductive justice framework can be further expanded to a queer-inclusive lens. It is crucial to acknowledge that many of the issues Black feminists identified in the early 1990s are still prominent in the lives of many cis queer women, trans men, and nonbinary individuals assigned female at birth. An expanded framework is needed to address rights to access alternative insemination, reproductive technologies, gender-affirming care, and rights related to sexual behavior and orientation. Some reproductive justice advocates and scholars assert a fourth tenet—the human right to disassociate sex from reproduction and that healthy sexuality and pleasure are essential to whole and full human life (NASEM, 2021c; Virginia Sexual and Domestic Violence Action Alliance, n.d.; Well Project, 2024; Welleck and Yeung, n.d.).

As a facilitator of health, Medicaid expansion is associated with lower rates of maternal mortality, especially among Black people (Eliason, 2020).

Sexually transmitted infection diagnoses among adolescent SMW are significantly lower in states with lower structural stigma (compared to states with higher structural stigma), and sexual orientation antidiscrimination laws have been linked to lower maternal hypertension among Black and White lesbian and bisexual women (Charlton et al., 2019; Everett and Agénor, 2023). In addition, Earned Income Tax Credit laws are associated with decreased low birthweight, especially among Black people (Komro et al., 2019). These findings underscore how targeted policy interventions can address sexual and reproductive health inequities and the need to research how policy impacts health outcomes.

Rights for SGM

Over the past decade, U.S. legislative and judiciary bodies have set policies that have both affirmed and denied the rights of SGM populations. These legal shifts, and the cultural shifts they represent, are relevant structures that produce needs for health care and manage the contexts in which it is sought. Laws and policies related to gender-affirming care and sexuality rights are the contexts in which women's health must be navigated. In addition, Supreme Court decisions, such as *Obergefell v. Hodges*,[6] resulting in the federal right to same-sex marriage, and *Bostock v. Clayton County*,[7] affirming that prohibiting sex discrimination in Title VII of the Civil Rights Act of 1964[8] protects employees against discrimination based on sexual orientation or transgender status, can affect women's health by reducing stigma and discrimination and increasing access to insurance and economic stability through spouses and employers (National Constitution Center, n.d.; U.S. Equal Employment Opportunity Commission, n.d.). Similarly, the Affordable Care Act Section 1557 names sexual orientation and gender identity as protected in public health insurance coverage (HHS, 2024).

Numerous laws and policies at the federal and state level affect TNB individuals' health, well-being, and health care quality and access. These include laws and policies that impede or protect TNB people's ability to participate in sports, use restrooms, update identification documents in accordance with their gender identity, access health care, particularly gender-affirming care, or maintain protection from discrimination in housing or other domains (Hohne, 2023; Movement Advancement Project, n.d.-a,b,c,d,e,f,g,h). Recent years have seen an increase in proposed state legislation aimed at limiting their rights, with over 560 such bills under consideration in 2023 (Hohne, 2023). Numerous bills have banned gender-affirming care for transgender

---

[6] Obergefell v. Hodges, No. 14–556, 576 U.S. (2015).
[7] Bostock v. Clayton County, No. 17–1618, 590 U.S. (2020).
[8] Public Law 88-352, 78 Stat. 241 (July 2, 1964).

youth, including banning medication and/or surgical care and sometimes making it a crime for clinicians to provide these (Movement Advancement Project, n.d.-a). Although these legislative efforts primarily restrict care for TNB youth, some state bills are restricting or attempting to restrict gender-affirming care for adults as well (Goldman, 2024). In 10 states, Medicaid policy explicitly excludes coverage of gender-affirming care for individuals of all ages (Movement Advancement Project, n.d.-g).

Conversely, some state laws protect access to health care for TNB people; 14 states and the District of Columbia (DC) have "shield" laws that aim to protect transgender individuals, their families, and medical providers traveling from a state where gender-affirming care is banned to provide or receive it (Movement Advancement Project, n.d.-h). Laws in 24 states and DC prohibit insurers from refusing to cover such care (Movement Advancement Project, n.d.-c). Other protective policies include the prohibition of health insurance discrimination based on gender identity and Medicaid policies that explicitly cover gender-affirming care (Movement Advancement Project, n.d.-c,g).

Summary of Structural Determinants of Health

Structures such as sexism, racism, colonialism, discrimination against SGM individuals, and laws and policies related to reproductive justice and SGM rights have important implications for women's health. Although many of these themes have traditionally been outside the scope of NIH's work, NIH is increasingly emphasizing the importance of this knowledge, particularly by creating the National Institute on Minority Health and Health Disparities. To advance health for all women, it is critical to understand how outcomes are affected by sex and gender and the range of additional identities and larger structural and policy contexts that shape women's experiences.

SDOH

Health Care Quality and Access

In Chapter 1, the committee introduced Heise and colleagues' (2019) framework on the gender system and health (see Figure 1-3), which reflects considerations that guided the committee. It also illustrates how health inequities and outcomes result from gendered pathways to health, including gendered impacts on care access and gender-biased health systems and health research, institutions, and data collection. Access to and use of the health care system, including insurance coverage and ability to pay, is gendered (Bertakis et al., 2000; KFF, 2023b; Lopes et al., 2024). Reports of negative experiences during health care encounters and with clinicians also vary by gender (Long et al., 2023). The knowledge with which clinicians and researchers operate to promote health and prevent and treat disease for women is also affected by the gendered health system (Mirin, 2021). Chapter 2 also discusses intersecting barriers to health care with differential effects on women.

Because of the lack of research on women's health and female physiology commensurate with that of men, it is not possible for clinicians to provide evidence-based care for women to the same degree. This problem exists across many diseases for which diagnoses and treatments have been fitted to the presentation and disease course in men, ranging from autism to many aspects of CVD, including aortic stenosis (D'Mello et al., 2022; Merone et al., 2022; Tribouilloy et al., 2021; Wenger et al., 2022). The deficit is more stark in diseases and conditions specific to women, which continue to receive comparatively little funding (Mirin, 2021) (see Chapter 4). Thus, the evidence base for diagnosis in women is limited at best. Similarly, more studies are needed on physical health disparities, chronic conditions, and access to preventive care for TNB people to ensure clinicians have the evidence for effective treatment and intervention. Failure to invest in women's health and sex differences research results in constrained choices for both women and clinicians, suboptimal care, and increased disease burden. Furthermore, studies indicate that the gaps in the knowledge base create an opportunity for high-impact science through funding of research on women's health (Baird et al., 2021a,b,c, 2022).

Despite the more limited evidence base for women's health care, women are more likely to use health care services than men and also play a central role in navigating health care services for themselves and their families (Bertakis et al., 2000; KFF, 2022b). This role of family caregiving and increased connectedness with the health care system may be an important facilitating factor for better health outcomes. While women are less likely to lack insurance coverage than men, they are more likely to have Medicaid (KFF, 2023b). Health insurance coverage is not the only indicator of health care access or quality of care. Access is also shaped by availability of care, timely appointments, geographic accessibility, affordable transportation, and health literacy to understand and carry out treatment plans (AHRQ, 2021; Cyr et al., 2019; Levy and Janke, 2016; NASEM, 2023b). The burden of health care costs is disproportionately felt by women, who spend over 18 percent more per year in out-of-pocket medical expenses than men, excluding pregnancy-related care, and more frequently delay medical care because of cost considerations (Deloitte, n.d.; Saad, 2023). Women are also more likely than men to report cost-related barriers to care, trouble paying deductibles, and medical debt (Lopes et al., 2024).

A higher share of women than men report negative experiences with a health care provider, at 38 and 32 percent, respectively (Long et al., 2023).

Among reports from women ages 18–64 who had seen a provider within the past 2 years, 29 percent had their concerns dismissed, 15 percent had a provider not believe them, and 13 percent had their doctor blame them for a health problem. Reports of negative experiences were higher among women who were low income, living with a disability or chronic condition, Black or Hispanic, and covered by Medicaid or uninsured (Long et al., 2023). Mistreatment during childbirth is common, particularly for racially and ethnically minoritized individuals, and may include loss of autonomy and being shouted at, ignored, or refused care (Vedam et al., 2019). Data illustrate significant racial inequities in maternal outcomes, often rooted in discrimination and clinician bias (Fernandez et al., 2024; Gunja et al., 2024; Tucker et al., 2007). For example, research shows that Black birthing people receive worse-quality care than White birthing people, including in measures of care process, outcomes, and perceptions (Gunja et al., 2024). In a 2023 study, 20 percent of those surveyed reported experiences of mistreatment during maternity care, with 30 percent of Black, 29 percent of Hispanic, and 27 percent of multiracial birthing people reporting mistreatment (Mohamoud et al., 2023). The most common types were receiving no response to requests for help, being shouted at or scolded, not having their physical privacy protected, being threatened with withholding treatment, and being made to accept unwanted treatment (Mohamoud et al., 2023).

How sexual orientation and gender identity affect access to care is also a critical consideration. For example, transgender people and cisgender bisexual women are almost twice as likely to report an unmet need for mental health care compared to cisgender heterosexual women (Steele et al., 2017). In addition, as discussed, laws and policies governing health care access for transgender individuals vary across the country, leaving them particularly vulnerable to lack of access to care and inequitable care. Discrimination is also a factor. Based on survey data from Lambda Legal (2010), about 70 percent of transgender and gender-nonconforming people report that they experienced one or more types of discriminatory acts in the health care setting: 26.7 percent were refused care, 20.9 percent were subjected to harsh or abusive language, and 20.3 percent were blamed for their health status (Figure 6-3). In addition, 73.0 percent reported that they believe medical personnel will treat them differently because they are transgender. These realities drive transgender people to delay or avoid care. Citing health care discrimination, more than 25 percent reported delaying or avoiding care when sick or injured, and 33 percent reported delaying preventive care. This can result in poorer health outcomes and increase the possibility of especially serious health consequences, such as late-stage cancer diagnoses, and complications of chronic conditions, such as heart disease and diabetes (Movement Advancement Project and Center for American Progress, 2024).

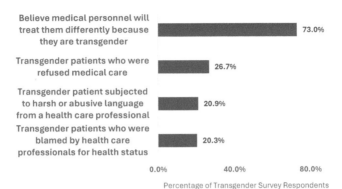

FIGURE 6-3 Transgender people report high rates of health care discrimination. SOURCE: Data from Lambda Legal, 2010. Adapted from Movement Advancement Project and Center for American Progress, 2024.

Data Gaps

While there are many data gaps related to social determinants for women's health in the health care realm, data gaps in pregnancy-related spheres are one striking example. A lack of robust measurements that help investigators tie community and structural drivers to pregnancy outcomes stymies advancement in understanding the upstream forces responsible for health outcomes inequities. For example, data and measures to capture domains of structural racism remain in their infancy (Headen et al., 2022). Novel approaches that combine qualitative or narrative data, geographic information systems technologies, machine learning, and social "big data" could help to fill data gaps surrounding environmental exposures, neighborhood conditions, and political and social capital that impact pregnancy and abortion outcomes. Understanding upstream social and community factors and their relationship to biological, genetic, and epigenetic processes can provide leverage points for intervention and policy change that could close gaps in pregnancy outcomes by race, ethnicity, income, or geography.

Economic Stability and Employment

Income and Poverty

Women in the United States experience persistent economic inequities that are further exacerbated among racially and ethnically minorized and SGM women (Badgett et al., 2019; Kochhar, 2023; Walker et al., 2021). Sex and gender bias result in systemic differences that leave women over-represented in certain occupations compared to men, such as caregiving and low-paid administrative positions (Frank et al., 2023). Poverty is more prevalent among women compared to men across all age groups (Shrider et al., 2023). Despite an overall trend toward narrowing the gender pay gap, White women still earn 83 percent of what their male counterparts do, while Asian, Black, and Hispanic women earn 93, 70, and 65 percent, respectively, of what White men do (Kochhar, 2023). Mothers and parents experience economic disparities most acutely, and 26.8 percent of female head-of-household families live in poverty (Creamer and Mohanty, 2019). Nationally, in 2021, working mothers of children under 18 earned 61.7 cents for every dollar made by working fathers (Institute for Women's Policy Research, 2023).

Poverty rates also vary by sexual orientation and gender identity. Rates are higher among cisgender bisexual women and transgender individuals, at 29.4 percent each, than cisgender straight or lesbian women, at 17.8 and 17.9 percent, respectively (Badgett et al., 2019). As discussed, *Bostock v. Clayton County* affirmed that Title VII of the Civil Rights Act of 1964 protects transgender people from employment discrimination (U.S. Equal Employment Opportunity Commission, n.d.). However, it only applies to employers with 15 or more employees. Laws in just 24 states, three territories, and DC provide additional protections, leaving transgender people especially at risk of being unfairly denied employment or forced out of jobs by harassment, mistreatment, or discrimination (Movement Advancement Project, n.d.-b; Movement Advancement Project and Center for American Progress, 2024).

A clear association exists between the effect of poverty on health arising from lack of insurance or access to care. However, poverty also affects physical and mental health through other mechanisms. For example, it can reduce access to other conditions that enable good health, including safe neighborhoods and housing and healthy food (OASH, n.d.-c). These gendered pathways link socioeconomic status and health across the life course, including for conditions such as chronic pain, depression, and cardiometabolic diseases (NASEM, 2024a).

Individuals' experiences with the criminal-legal system can also affect their economic standing. For example, incarceration is associated with a 52 percent reduction in annual earnings and with employment in low-paying jobs, which affects earnings growth for life (Craigie et al., 2020; NASEM, 2023b). Women face distinct economic challenges during and after incarceration, including specific financial issues that affect their success during reentry; for example, low and stagnant wages are a major financial barrier (Callahan et al., 2016). These data have particularly important implications for transgender individuals, who are overrepresented among incarcerated individuals because of vulnerabilities, such as family rejection and homelessness, unfair school disciplinary policies, and employment and housing discrimination, and laws and policies such as the criminalization of sex work, drug laws, police profiling, and inaccurate/misgendering identity documents (Center for American Progress, 2016b).

Employment and the Workplace

Workplace factors, such as employer benefits and sex and age discrimination, also affect health (Goodman et al., 2021; Rochon et al., 2021). Age discrimination in the workplace is more prominent for women and can have negative consequences, including on recruitment, access to career opportunities, and pensions. Across the life course, inequity in opportunity and policies such as loss of pension contributions during maternity leave have resulted in women receiving 27 percent fewer annual pension payments than men in Organization for Economic Co-operation and Development countries (Rochon et al., 2021).

Access to workforce support and protection, such as paid sick leave, health insurance, other benefits, and minimum wage and overtime laws, is an important consideration for women's health. Women are more likely than men to stay home to care for sick children and hold part-time jobs, which are less likely to offer paid sick leave (KFF, 2021). According to the Department of Labor, mothers provide an average of $295,000 of unpaid care for children and adults throughout their lifetime, based on the 2021 U.S. dollar value (DOL, 2023). Paid parental leave offers several economic and health benefits, including reducing the risk of poverty, especially among single mothers with lower income and education (Goodman et al., 2021). In addition, a recent analysis of state-level paid sick leave policies in three states found that it reduced the days that women experienced poor physical and mental health (Slopen, 2023).

There are also racial and ethnic inequities in employment benefits and protections, with non-Hispanic Black and Hispanic women receiving fewer weeks of paid family leave on average and less access to it through both their employers and government programs in comparison to non-Hispanic White and Asian women (Goodman et al., 2021). Racially and ethnically minoritized women are also overrepresented in some low-wage occupations that lack benefits. For example, they make up approximately two-thirds of home health workers (Yearby, 2022). Historically, laws both segregated these women, especially Black women, into these occupations and excluded them from efforts to improve worker conditions (e.g., the Fair Labor Standards Act of 1938 [FLSA][9] and the Social Security Act of 1935[10]). Although FLSA and the Social Security Act were amended to include domestic workers

---

[9] 29 U.S.C. §201 *et seq.*
[10] 42 U.S.C. §301 *et seq.*

in 1974 and 1950, respectively, policies allowing home health workers to be labeled as independent contractors excludes many from FLSA protections (Kijakazi et al., 2019; Yearby, 2022).

Scholars and advocates of law reform and policies to improve economic well-being and justice for women have focused on policies such as wage equity, paid family leave, childcare, and social safety net programs, such as the Supplemental Nutrition Assistance Program, Temporary Assistance for Needy Families, the Children's Health Insurance Program, and the Earned Income Tax Credit (NASEM, 2019a,b, 2024d). Despite progress, significant financial insecurity remains for many women and families with young children, including lack of support for those who stay home to care for children and a lack of affordable childcare and early childhood education options. In addition, the control of paid family, medical, and sick leave policies at the state and local rather than federal level introduces inequities (Goodman et al., 2021; KFF, 2021; Slopen, 2023). Consideration of factors such as poverty and the workplace in WHR, and how these policies might be improved and expanded, is needed to support the health of working women and their families.

Caregiving

While many workplace family leave policies have improved support for childcare (e.g., childbearing, childrearing), support for informal caregiving and eldercare has lagged. Because many leave policies are structured to require time to be taken consecutively, they do not account for the often acute and unanticipated needs of informal caregiving and eldercare, resulting in lost wages. Informal caregivers provide uncompensated care to ill or disabled family members and friends (Rennels et al., 2024). Women are disproportionately represented, accounting for two of every three caregivers (Sosa and Mangurian, 2023). Based on data from the Behavioral Risk Factor Surveillance System, one in four women are caregivers compared to one in five men. The data also illustrate the physical and emotional toll of caregiving, with 14.5 and 17.6 percent of caregivers reported experiencing 14 or more mentally or physically unhealthy days in the past 30 days, respectively. In addition, 36.7 percent of caregivers reported getting insufficient sleep, defined as fewer than 7 hours in a 24-hour period (CDC, n.d.-c).

Caregiving also has unique effects on racially and ethnically minoritized women. The Centers for Disease Control and Prevention estimates that one-third of AIAN adults are caregivers, and 60 percent of them are women (CDC, n.d.-b). Data from the American Association of Retired Persons shows that non-White caregivers (both men and women) provide more hours of care each week than White caregivers and experience a higher burden of high-intensity care (AARP and National Alliance for Caregiving, 2020). For example, Black and Hispanic cancer caregivers (both men and women) spend more time, take on more tasks, and face greater financial burdens compared to their non-Hispanic White counterparts. However, they report similar or lower levels of social, emotional, and health-related burdens. Differences in social support and caregiving preparedness between racial groups partially account for the inequities in burden. To address these inequities, research and policy need to focus on alleviating the financial strain experienced by Black and Hispanic caregivers and on the lack of support services (Fenton et al., 2022).

Nurses and other health care providers often take on unpaid caregiving for family members, resulting in negative health consequences, such as shorter sleep duration and poorer sleep quality (DePasquale et al., 2019). Women working in nursing homes also experience higher perceived stress, poorer psychological well-being, and more family–work conflict than those without additional unpaid caregiving responsibilities, whether for children or elders (DePasquale et al., 2016). For conditions with a high caregiving burden, such as dementia, women reduce their work hours or tend to leave the workforce altogether because of the time required, reducing the gross domestic product (Kubendran et al., 2016). Lack of policies to support informal caregiving and eldercare also negatively affects the physician workforce caring for and conducting research on women's health (see Chapter 8).

Social and Community Context

The social and community context influences women's health in a number of ways. For example, strong social networks provide emotional support and practical help, such as childcare or transportation, which can alleviate stress and improve health outcomes. Women with robust social ties often experience better mental health and can better manage chronic conditions (NASEM, 2024a).

Safe neighborhoods with supportive community structures contribute to overall well-being. Civic engagement and active participation in community activities and organizations can enhance a sense of belonging and social support, leading to better mental health and overall well-being (NASEM, 2023a,b; Rippel Foundation, n.d.). Social norms and expectations regarding gender roles can affect women's health by influencing access to health care, autonomy, and opportunities for education and employment. Conversely, norms that restrict women's choices or access to resources can contribute to poorer health outcomes. Another crucial aspect of the social and community context is violence, which profoundly affects women's health and is explored next.

Violence Against Women

Violence against women is common worldwide, with over 35 percent of women reporting experiences of domestic violence, abuse, and intimate and non-intimate partner sexual violence. Women experiencing violence are three-, four-, and seven-fold more likely to suffer from depression, anxiety disorders, and post-traumatic stress disorder, respectively (Oram et al., 2017).

Violence and abuse that starts in childhood can have lifelong, negative effects on a woman's health. *Advancing Research on Chronic Conditions in Women* describes how early experiences of trauma, also called adverse childhood experiences (ACEs) or early life adversity and which encompass verbal, emotional, physical, and sexual abuse, lead to physiological changes that affect the development of chronic conditions in women (NASEM, 2024a). Research has described associations between such traumatic experiences and seemingly disparate conditions such as endometriosis, vulvodynia, and fibroids, which are female specific, and depression, chronic pain, heart disease, stroke, and autoimmune disease, which occur predominantly or differently in women (Felitti et al., 1998; NASEM, 2024a). Research has identified sex and gender differences in the frequency and type of trauma experienced, with women experiencing more ACEs than men (Haahr-Pedersen et al., 2020). Other studies have reported higher prevalence of ACEs in women compared to men (Haahr-Pedersen et al., 2020; Hurley et al., 2022). Further research is needed to understand precisely how trauma alters women's mental and physical health across the life course, how gender-related social factors make women vulnerable to trauma, and how to mitigate trauma risks and the later detrimental health consequences in women (NASEM, 2024c).

Intimate partner violence (IPV) is the leading cause of injury among women and is associated with physical injuries (NASEM, 2024b). Furthermore, IPV is associated with adverse outcomes in sexual and reproductive health (including gynecologic infections, HIV/AIDS and other sexually transmitted infections, and unintended pregnancies) and mental health (such as anxiety, post-traumatic stress disorder, depression, substance misuse, suicidality, and eating disorders). Essential health care services for IPV can include universal screening paired with education, enduring safety planning centered on women's needs, and referrals to care and support services (NASEM, 2024b).

Violence against women and Two-Spirit individuals is of large concern among AIAN people. Homicide is the seventh leading cause of death among AIAN females aged 1–54 (Petrosky et al., 2021). Native women are also 2.5 times more likely to be raped than non-Native women (Urban Indian Health Institute, n.d.). A 2011 study by the National Gay & Lesbian Task Force found that 45 percent of Two-Spirit people reported family violence, 55 percent were harassed by shelter staff while at a shelter, and 22 percent were sexually assaulted by shelter residents or staff (Tribal Information Exchange, n.d.). Moreover, violence against AIAN women and Two-Spirit individuals is often underreported, given the lack of trust in law enforcement and jurisdictional complexities. The interplay between tribal, federal, and state jurisdictions can complicate legal responses and justice.

Transgender individuals also face high rates of violence victimization, including IPV and bias-motivated murder and violence, which has important implications for their health and well-being (Coston, 2023). Data from the 2017 and 2018 National Crime Victimization Survey demonstrate that transgender people experience nearly four times more violence than cisgender people at 86.2 victimizations per 1,000 persons compared to 21.7, and households with a transgender person have higher rates of property victimization than cisgender households at 214.1 per 1,000 households versus 108 (Flores et al., 2021). Of reported hate violence in 2017, 17 percent involved anti-transgender bias. Of 52 reports of hate violence homicides in 2017, 52 percent were against transgender or gender-nonconforming people (National Coalition of Anti-Violence Programs, 2018). Furthermore, a 2020 systematic review and meta-analysis found that transgender individuals were 2.2 and 2.5 times more likely to experience physical and sexual IPV, respectively (Peitzmeier et al., 2020). Factors such as social isolation and economic vulnerability can leave them dependent on abusive partners. The National Coalition of Anti-Violence Programs found that 33 percent of violence reported as IPV, rather than as bias motivated, involved anti-transgender bias (Coston, 2023; National Coalition of Anti-Violence Programs, 2018). It is also common for transgender individuals to experience discrimination when seeking assistance from domestic violence shelters, police, or health care providers (Center for American Progress, 2016a; Peitzmeier et al., 2020).

Women with a disability are more likely to experience IPV, including sexual and physical violence, stalking, psychological aggression, and control of reproductive or sexual health, compared to women without a disability (CDC, 2023b). Disabilities can lead to social isolation, limiting women's access to supportive networks or resources. This isolation can make it harder for them to seek help or escape abusive situations (Anyango et al., 2023).

Violence against women profoundly affects their health outcomes, leading to both immediate and long-term consequences. The resulting physical injuries and psychological trauma contribute to a range of health issues, including chronic pain, mental health disorders, and increased susceptibility to other illnesses (Uvelli et al., 2023; Wuest et al., 2009, 2010). Systemic barriers, such as limited access to health care, stigma, and discrimination, exacerbate the effects. Addressing these challenges requires a comprehensive approach that includes improving access to support services, enhancing legal protections, and addressing the broader SDOH that contribute to the vulnerability of affected individuals (Arcaya et al., 2024; Gehris et al., 2023; Robinette et al., 2021).

Neighborhood and Built Environment

The neighborhood and built environment significantly affect women's health outcomes through a variety of mechanisms, encompassing both physical and social aspects (OASH, n.d.-d). For example, neighborhoods with closer proximity to health care services have improved access to preventive care, screenings, and treatment and more specialized services, such as maternal care, mental health support, or reproductive health services, and this can greatly affect women's health (OASH, n.d.-b). In general, people in unsafe neighborhoods may experience higher levels of anxiety and stress, and the perception of safety may affect women's willingness to engage in physical activity, seek health care, or use community resources (Gehris et al., 2023; Robinette et al., 2021). Environmental exposures and geography are additional factors with critical impacts on women's health and will be further explored in the following sections.

Geography

Geographic location can have critical impacts on women's health. For example, as discussed, laws and policies that affect TNB people's health, such as those that impede or protect their ability to participate in sports, use restrooms, update identification documents in accordance with their gender identity, access health care, particularly gender-affirming care, or maintain protection from discrimination in housing or other domains, vary by state (Hohne, 2023; Movement Advancement Project, n.d.-a,b,c,d,e,f,g,h). Other examples include the effects of state-level structural sexism and variability in the expansion of Medicaid and access to abortion services on women's health (Homan, 2019; KFF, 2023a; Margerison et al., 2020) (see Chapter 7 for more information).

In considering the impact of geography on women's health, rurality in particular is an important factor. For rural residents, high poverty and lack of opportunity can create challenges to staying healthy, causing difficulty accessing housing, education, jobs, health care, transportation, and healthy food. Low physician density and the small scale, limited staff, and limited resources of health systems pose challenges to the management of chronic conditions, access to timely care, and access to subspecialists. Furthermore, transportation challenges can create difficulties accessing even this limited available health care (NASEM, 2017, 2021b). Data suggest that fewer rural residents participate in clinical trials than urban residents, and they travel further to do so (Bharucha et al., 2021).

Rural women experience significant inequities compared to urban women, including higher rates of fair or poor self-reported health, unintentional injury and motor vehicle–related deaths, cerebrovascular disease deaths, suicide, cigarette smoking, obesity, difficulty with basic actions or limitation of complex activities, and incidence of cervical cancer. Additionally, fewer rural women receive recommended preventive screenings for breast and cervical cancer (ACOG Committee on Health Care for Underserved Women, 2014). In addressing gaps in women's health, it is critical to consider these and other ways they are affected by place.

Environmental Factors and Women's Health

Women may be at increased risk for some diseases associated with environmental exposures because of biological or behavioral differences. Health conditions such as endometriosis and uterine fibroids, reproductive health outcomes, female-specific cancers, and autoimmune diseases all have links to environmental causes (Corbett et al., 2022; Giudice, 2021; Haggerty et al., 2021; Hassan et al., 2024; Katz et al., 2016; Mallozzi et al., 2017; McCue and DeNicola, 2019; Rickard et al., 2022; Rudel et al., 2014; Stiel et al., 2016; Vallée et al., 2024; Van Loveren et al., 2001; Zlatnik, 2016).

Physiological differences between women and men significantly affect exposure, uptake, metabolism, and retention of toxic chemicals. Women's higher body fat content facilitates the accumulation of lipophilic chemicals, which can be released during weight fluctuations or lactation. Gender-specific metabolic pathways and enzyme activity differences can result in varying internal doses and toxic chemical responses (Silbergeld and Flaws, 2002). In addition, hormonal variations influence metabolic pathways and bone physiology, altering chemical processing and storage. For example, women's reproductive stages affect enzyme activity and bone mineral metabolism, influencing the body's interaction with toxic substances, such as lead and mercury. These factors underscore the crucial importance of gender-specific considerations in toxicology research and risk assessment, a complexity that is often overlooked (Silbergeld and Flaws, 2002).

As a result of socioeconomic factors and traditional gender roles, women experience environmental health risks disproportionately and uniquely (Moss, 2002). For example, exposure to air pollution increases the risk of adverse outcomes in pregnancy, such as preterm birth, low birthweight, and stillbirth. Moreover, data illustrate that racially and ethnically minoritized individuals are exposed to disproportionately high levels of air pollution, including Hispanic, African American, and Asian/Pacific Islander mothers, with more adverse pregnancy outcomes related to such exposure among Black and Hispanic people than Non-Hispanic White people (Dzekem et al., 2024). Additionally, while Black people are overall 40 percent more likely to have asthma than White people, Black women are 84 percent more likely to have asthma than Black men (NHLBI, 2023).

Additionally, spending more time at home can increase women's exposure to contaminants in drinking water (Silbergeld and Flaws, 2002). Despite evolving gender roles, women are still more likely to be primary caregivers and homemakers, placing them at risk of exposure to indoor pollutants from various sources, including household products, building materials, and outdoor air infiltration (Folletti et al., 2017; Rousseau et al., 2022). Cooking can increase exposure to particulate matter and gases (Kashtan et al., 2024). Hobbies such as arts and crafts can also increase women's exposure to metals in paints or jewelry-making materials (Silbergeld and Flaws, 2002).

Beauty and personal care products are known sources of potential exposure to toxic chemicals, and understanding the exposure pathway and disease risks requires further elucidation. For example, a study found toxic chemicals, such as lead and arsenic, in tampons, though some researchers have stated that these cannot leach out during use (Shearston et al., 2024). Phthalates and talc in vaginal douches and other feminine care products are associated with gynecological cancers (Zota and Shamasunder, 2017). Others have also documented the potentially carcinogenic effects of cosmetics, highlighting the need for additional research, particularly per- and polyfluoroalkyl substances in cosmetics (Balwierz et al., 2023; FDA, n.d.).

Products marketed to women for beauty, feminine hygiene, or other aspects of personal care may also contribute to racial and ethnic health disparities. Colorism, hair texture preferences, and odor discrimination can increase toxicant exposure (Zota and Shamasunder, 2017). For example, mercury in skin-lightening creams is associated with poisoning, neurotoxicity, and kidney damage. Parabens, a common ingredient in hair relaxers, are associated with precocious puberty and fibroids. Chemicals in hair relaxers marketed to Black women appear to be associated with both harmful exposures and disease risks (Zota and Shamasunder, 2017). One study that measured chemicals in hair products marketed to Black women found that root stimulators, hair lotions, and relaxers frequently contained nonylphenols and parabens, which were not always listed on the product label (Helm et al., 2018). Studies have shown a correlation between frequent and long-term use of these products and an increased risk of uterine cancer, an increased risk of breast cancer with lye-based relaxers, and increased risk of earlier menarche (Chang et al., 2022; Coogan et al., 2021; James-Todd et al., 2011; Wise et al., 2023).

Occupational hazards experienced by women include repetitive stress, exposure to violence, and exposure to solvents used in cleaning and sterilization. Women may be at increased risk for workplace-related mus-culoskeletal disorders such as sprains, strains, carpal tunnel syndrome, and tendonitis (CDC, n.d.-e). In addition, in 2020, 73 percent of victims who experienced trauma from nonfatal workplace violence were women (CDC, n.d.-a). Some occupational exposures linked to jobs with a higher percent-age of women are also associated with cancers that are female specific or more common in women. For example, hospital workers who sterilize medical equipment may be exposed to ethylene oxide, which is associated with breast cancer. Perchloroethylene, the main solvent in dry cleaning, may increase cervical cancer risk (CDC, n.d.-e). Women may also be less pro-tected when they participate in traditionally male-dominated fields because of ill-fitting personal protective equipment and can face additional stressors, such as sexual harassment (CDC, n.d.-e).

Despite growing evidence linking environmental exposures to wom-en's health issues, significant gaps remain in understanding these complex relationships. While epidemiological studies suggest associations between environmental exposures and various health conditions in women, more research is needed to establish causal links. Multiple factors are associated with most outcomes, and the timing of the exposure, intensity, and duration also contribute. A deeper understanding of how environmental exposures at different life stages (prenatal, puberty, pregnancy, menopause transi-tion) affect women's health across the life-span is needed. This includes investigating potential long-term consequences of exposures during critical developmental windows. Research also needs to explore how interactions between chemicals and pollutants influence women's health outcomes; NIH could fund this type of research.

Gaps also exist concerning the specific vulnerabilities faced by racially and ethnically minoritized, low-income, and immigrant women. These groups may experience heightened risks arising from factors such as resi-dential segregation near pollution sources, limited access to health care, and cultural practices that increase exposure (NASEM, 2023b).

Developing and promoting safer alternatives to potentially harmful chemicals in consumer products, building materials, and personal care items is crucial to reduce women's exposure risks. Although many are marketed as safer or greening cleaning products, few studies have confirmed that they effectively reduce exposure to toxic chemicals (Sieck et al., 2024).

Education Access and Quality

Education, as an SDOH, has an effect on health in a number of ways, including improving health literacy, access to health care, economic stabil-ity, and health behaviors. Education can drive opportunity and reproduce inequality (Zajacova and Lawrence, 2018). For example, individuals with higher education levels generally have greater health literacy, leading to a better understanding of health information and more informed medical choices (Coughlin et al., 2020; NASEM, 2021a). Higher levels of education often correlate with increased use of preventive health services, such as screenings and vaccinations, which can lead to earlier detection and better management of conditions, better employment opportunities, and access to health insurance, improving overall health outcomes (NASEM, 2017). Conversely, poor health not only results from lower educational attainment but also can cause educational setbacks and diminished success because of recurrent absences and difficulty concentrating in class.

Associations between education and health and survival are well documented, but whether their strength depends on gender is not, with few studies on U.S. populations (Montez and Cheng, 2022; NASEM, 2017, 2019b; Raghupathi and Raghupathi, 2020). A study found that effects of education on perceived health and survival vary by gender but in contrasting ways: it significantly improves women's self-rated health more than men's, yet it has a greater effect on reducing men's mortality rates (Ross et al., 2012). Some studies have pointed to important health outcomes correlated with education for women. Globally, women with higher levels of education are more likely to have better mental and physical health, including lower rates of anxiety and depression (Kondirolli and Sunder, 2022). Studies have found that enhancing women's education leads to a decrease in their short- and long-term likelihood of psychological, physical, and sexual violence. It also reduced their chances of encountering any form of IPV and multiple forms of victimization (Villardón-Gallego et al., 2023; Weitzman, 2018).

In the United States, women are more likely than men to hold a bachelor's degree or higher. In 2022, 39 percent of women aged 25 and older had a bachelor's degree, compared to 36.2 percent of men in the same age group. Women also have a higher graduation rate from 4-year institutions, with 66.4 percent graduating within 4–6 years between 2015 and 2021, compared to 60.4 percent of men (WIA Report, 2022). Nevertheless, men continue to have an edge in certain professional fields, such as law, medicine, and dentistry (Nguyen Le et al., 2017). In 2022, men earned 1,869,000 professional degrees, while women earned 1,584,000 (Census Bureau, 2023). In addition, women with bachelor's degrees in social science or business earn over $1 million less than their male counterparts over their lifetimes. This gap widens to $1.6 million for business majors with graduate degrees and exceeds $1 million for women in law and public policy with advanced degrees (Carnevale et al., 2018).

Research is required to elucidate the specific pathways and mechanisms through which education influences women's health outcomes, including how it interacts with other SDOH and demographic factors, such as race, ethnicity, socioeconomic status, and geography.

Health Behaviors and SDOH

Another important consideration for women's health is the interaction of SDOH and health behaviors. SDOH create the conditions that shape health behaviors, and these behaviors can influence overall health outcomes. For example, poverty can limit access to healthful food, making eating less about an individual's choices and more about what choices are available. In addition, poverty restricts access to safe neighborhoods, potentially limiting the ability to be physically active (OASH, n.d.-c). Additionally, the built environment can significantly influence healthy behaviors and adherence to disease prevention guidelines. Factors such as access to supermarkets or grocery stores and to safe, walkable spaces for physical activity can facilitate or hinder healthy practices (Feskens et al., 2022). These challenges often disproportionately affect racially and ethnically minoritized women (Hilmers et al., 2012; NASEM, 2017; Pichardo et al., 2023). Health behaviors such as lack of physical inactivity, smoking, alcohol consumption, and poor diet can increase the risk of chronic conditions, such as diabetes, heart disease, and lung disease, thereby accounting for a significant portion of the country's burden of chronic illness (American Public Health Association, n.d.).

There are clear differences in health behaviors between men and women. Although women have lower rates of smoking, they engage in less regular physical activity, defined as more than 75 minutes per week. In the United States, 10.1 percent of women versus 13.1 percent of men smoke tobacco, 28.3 percent of women versus 38.9 percent of men engage regularly in vigorous physical activity, and 5.2 percent of women versus 8.1 percent of men report a moderate to severe alcohol use disorder in their lifetime (CDC, n.d.-d; Grant et al., 2016; Ji et al., 2024). Although the prevalence of alcohol use disorder is lower in women, alcohol-associated liver disease is often more severe in women, and they tend to develop it with less exposure to alcohol (Kezer et al., 2021). Moreover, data suggest that SMW may exhibit poorer health behaviors, such as heavy drinking and smoking, compared to heterosexual women (Baptiste-Roberts et al., 2017).

Societal factors can heavily affect women's health-promoting behaviors. For example, gender norms and cultural expectations uniquely shape women's health behaviors. As noted, caregiving responsibilities often fall more heavily on women, limiting time for self-care and health-promoting activities, such as exercise, and women in lower-wage jobs often have less access to workplace wellness programs and paid sick leave, impacting health behaviors (Kelley and Gilbert, 2023). Lower education levels have been linked to higher rates of obesity and smoking in women specifically (Baheiraei et al., 2015).

In general, the effects of health behaviors and programs to modify lifestyles in women have been understudied; as noted in Chapter 5, sex differences in the levels at which specific health behaviors are most beneficial remain understudied as well. More attention to understanding the crucial role of modifiable behaviors among women is needed within WHR. Integrating the structural and social determinants of health when studying mechanisms to improve health behaviors is needed to identify actionable interventions to improve health outcomes for women. At NIH, work on women's health would benefit from coordination with the NIH Office of Behavioral and Social Sciences Research.

Summary of SDOH

Social factors, such as health care quality and access, economic stability and employment, violence, and environment, all uniquely impact women's health outcomes. Without examining these factors and understanding the mechanisms by which they do so, the nation's WHR agenda will not be adequately prepared to achieve health equity for women.

RESILIENCE

Despite the barriers that inequities pose, women have worked to improve their social and health outcomes. Resilience among women, including racially and ethnically minoritized, transgender, and SGM individuals, often manifests in various ways. For example, many racially and ethnically minoritized and LGBTQIA+ women build and rely on strong community networks that provide emotional support, advocacy, and practical resources. These networks often help individuals navigate health care systems, access services, and share information about health resources (Ceatha et al., 2021; Hudson and Romanelli, 2020). Women from minoritized communities frequently engage in advocacy and activism to address health care disparities and push for policy changes (Kumanyika et al., 2001). For example, LGBTQ activists have fought for rights such as access to gender-affirming care and protection from discrimination (Center for American Progress, 2021). Transgender and gender minority individuals often develop coping strategies and resilience through mental health support groups, therapy, and peer support (DeBower, 2024). These resources help them manage the stress of discrimination and navigate the complexities of gender-affirming care. Moreover, data suggest that SMW in states with policy protections for lesbian, gay, and bisexual individuals may have better outcomes even relative to heterosexual women (Everett et al., 2022b, 2024a).

Culture as protection for health conditions is a concept gaining widespread traction in Western research, although it has always been known to AIAN people. If colonialism is at the root of negative health outcomes, then culture is needed to heal (University of Arizona Health Sciences, n.d.). Indigenous women and communities often draw on cultural traditions and

practices to maintain health and resilience. This can include traditional healing practices, community-based health initiatives, and cultural ceremonies
that promote mental and physical well-being. For example, the connection
to traditional foods can be an important aspect of cultural identity and resilience (Britwum and Demont, 2022; Wehi et al., 2023). Indigenous and other
researchers have pointed to asset models in research and health care that
emphasize the importance of community strengths and traditional health
practices as vital components of well-being (Kennedy et al., 2022; O'Keefe
et al., 2023). By focusing on these assets, researchers and practitioners can
leverage existing resources, cultural knowledge, and community networks to
enhance health outcomes. This approach recognizes the value of traditional
health practices and local expertise, fostering more inclusive and effective
health care solutions that build on the resilience and resources within communities. Integrating these strengths into health research and practice at
NIH can lead to more culturally relevant and sustainable interventions.

Many individuals from minoritized communities share their personal
stories of overcoming health barriers through platforms such as social
media, advocacy groups, and public speaking (Endometriosis Coalition,
n.d.; Fibroid Foundation, n.d.; National Menopause Foundation, n.d.;
PCOS Challenge, n.d.; Tight Lipped, n.d.). These stories highlight the
strength and resilience within these communities.

These examples underscore the diverse and resourceful ways women
demonstrate resilience in overcoming barriers to health and not only illustrate successful strategies for advancing women's health despite adversity
but also offer valuable insights for research to further enhance efforts to
improve women's health.

CONCLUDING OBSERVATIONS

The interplay among women, health, and society highlights the intri-
cate ways social structures, cultural norms, and systemic inequalities shape
women's health outcomes. Understanding it is essential for developing
evidence-based, effective interventions and policies that address not only
individual health needs but also the broader societal factors that influence
health. By recognizing and addressing these interconnected issues—ranging
from gender-based discrimination and economic disparities to access to
health care and social support—society can work toward creating structures
that support women's health needs, including filling the many research gaps
highlighted in this chapter. Understanding these underlying mechanisms
and how they affect health will increase the ability to achieve health equity
for women. The committee's recommendations for priority research areas,
including social and structural determinants of women's health, are in
Chapter 9—see Recommendation 8.

REFERENCES

AARP (American Association of Retired Persons) and National Alliance for Caregiving. 2020. *Caregiving in the United States 2020.* Washington, DC: American Association of Retired Persons.

ACOG (American College of Obstetricians and Gynecologists) Committee on Health Care for Underserved Women. 2014. ACOG committee opinion no. 586: Health disparities in rural women. *Obstetrics & Gynecology* 123(2 Pt 1):384–388.

Adoption History Project. n.d. *Indian Adoption Project.* https://pages.uoregon.edu/adoption/topics/IAP.html (accessed August 23, 2024).

Agénor, M., A. E. Pérez, A. Wilhoit, F. Almeda, B. M. Charlton, M. L. Evans, S. Borrero, and S. B. Austin. 2021. Contraceptive care disparities among sexual orientation identity and racial/ethnic subgroups of U.S. women: A national probability sample study. *Journal of Women's Health* 30(10):1406–1415.

Ahmed, A., D. P. Evans, J. Jackson, B. M. Meier, and C. Tomori. 2023. Dobbs v. Jackson Women's Health: Undermining public health, facilitating reproductive coercion. *Journal of Law, Medicine, & Ethics* 51(3):485–489.

AHRQ (Agency for Healthcare Research and Quality). 2021. *National healthcare quality & disparities reports 2021.* Rockville, MD: Agency for Healthcare Research and Quality.

American Cancer Society. 2024. *Cancer Facts for Lesbian and Bisexual Women.* https://www.cancer.org/cancer/risk-prevention/understanding-cancer-risk/cancer-facts/cancer-facts-for-lesbian-and-bisexual-women.html (accessed August 26, 2024).

American Heart Association. 2023. *Heart Health Is Sub-Optimal Among American Indian/Alaska Native Women, Supports Needed.* https://newsroom.heart.org/news/heart-health-is-sub-optimal-among-american-indianalaska-native-women-supports-needed (accessed August 26, 2024).

American Public Health Association. n.d. *Encourage Healthy Behaviors and Choices.* https://www.apha.org/what-is-public-health/generation-public-health/our-work/healthy-choices (accessed August 26, 2024).

Anyango, C., I. Goicolea, and F. Namatovu. 2023. Women with disabilities' experiences of intimate partner violence: A qualitative study from Sweden. *BMC Women's Health* 23(1):381.

Arcaya, M. C., I. G. Ellen, and J. Steil. 2024. Neighborhoods and health: Interventions at the neighborhood level could help advance health equity. *Health Affairs* 43(2):156–163.

Badgett, M., S. K. Choi, and B. D. Wilson. 2019. *LGBT poverty in the United States: A study of differences between sexual orientation and gender identity groups.* Los Angeles, CA: Williams Institute.

Baheiraei, A., F. Bakouei, E. Mohammadi, A. Montazeri, and M. Hosseni. 2015. The social determinants of health in association with women's health status of reproductive age: A population-based study. *Iranian Journal of Public Health* 44(1):119–129.

Baird, M. D., M. A. Zaber, A. Chen, A. W. Dick, C. E. Bird, M. Waymouth, G. Gahlon, D. D. Quigley, H. Al-Ibrahim, and L. Frank. 2021a. *The WHAM report: The case to fund women's health research: An economic and societal impact analysis.* Santa Monica, CA: RAND Corporation.

Baird, M. D., M. A. Zaber, A. W. Dick, C. E. Bird, A. Chen, M. Waymouth, G. Gahlon, D. D. Quigley, H. Al-Ibrahim, and L. Frank. 2021b. *Societal impact of research funding for women's health in Alzheimer's disease and Alzheimer's disease-related dementias.* Santa Monica, CA: RAND Corporation.

Baird, M. D., M. A. Zaber, A. W. Dick, C. E. Bird, A. Chen, M. Waymouth, G. Gahlon, D. D. Quigley, H. Al-Ibrahim, and L. Frank. 2021c. *Societal impact of research funding for women's health in coronary artery disease.* Santa Monica, CA: RAND Corporation.

Baird, M. D., M. A. Zaber, A. Chen, A. W. Dick, C. E. Bird, M. Waymouth, G. Gahlon, D. D. Quigley, H. Al-Ibrahim, and L. Frank. 2022. *Societal impact of research funding for women's health in rheumatoid arthritis.* Santa Monica, CA: RAND Corporation.

Balistreri, K. S. 2024. Structural sexism and breastfeeding in the United States, 2016–2021. *Maternal and Child Health Journal* 28(3):431–437.

Balwierz, R., P. Biernat, A. Jasińska-Balwierz, D. Siodłak, A. Kusakiewicz-Dawid, A. Kurek-Górecka, P. Olczyk, and W. Ochędzan-Siodłak. 2023. Potential carcinogens in makeup cosmetics. *International Journal of Environmental Research and Public Health* 20(6).

Baptiste-Roberts, K., E. Oranuba, N. Werts, and L. V. Edwards. 2017. Addressing health care disparities among sexual minorities. *Obstetrics and Gynecology Clinics of North America* 44(1):71–80.

Beccia, A. L., S. B. Austin, J. Baek, M. Agénor, S. Forrester, E. Y. Ding, W. M. Jesdale, and K. L. Lapane. 2022. Cumulative exposure to state-level structural sexism and risk of disordered eating: Results from a 20-year prospective cohort study. *Social Science & Medicine* 301:114956.

Beccia, A. L., M. Agénor, J. Baek, E. Y. Ding, K. L. Lapane, and S. B. Austin. 2024. Methods for structural sexism and population health research: Introducing a novel analytic framework to capture life-course and intersectional effects. *Social Science & Medicine* 351:116804.

Berger, M., and Z. Sarnyai. 2015. "More than skin deep": Stress neurobiology and mental health consequences of racial discrimination. *Stress* 18(1):1–10.

Bertakis, K. D., R. Azari, L. J. Helms, E. J. Callahan, and J. A. Robbins. 2000. Gender differences in the utilization of health care services. *Journal of Family Practice* 49(2):147–152.

Bharucha, A. E., C. I. Wi, S. G. Srinivasan, H. Choi, P. H. Wheeler, J. R. Stavlund, D. A. Keller, K. R. Bailey, and Y. J. Juhn. 2021. Participation of rural patients in clinical trials at a multisite academic medical center. *Journal of Clinical and Translational Science* 5(1):e190.

Biggs, M. A., R. Schroeder, M. T. Casebolt, B. I. Laureano, R. L. Wilson-Beattie, L. J. Ralph, S. Kaller, A. Adler, and M. W. Gichane. 2023. Access to reproductive health services among people with disabilities. *JAMA Network Open* 6(11):e2344877.

Bleich, S. N., J. F. Figueroa, and M. Minow. 2024. Institutional efforts to address legacies of slavery—implications for the health care system. *JAMA Health Forum* 5(3):e240785.

Britwum, K., and M. Demont. 2022. Food security and the cultural heritage missing link. *Global Food Security* 35:100660.

Brooks, V. R. 1981. *Minority stress and lesbian women.* Lexington, MA: Lexington Books.

Brown-Rice, K. 2013. Examining the theory of historical trauma among Native Americans. *Professional Counselor* 3(3):117–130.

Brydon, M. 2022. Weight bias: A consideration for medical radiation sciences. *Journal of Medical Imaging and Radiation Sciences* 53(4):534–537.

Callahan, S., L. A. Jason, and L. Robinson. 2016. Reducing economic disparities for female offenders: The Oxford House model. *Alcoholism Treatment Quarterly* 34(3):292–302.

Carnevale, A. P., N. Smith, and A. Gulish. 2018. *Women can't win: Despite making educational gains and pursuing high-wage majors, women still earn less than men.* Washington, DC: Georgetown University McCourt School of Public Policy.

Carroll, S. R., M. Suina, M. B. Jäger, J. Black, S. Cornell, A. A. Gonzales, M. Jorgensen, N. L. Palmanteer-Holder, J. S. De La Rosa, and N. I. Teufel-Shone. 2022. Reclaiming Indigenous health in the U.S.: Moving beyond the social determinants of health. *International Journal of Environmental Research and Public Health* 19(12).

CDC (Centers for Disease Control and Prevention). n.d.-a. *About Workplace Violence.* https://www.cdc.gov/niosh/violence/about/index.html (accessed October 21, 2024).

CDC. n.d.-b. *Caregiving Among American Indian/Alaska Native Adults.* https://www.cdc.gov/aging/data/infographic/2018/american-indian-adults-caregiving.html (accessed August 23, 2024).

CDC. n.d.-c. *Caregiving for Family and Friends—A Public Health Issue.* https://www.cdc.gov/aging/caregiving/pdf/caregiver-brief-508.pdf (accessed August 9, 2024).

CDC. n.d.-d. *Current Cigarette Smoking Among Adults in the United States.* https://www. cdc.gov/tobacco/data_statistics/fact_sheets/adult_data/cig_smoking/index.htm (accessed August 26, 2024).

CDC. n.d.-e. *Women's Safety and Health Issues at Work.* https://www.cdc.gov/niosh/ docs/2001–123/default.html (accessed August 26, 2024).

CDC. 2023a. *Cancer in American Indian and Alaska Native people.* https://www.cdc.gov/ cancer/research/cancer-in-american-indian-and-alaska-native-people.html (accessed August 26, 2024).

CDC. 2023b. *Supporting Women with Disabilities to Achieve Optimal Health.* https://www. cdc.gov/womens-health/features/women-disabilities.html (accessed August 26, 2024).

CDC. 2024. *Pregnancy-Related Deaths Among American Indian or Alaska Native Persons: Data from Maternal Mortality Review Committees in 38 U.S. States, 2020.* https://www. cdc.gov/maternal-mortality/php/data-research/aian-mmrc/index.html (accessed August 22, 2024).

Ceatha, N., A. C. C. Koay, C. Buggy, O. James, L. Tully, M. Bustillo, and D. Crowley. 2021. Protective factors for LGBTI+ youth wellbeing: A scoping review underpinned by recognition theory. *International Journal of Environmental Research and Public Health* 18(21).

Census Bureau. 2023. *Educational Attainment in the United States: 2022, Table 2.* https:// www.census.gov/data/tables/2022/demo/educational-attainment/cps-detailed-tables.html (accessed August 26, 2024).

Center for American Progress. 2016a. *Discrimination Against Transgender Women Seeking Access to Homeless Shelters.* https://www.americanprogress.org/article/discrimination-against-transgender-women-seeking-access-to-homeless-shelters/ (accessed August 23, 2024).

Center for American Progress. 2016b. *Unjust: How the broken criminal justice system fails LGBT people of color.* Washington, DC: Center for American Progress.

Center for American Progress. 2021. *Improving the lives and rights of LGBTQ people in America: A road map for the Biden administration.* Washington, DC: Center for American Progress.

Chang, C.-J., K. M. O'Brien, A. P. Keil, S. A. Gaston, C. L. Jackson, D. P. Sandler, and A. J. White. 2022. Use of straighteners and other hair products and incident uterine cancer. *Journal of the National Cancer Institute* 114(12):1636–1645.

Charlton, B. M., M. L. Hatzenbuehler, H. J. Jun, V. Sarda, A. R. Gordon, J. R. G. Raifman, and S. B. Austin. 2019. Structural stigma and sexual orientation-related reproductive health disparities in a longitudinal cohort study of female adolescents. *Journal of Adolescence* 74:183–187.

Charlton, B. M., B. G. Everett, A. Light, R. K. Jones, E. Janiak, A. J. Gaskins, J. E. Chavarro, H. Moseson, V. Sarda, and S. B. Austin. 2020. Sexual orientation differences in pregnancy and abortion across the lifecourse. *Women's Health Issues* 30(2):65–72.

Chen, S., and A. B. Mallory. 2021. The effect of racial discrimination on mental and physical health: A propensity score weighting approach. *Social Science & Medicine* 285:114308.

Chinn, J. J., I. K. Martin, and N. Redmond. 2021. Health equity among Black women in the United States. *Journal of Women's Health* 30(2):212–219.

Coogan, P. F., L. Rosenberg, J. R. Palmer, Y. C. Cozier, Y. M. Lenzy, and K. A. Bertrand. 2021. Hair product use and breast cancer incidence in the Black Women's Health study. *Carcinogenesis* 42(7):924–930.

Corbett, G. A., S. Lee, T. J. Woodruff, M. Hanson, M. Hod, A. M. Charlesworth, L. Giudice, J. Conry, and F. M. McAuliffe. 2022. Nutritional interventions to ameliorate the effect of endocrine disruptors on human reproductive health: A semi-structured review from FIGO. *International Journal of Gynecology & Obstetrics* 157(3):489–501.

Coston, B. E. 2023. Looking back: Intimate partner violence in transgender populations. *American Journal of Public Health* 113(5):474–476.

Coughlin, S. S., M. Vernon, C. Hatzigeorgiou, and V. George. 2020. Health literacy, social determinants of health, and disease prevention and control. *Journal of Environmental Health Science* 6(1).

Craigie, T. A., A. Grawert, and C. Kimble. 2020. *Conviction, imprisonment, and lost earnings: How involvement with the criminal justice system deepens inequality.* New York: Brennan Center for Justice.

Creamer, J., and A. Mohanty. 2019. *Poverty Rate for People in Female-Householder Families Lowest on Record—U.S. Poverty Rate Drops to 11.8% in 2018.* https://www.census.gov/library/stories/2019/09/poverty-rate-for-people-in-female-householder-families-lowest-on-record.html (accessed August 23, 2024).

Cree, R. A., C. A. Okoro, M. M. Zack, and E. Carbone. 2020. Frequent mental distress among adults, by disability status, disability type, and selected characteristics—United States, 2018. *MMWR* 69(36):1238–1243.

Cunningham, G. B., and P. Wicker. 2024. Sexual harassment and implicit gender-career biases negatively impact women's life expectancy in the U.S.: A state-level analysis, 2011–2019. *BMC Public Health* 24(1):1115.

Cyr, M. E., A. G. Etchin, B. J. Guthrie, and J. C. Benneyan. 2019. Access to specialty healthcare in urban versus rural U.S. populations: A systematic literature review. *BMC Health Services Research* 19(1):974.

D'Mello, A. M., I. R. Frosch, C. E. Li, A. L. Cardinaux, and J. D. E. Gabrieli. 2022. Exclusion of females in autism research: Empirical evidence for a "leaky" recruitment-to-research pipeline. *Autism Research* 15(10):1929–1940.

Daniel, M. 2021. The social movement for reproductive justice: Emergence, intersectional strategies, and theory building. *Sociology Compass* 15(8):e12907.

DeBower, J. 2024. *Worldbuilding: A theory of resilience in transgender and gender expansive young people.* New York: Social Welfare, City University of New York.

Deloitte. n.d. *Closing the Cost Gap: Strategies to Advance Women's Health Equity.* https://www2.deloitte.com/us/en/pages/life-sciences-and-health-care/articles/womens-health-equity-disparities.html?utm_source=newsletter&utm_medium=email&utm_campaign=newsletter_axiosvitals&stream=top (accessed August 23, 2024).

DePasquale, N., K. D. Davis, S. H. Zarit, P. Moen, L. B. Hammer, and D. M. Almeida. 2016. Combining formal and informal caregiving roles: The psychosocial implications of double- and triple-duty care. *Journals of Gerontology: Psychological Sciences* 71(2):201–211.

DePasquale, N., M. J. Sliwinski, S. H. Zarit, O. M. Buxton, and D. M. Almeida. 2019. Unpaid caregiving roles and sleep among women working in nursing homes: A longitudinal study. *Gerontologist* 59(3):474–485.

Diaz-Thomas, A. M., S. H. Golden, D. M. Dabelea, A. Grimberg, S. N. Magge, J. D. Safer, D. E. Shumer, and F. C. Stanford. 2023. Endocrine health and health care disparities in the pediatric and sexual and gender minority populations: An Endocrine Society scientific statement. *Journal of Clinical Endocrinology & Metabolism* 108(7):1533–1584.

DOL (Department of Labor). 2023. *Readout: U.S. Department of Labor Report Finds Impact of Caregiving on Mother's Wages Reduces Lifetime Earnings by 15 Percent.* https://www.dol.gov/newsroom/releases/wb/wb20230511#:~:text=The%20estimated%20employment-related%20costs%20for%20mothers%20providing%20unpaid,which%20also%20creates%20a%20reduction%20in%20retirement%20income. (accessed August 23, 2024).

Dolezsar, C. M., J. J. McGrath, A. J. M. Herzig, and S. B. Miller. 2014. Perceived racial discrimination and hypertension: A comprehensive systematic review. *Health Psychology* 33(1):20–34.

Dongarwar, D., V. Mercado-Evans, S. Adu-Gyamfi, M.-L. Laracuente, and H. M. Salihu. 2022. Racial/ethnic disparities in infertility treatment utilization in the U.S., 2011–2019. *Systems Biology in Reproductive Medicine* 68(3):180–189.

Dore, E. C., S. Shrivastava, and P. Homan. 2024. Structural sexism and preventive health care use in the United States. *Journal of Health and Social Behavior* 65(1):2–19.

Dzekem, B. S., B. Aschebrook-Kilfoy, and C. O. Olopade. 2024. Air pollution and racial disparities in pregnancy outcomes in the United States: A systematic review. *Journal of Racial and Ethnic Health Disparities* 11(1):535–544.

Edwards-Gayfield, P. n.d. *Weight Stigma.* https://www.nationaleatingdisorders.org/weight-stigma/ (accessed October 20, 2024).

Eliason, E. L. 2020. Adoption of Medicaid expansion is associated with lower maternal mortality. *Women's Health Issues* 30(3):147–152.

Eltoukhi, H. M., M. N. Modi, M. Weston, A. Y. Armstrong, and E. A. Stewart. 2014. The health disparities of uterine fibroid tumors for African American women: A public health issue. *American Journal of Obstetrics & Gynecology* 210(3):194–199.

Endometriosis Coalition. n.d. *The Endo Co: What We Do.* https://www.theendo.co/what-we-do (accessed August 27, 2024).

Everett, B. G., and M. Agénor. 2023. Sexual orientation-related nondiscrimination laws and maternal hypertension among Black and White U.S. Women. *Journal of Women's Health* 32(1):118–124.

Everett, B. G., M. A. Kominiarek, S. Mollborn, D. E. Adkins, and T. L. Hughes. 2019. Sexual orientation disparities in pregnancy and infant outcomes. *Maternal and Child Health Journal* 23(1):72–81.

Everett, B. G., A. Limburg, P. Homan, and M. M. Philbin. 2022a. Structural heteropatriarchy and birth outcomes in the United States. *Demography* 59(1):89–110.

Everett, B. G., A. Limburg, S. McKetta, and M. L. Hatzenbuehler. 2022b. State-level regulations regarding the protection of sexual minorities and birth outcomes: Results from a population-based cohort study. *Psychosomatic Medicine* 84(6):658–668.

Everett, B. G., Z. Bergman, B. M. Charlton, and V. Barcelona. 2024a. Sexual orientation-specific policies are associated with prenatal care use in the first trimester among sexual minority women: Results from a prospective cohort study. *Annals of Behavioral Medicine* 58(9):594–602.

Everett, B. G., M. M. Philbin, and P. Homan. 2024b. Structural heteropatriarchy and maternal cardiovascular morbidities. *Social Science & Medicine* 351:116434.

FDA (Food and Drug Administration). n.d. *Per and Polyfluoroalkyl Substances (PFAS) in Cosmetics.* https://www.fda.gov/cosmetics/cosmetic-ingredients/and-polyfluoroalkyl-substances-pfas-cosmetics (accessed August 26, 2024).

Felitti, V. J., R. F. Anda, D. Nordenberg, D. F. Williamson, A. M. Spitz, V. Edwards, M. P. Koss, and J. S. Marks. 1998. Relationship of childhood abuse and household dysfunction to many of the leading causes of death in adults. The Adverse Childhood Experiences (ACE) study. *American Journal of Preventive Medicine* 14(4):245–258.

Fenton, A., K. A. Ornstein, P. Dilworth-Anderson, N. L. Keating, E. E. Kent, K. Litzelman, A. C. Enzinger, J. H. Rowland, and A. A. Wright. 2022. Racial and ethnic disparities in cancer caregiver burden and potential sociocultural mediators. *Supportive Care in Cancer* 30(11):9625–9633.

Fernandez, H., M. Ayo Vaughan, L. C. Zephyrin, and R. Block, Jr. 2024. *Revealing disparities: Health care workers' observations of discrimination against patients.* New York: The Commonwealth Fund.

Feskens, E. J. M., R. Bailey, Z. Bhutta, H. K. Biesalski, H. Eicher-Miller, K. Krämer, W. H. Pan, and J. C. Griffiths. 2022. Women's health: Optimal nutrition throughout the lifecycle. *European Journal of Nutrition* 61(Suppl 1):1–23.

Fibroid Foundation. n.d. *Fibroid Foundation: About Us.* https://www.fibroidfoundation.org/about/ (accessed August 27, 2024).

Flores, A. R., I. H. Meyer, L. Langton, and J. L. Herman. 2021. Gender identity disparities in criminal victimization: National crime victimization survey, 2017–2018. *American Journal of Public Health* 111(4):726–729.

Folletti, I., A. Siracusa, and G. Paolocci. 2017. Update on asthma and cleaning agents. *Current Opinion in Allergy and Clinical Immunology* 17(2):90–95.

Frank, J., C. Mustard, P. Smith, A. Siddiqi, Y. Cheng, A. Burdorf, and R. Rugulies. 2023. Work as a social determinant of health in high-income countries: Past, present, and future. *Lancet* 402(10410):1357–1367.

Friedman, C. 2024. Disparities in social determinants of health amongst people with disabilities. *International Journal of Disability, Development and Education* 71(1):101–117.

Gehris, J. S., A. L. Oyeyemi, M. L. Baishya, S. C. Roth, and M. Stoutenberg. 2023. The role of physical activity in the relationship between exposure to community violence and mental health: A systematic review. *Preventive Medicine Reports* 36:102509.

Geronimus, A. T., M. Hicken, D. Keene, and J. Bound. 2006. "Weathering" and age patterns of allostatic load scores among Blacks and Whites in the United States. *American Journal of Public Health* 96(5):826–833.

Giudice, L. C. 2021. Environmental impact on reproductive health and risk mitigating strategies. *Current Opinion in Obstetrics and Gynecology* 33(4):343–349.

Goldman, M. 2024. *States Are Limiting Gender-Affirming Care for Adults, Too.* https://www.axios.com/2024/01/10/trans-care-adults-red-states (accessed August 23, 2024).

Gonzalo-Encabo, P., N. Sami, R. L. Wilson, D. W. Kang, S. Ficarra, and C. M. Dieli-Conwright. 2023. Exercise as medicine in cardio-oncology: Reducing health disparities in Hispanic and Latina breast cancer survivors. *Current Oncology Reports* 25(11):1237–1245.

Goodman, J. M., C. Williams, and W. H. Dow. 2021. Racial/ethnic inequities in paid parental leave access. *Health Equity* 5(1):738–749.

Grant, B. F., T. D. Saha, W. J. Ruan, R. B. Goldstein, S. P. Chou, J. Jung, H. Zhang, S. M. Smith, R. P. Pickering, B. Huang, and D. S. Hasin. 2016. Epidemiology of DSM-5 drug use disorder: Results from the National Epidemiologic Survey on Alcohol and Related Conditions—III. *JAMA Psychiatry* 73(1):39–47.

Greer, T., and J. L. Lemacks. 2024. The medicine wheel as a public health approach to lifestyle management interventions for indigenous populations in North America. *Frontiers in Public Health* 12:1392517.

Gunja, M. Z., E. D. Gumas, R. Masitha, and L. C. Zephyrin. 2024. *Insights into the U.S. maternal mortality crisis: An international comparison.* New York: The Commonwealth Fund.

Haahr-Pedersen, I., C. Perera, P. Hyland, F. Vallières, D. Murphy, M. Hansen, P. Spitz, P. Hansen, and M. Cloitre. 2020. Females have more complex patterns of childhood adversity: Implications for mental, social, and emotional outcomes in adulthood. *European Journal of Psychotraumatology* 11(1):1708618.

Haggerty, D. K., K. Upson, D. C. Pacyga, J. E. Franko, J. M. Braun, and R. S. Strakovsky. 2021. Reproductive toxicology: Pregnancy exposure to endocrine disrupting chemicals: Implications for women's health. *Reproduction* 162(5):F169–F180.

Harlow, S. D., S.-A. M. Burnett-Bowie, G. A. Greendale, N. E. Avis, A. N. Reeves, T. R. Richards, and T. T. Lewis. 2022. Disparities in reproductive aging and midlife health between Black and White women: The study of Women's Health Across the Nation (SWAN). *Women's Midlife Health* 8(1):3.

Hassan, S., A. Thacharodi, A. Priya, R. Meenatchi, T. A. Hegde, T. R, H. T. Nguyen, and A. Pugazhendhi. 2024. Endocrine disruptors: Unravelling the link between chemical exposure and women's reproductive health. *Environmental Research* 241:117385.

Hatzenbuehler, M. L., and K. A. McLaughlin. 2014. Structural stigma and hypothalamic-pituitary-adrenocortical axis reactivity in lesbian, gay, and bisexual young adults. *Annals of Behavioral Medicine* 47(1):39–47.

Headen, I. E., M. A. Elovitz, A. N. Battarbee, J. O. Lo, and M. P. Debbink. 2022. Racism and perinatal health inequities research: Where we have been and where we should go. *American Journal of Obstetrics & Gynecology* 227(4):560–570.

Heise, L., M. E. Greene, N. Opper, M. Stavropoulou, C. Harper, M. Nascimento, D. Zewdie, G. L. Darmstadt, M. E. Greene, S. Hawkes, L. Heise, S. Henry, J. Heymann, J. Klugman, R. Levine, A. Raj, and G. Rao Gupta. 2019. Gender inequality and restrictive gender norms: Framing the challenges to health. *Lancet* 393(10189):2440–2454.

Helm, J. S., M. Nishioka, J. G. Brody, R. A. Rudel, and R. E. Dodson. 2018. Measurement of endocrine disrupting and asthma-associated chemicals in hair products used by Black women. *Environmental Research* 165:448–458.

HHS (Department of Health and Human Services). 2024. *Section 1557 of the Patient Protection and Affordable Care Act.* https://www.hhs.gov/civil-rights/for-individuals/section-1557/index.html (accessed August 27, 2024).

Hicken, M. T., H. Lee, J. Morenoff, J. S. House, and D. R. Williams. 2014. Racial/ethnic disparities in hypertension prevalence: Reconsidering the role of chronic stress. *American Journal of Public Health* 104(1):117–123.

Higgins, J. A., E. Carpenter, B. G. Everett, M. Z. Greene, S. Haider, and C. E. Hendrick. 2019. Sexual minority women and contraceptive use: Complex pathways between sexual orientation and health outcomes. *American Journal of Public Health* 109(12):1680–1686.

Hilmers, A., D. C. Hilmers, and J. Dave. 2012. Neighborhood disparities in access to healthy foods and their effects on environmental justice. *American Journal of Public Health* 102(9):1644–1654.

Hing, A. K., T. Chantarat, S. Fashaw-Walters, S. L. Hunt, and R. R. Hardeman. 2024. Instruments for racial health equity: A scoping review of structural racism measurement, 2019–2021. *Epidemiologic Reviews* 46(1):1–26.

Hohne, S. 2023. How to win the war on 100 fronts: What caused the rise of anti-trans bills and how to defeat them. *Georgetown Journal of Gender and the Law* XXV(1).

Homan, P. 2019. Structural sexism and health in the United States: A new perspective on health inequality and the gender system. *American Sociological Review* 84(3):486–516.

Homan, P. 2021. Sexism and health: Advancing knowledge through structural and intersectional approaches. *American Journal of Public Health* 111(10):1725–1727.

Howell, E. A. 2018. Reducing disparities in severe maternal morbidity and mortality. *Clinical Obstetrics and Gynecology* 61(2):387–399.

Hudson, K. D., and M. Romanelli. 2020. "We are powerful people": Health-promoting strengths of LGBTQ communities of color. *Qualitative Health Research* 30(8):1156–1170.

Hurley, L., A. Stillerman, J. Feinglass, and C. Percheski. 2022. Adverse childhood experiences among reproductive age women: Findings from the 2019 Behavioral Risk Factor Surveillance System. *Women's Health Issues* 32(5):517–525.

Institute for Women's Policy Research. 2023. *State by state, mothers are paid much less than fathers: The gender wage gap between mothers and fathers by state and by race and ethnicity.* Washington, DC: Institute for Women's Policy Research.

IOM (Institute of Medicine). 2013. *Leveraging culture to address health inequalities: Examples from Native communities: Workshop summary.* Edited by K. M. Anderson and S. Olson. Washington, DC: The National Academies Press.

Ives-Rublee, M., and A. Neal. 2024. *Eliminating Barriers to Employment for Disabled Women.* https://www.americanprogress.org/article/playbook-for-the-advancement-of-women-in-the-economy/eliminating-barriers-to-employment-for-disabled-women/#:~:text=Disabled%20women%20face%20employment%20gaps,disabled%20men%2C%20at%2024.8%20percent (accessed August 26, 2024).

Jahn, J. L., D. Zubizarreta, J. T. Chen, B. L. Needham, G. Samari, A. J. McGregor, M. Daugherty, Douglas, S. B. Austin, and M. Agénor. 2023. Legislating inequity: Structural racism in groups of state laws and associations with premature mortality rates. *Health Affairs* 42(10):1325–1333.

James-Todd, T., M. B. Terry, J. Rich-Edwards, A. Deierlein, and R. Senie. 2011. Childhood hair product use and earlier age at menarche in a racially diverse study population: A pilot study. *Annals of Epidemiology* 21(6):461–465.

Ji, H., M. Gulati, T. Y. Huang, A. C. Kwan, D. Ouyang, J. E. Ebinger, K. Casaletto, K. L. Moreau, H. Skali, and S. Cheng. 2024. Sex differences in association of physical activity with all-cause and cardiovascular mortality. *Journal of the American College of Cardiology* 83(8):783–793.

Kashtan, Y., M. Nicholson, C. J. Finnegan, Z. Ouyang, A. Garg, E. D. Lebel, S. T. Rowland, D. R. Michanowicz, J. Herrera, K. C. Nadeau, and R. B. Jackson. 2024. Nitrogen dioxide exposure, health outcomes, and associated demographic disparities due to gas and propane combustion by U.S. stoves. *Science Advances* 10(18):eadm8680.

Katon, J. G., T. C. Plowden, and E. E. Marsh. 2023. Racial disparities in uterine fibroids and endometriosis: A systematic review and application of social, structural, and political context. *Fertility and Sterility* 119(3):355–363.

Katz, T. A., Q. Yang, L. S. Treviño, C. L. Walker, and A. Al-Hendy. 2016. Endocrine-disrupting chemicals and uterine fibroids. *Fertility and Sterility* 106(4):967–977.

Kelley, J. A., and M. Gilbert. 2023. Structural sexism across the life course: How social inequality shapes women's later-life health. In *A Life Course Approach to Women's Health*, edited by G. Mishra, R. Hardy, and D. Kuh. Oxford, UK: Oxford University Press. Pp. 327–342.

Kennedy, A., A. Sehgal, J. Szabo, K. McGowan, G. Lindstrom, P. Roach, L. L. Crowshoe, and C. Barnabe. 2022. Indigenous strengths-based approaches to healthcare and health professions education—recognising the value of elders' teachings. *Health Education Journal* 81(4):423–438.

Kezer, C. A., D. A. Simonetto, and V. H. Shah. 2021. Sex differences in alcohol consumption and alcohol-associated liver disease. *Mayo Clinic Proceedings* 96(4):1006–1016.

KFF. n.d. *How History Has Shaped Racial and Ethnic Health Disparities.* https://www.kff.org/how-history-has-shaped-racial-and-ethnic-health-disparities-a-timeline-of-policies-and-events/ (accessed August 25, 2024).

KFF. 2021. *Paid Leave in the U.S.* https://www.kff.org/womens-health-policy/fact-sheet/paid-leave-in-u-s/ (accessed August 23, 2024).

KFF. 2022a. *Racial Disparities in Maternal and Infant Health: Current Status and Efforts to Address Them.* https://www.kff.org/racial-equity-and-health-policy/issue-brief/racial-disparities-in-maternal-and-infant-health-current-status-and-efforts-to-address-them/ (accessed August 22, 2024).

KFF. 2022b. *Workplace Benefits and Family Health Care Responsibilities: Key Findings from the 2022 KFF Women's Health Survey.* https://www.kff.org/womens-health-policy/issue-brief/workplace-benefits-and-family-health-care-responsibilities-key-findings-from-the-2022-kff-womens-health-survey/ (accessed August 25, 2024).

KFF. 2023a. *What Does the Recent Literature Say About Medicaid Expansion?: Impacts on Sexual and Reproductive Health.* https://www.kff.org/medicaid/issue-brief/what-does-the-recent-literature-say-about-medicaid-expansion-impacts-on-sexual-and-reproductive-health/ (accessed October 17, 2024).

KFF. 2023b. *Women's Health Insurance Coverage.* https://www.kff.org/womens-health-policy/fact-sheet/womens-health-insurance-coverage/ (accessed August 25, 2024).

KFF. 2024. *Abortion in the United States Dashboard.* https://www.kff.org/womens-health-policy/dashboard/abortion-in-the-u-s-dashboard/ (accessed August 15, 2024).

Kijakazi, K., K. Smith, and C. Runes. 2019. *African American economic security and the role of Social Security.* Washington, DC: Urban Institute.

Kochhar, R. 2023. *The Enduring Grip of the Gender Pay Gap.* https://www.pewresearch.org/social-trends/2023/03/01/the-enduring-grip-of-the-gender-pay-gap/#:~:text=Gender%20pay%20gap%20differs%20widely%20by%20race%20and%20ethnicity,-Looking%20across%20racial&text=In%202022%2C%20Black%20women%20earned,%2C%20making%2 (accessed August 23, 2024).

Komro, K. A., S. Markowitz, M. D. Livingston, and A. C. Wagenaar. 2019. Effects of state-level earned income tax credit laws on birth outcomes by race and ethnicity. *Health Equity* 3(1):61–67.

Kondirolli, F., and N. Sunder. 2022. Mental health effects of education. *Health Economics* 31(Suppl 2):22–39.

Krieger, N. 2001. Theories for social epidemiology in the 21st century: An ecosocial perspective. *International Journal of Epidemiology* 30(4):668–677.

Krieger, N. 2014. Discrimination and health inequities. *International Journal of Social Determinants of Health and Health Services* 44(4):643–710.

Kubendran, S., R. DeVol, and A. Chatterjee. 2016. *The price women pay for dementia: Strategies to ease gender disparity and economic costs.* Santa Monica, CA: Milken Institute.

Kukielka, E. 2020. How safety is compromised when hospital equipment is a poor fit for patients who are obese. *Patient Safety* 2(1):48–56.

Kumanyika, S. K., C. B. Morssink, and M. Nestle. 2001. Minority women and advocacy for women's health. *American Journal of Public Health* 91(9):1383–1388.

Kwon, S. C., R. Kabir, and A. Saadabadi. 2024. Mental health challenges in caring for American Indians and Alaska Natives. In *Statpearls.* Treasure Island, FL: StatPearls Publishing.

Lambda Legal. 2010. *When Health Care Isn't Caring: Lambda Legal's Survey of Discrimination Against LGBT People and People with HIV.* http://www.lambdalegal.org/sites/default/files/publications/downloads/whcic-report_when-health-care-isnt-caring.pdf (accessed November 18, 2024).

Larson, K. C. 2021. Mississippi appendectomy. In *Walk with me: A biography of Fannie Lou Hamer.* Oxford, UK: Oxford University Press. Pp. 35–49.

Lawrence, B. J., D. Kerr, C. M. Pollard, M. Theophilus, E. Alexander, D. Haywood, and M. O'Connor. 2021. Weight bias among health care professionals: A systematic review and meta-analysis. *Obesity* 29(11):1802–1812.

Lawrence, J. 2000. The Indian Health Service and the sterilization of Native American women. *American Indian Quarterly* 24(3):400–419.

Levy, H., and A. Janke. 2016. Health literacy and access to care. *Journal of Health Communication* 21(Suppl 1):43–50.

Long, M., B. Frederiksen, U. Ranji, K. Diep, and A. Salganicoff. 2023. *Women's Experiences with Provider Communication and Interactions in Health Care Settings: Findings from the 2022 KFF Women's Health Survey.* https://www.kff.org/womens-health-policy/issue-brief/womens-experiences-with-provider-communication-interactions-health-care-settings-findings-from-2022-kff-womens-health-survey/ (accessed August 20, 2024).

Lopes, L., A. Montero, M. Presiado, and L. Hamel. 2024. *Americans' Challenges with Health Care Costs.* https://www.kff.org/health-costs/issue-brief/americans-challenges-with-health-care-costs/ (accessed August 8, 2024).

Lopez, I. 2008. *Matters of choice: Puerto Rican women's struggle for reproductive freedom.* New Brunswick, NJ and London: Rutgers University Press.

Mallozzi, M., C. Leone, F. Manurita, F. Bellati, and D. Caserta. 2017. Endocrine disrupting chemicals and endometrial cancer: An overview of recent laboratory evidence and epidemiological studies. *International Journal of Environmental Research and Public Health* 14(3).

Margerison, C. E., C. L. MacCallum, J. Chen, Y. Zamani-Hank, and R. Kaestner. 2020. Impacts of Medicaid expansion on health among women of reproductive age. *American Journal of Preventive Medicine* 58(1):1–11.

Mason, A., E. Crowe, B. Haragan, S. Smith, and A. Kyriakou. 2023. Gender dysphoria in young people: A model of chronic stress. *Hormone Research in Paediatrics* 96(1): 54–65.

Matin, B. K., H. J. Williamson, A. K. Karyani, S. Rezaei, M. Soofi, and S. Soltani. 2021. Barriers in access to healthcare for women with disabilities: A systematic review in qualitative studies. *BMC Women's Health* 21(1):44.

McCue, K., and N. DeNicola. 2019. Environmental exposures in reproductive health. *Obstetrics & Gynecology Clinics of North America* 46(3):455–468.

Merone, L., K. Tsey, D. Russell, and C. Nagle. 2022. Sex inequalities in medical research: A systematic scoping review of the literature. *Women's Health Reports* 3(1):49–59.

Meyer, I. H. 2003. Prejudice, social stress, and mental health in lesbian, gay, and bisexual populations: Conceptual issues and research evidence. *Psychological Bulletin* 129(5):674–697.

Mirin, A. A. 2021. Gender disparity in the funding of diseases by the U.S. National Institutes of Health. *Journal of Women's Health* 30(7):956–963.

Mohamoud, Y. A., E. Cassidy, E. Fuchs, L. S. Womack, L. Romero, L. Kipling, R. Oza-Frank, K. Baca, R. R. Galang, A. Stewart, S. Carrigan, J. Mullen, A. Busacker, B. Behm, L. M. Hollier, C. Kroelinger, T. Mueller, W. D. Barfield, and S. Cox. 2023. Vital signs: Maternity care experiences—United States, April 2023. *MMWR* 72(35):961–967.

Montez, J. K., and K. J. Cheng. 2022. Educational disparities in adult health across U.S. states: Larger disparities reflect economic factors. *Frontiers in Public Health* 10:966434.

Moss, M. 2019. *Trauma Lives on in Native Americans by Making Us Sick—While the U.S. Looks Away.* https://www.theguardian.com/commentisfree/2019/may/09/trauma-lives-on-in-native-americans-while-the-us-looks-away (accessed March 6, 2023).

Moss, N. E. 2002. Gender equity and socioeconomic inequality: A framework for the patterning of women's health. *Social Science & Medicine* 54(5):649–661.

Movement Advancement Project. n.d.-a. *Bans on Best Practice Medical Care for Transgender Youth.* https://www.lgbtmap.org/equality-maps/healthcare/youth_medical_care_bans (accessed August 23, 2024).

Movement Advancement Project. n.d.-b. *Equality Maps: Employment Nondiscrimination Laws.* https://www.lgbtmap.org/equality_maps/employment_non_discrimination_laws (accessed August 25, 2024).

Movement Advancement Project. n.d.-c. *Healthcare Laws and Policies.* https://www.lgbtmap.org/equality-maps/healthcare_laws_and_policies (accessed August 23, 2024).

Movement Advancement Project. n.d.-d. *Identity Document Laws and Policies—Birth Certificate.* https://www.lgbtmap.org/equality-maps/identity_documents/birth_certificate (accessed August 23, 2024).

Movement Advancement Project. n.d.-e. *Identity Document Laws and Policies—Driver's License.* https://www.lgbtmap.org/equality-maps/identity_documents (accessed August 23, 2024).

Movement Advancement Project. n.d.-f. *Identity Document Laws and Policies—Name Change.* https://www.lgbtmap.org/equality-maps/identity_documents/name_change (accessed August 23, 2024).

Movement Advancement Project. n.d.-g. *Medicaid Coverage of Transgender-Related Health Care.* https://www.lgbtmap.org/equality-maps/healthcare/medicaid (accessed August 23, 2024).

Movement Advancement Project. n.d.-h. *Transgender Healthcare "Shield" Laws.* https://www.lgbtmap.org/equality-maps/healthcare/trans_shield_laws (accessed August 23, 2024).

Movement Advancement Project and Center for American Progress. 2024. *Paying an Unfair Price: The Financial Penalty for Being Transgender in America.* Washington, DC: Center for American Progress.

Nagle, A., and G. Samari. 2021. State-level structural sexism and cesarean sections in the United States. *Social Science & Medicine* 289:114406.

NASEM (National Academies of Sciences, Engineering, and Medicine). 2017. *Communities in action: Pathways to health equity.* Washington, DC: The National Academies Press.

NASEM. 2019a. *A roadmap to reducing child poverty.* Washington, DC: The National Academies Press.

NASEM. 2019b. *Vibrant and healthy kids: Aligning science, practice, and policy to advance health equity.* Washington, DC: The National Academies Press.

NASEM. 2020a. *Birth settings in America: Outcomes, quality, access, and choice.* Washington, DC: The National Academies Press.

NASEM. 2020b. *Understanding the well-being of LGBTQI+ populations.* Washington, DC: The National Academies Press.

NASEM. 2021a. *Exploring the role of critical health literacy in addressing the social determinants of health: Proceedings of a workshop—in brief.* Edited by R. M. Martinez and K. McHugh. Washington, DC: The National Academies Press.

NASEM. 2021b. *Population health in rural America in 2020: Proceedings of a workshop.* Edited by A. Nicholson. Washington, DC: The National Academies Press.

NASEM. 2021c. *Sexually transmitted infections: Adopting a sexual health paradigm.* Washington, DC: The National Academies Press.

NASEM. 2023a. *Civic engagement and civic infrastructure to advance health equity: Proceedings of a workshop.* Edited by A. Baciu and A. Andrada. Washington, DC: The National Academies Press.

NASEM. 2023b. *Federal policy to advance racial, ethnic, and tribal health equity.* Washington, DC: The National Academies Press.

NASEM. 2024a. *Advancing research on chronic conditions in women.* Washington, DC: The National Academies Press.

NASEM. 2024b. *Essential health care services addressing intimate partner violence.* Washington, DC: The National Academies Press.

NASEM. 2024c. *Overview of research gaps for selected conditions in women's health research at the National Institutes of Health: Proceedings of a workshop—in brief.* Washington, DC: The National Academies Press.

NASEM. 2024d. *Reducing intergenerational poverty.* Washington, DC: The National Academies Press.

National Coalition of Anti-Violence Programs. 2018. *Lesbian, gay, bisexual, transgender, queer and HIV-affected hate and intimate partner violence in 2017.* New York: National Coalition of Anti-Violence Programs.

National Constitution Center. n.d. *Obergefell v. Hodges (2015).* https://constitutioncenter.org/the-constitution/supreme-court-case-library/obergefell-v-hodges (accessed August 27, 2024).

National Library of Medicine. n.d. *Medicine Ways: Traditional Healers and Healing.* https://www.nlm.nih.gov/nativevoices/exhibition/healing-ways/medicine-ways/medicine-wheel.html (accessed August 26, 2024).

National Menopause Foundation. n.d. *National Menopause Foundation: About Us.* https://nationalmenopausefoundation.org/about/ (accessed August 27, 2024).

Newland, B. 2022. *Federal Indian Boarding School Initiative investigative report.* Washington, DC: The Office of the Assistant Secretary—Indian Affairs.

Nguyen Le, T. A., A. T. Lo Sasso, and M. Vujicic. 2017. Trends in the earnings gender gap among dentists, physicians, and lawyers. *Journal of the American Dental Association* 148(4):257–262.e252.

NHLBI (National Heart, Lung, and Blood Institute). 2023. *Asthma in the Black Community.* https://www.nhlbi.nih.gov/sites/default/files/publications/asthma_in_black_community_fact_sheet.pdf (accessed October 21).

NIH (National Institutes of Health). n.d. *Reporter Search Results for "Two-Spirit."* https://reporter.nih.gov/search/WnMXFzqBiEa88HOf_3lrpw/projects (accessed October 22, 2024).

Novak, N. L., N. Lira, K. E. O'Connor, S. D. Harlow, S. L. R. Kardia, and A. M. Stern. 2018. Disproportionate sterilization of Latinos under California's eugenic sterilization program, 1920–1945. *American Journal of Public Health* 108(5):611–613.

O'Keefe, V. M., T. L. Maudrie, A. B. Cole, J. S. Ullrich, J. Fish, K. X. Hill, L. A. White, N. Redvers, V. B. B. Jernigan, J. P. Lewis, A. E. West, C. A. Apok, E. J. White, J. D. Ivanich, K. Schultz, M. E. Lewis, M. C. Sarche, M. B. Gonzalez, M. Parker, S. E. Neuner Weinstein, C. J. McCray, D. Warne, J. C. Black, J. R. Richards, and M. L. Walls. 2023. Conceptualizing Indigenous strengths-based health and wellness research using group concept mapping. *Archives of Public Health* 81(1):71.

OASH (Office of the Assistant Secretary for Health). n.d.-a. *Healthy People 2030*. https://health. gov/healthypeople/objectives-and-data/social-determinants-health (accessed July 18, 2024).

OASH. n.d.-b. *Healthy People 2030—Access to Health Services*. https://health.gov/healthypeople/ priority-areas/social-determinants-health/literature-summaries/access-health-services (accessed August 26, 2024).

OASH. n.d.-c. *Healthy People 2030—Poverty*. https://health.gov/healthypeople/priority-areas/ social-determinants-health/literature-summaries/poverty (accessed August 23, 2024).

OASH. n.d.-d. *Healthy People 2030: Neighborhood and Built Environment*. https://odphp. health.gov/healthypeople/objectives-and-data/browse-objectives/neighborhood-and-built-environment (accessed October 21, 2024).

Office of Disability Employment Policy. 2021. *Spotlight on women with disabilities*. Washington, DC: Department of Labor.

OMH (Office of Minority Health). 2024a. *Obesity and African Americans*. https://minority-health.hhs.gov/obesity-and-african-americans (accessed October 22, 2024).

OMH. 2024b. *Obesity and Hispanic Americans*. https://minorityhealth.hhs.gov/obesity-and-hispanic-americans (accessed October 22, 2024).

Oram, S., H. Khalifeh, and L. M. Howard. 2017. Violence against women and mental health. *Lancet Psychiatry* 4(2):159–170.

Ordway, D.-M. 2023. *Weight Bias, Common in Health Care, Can Drive Weight Gain and Prompt People with Obesity to Avoid Doctors, Research Finds*. https://journalistsresource. org/health/weight-bias-health-care-obesity-research/ (accessed August 26, 2024).

Paz, K., and K. P. Massey. 2016. Health disparity among Latina women: Comparison with non-Latina women. *Clinical Medical Insights: Women's Health* 9(Suppl 1):71–74.

PCOS Challenge. n.d. *About PCOS Challenge*. https://pcoschallenge.org/about-pcos-challenge/ (accessed August 27, 2024).

Peitzmeier, S. M., M. Malik, S. K. Kattari, E. Marrow, R. Stephenson, M. Agénor, and S. L. Reisner. 2020. Intimate partner violence in transgender populations: Systematic review and meta-analysis of prevalence and correlates. *American Journal of Public Health* 110(9):e1–e14.

Pendergrass, D. C., and M. Y. Raji. 2017. *The Bitter Pill: Harvard and the Dark History of Birth Control*. https://www.thecrimson.com/article/2017/9/28/the-bitter-pill/ (accessed October 21, 2024).

Perry, B. L., K. L. Harp, and C. B. Oser. 2013. Racial and gender discrimination in the stress process: Implications for African American women's health and well-being. *Sociological Perspectives* 56(1):25–48.

Petrosky, E., L. M. Mercer Kollar, M. C. Kearns, S. G. Smith, C. J. Betz, K. A. Fowler, and D. E. Satter. 2021. Homicides of American Indians/Alaska Natives—National Violent Death Reporting System, United States, 2003–2018. *MMWR Surveillance Summaries* 70(8):1–19.

Philbin, M. M., B. G. Everett, and J. D. Auerbach. 2024. Gender(ed) science: How the institutionalization of gender continues to shape the conduct and content of women's health research. *Social Science & Medicine* 351:116456.

Pichardo, M. S., L. M. Ferrucci, Y. Molina, D. A. Esserman, and M. L. Irwin. 2023. Structural racism, lifestyle behaviors, and obesity-related cancers among Black and Hispanic/Latino adults in the United States: A narrative review. *Cancer Epidemiology Biomarkers and Prevention* 32(11):1498–1507.

Presumey-Leblanc, G., and M. Sandel. 2024. The legacy of slavery and the socialization of Black female health and human services workforce members in addressing social determinants of health. *Journal of Racial and Ethnic Health Disparities* 11(1):192–202.

Price, G. N., and W. A. Darity. 2010. The economics of race and eugenic sterilization in North Carolina: 1958–1968. *Economics & Human Biology* 8(2):261–272.

Puhl, R. M., and C. A. Heuer. 2010. Obesity stigma: Important considerations for public health. *American Journal of Public Health* 100(6):1019–1028.

Raghupathi, V., and W. Raghupathi. 2020. The influence of education on health: An empirical assessment of OECD countries for the period 1995–2015. *Archives of Public Health* 78:20.

Ransohoff, J. I., P. Sujin Kumar, D. Flynn, and E. Rubenstein. 2022. Reproductive and pregnancy health care for women with intellectual and developmental disabilities: A scoping review. *Journal of Applied Research in Intellectual Disabilities* 35(3):655–674.

Rapp, K. S., V. V. Volpe, and H. Neukrug. 2021. State-level sexism and women's health care access in the United States: Differences by race/ethnicity, 2014–2019. *American Journal of Public Health* 111(10):1796–1805.

Redd, S. K., W. S. Rice, M. S. Aswani, S. Blake, Z. Julian, B. Sen, M. Wingate, and K. S. Hall. 2021. Racial/ethnic and educational inequities in restrictive abortion policy variation and adverse birth outcomes in the United States. *BMC Health Services Research* 21(1):1139.

Rennels, C., S. G. Murthy, M. A. Handley, M. D. Morris, B. K. Alldredge, P. Dahiya, R. Jagsi, J. L. Kerns, and C. Mangurian. 2024. Informal caregiving among faculty at a large academic health sciences university in the United States: An opportunity for policy changes. *Academic Psychiatry* 48(4):320–328.

Rickard, B. P., I. Rizvi, and S. E. Fenton. 2022. Per- and poly-fluoroalkyl substances (PFAS) and female reproductive outcomes: PFAS elimination, endocrine-mediated effects, and disease. *Toxicology* 465:153031.

Rippel Foundation. n.d. *Vital Conditions for Health and Well-Being*. https://rippel.org/vital-conditions/ (accessed August 26, 2024).

Robinette, J. W., J. R. Piazza, and R. S. Stawski. 2021. Neighborhood safety concerns and daily well-being: A national diary study. *Wellbeing, Space, and Society* 2: 100047.

Robinson, M. 2022. Recent insights into the mental health needs of Two-Spirit people. *Current Opinion in Psychology* 48:101494.

Rochon, P. A., S. Kalia, and P. Higgs. 2021. Gendered ageism: Addressing discrimination based on age and sex. *Lancet* 398(10301):648–649.

Ross, C. E., R. K. Masters, and R. A. Hummer. 2012. Education and the gender gaps in health and mortality. *Demography* 49(4):1157–1183.

Rousseau, M., C. Rouzeau, J. Bainvel, and F. Pelé. 2022. Domestic exposure to chemicals in household products, building materials, decoration, and pesticides: Guidelines for interventions during the perinatal period from the French National College of Midwives. *Journal of Midwifery and Women's Health* 67(Suppl 1):S113–S134.

RRC Polytech. 2024. *Gender and Sexual Diversity—Two-Spirit People*. https://library.rrc.ca/2SLGBTQIA/2spirit (accessed August 26, 2024).

Rudel, R. A., J. M. Ackerman, K. R. Attfield, and J. G. Brody. 2014. New exposure biomarkers as tools for breast cancer epidemiology, biomonitoring, and prevention: A systematic approach based on animal evidence. *Environmental Health Perspectives* 122(9):881–895.

Saad, L. 2023. *7 Insights Into Women's Lives in the U.S.* https://news.gallup.com/opinion/gallup/471242/insights-women-lives.aspx (accessed August 23, 2024).

Sattler, K. M., F. P. Deane, L. Tapsell, and P. J. Kelly. 2018. Gender differences in the relationship of weight-based stigmatisation with motivation to exercise and physical activity in overweight individuals. *Health Psychology Open* 5(1):2055102918759691

Seven Directions: A Center for Indigenous Public Health. 2023. *Indigenous Social Determinants of Health*. https://cdn.prod.website-files.com/5d4b3177c03a6439be501a14/65fdf 6eea8be02b9051d9a86_Module-Report-Compressed.pdf (accessed October 18, 2024).

Shearston, J. A., K. Upson, M. Gordon, V. Do, O. Balac, K. Nguyen, B. Yan, M.-A. Kioumourtzoglou, and K. Schilling. 2024. Tampons as a source of exposure to metal(loid)s. *Environment International*:108849.

Shrider, E. A., M. Kollar, F. Chen, and J. Semega. 2023. *Income and Poverty in the United States: 2020*. https://www.census.gov/library/publications/2021/demo/p60-273.html (accessed August 27, 2024).

Sieck, N. E., M. Bruening, I. v. Woerden, C. Whisner, and D. C. Payne-Sturges. 2024. Effects of behavioral, clinical, and policy interventions in reducing human exposure to bisphenols and phthalates: A scoping review. *Environmental Health Perspectives* 132(3):036001.

Silbergeld, E. K., and J. A. Flaws. 2002. Environmental exposures and women's health. *Clinical Obstetrics and Gynecology* 45(4).

Simons, R. L., M. K. Lei, E. Klopack, Y. Zhang, F. X. Gibbons, and S. R. H. Beach. 2021. Racial discrimination, inflammation, and chronic illness among African American women at midlife: Support for the weathering perspective. *Journal of Racial and Ethnic Health Disparities* 8(2):339–349.

SisterSong. n.d. *Reproductive Justice.* https://www.sistersong.net/reproductive-justice/ (accessed August 23, 2024).

Slopen, M. 2023. The impact of paid sick leave mandates on women's health. *Social Science & Medicine* 323:115839.

Sosa, J. A., and C. Mangurian. 2023. Addressing eldercare to promote gender equity in academic medicine. *JAMA* 330(23):2245–2246.

Statista. n.d. *Distribution of the Leading Causes of Death for American Indians or Alaska Natives in the United States in 2019, by Gender.* https://www.statista.com/statistics/1285749/aian-leading-causes-of-death-by-gender/ (accessed August 22, 2024).

Steele, L. S., A. Daley, D. Curling, M. F. Gibson, D. C. Green, C. C. Williams, and L. E. Ross. 2017. LGBT identity, untreated depression, and unmet need for mental health services by sexual minority women and trans-identified people. *Journal of Women's Health* 26(2):116–127.

Stern, A. M. 2005. Sterilized in the name of public health: Race, immigration, and reproductive control in modern California. *American Journal of Public Health* 95(7):1128–1138.

Stern, A. M. 2020. *Forced Sterilization Policies in the U.S. Targeted Minorities and Those with Disabilities—and Lasted into the 21st Century.* https://ihpi.umich.edu/news/forced-sterilization-policies-us-targeted-minorities-and-those-disabilities-and-lasted-21st (accessed March 18, 2023).

Stiel, L., P. B. Adkins-Jackson, P. Clark, E. Mitchell, and S. Montgomery. 2016. A review of hair product use on breast cancer risk in African American women. *Cancer Medicine* 5(3):597–604.

Strings, S. 2019. *Fearing the Black body: The racial origins of fat phobia.* New York: NYU Press.

Thornburg, B., A. Kennedy-Hendricks, J. D. Rosen, and M. D. Eisenberg. 2024. Anxiety and depression symptoms after the Dobbs abortion decision. *JAMA* 331(4):294–301.

Tight Lipped. n.d. *Tight Lipped.* https://www.tightlipped.org/ (accessed August 27, 2024).

Tribal Information Exchange. n.d. *Walking in Two Worlds: Supporting the Two Spirit and Native LGBTQ Community.* https://tribalinformationexchange.org/files/resources/twospiritbrochure.pdf (accessed August 26, 2024).

Tribouilloy, C., Y. Bohbot, D. Rusinaru, K. Belkhir, M. Diouf, A. Altes, Q. Delpierre, S. Serbout, M. Kubala, F. Levy, S. Maréchaux, and M. Enriquez Sarano. 2021. Excess mortality and undertreatment of women with severe aortic stenosis. *Journal of the American Heart Association* 10(1):e018816.

Trost, S., J. Beauregard, G. Chandra, F. Njie, A. Harvey, J. Berry, and D. A. Goodman. 2022. *Pregnancy-related deaths among American Indian or Alaska Native persons: Data from maternal mortality review committees in 36 US states, 2017–2019.* Atlanta, GA: Centers for Disease Control and Prevention.

Tucker, M. J., C. J. Berg, W. M. Callaghan, and J. Hsia. 2007. The Black-White disparity in pregnancy-related mortality from 5 conditions: Differences in prevalence and case-fatality rates. *American Journal of Public Health* 97(2):247–251.

University of Arizona Health Sciences. n.d. *"Winter Institute" to Focus on Health and Research Issues Relevant to Native Americans, Feb. 17–20 at UA Health Sciences.* https:// azpride.uahs.arizona.edu/news/winter-institute%E2%80%99-focus-health-and-research-issues-relevant-native-americans-feb-17–20-ua (accessed August 26, 2024).

Urban Indian Health Institute. n.d. *Our bodies, our stories: Sexual violence among native women in Seattle, WA.* Washington, DC: Urban Indian Health Institute.

U.S. Equal Employment Opportunity Commission. n.d. *Sexual Orientation and Gender Identity (SOGI) Discrimination.* https://www.eeoc.gov/sexual-orientation-and-gender-identity-sogi-discrimination (accessed August 24, 2024).

Uvelli, A., C. Duranti, G. Salvo, A. Coluccia, G. Gualtieri, and F. Ferretti. 2023. The risk factors of chronic pain in victims of violence: A scoping review. *Healthcare* 11(17).

Vallée, A., P. F. Ceccaldi, M. Carbonnel, A. Feki, and J. M. Ayoubi. 2024. Pollution and endometriosis: A deep dive into the environmental impacts on women's health. *BJOG* 131(4):401–414.

Van Loveren, H., J. G. Vos, D. Germolec, P. P. Simeonova, G. Eijkemanns, and A. J. McMichael. 2001. Epidemiologic associations between occupational and environmental exposures and autoimmune disease: Report of a meeting to explore current evidence and identify research needs. *International Journal of Hygiene and Environmental Health* 203(5–6):483–495.

Vedam, S., K. Stoll, T. K. Taiwo, N. Rubashkin, M. Cheyney, N. Strauss, M. McLemore, M. Cadena, E. Nethery, E. Rushton, L. Schummers, and E. Declercq. 2019. The Giving Voice to Mothers study: Inequity and mistreatment during pregnancy and childbirth in the United States. *Reproductive Health* 16(1):77.

Vigod, S. N., and P. A. Rochon. 2020. The impact of gender discrimination on a woman's mental health. *eClinicalMedicine* 20.

Villardón-Gallego, L., A. García-Cid, A. Estévez, and R. García-Carrión. 2023. Early educational interventions to prevent gender-based violence: A systematic review. *Healthcare* 11(1).

Virginia Sexual and Domestic Violence Action Alliance. n.d. *What Is Reproductive Justice?* https://vsdvalliance.org/wp-content/uploads/2022/07/Part-1-What-is-Reproductive-Justice.pdf (accessed August 26, 2024).

Voges, M. M., H. L. Quittkat, B. Schöne, and S. Vocks. 2022. Giving a body a different face—how men and women evaluate their own body vs. that of others. *Frontiers in Psychology* 13:853398.

Walker, R. J., E. Garacci, A. Z. Dawson, J. S. Williams, M. Ozieh, and L. E. Egede. 2021. Trends in food insecurity in the United States from 2011–2017: Disparities by age, sex, race/ethnicity, and income. *Populational Health Management* 24(4):496–501.

Wallerstein, N. B., and B. Duran. 2006. Using community-based participatory research to address health disparities. *Health Promotion Practice* 7(3):312–323.

Washington, H. A. 2006. The Black stork: The eugenic control of African American reproduction. In *Medical Apartheid: The Dark History of Medical Experimentation on Black Americans from Colonial Times to the Present.* New York: Harlem Moon. Pp. 189–215.

Wehi, P. M., M. P. Cox, H. Whaanga, and T. Roa. 2023. Tradition and change: Celebrating food systems resilience at two Indigenous Māori community events. *Ecology and Society* 28(1).

Weiss, M. S., and E. E. Marsh. 2023. Navigating unequal paths: Racial disparities in the infertility journey. *Obstetrics & Gynecology* 142(4):940–947.

Weitzman, A. 2018. Does increasing women's education reduce their risk of intimate partner violence? Evidence from an education policy reform. *Criminology* 56(3):574–607.

Well Project. 2024. *Sexual and Reproductive Health, Rights, Justice, Pleasure, and HIV.* https://www.thewellproject.org/hiv-information/sexual-and-reproductive-health-rights-justice-pleasure-and-hiv (accessed August 26, 2024).

Welleck, A., and M. Yeung. n.d. *Reproductive Justice and Lesbian, Gay, Bisexual, and Transgender Liberation.* https://www.protectchoice.org/article.php?id=135 (accessed August 26, 2024).

Wenger, N. K., D. M. Lloyd-Jones, M. S. V. Elkind, G. C. Fonarow, J. J. Warner, H. M. Alger, S. Cheng, C. Kinzy, J. L. Hall, V. L. Roger, and American Heart Association. 2022. Call to action for cardiovascular disease in women: Epidemiology, awareness, access, and delivery of equitable health care: A presidential advisory from the American Heart Association. *Circulation* 145(23):e1059–e1071.

WHO (World Health Organization). n.d. *Health Equity.* https://www.who.int/health-topics/health-equity#tab=tab_1 (accessed August 25, 2024).

WIA Report. 2022. *The Significant Gender Gap in College Graduation Rates.* https://www.wiareport.com/2022/11/the-significant-gender-gap-in-college-graduation-rates/ (accessed October 22, 2024).

Wise, L. A., T. R. Wang, C. N. Ncube, S. M. Lovett, J. Abrams, R. Boynton-Jarrett, M. R. Koenig, R. J. Geller, A. K. Wesselink, C. M. Coleman, E. E. Hatch, and T. James-Todd. 2023. Use of chemical hair straighteners and fecundability in a North American preconception cohort. *American Journal of Epidemiology* 192(7):1066–1080.

Wuest, J., M. Ford-Gilboe, M. Merritt-Gray, C. Varcoe, B. Lent, P. Wilk, and J. Campbell. 2009. Abuse-related injury and symptoms of posttraumatic stress disorder as mechanisms of chronic pain in survivors of intimate partner violence. *Pain Medicine* 10(4):739–747.

Wuest, J., M. Ford-Gilboe, M. Merritt-Gray, P. Wilk, J. C. Campbell, B. Lent, C. Varcoe, and V. Smye. 2010. Pathways of chronic pain in survivors of intimate partner violence. *Journal of Women's Health* 19(9):1665–1674.

Yearby, R. 2022. The social determinants of health, health disparities, and health justice. *Journal of Law, Medicine, & Ethics* 50(4):641–649.

Yu, S. 2018. Uncovering the hidden impacts of inequality on mental health: A global study. *Translational Psychiatry* 8(1):98.

Zajacova, A., and E. M. Lawrence. 2018. The relationship between education and health: Reducing disparities through a contextual approach. *Annual Review of Public Health* 39:273–289.

Zhao, J., A. Zahn, S. C. Pang, T. S. Quang, J. Campbell, and P. N. Halkitis. 2024. Early national trends in non-abortion reproductive care access after Roe. *Frontiers in Public Health* 12:1309068.

Zhu, D. T., L. Zhao, T. Alzoubi, N. Shenin, T. Baskaran, J. Tikhonov, and C. Wang. 2024. Public health and clinical implications of Dobbs v. Jackson for patients and healthcare providers: A scoping review. *PLoS One* 19(3):e0288947.

Zlatnik, M. G. 2016. Endocrine-disrupting chemicals and reproductive health. *Journal of Midwifery and Women's Health* 61(4):442–455.

Zota, A. R., and B. Shamasunder. 2017. The environmental injustice of beauty: Framing chemical exposures from beauty products as a health disparities concern. *American Journal of Obstetrics and Gynecology* 217(4):418.e411–418.e416.

Zubizarreta, D., A. L. Beccia, J. T. Chen, J. L. Jahn, S. B. Austin, and M. Agénor. 2024. Structural racism-related state laws and healthcare access among Black, Latine, and White U.S. adults. *Journal of Racial and Ethnic Health Disparities* [Epub ahead of print].

7

Overview of Selected Women's Health Conditions

A wide range of conditions are specific to females,[1] more prevalent among women, or affect women differently than men (see Table 7-1). Moreover, as a result of insufficient research and measurement, it remains unclear the full extent of conditions that uniquely affect women. While it was not possible for the committee to review every women's health condition in depth, it presents a framework in this chapter for quantifying and categorizing health conditions that affect women's morbidity, mortality, and quality of life in different ways and selects exemplar conditions to illustrate pressing needs for further research investment in women's health scientific investigation. Together, the examples across the life course highlighted in this chapter represent those that are present in women and men but progress differently in and cause greater disability in women (e.g., mood disorders) or cause more premature mortality in women compared to men (e.g., cardiometabolic diseases, autoimmune disease, and Alzheimer's disease [AD]); are female specific and leading causes of death (e.g., gynecological cancers); and are female specific and a leading cause of reduced quality of life and disability (e.g., endometriosis, fibroids, and perinatal and menopause-related depression). Because pregnancy influences the trajectory of cardiometabolic and cognitive disease later in life, the chapter also summarizes its effects across the life course.

---

[1] The terms "female" and "woman" are used differently according to context and perspective, which may cause confusion (see Chapter 1). In this chapter, the committee uses "female" when discussing specific sex traits related to a specific condition and "woman" when discussing the population more generally (the latter includes all people who identify as a woman or girl, solely or in addition to other gender identities and regardless of biological sex traits).

Two recent National Academies of Sciences, Engineering, and Medicine (National Academies) reports comprehensively reviewed and identified research gaps for two pressing women's health topics: autoimmune disease and chronic conditions (see Box 7-1 for a summary of the conditions). The findings of those reports corroborate the research needs this committee identified; it relied upon and attempted not to duplicate the effort of these reports. Boxes 7-2 and 7-3 provide a summary of key recommendations to address research gaps from those reports.

BOX 7-1
Women's Health Conditions Reviewed in *Enhancing National Institutes of Health Research on Autoimmune Disease* and *Advancing Research on Chronic Conditions in Women*

Conditions reviewed in *Enhancing NIH Research on Autoimmune Disease (2022)*
- Sjögren's disease
- Systemic lupus erythematosus
- Antiphospholipid syndrome
- Rheumatoid arthritis
- Psoriasis
- Inflammatory bowel disease
- Celiac disease
- Primary biliary cholangitis
- Multiple sclerosis
- Type 1 diabetes
- Autoimmune thyroid diseases

Conditions reviewed in *Advancing Research on Chronic Conditions in Women (2024)*
- Endometriosis/dysmenorrhea/chronic pelvic pain
- Uterine fibroids
- Infertility
- Vulvodynia
- Pelvic floor disorders (including urinary incontinence and pelvic organ prolapse)
- Menopausal symptoms (including exogenous hormone use)
- Systemic lupus erythematosus
- Multiple sclerosis (also affects the neurocognitive system)
- Osteoporosis
- Sarcopenia
- Alzheimer's disease
- Migraine/headache
- Chronic pain

BOX 7-1 Continued

- Fibromyalgia
- Myalgic encephalomyelitis/chronic fatigue syndrome
- Cardiovascular disease
- Stroke
- Metabolic conditions (Type 2 diabetes, metabolic syndrome)
- Depression
- Substance use disorder
- Human immunodeficiency virus

SOURCES: NASEM, 2022, 2024b.
NOTE: These are a combination of conditions that are female specific, are more common in women, or impact women differently.

BOX 7-2
***Enhancing National Institutes of Health Research on Autoimmune Disease*: Summary of Recommended Research Priorities**

This report identified several crosscutting research needs for autoimmune disease and recommended research to address gaps in knowledge, including to

- Dissect heterogeneity across and within autoimmune diseases to decipher common and disease-specific pathogenic mechanisms.
- Study rare autoimmune diseases and develop supporting animal models.
- Define autoantibodies and other biomarkers that can diagnose and predict the initiation and progression of autoimmune diseases.
- Determine the biologic functions of genetic variants and gene–environment interactions within and across autoimmune diseases using novel, cutting-edge technologies.
- Examine the role of environmental exposures and social determinants of health in autoimmune diseases across the life-span.
- Determine the impact of coexisting morbidities, including co-occurring autoimmune diseases and complications of autoimmune diseases, across the life-span, and develop and evaluate interventions to improve patient outcomes.
- Foster research to advance health equity for all autoimmune disease patients.

SOURCE: NASEM, 2022.

BOX 7-3
Advancing Research on Chronic Conditions in Women:
Summarized Research Agenda

The report identified key research gaps that the National Institutes of Health and other relevant agencies that fund research should support to advance the understanding of chronic conditions in women. The following areas of research were recommended to help fill those research gaps.

Recommendation 1: Impact—improve estimates and support national surveillance and population-based studies; expand data collection activities to include female-specific and gynecologic and female-predominant conditions not currently included.

Recommendation 2: Biology and Pathophysiology—understand how gonadal hormones and sex chromosome genes interact to cause sex differences, role of inflammation and immune system, and genetic heterogeneity of conditions (e.g., endometriosis); improve animal and preclinical models.

Recommendation 3: Female-Specific Risk Factors—the specific role of reproductive milestones across the life course (e.g., menarche, pregnancy, perimenopause, menopause, and postmenopause) and address symptoms.

Recommendations 4–6: Disparities and Life Experiences—interaction of multiple social identities with structural and social determinants of health; role of traumatic experiences; role of lifestyle behaviors.

Recommendation 7: Diagnosis and Treatment—improve early and accurate detection and diagnosis of chronic conditions; develop sex- and gender-specific tools; establish better diagnostic tools of conditions that share similar symptoms (e.g., chronic pain, fibromyalgia).

Recommendation 8: Multiple Chronic Conditions—understand biological mechanisms, diagnosis, and treatment and care for women with multiple chronic conditions; develop research approaches to appropriately study and include women with multiple chronic conditions.

Recommendation 9 & 10: Inequities and Women-Centered Research—develop methods for assessing structural determinants of health such as sexism and ageism; recruit women from different backgrounds and use novel techniques for engaging women; account for sex and gender in studies.

SOURCE: NASEM, 2024b.

A FRAMEWORK FOR QUANTIFYING DISEASE
BURDEN TO ILLUSTRATE WHR GAPS

This section illustrates the annual burden of disease experienced by women in the United States in terms of years of life lost (YLLs), years lived with disability (YLDs), and disability-adjusted life years (DALYs). Further, it demonstrates through simplified examples how such analyses can help in setting priorities for women's health research (WHR) by identifying imbalances in health research investments. The committee used this analytic approach to frame the discussion of key exemplar conditions affecting women's health later in this chapter.

The Value of Research Investment and Metrics
for Quantifying Disease Burden

The burden of different health conditions and the opportunities for research to alleviate it (i.e., the expected health return on research investment) are important factors in decisions about allocating a limited pool of funding. Both are difficult to quantify and involve substantial uncertainty; in particular, the latter requires assumptions about potential advancements and breakthroughs. This section describes available metrics to quantify disease burden and explores their application to funding allocation decisions. The committee assumes that investments in women's health would have at least as much potential for health returns as investments in other areas, which is conservative given the historical underinvestment in WHR described in Chapters 2 and 4. The analysis therefore focuses on quantifying the burden of disease that could be addressed by WHR. In practice, such analyses would ideally consider both of these metrics and other factors, including expected research returns, explicit investment in historically neglected areas, and the minimum threshold needed to ensure progress across a range of areas.

A key challenge for quantifying the burden of disease and comparing the health effects of different conditions is determining comparable outcomes across disease areas. For example, health effects can be measured in terms of people affected using metrics such as incidence (the number of new cases per unit of time, often annually) and prevalence (the number of individuals affected in some time period). Other metrics, such as annual deaths, also reflect disease severity. In comparing diseases, qualitative differences in burden across health problems present critical challenges, such as how to compare the societal health effect of endometriosis, a condition affecting roughly 11 percent of reproductive-age women—approximately 1 in 26 U.S. women—that can cause severe abdominal pain; persistent or recurring genital pain before, during, or after intercourse (dyspareunia); and infertility, to that of gynecological cancers, which affect approximately 1 in 168 U.S. women but more frequently cause mortality (Buck Louis et al., 2011; Ellis et al., 2022; IHME, n.d.-a; Stewart et al., 2013). A similar challenge is how to compare the effect of a chronic illness, such as asthma, to that of a brief but severe episode of acute illness, such as influenza or COVID-19.

The committee drew on the validated approach of aggregated health metrics, which include both DALYs and related measures, such as quality-adjusted life years. These standardized methods are widely used both nationally and internationally and aggregate nonfatal and fatal health effects into comparable measures (Augustovski et al., 2018; NCCID, 2015; Sassi, 2006). Furthermore, they integrate the type and duration of health effects to quantify burden in a way that can be easily compared across disease areas. Although these measures have limitations, discussed later, such analyses can nevertheless provide insights into comparisons among all women's health conditions.

Understanding DALYs

In this chapter, burden of disease is quantified in terms of DALYs, which measure the loss of health resulting from disease or injury, where a year lived in perfect health is denoted as 0 and a year of life lost is denoted as 1. In general, health interventions seek to avert or reduce DALYs. Because health conditions may cause impaired quality of life or loss of life, DALYs are the sum of YLLs and YLDs (Salomon et al., 2012). Figure 7-1 displays this breakdown, with YLDs, marked in orange, accruing both as a result of temporary and chronic conditions and YLLs, marked in beige, showing years of life lost compared to a full healthy life expectancy.

To calculate YLLs, researchers compare an estimate of the average age at death for a particular condition to an estimate of an average full healthy life expectancy. To calculate YLDs, researchers use weights that convert the health burden of different conditions into a number of effective years lost. Usually, standardized DALY weights come from the Global Burden of Disease (GBD) study that presented an international sample of individuals with two descriptions of health states and asked which scenario described a healthier individual (Salomon et al., 2012, 2015). Using another series of questions, these ratings were anchored onto the 0–1 scale described. Given the extremely high correlations across nations,[2] researchers designed only one scale of DALY weights, which are regularly updated, calculated in a standard way across conditions, and applied broadly. The weights are publicly available (IHME, n.d.-c; Salomon et al., 2012).

---

[2] Nations included Indonesia, Peru, Bangladesh, Tanzania, and the United States in 2009–2010, and Hungary, Italy, the Netherlands, and Sweden were added in 2013 GBD analysis (Salomon et al., 2015).

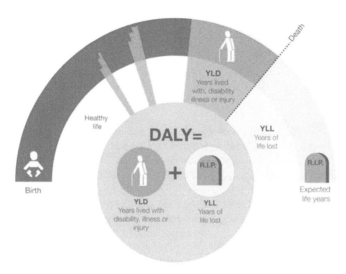

FIGURE 7-1 The components used to calculate disability-adjusted life years (DALYs). SOURCE: U.K. Health Security Agency, 2015; licensed by Open Government Licence v3.0 (https://www.nationalarchives.gov.uk/doc/open-government-licence/version/3/).

Analyses

This section provides descriptive statistics for the burden of female diseases in estimates from the GBD study, characterizing the burden's distribution across conditions and comparing it to the male burden. Second, this section uses stylized benchmarking analyses to explore how decision makers may use data that measure the burden of illness in a standardized to inform funding allocation and priority setting decisions in WHR.

Descriptive Statistics

Data   The GBD study regularly provides publicly available and comprehensive estimates of the frequency and burden of all health conditions in the United States by sex. The concept of DALYs is organized into a hierarchical structure with multiple levels to provide a comprehensive view of health loss (see Box 7-4). The committee extracted annual prevalence, incidence, DALYs, YLLs, and YLDs across all available disease areas by sex from GBD 2021 U.S. estimates, the most recent year available, for Level 3 causes, the most granular comprehensive level in the GBD database (IHME, n.d.-a). For outcomes of particular women's health interest, annual incidence and prevalence, the committee benchmarked estimates against external, independent estimates from the peer-reviewed literature, generally finding equivalence, with limitations as noted. The committee excluded COVID-19

BOX 7-4
Disability-Adjusted Life Year Categories

The DALY hierarchical framework has three or four levels, depending on the level of analysis:

Level 1 is the highest level of aggregation and includes noncommunicable diseases; injuries; and a group of infectious diseases, maternal and neonatal disorders, and nutritional deficiencies. This level provides a broad overview of the major types of health issues affecting populations.

Level 2 breaks down the Level 1 categories into more specific risk categories: 22 disease and injury aggregate categories, such as respiratory infections and tuberculosis, cardiovascular diseases, and transport injuries.

Level 3 further refines the risk categories into more specific causes, such as tuberculosis, stroke, and road injuries. In some cases, Level 3 causes are the most detailed classification, while for others, a more detailed category is specified at Level 4.

Level 4 is not consistently defined across conditions, and its use varies depending on the study and level of detail required.

SOURCES: GBD 2021 Diseases and Injuries Collaborators, 2024; IHME, n.d.-b.

---

from the analysis given its anomalous burden in 2021; burden estimates were otherwise comparable to 2019.

Methods For reporting and display purposes, the committee aggregated 175 Level 3 conditions into 17 categories, adjusting standardized Level 2 categories to highlight outcomes of interest, such as separating out female-specific cancers. Outcomes are presented by sex, condition, and type in terms of DALYs, YLLs, and YLDs.

Burden of Female Disease

Figure 7-2 summarizes estimated 2021 DALYs by disease category, sex (top panel), and type (bottom panel). Overall, men have a higher number of DALYs than women (who were 49 percent), but women experienced a disproportionate share of disability (55 percent of YLDs). For both, mental health and substance use disorders were the most common DALY categories,

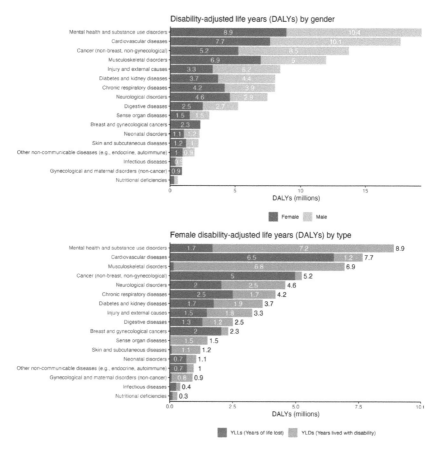

FIGURE 7-2 Disability-adjusted life year (DALY) burden by sex, condition, and type, United States 2021.
NOTES: The top panel displays DALYs by sex. The bottom panel displays only female-specific DALYs, decomposed into years of life lost (YLLs) and years lived with disability (YLDs).

followed by cardiovascular disease (CVD) and cancer, with men experiencing a majority of DALYs in these conditions. By contrast, among conditions experienced by both men and women, women had a majority of DALYs related to musculoskeletal, chronic respiratory, and neurological conditions.

The bottom panel of Figure 7-2 further breaks down contributions of disability and mortality to the female DALY burden. The dark blue portion of each bar shows the YLLs attributable to each condition. The light blue portion shows DALYs resulting from time spent with disability, such as loss of quality of life through physical or mental health limitations or discomfort. CVD and cancers are the main drivers of YLLs among women. In contrast, for mental health, substance use, and musculoskeletal disorders, DALYs from mental health conditions are attributable primarily to disability. The former may be, in part, an artifact of GBD coding—several mental health conditions, such as depression leading to suicide and schizophrenia, are also associated with premature mortality (Schoenbaum et al., 2017; Vigo et al., 2022). Some women-specific health conditions, such as female-specific cancers, gynecological problems, and female sexually transmitted infections, constitute a smaller total DALY burden compared to other categories, though female-specific cancers are the fourth-leading cause of premature mortality among women through YLLs. The next section discusses the challenge of connecting the burden of female disease and disability to WHR.

Benchmarking

While these descriptive results characterize the overall burden of disease in women, further analysis would be required to inform funding allocation with disease burden. The following presents two stylized examples of how burden data could inform resource allocation.

Cancer funding is considered as a simplified example of within–National Institutes of Health (NIH) Institute and Center (IC) prioritization; in this case, comparing spending on female-specific and non-female-specific cancers. Approaches to delineating the total burden of disease that research on women-specific diseases and those that affect women disproportionately or differently might address are then explored.

1. **Cancer spending** This is a discrete, well-defined case study that allows comparing investments in female-specific or predominant disease subtypes, including breast, uterine, cervical, and uterine/endometrial, to cancers affecting both men and women. National Cancer Institute (NCI) data were extracted on estimated 2021 spending across 17 cancer types (NCI, 2024e). For each type, spending was divided by total 2019 burden measures (e.g., DALYs, YLLs, YLDs), summed over both sexes, to understand how research investment compared each type's health burden. Although this exercise is simplified by considering only 1 year of data and crudely comparing female-specific to non-female-specific cancers, this approach can highlight areas of underinvestment relative to disease effects.

2. **WHR portfolio** Next, a more challenging question is considered—the fraction of the total U.S. disease burden falling under the purview of WHR, defined as encompassing conditions that are female specific, are disproportionately female, or affect women

differently. Most people would not consider research on any disease affecting women to be "WHR," since that would encompass nearly all modern clinical research, be so overly broad as to obscure the gaps and barriers discussed in this report, and overlook the value of research that studies two sexes. Nevertheless, as this report elucidates, adequately addressing women's health issues requires understanding sex differences in disease pathways and presentation. Such research is critical for women's health and well-being, including in domains such as CVD, for which women experience 43 percent of the overall DALY burden.

To provide a simplified schematic that addresses this balance, the committee divided the 175 level 3 GBD categories by those disproportionately occurring in women (more than 67 percent of DALYs); those more common in women (51–67 percent of DALYs); and other conditions (50 percent or fewer DALYs but often occurring differently in women). Next, the committee estimated the proportion of WHR-related DALYs, attributing 100 percent of female DALYs in the first category to women's health, 50 percent in the second, and 33 percent in the third. This was intended to include contributions of both domains that traditionally fall entirely under the purview of WHR, such as gynecological conditions, and conservatively estimate the need for research powered to detect or focused specifically on sex differences. DALYs were reported by condition, category, and percentage of overall disease burden falling in this category.

Cancer spending

Figure 7-3 summarizes spending per unit of disease burden across cancer types, summarizing the ratio of fiscal year (FY) 2021 NCI reported spending to 2019 cancer incidence, prevalence, deaths, DALYs, YLLs, and YLDs in males and females. In each case, some female-specific cancers (blue bars) receive less NIH funding than many other cancers. In particular, uterine cancer ($57 per DALY) receives markedly lower funding per DALY compared to conditions such as non-Hodgkin's lymphoma ($2,794), brain cancer ($444), and pancreatic cancer ($190).

WHR portfolio

Figure 7-4 presents estimates related to a potential WHR portfolio. It highlights important contributions of both female-dominant and specific conditions, such as breast and gynecological cancers and gynecological and maternal disorders, and other conditions (e.g., musculoskeletal, mental health, and substance use disorders) relevant to women's health.

Overall, this classification encompasses 34 percent of all female DALYs and 16 percent of U.S. DALYs across both men and women. This framework

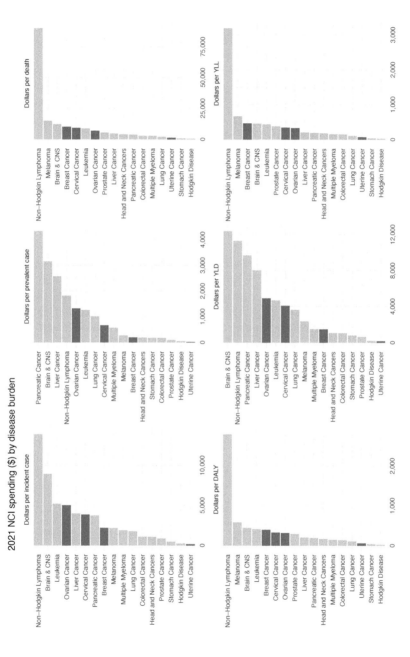

FIGURE 7-3 National Cancer Institute (NCI) 2021 spending by measures of cancer disease burden. NOTE: Blue bars indicate female-specific cancers.

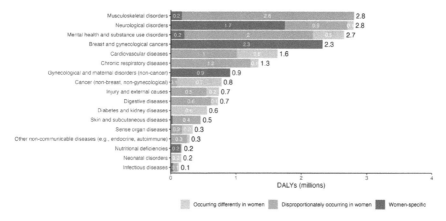

FIGURE 7-4 Disability-adjusted life years (DALYs) for conditions that impact women's health.
NOTE: These include all female DALYs for female-specific conditions (more than 67 percent of DALY disease burden in women) and a fraction of female DALYs for conditions experienced disproportionately in women (50 percent) or differently in women (33 percent).

is simplified and likely conservative: DALY estimates may be underestimates of the true prevalence of women's disease burden due to underdiagnosis (see Box 7-5), and as noted, this analysis does not account for lack of investment in basic science related to women's health (see Chapter 5), which would likely increase relative returns on investment. This rough estimate nevertheless provides a striking benchmark in comparison to the committee's funding analysis in Chapter 4—for NIH funding on WHR (which averaged 8.8 percent from FY 2013 to FY 2023) to reach this 16.5 percent burden estimate, it would need to increase by nearly twofold (87.5 percent). These burden estimates guide the discussion of conditions in this chapter.

Rare Diseases

One concern is that metrics focusing on population prevalence overlook rare diseases; funding research in proportion to DALYs would risk stunting progress toward preventing and treating rare illnesses.[3] In practice, there is a strong societal preference for investment in serious disabling conditions, even if they affect only a small number of people. Furthermore, making therapeutic progress for any condition requires a minimum threshold of investment, which may require funding rare conditions disproportionately to burden.

---

[3] According to the Orphan Drug Act, a disease or condition is considered rare if it affects fewer than 200,000 Americans (Public Law 97–414). *[This footnote was changed after release of the report to clarify the source of the definition.]*

DALYs per affected individual may also be considered to illustrate the concentration of disease burden. Nevertheless, tradeoffs remain challenging: how is a rare, severe neurological condition, such as Rett syndrome, which affects only one in 10,000 female individuals, weighted against a much more common but less debilitating condition, such as endometriosis or osteoarthritis?

A Framework for Selecting Exemplar Conditions Illustrating WHR Gaps

Several limitations to these analyses—and the use of DALYs or aggregated metrics more broadly—may merit consideration or further study when using disease burden analysis to identify research gaps and support funding decisions (see Box 7-5). Although DALYs are an imperfect metric, they

---

BOX 7-5
Limitations of Disability-Adjusted Life Years and
Future Directions for Health Metrics

DALYs and other aggregated health metrics can only provide insight related to the burden of disease for specific conditions. This approach is less useful for informing less-targeted basic science research or research focused on health-promotion, such as supporting contraceptive use.

There are also several limitations specific to the GBD study calculation of DALY weights.

- Weights were calculated by soliciting paired comparisons about the "health" of individuals experiencing various conditions. Some conditions, such as infertility, may substantially affect quality of life but have a low disability weight due to perceptions that the impact does not fall into the category of "unhealthy."
- GBD weights are being updated, particularly to account for women's health conditions. For example, new weights for dyspareunia and chronic conditions will be in a forthcoming update.
- In some cases, GBD burden estimates differ from those in other sources. For example, GBD reports a much lower prevalence of endometriosis than other estimates. This may arise because GBD prevalence estimates are differentially affected by diagnosis. For example, estimates of premenstrual disorder include self-reported survey responses, while endometriosis requires surgical diagnosis.

Additional research to contextualize DALYs to account for differential circumstances in which disability is experienced, such as social support and economic resources, would be valuable.

remain a widely applied measure that allow comparisons across diseases and sequelae. Therefore, despite these limitations, the committee found this to be a useful framework for identifying exemplar conditions to illustrate WHR needs and create a matrix of women's health conditions (see Table 7-1). Some conditions could fit into two categories, but for this overview, conditions are discussed in the DALY category based on the committee's analysis.

EXEMPLAR WOMEN'S HEALTH CONDITIONS

In this section, the committee provides a brief overview of some of the research gaps that fall into the categories identified in the matrix in the DALYs section (see Table 7-1).

FEMALE-SPECIFIC CONDITIONS WITH INCREASED DALYS RESULTING FROM DISABLING CONDITIONS

The 2024 National Academies report *Advancing Research on Chronic Conditions in Women* reviewed several female-specific conditions that increase DALYs as a result of disability and affect a significant proportion of women (NASEM, 2024b). This section highlights and summarizes several of these conditions, including uterine fibroids (leiomyomas), endometriosis, pelvic floor disorders, and female-specific mental health conditions (see NASEM, 2024b for an in-depth overview of these conditions).

Gynecological Conditions

Fibroids

Fibroids are the most common solid tumor of the pelvis and the leading cause of hysterectomy in the United States (Bulun, 2016; Marsh et al., 2024). While benign, they can lead to significant symptoms, including irregular and excessive uterine bleeding, lower abdominal pressure, dyspareunia, pelvic pain, recurrent pregnancy loss (RPL), infertility, and adjacent organ compression (Bulun, 2016; Marsh et al., 2024; NASEM, 2024b). Fibroids are more common in African American and Black females (Eltoukhi et al., 2014), who are also more likely to develop uterine fibroids at an earlier age, have larger-sized and greater number of fibroids, and experience more severe symptoms (Marsh et al., 2024). Despite their high prevalence, little is known about their pathophysiology. While researchers have studied estrogen as a mitogen for myoma growth, little research has been done to understand the role of other hormonal and non-hormonal factors in fibroid development and why they are more prevalent in Black females (Bulun, 2016; Cetin et al., 2020; NASEM, 2024c; Reis et al., 2016; Sefah et al., 2022). Given the high prevalence and morbidity, additional research

TABLE 7-1 Matrix of Women's Health Conditions

Affect only females			Differentially or disproportionately affect women		
DALYs resulting from disabling conditions Large population effect on females	DALYs resulting from early mortality	DALYs resulting from disabling conditions AND early mortality	DALYs resulting from disabling conditions	DALYs resulting from early mortality in women, and/or mortality in women versus men	DALYs resulting from disabling conditions AND early mortality in women, and/or early mortality in women versus men
• Endometriosis • Fibroids • Polycystic ovary syndrome • Pelvic floor disorders	• Female-specific cancers (uterine, cervical, ovarian, endometrial cancer)	• Breast cancer* • Maternal disorders/ pregnancy complications • Perinatal depression • Premenstrual dysphoric disorder • Menopause-related depression	• Mood disorders (depressive and anxiety disorders) • Musculoskeletal conditions, such as osteoarthritis	• Cardiovascular disease • Mental health disorders (mood disorders, cognition and dementia)	• Alzheimer's disease and dementias • Autoimmune disorders

NOTES: This table does not cover all conditions that affect only females or disproportionally or differentially affect women; it is a selection of conditions based on the committee's DALY analysis. For example, additional important female-specific conditions include vulvar and vaginal cancers and vulvodynia. DALY = disability-adjusted life year; * Breast cancer does affect men, but less than 1 percent of all U.S. breast cancer diagnoses are in men.

is needed across the entire translational spectrum to better understand the pathophysiology so that novel targeted medical and surgical treatments can be developed and disseminated (NASEM, 2024b).

Endometriosis

Despite endometriosis being one of the most common causes of infertility and chronic pelvic pain, its cause, risk factors, and true incidence remain uncertain (NASEM, 2024b; Young, 2024). It has no nonsurgical approach to diagnosis, and surgical treatments requiring hysterectomy and hormonal medical treatments are incompatible with fertility and fecundity (Young, 2024). It is also a risk factor for development of ovarian cancer and other chronic pain conditions, including irritable bowel syndrome (Barnard et al., 2024; Nabi et al., 2022). A population-based study found that those who developed endometriosis were 4.2 times more likely to develop ovarian cancer compared to those without endometriosis (Barnard et al., 2024). Additional research is needed to understand the pathophysiology and develop fertility-sparing approaches to treat this debilitating condition.

Pelvic Floor Disorders

Pelvic floor disorders, which are also common and significantly affect quality of life, lead to pelvic organ prolapse, urinary and fecal incontinence, recurrent urinary tract infections, bladder pain syndrome, and myofascial pelvic pain. Pelvic organ prolapse specifically occurs in up to 50 percent of female patients, but there are significant knowledge gaps in the basic science understanding of normal and abnormal pelvic floor function and the structural aspects of pelvic floor support (Aboseif and Liu, 2022; Swenson, 2024). A better understanding of pelvic floor function and its hormonal, structural, and functional determinants will enable more effective interventions. These are sorely needed given the high surgical treatment failure rate, impairing female quality of life (Swenson, 2024).

Polycystic Ovary Syndrome (PCOS)

PCOS is the most common endocrine disease in female patients and a leading cause of female impaired fecundity (Akre et al., 2022). It is a complex hormonal, metabolic, and reproductive disorder affecting multiple organ systems and afflicting approximately 4–18 percent of reproductive-age females (Bozdag et al., 2016; Dennett and Simon, 2015). Research has yet to fully elucidate the etiology, although in the majority of patients, it appears to be linked to some combination of polycystic ovarian morphology, hyperandrogenism, and ovulatory dysfunction. Many people are unaware they have it, as it is often characterized by myriad heterogeneous signs and symptoms. The Rotterdam diagnostic criteria are the most accepted, requiring two of the following three features: hyperandrogenism, oligo- or anovulation causing missed or irregular periods, or polycystic ovaries (Christ and Cedars, 2023). The hyperandrogenic state is proposed to contribute to insulin resistance and hyperglycemia and ultimately adiposity, or excessive body fat accumulation. PCOS can lead to significant medical conditions, including CVD, Type 2 diabetes, impaired fecundity, fatty liver disease, endometrial hyperplasia, and endometrial cancer, some of which may develop as a function of higher levels of body fat. It has no cure and no Food and Drug Administration (FDA)–approved therapies (Allen et al., 2022; Dennett and Simon, 2015; NASEM, 2024c).

Additional research is needed to better delineate the underlying cause; understand the complex interplay of genetic, epigenetic, and environmental factors associated with PCOS; identify curative therapies; assess long-term cardiovascular, metabolic, and cognitive decline risks; and identify mitigation strategies to prevent comorbid conditions (Che et al., 2023; Christ and Cedars, 2023). Recent research has also highlighted the need for further investigations on PCOS and its relationship to brain health during midlife (Huddleston et al., 2024). Despite its prevalence among females and substantial research gaps, PCOS also ranks near the bottom among NIH-funded conditions, according to the committee's funding analysis (see Chapter 4).

Additional gynecological conditions that take a significant toll on the lives of women and lead to disability are discussed in the 2024 report, including vulvodynia (NASEM, 2024b). The committee heard from many brave individuals who shared their experiences with gynecological conditions during the committee's information-gathering stage; see Box 7-6 for some of their experiences.

Funding Shortfall

A significant challenge to advancing research on these female-specific conditions is that noncancer gynecological conditions lack an NIH funding home among the current ICs. Figure 7-5 illustrates this contrast—even though more females are affected by endometriosis and PCOS than breast cancer, there is a paucity of funding for these conditions relative to breast cancer. Without a dedicated funding stream and NIH study sections that include the proper scientific expertise to review grants submitted on these conditions, there is a missed opportunity to advance scientific discoveries and treatments that will significantly improve quality of life and productivity for a significant proportion of the female population. It is critical to increase funding for these conditions to be on par with female-specific cancers.

BOX 7-6
In Their Own Words: Excerpts from Patients and Patient Advocates on Gynecologic Conditions During Public Comments at Committee Meetings

Polycystic Ovary Syndrome (PCOS)
- There isn't enough funding for research across women's health, but PCOS is an interesting case where it's a really prevalent disorder globally impacting 8 to 13 percent of women. Yet PCOS wasn't even listed in NIH's Research Condition Diseases Category reporting, the RCDC, until our organization's advocacy work. And so, this highlights that there are certain aspects of women's health which haven't been prioritized even though it impacts so many of us.
- We need to implement policies to ensure equitable funding and focus across diseases affecting women of all backgrounds. PCOS disproportionately impacts women of color and their metabolic health, mental health, et cetera, yet there is very little funding in this area, and very few Black researchers who are getting funded. So, thinking about not only who we are studying but who's doing the research and care as well.

Pelvic Floor Disorders
- Pelvic floor disorders cause musculoskeletal dysfunction, pain, loss of productivity, decline in self-esteem, relationship difficulties, mental health issues, just to name a few. Frequently, for pelvic floor research, we may see a study done with 30 subjects or a case study done with 1–3 people simply because NIH has not funded or prioritized research in this area. The data are shocking.
- Pelvic floor research is divided throughout NIH, and it has not focused on women's pelvic health through the life-span. The result is, without research data, the diagnostic criteria is variable. We don't have well-researched treatment options. Therefore, women cannot get the treatment and the services they need covered by health care.

Fibroids
- The lived experience of women with uterine fibroids is, I believe, a societally dismissed experience in communities worldwide that is steeped in a millennia old stigma that is expected that women will endure immense pain. Today in many countries women are still community outcast during their menstrual cycles.

(continued)

BOX 7-6 Continued

Endometriosis

- I'm not being alarmist when I say the lives of more than 6 million women nationwide quite literally depends on [more research]. Endometriosis has affected every single aspect of my life. It has ravaged my body beyond repair, destroyed relationships, stripped me of identity.
- At just 27 years old, it forced me to go on medical disability from work for over a year. It forced me to drop out of graduate school, just one class short of earning a master's degree. And I wish my story of turmoil and loss due to endometriosis were unique, but sadly, it is just one of millions.
- Despite my medical background and knowledge, it still took me over 4 years and 10 specialists ranging from pulmonology to cardiothoracic surgery to gastroenterology to be officially diagnosed with diaphragmatic endometriosis.

Vulvodynia

- Despite how common this condition is, it took years of going from doctor to doctor to get diagnosed. Clinicians told me to drink wine to relax before sex and seemed to incorrectly attribute my pain to something psychological. Meanwhile, I was trying to figure out how to sit and move without hurting. This was one of the most upsetting and isolating periods of my life, trying to find out why I was having this severe and terrifying pain, and why no provider seemed to take it seriously.
- Diagnosis was half the battle; treatment is another. I spent years trying every imaginable treatment and medication. Everything I have tried was off-label since there is no FDA-approved drug for any kind of chronic vulvovaginal pain. There is an effective surgery but it's only done by a few surgeons in the country and can cost tens of thousands of dollars out of pocket.
- It's daunting to stare down a lifetime of chronic pain, and it is made so much worse by the fact that most doctors, even OB-GYNs, have not heard of this issue. We need hope that some attention is going to be paid to finding effective treatments for this devastating diagnosis.

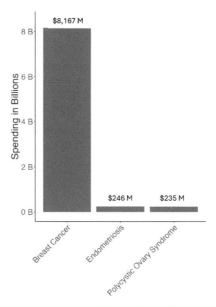

FIGURE 7-5 National Institutes of Health funding of breast cancer, endometriosis, and polycystic ovary syndrome, 2013–2023.
SOURCE: Committee's funding analysis (see Chapter 4).

Mental Health Conditions

Perinatal Depression

Perinatal depression, a major depressive disorder that occurs during pregnancy or in the first 12 months following childbirth, appears in approximately 10–20 percent of pregnancies in the United States and, along with other mental health conditions, is the leading cause of maternal mortality, accounting for 23 percent of maternal deaths (Dagher et al., 2021; Payne and Maguire, 2019; Sayres Van Niel and Payne, 2020; Trost et al., 2022). Specifically, 1 in every 7–10 pregnant people and 1 in every 5–8 postpartum people develop a depressive disorder, which translates to more than a half million cases each year, approximately the same number diagnosed with diabetes (Sayres Van Niel and Payne, 2020). Like diabetes, perinatal depression is a costly and potentially fatal condition, with its annual cost totaling at least $15 billion, or more than $22,600 per mother and infant, yet unlike diabetes, 91–93 percent of those with perinatal depression do not receive effective treatment (Cox et al., 2016), an enormous gap in clinical care.

As discussed in Chapter 5, NIH investment in research to understand the neuroendocrine mechanisms of perinatal depression resulted in two FDA-approved, highly effective treatments using allopregnanolone, a neuro-receptor modulator. It took over 80 years, however, from compound discovery to translation to treatment, and despite the advances, research funding for allopregnanolone and perinatal stress and depression remained much lower than other chronic conditions, such as breast cancer, afflicting a similarly large segment of the U.S. population (Deligiannidis, 2024; Pinna, 2020; Reddy et al., 2023). This funding trend has persisted (see Chapter 4 for more information), and important barriers to care, including a lack of screening and diagnosis, prevent most women from receiving effective treatment.

Psychotherapy is the first-line treatment for perinatal depression (Cuijpers and Karyotaki, 2021), and 92 percent of pregnant people prefer individual therapy to group treatment or medication (Goodman, 2009). However, only 7 percent of those with perinatal depression receive effective treatment because of systemic barriers to care (Cox et al., 2016), including cost, limited numbers of mental health specialists, geographic distance from specialty clinics, scheduling challenges arising from work-related and childcare demands, and stigma associated with seeking mental health care (Byatt et al., 2012; Dagher et al., 2021; Hellberg et al., 2023).

Moreover, although the new fast-acting, FDA-approved medications reduce depressive symptoms more rapidly and to a greater degree than earlier medications, they are not effective for about one-third of females; can only be used in the postpartum period, even though most cases of perinatal depression begin during pregnancy; have not been tested in lactating women; cannot be used as a prophylactic; and may be difficult to access given the cost and need for specialist prescribers and specialized treatment facilities that can provide inpatient hospitalization in facilities with 1:1 nursing supervision, for example (Meltzer-Brody et al., 2018; Patterson et al., 2024; Reddy et al., 2023). Of all the reproductive-related mood disorders, perinatal depression has received the most funding and has the strongest scientific foundation upon which to build rapid advances in identifying neurobiological mechanisms, objective diagnostics, novel treatments, and prevention, but realizing that potential still requires substantial monetary investment (Deligiannidis, 2024).

Menopause-Related Depression

The transition to menopause, or perimenopause, is characterized by irregular menses, vasomotor symptoms, sleep and sexual disturbances, weight gain, lassitude, cognitive dysfunction, vaginal dryness, urinary symptoms, and mood symptoms (Woods and Mitchell, 2005). The most commonly studied mood symptom is depression, but other common ones include irritability and anxiety (de Wit et al., 2021; Rössler et al., 2016; Seritan et al., 2010). Depression risk increases up to 14-fold in the 2 years surrounding the menopause transition (Schmidt et al., 2004), implicating ovarian hormone change as a trigger. Prospective longitudinal studies indicate this transition as a period of increased risk for both depressive symptoms and depressive disorders (Schmidt et al., 2004). With approximately 73 million U.S. women over age 45 (Statista, 2023), more than 1 million women reach menopause every year, and up to 70 percent will experience psychogenic symptoms associated with perimenopause and postmenopause (including anger/irritability, anxiety/tension, and depression) (NIA, 2022; Peacock et al., 2023). Depression (and anxiety) reduce health-related quality of life more than any of the other symptoms related to mental health (Wariso et al., 2017; Whiteley et al., 2013), contributing to the $326.2 billion annual cost associated with depression in the United States (Greenberg et al., 2021).

While research has shown that hormonal changes during perimenopause can affect mood, the precise mechanisms by which these fluctuations lead to depression are not fully understood, and studies are needed to elucidate the roles of estrogen, progesterone (PG), and other hormones in mood regulation during this time (Alblooshi et al., 2023; Bromberger and Epperson, 2018). In addition, factors such as stressful life events, social support, and attitudes toward aging and the menopause transition can influence the onset of depression. However, the interplay between these psychosocial factors and biological changes is not well characterized, representing a major research gap (Bromberger and Epperson, 2018). Although hormone therapy is commonly used to treat menopausal symptoms, its effectiveness as a monotherapy and use in combination with other treatments, specifically for menopause-related depression, merits more robust research (Gnanasegar et al., 2024; Maki et al., 2019). Studies on the long-term effects and safety of hormone therapy for mental health are needed as well. Without a clear understanding of the biological mechanisms driving menopause-related depression or well-powered studies to identify efficacious treatments, clinicians lack the evidence base needed to guide patient care.

FEMALE-SPECIFIC CONDITIONS WITH INCREASED DALYS RESULTING FROM EARLY MORTALITY

This section discusses female-specific cancers that are leading causes of early mortality in women and their variable progress based on NIH investment in research funding. Although breast cancer could fit in this category, it is discussed in the increased DALYs resulting from disability and early mortality section.

Uterine Malignancies

Uterine malignancies, including endometrial carcinomas and uterine sarcomas, are the most common and leading cause of gynecologic cancer. Over the past 2 decades, incidence and mortality rates for uterine cancers have risen alarmingly (Clarke et al., 2019; NASEM, 2024c; NCI, n.d.-d; Whetstone et al., 2022). It is estimated there will be 67,880 new cases and 13,250 deaths from uterine malignancies in 2024, representing 3.4 percent of all new cancer cases, with significant race-related survival disparities (NCI, n.d.-d; Siegel et al., 2024). The 5-year relative survival rate is 84 percent for White women and 63 percent for Black women (Whetstone et al., 2022).

The increasing rates of this disease, rising mortality, and alarming race-related disparities in endometrial cancer necessitate identifying and addressing research gaps (Siegel et al., 2024). Specifically, research is needed to understand the relationship between sex hormones, body weight, inflammation, environmental factors, and social determinants of health (SDOH) in disease etiology; develop prevention strategies and better diagnostic tools; and develop novel FDA-approved treatments. Prevention efforts will need to focus on balancing hormones, weight management, and physical activity (Bae-Jump, 2024). The advent of immunotherapy has seen a dramatic improvement in survival rates for individuals diagnosed with advanced disease, but an approach is lacking for identifying women most likely to benefit from these treatments (Tillmanns et al., 2024). Additional research is needed to assess and validate novel biomarkers of molecular classification to identify patients most likely to respond to therapy and elucidate resistance mechanisms for those who fail to respond to chemotherapy, immunotherapy, and the emerging antibody-drug conjugates.

Ovarian Cancer

Ovarian, tubal, and peritoneal cancer, collectively called "ovarian cancer," is an often lethal gynecologic malignancy, with 19,680 new cases and 12,740 deaths anticipated in 2024 (NCI, n.d.-c). Screening and early detection of ovarian cancer are challenging, and efforts to improve that have been unsuccessful and did not reduce mortality; it is therefore most common for cancer to be in a late stage at diagnosis (Buys et al., 2011; Karlan, 2024; Menon et al., 2021; NASEM, 2024c). While the incidence and mortality rates are declining, successful cures for this lethal disease remain elusive (American Cancer Society, 2024a). The landscape of ovarian cancer treatment shifted dramatically for high-grade serous—the most common type—and endometrioid cancers with the incorporation of maintenance poly(ADP-ribose) polymerase (PARP) inhibitor therapy. Since the approval of olaparib in 2018, several other PARP inhibitors have been approved to treat epithelial ovarian cancer or undergone evaluation (Coleman et al., 2017, 2019; González-Martín et al., 2019; Moore et al., 2018). Maintenance PARP inhibitor therapy for newly diagnosed ovarian cancer patients improved progression-free survival significantly, with the greatest benefit seen for those with *BRCA*-mutated cancers, followed by those with cancer that is homologous recombination deficient (Karlan, 2024; NCCN, 2024). Identifying active treatment options for patients with non-homologous-recombination-deficient epithelial ovarian cancers and primary platinum resistant disease is an important research need (Karlan, 2024).

Specific critical gaps in ovarian cancer include screening, understanding mechanisms of resistance to platinum-based chemotherapy and PARP inhibitor therapy, identification of treatment options for patients who progress on PARP inhibitor therapy, biomarkers to better identify homologous recombination deficiency, and identification of novel therapies beyond PARP inhibitors and emerging antibody-drug conjugates. Gaps to address for rare ovarian cancers, such as nonserous epithelial cancer, germ cell tumors, and stromal tumors, which tend to occur in younger women (Al Harbi et al., 2021; Berek et al., 2021), include developing representative animal models to understand pathophysiology and guide innovative therapies.

Cervical, Vulvar, and Vaginal Cancers

Most cervical, vulvar, and vaginal cancers are caused by human papillomavirus (HPV). Other risk factors include immune system suppression, long-term use of oral contraceptives, cigarette smoking, and prenatal exposure to diethylstilbestrol. In 2024, there will be an estimated 13,820 new cases of cervical cancer and 6,900 cases of vulvar cancer, accounting for 4,360 and 1,630 deaths, respectively (Siegel et al., 2024). The NCI "Last Mile" Initiative Self-Collection for HPV Testing to Improve Cervical Cancer Prevention Trial is assessing HPV self-collection for testing to prevent cervical cancer (NCI, n.d.-a). While this study will help address screening barriers, gaps remain regarding the multifactorial issues that negatively affect follow-up assessment of patients with abnormal screening results, access to care, and improving cure rates (NCI, n.d.-a; Rimel et al., 2022). Additional gaps in research remain regarding the role of induction immunotherapy, radiotherapy sequencing, optimal radiation therapy techniques, understanding mechanisms of resistance to immunotherapy and other novel therapies, and treatment of non-HPV-associated aggressive cervical, vulvar, and vaginal cancers.

Benefits of Funding Research on Female-Specific Cancers

There have been repeated calls to increase funding for research in gynecological cancers. As noted, uterine cancer ranks particularly low in NCI funding across a range of metrics that benchmark funding against population health impact. In 2021, for example, it ranked last in spending per YLDs and third to last in spending per YLLs. Cervical and ovarian cancer also rank below several cancers—including prostate, brain/central nervous system, and leukemia—in spending per YLL. Furthermore, although gynecologic cancers are rarer than, for example, breast, lung, prostate, and colorectal cancer and contribute to a smaller number of total DALYs and YLLs, prognosis remains poor, as quantified in recent gynecological oncology studies that measured YLL per incident case (described as "funding to lethality scores") (Guevara et al., 2023; Spencer et al., 2019). Greater investment in treatment for gynecological cancers may therefore substantially reduce dire health consequences experienced by many people with these conditions.

The benefits of funding research for female-specific cancers are illustrated by the congressionally directed Department of Defense Ovarian Cancer Research Program (OCRP), initiated in 1997 to support high-impact, cutting-edge research to address the unmet needs in ovarian cancer (CDMRP, 2024). From 1997 to 2022, it funded 633 awards, and 2023 had 298 applicants for awards, of which 42 were funded. Over the 27 years since the inception of OCRP, ovarian cancer incidence and mortality rates have declined (NCI, n.d.-c), and it is easy to speculate that OCRP's investment of over $496 million in ovarian cancer research was pivotal. For example, OCRP-funded studies have yielded transformative research tools, preventive tests, biomarkers to direct therapy, and novel treatments in the scientific and clinical arena. This includes several distinct novel ovarian cancer animal models; genetic testing guidelines; genetic risk test kits for RAD51D, PALB2, and BARD1 mutations; algorithms to diagnose precursor serous tubal intraepithelial carcinoma lesions; companion biomarker tests to direct PARP inhibitor therapy; and novel therapies (CDMRP, n.d.).[4] In contrast, lack of investment in other gynecologic cancers has coincided with rising incidence and mortality of endometrial cancer and stagnant mortality rates in cervical cancer, with disproportionately worse survival outcomes in Hispanic and non-White women and the greatest burden on Black women (NASEM, 2024c; NCI, n.d.-b,d; Siegel et al., 2024).

---

[4] One such novel therapy is rucaparib, which received accelerated FDA approval for treating patients with *BRCA*-mutated recurrent ovarian cancer in 2016 and later for maintenance treatment for select patients with platinum-sensitive disease. FDA has approved it for *BRCA*-mutated metastatic castration-resistant prostate cancer (FDA, 2016).

FEMALE-SPECIFIC CONDITIONS WITH INCREASED DALYS RESULTING FROM DISABLING CONDITIONS AND EARLY MORTALITY

Breast Cancer[5]

Breast cancer rates have increased by approximately 0.6 percent per year since the mid-2000s, with a slightly steeper incidence in women younger than age 50. It is the most common cancer in women other than skin cancers. The American Cancer Society estimates that 2024 will have approximately 310,720 new cases of invasive breast cancer and 56,500 new cases of ductal carcinoma in situ, and 42,250 women will die from breast cancer (American Cancer Society, 2024b).

Despite significant gaps in breast cancer research, investment has significantly affected mortality rates, with striking improvements in mortality over past decades that reflect multiple moderate gains from screening and treatment improvements (Jagsi, 2024). Increased NIH funding has led to breakthroughs in early detection methods, such as improved mammography and the development of genetic testing, allowing for earlier diagnosis and intervention, as well as improved medications that reduce breast cancer mortality and recurrence (see Box 7-7). Surgical techniques have evolved from radical mastectomies to more conservative approaches, such as lumpectomies and focused and targeted lymphadenectomy, minimizing the physical and emotional impact while maintaining efficacy (Jagsi, 2024). Radiation therapy has also seen progress with more precise targeting methods, reducing damage to healthy tissue and improving outcomes. Chemotherapy has become more effective with the introduction of targeted therapies and less toxic drug regimens, allowing for more personalized and effective treatment plans (Jagsi, 2024). NIH-funded studies have advanced the understanding of how the immune system interacts with breast cancer, which has contributed to developing immunotherapeutic approaches, including checkpoint inhibitors and vaccine therapies, that are now being explored in clinical trials (Al-Hawary et al., 2023; Morrison et al., 2024; Nordin et al., 2023; Pallerla et al., 2021).

Although these investments have paid off in terms of decreasing morbidity and mortality, the journey to preventing and treating breast cancer is not over. Gaps remain in translating many of these discoveries into practice. For example, the U.S. Preventive Services Task Force has concluded there is insufficient evidence to determine the benefits and harms of screening mammography among women aged 75 and older and of supplemental screening

---

[5] Although breast cancer does affect men, less than 1 percent of all U.S. breast cancer diagnoses are in men (NCI, 2020).

BOX 7-7
NIH-Funded Breast Cancer Prevention and
Treatment Discoveries

- In 1958, chemotherapy drugs were used at the NIH Clinical Center to treat solid tumor cancers (including breast cancer), which is now a standard treatment.
- Breakthroughs in imaging technologies (e.g., 3-D mammography) and new biomarker-based tests have improved early detection and diagnosis, allowing for earlier and more precise intervention.
- Research helped identify breast cancer subtypes based on tumor molecular features, which allows for more targeted treatments, contributing to a 41 percent decrease in death rates from 1990–2019.
- In 2012, an NIH-funded study found that a combination of two drugs can lengthen the lives of postmenopausal women with the most common type of metastatic breast cancer.
- Research that identified and characterized the *BRCA* gene mutations in breast, ovarian, prostate, and pancreatic cancer, which allows individuals with a family history of these cancers to use genetic test results to inform decision making for screening, prevention, and treatments.
- Research has led to developing new drugs that target specific aspects of breast cancer biology. For example, aromatase inhibitors are a standard treatment for postmenopausal women with hormone receptor–positive breast cancer, and CDK4/6 inhibitors have also improved treatment options for this type of breast cancer.
- NIH research led to the discovery and clinical use of drugs such as trastuzumab (Herceptin) for HER2-positive breast cancer and significantly improved outcomes for patients with this subtype.

SOURCES: Early Breast Cancer Trialists' Collaborative Group, 2015; Morrison et al., 2024; NIH, 2013, n.d.-a; Santen et al., 2009; Ulm et al., 2019.

with ultrasonography or magnetic resonance imaging in women with dense breasts (USPSTF, 2024). Additionally, although robust evidence shows some women can safely avoid potentially toxic treatments, that does not always translate into practice, and many women pursue unnecessarily aggressive treatments, leading to worsened quality of life, second malignancies after unnecessary radiation, and other side effects, such as cardiac toxicity, cognitive decline, and financial toxicity (Jagsi et al., 2017; NASEM, 2024c). Additional research is needed to prevent and treat metastatic breast cancer and to elucidate the biological mechanisms driving metastasis, including how cancer cells evade the immune system and survive in distant organs.

Racial and Ethnic Survival Disparities in Breast and Gynecologic Cancers

Significant racial and ethnic survival disparities for individuals diagnosed with breast and gynecologic cancers have been reported since the 1970s (Towner et al., 2022). Despite this knowledge, gaps in care have not been completely addressed, leading to persistent and detrimental survival disparities. Overall, the age-standardized death rate for all cancers is highest for non-Hispanic Black patients compared to all other racial and ethnic groups (Cronin et al., 2022). Survival disparities are most striking for uterine cancer, the only cancer for which mortality rates have increased over the past 4 decades (Siegel et al., 2024). Its increased incidence is most pronounced among those who identify as Black, Asian American, Pacific Islander, and/or Hispanic, with a greater than 2 percent increase since the mid-2000s (Siegel et al., 2024). The most alarming racial survival disparity is between Black and White patients; Black people with uterine cancers have a twofold increased risk of death (Siegel et al., 2024). In 2018, the 3-year survival rates were only 69.1 percent in Black patients compared to 86.5 percent in White patients (NCI, 2024d).

Conversely, since about 2000, death rates for breast and ovarian cancer have decreased, while mortality rates have remained stagnant for cervical cancer patients (Siegel et al., 2024). However, Black people with breast, ovarian, and cervical cancers also have worse outcomes compared to White people for every stage of diagnosis (Siegel et al., 2024). For breast cancer, the 3-year relative survival rates in 2018 were 94.8 versus 88.8 percent for White and Black patients, respectively (NCI, 2024a,b). Similar trends were reported for ovarian cancer in 2018, with 3-year relative survival rates of 61.5 versus 55.5 percent for White and Black patients, respectively (NCI, 2024f). For cervical cancer, Black, Hispanic, and American Indian/Alaska Native patients still have the highest incidence and mortality rates compared to White and non-Hispanic patients (AARC, 2024; NCI, n.d.-b; Siegel et al., 2024). Furthermore, screening tests are less likely to be obtained for Hispanic patients compared to White and Black patients (AARC, 2024). The 3-year relative survival rates for cervical cancer are 74.4 versus 64.8 percent for White and Black patients, respectively (NCI, 2024c).

Additionally, Black and Hispanic women with breast, ovarian, cervical, and endometrial cancer are less likely to receive care that adheres to current guidelines (AARC, 2024; Hinchcliff et al., 2019; Siegel et al., 2024; Zhang et al., 2020a). Marginalized patient populations are also less likely to be represented in clinical trials (Scalici et al., 2015); including them is imperative to ensure improved understanding of racial and ethnic differences in tumor biology, biomarkers, response to therapy, and survival outcomes. Cancer survivors who identify as Black and Hispanic/Latina have poorer quality of life and mental health compared to White or other racial and ethnic groups, respectively (AARC, 2024).

Research has improved understanding of the underlying molecular biology of disease. However, significant gaps remain. More research is needed to understand the underlying etiology of racial and ethnic survival disparities and intersections with SDOH. Dedicated funding to address cancer disparities for female-specific cancers are critical to mitigate racial and ethnic survival disparities and ensure equitable care for all patients.

Maternal Disorders/Pregnancy-Related Complications

Each year, there are 5.5–6.5 million pregnancies in the United States. Despite the incredibly common nature of pregnancy, its understanding along the translational science spectrum from basic science to population health outcomes and policy impact remains poor. In fact, even the precise number of pregnancies in any given year remains elusive, largely because of data collection gaps (NASEM, 2024a; Rossen et al., 2023). Pregnancy and childbirth are often relational experiences, with effects on not only the pregnant person but also partners, families, and communities.

Adverse pregnancy outcomes most often have multiple contributing factors, including genetic, epigenetic, environmental, and behavioral factors; quality of care; and structural causes. As with many health outcomes, inequities in pregnancy exist across and between multiple axes of social risk, including education, access to care, and geographic location. Data are limited on how structural drivers of health, such as racism, discrimination, classism, and sexism, manifest in the body to change biological process and impact pregnancy outcomes. However, epidemiologic data demonstrate that Black, American Indian and Alaska Native (AIAN), and Native Hawaiian and Pacific Islander (NHPI) mothers and infants, for example, experience two- to threefold higher rates of adverse outcomes compared to their White counterparts (CDC, n.d.-c; Hill et al., 2022; NASEM, 2020; Petersen et al., 2019). The gaps in these outcomes, which include stillbirth, low birthweight, infant mortality, and maternal mortality, have remained nearly unchanged for over a century despite medical, technical, and public health advances that have reduced overall rates. This suggests that structural factors—in this case, structural racism—play a role in distributing access to opportunities for health improvement inequitably across social axes (Hill et al., 2022; NASEM, 2019, 2020, 2023).

This section provides examples of pregnancy-related conditions for which research investment could significantly improve treatment and prevention or close gaps in maternal health morbidity and mortality. For many of these conditions, different pathophysiologic pathways may lead to the same downstream consequences, but current scientific knowledge lacks the detail and precision to differentiate these, which also results in ineffective treatments, as heterogenous processes are often lumped together and treated similarly.

Maternal Mortality

Maternal mortality is generally defined as death while pregnant or within 42 days of the end of the pregnancy, and the Centers for Disease Control and Prevention (CDC) use the phrase "pregnancy-related mortality" to include deaths that occur during or within 1 year of the end of pregnancy from any cause related to or aggravated by the pregnancy (CDC, n.d.-b; WHO, n.d.). In 2022, 817 people died of pregnancy-related causes in the United States, resulting in a maternal mortality ratio of 22 per 100,000 live births (Hoyert, 2024). This has earned the United States the unenviable rank of the highest maternal mortality ratio among high-income countries (Gunja et al., 2024).[6] Its maternal mortality is also characterized by stark racial disparities, with NHPI, Black, and AIAN people having the highest rates (CDC, n.d.-b). In 2022, the rate was 49.5 per 100,000 live births among Black patients, which is nearly threefold higher than the 19 per 100,000 among White birthing people (Hoyert, 2024). Geographical disparities also exist, with the highest rates in Arkansas and Mississippi (CDC, n.d.-a).

A review of maternal deaths from 2017 to 2019 in 36 states showed that pregnancy-related deaths occurred during pregnancy, birth, and up to 1 year postpartum, with 53 percent occurring from 7 days to 1 year postpartum (Trost et al., 2022). Moreover, over 80 percent of these deaths were determined to be preventable (Trost et al., 2022).

The etiology of maternal mortality is multifaceted and includes direct and indirect causes. The CDC analysis showed that the six most frequent direct causes were mental health conditions (22.7 percent), hemorrhage (13.7 percent), cardiac and coronary conditions (12.8 percent), infection (9.2 percent), thrombotic embolism (8.7 percent), and cardiomyopathy (8.5 percent), accounting for over 75 percent of these deaths (Trost et al., 2022). The leading underlying cause of death varied by race and ethnicity, with cardiac and coronary conditions most common among non-Hispanic Black persons; mental health conditions most common among Hispanic and non-Hispanic White persons; and hemorrhage most common among non-Hispanic Asian people (Trost et al., 2022).

---

[6] High-income countries have data collection, reporting, definitional, and population differences, making this comparison complex.

Indirect causes of maternal mortality include structural racism, economic inequities, public policies, such as a lack of access to insurance or parental leave, and other social drivers, including food, housing, and transportation instability, that culminate in inequities in the longitudinal provision of preconception, antenatal, intrapartum, and postpartum care at the system, provider, and patient levels (Crear-Perry et al., 2021; Howell, 2018). The effect of state abortion bans enabled by the Supreme Court overturning *Roe v. Wade* may also affect maternal deaths. There have numerous reports and litigation on the effect of the denial of care that includes abortion or miscarriage management care to women experiencing potentially life-threatening pregnancy-related emergencies (Grossman et al., 2023).[7,8,9] Research conducted before the *Dobbs v. Jackson Women's Health Organization* decision found a higher likelihood of maternal mortality in states with restrictive abortion policies (Vilda et al., 2021). Recent news reports have begun to identify cases of maternal deaths that have been attributed to denial of appropriate care due to abortion bans, but initial research from national vital statistics data for the year following the decision has not noted such an effect (Stevenson and Root, 2024; Surana, 2024a,b). A landmark prospective study on the effect of abortion denial found that women who were denied abortions and who gave birth had higher rates of pregnancy-related complications, including, eclampsia, postpartum hemorrhage, and gestational hypertension, compared to those who were able to obtain a wanted abortion (ANSIRH, n.d.; Gerdts et al., 2016; Ralph et al., 2019).

Gaps in maternal mortality and morbidity research include difficulties in case ascertainment for maternal mortality from death records and potential misclassification in current coding methods and systems (Collier and Molina, 2019; Joseph et al., 2024; MacDorman and Declercq, 2018; van den Akker et al., 2017). Each U.S. state may choose to participate in Maternal Mortality Review Committee efforts; a multidisciplinary committee reviews the circumstances of maternal deaths to adjudicate pregnancy relatedness and opportunities for prevention or intervention (Collier and Molina, 2019; St. Pierre et al., 2018). Funding for this remains limited, as does the ability for any central authority to combine and synthesize recommendations for prevention or intervention to develop programs to reduce maternal mortality and morbidity (St. Pierre et al., 2018). In addition, granular analyses that provide insight into community or population experience are hampered by low numbers (e.g., lack of granular race data for NHPI individuals) (Trost et al., 2022).

---

[7] Blackmon v. State of Tennessee (2023).
[8] Adkins v. State of Idaho (2023).
[9] Zurawski v. State of Texas (2023).

A leading cause of maternal mortality is death from suicide or overdose—that is, perinatal mental health concerns and substance use disorders (Chin et al., 2022; Han et al., 2024). Though a monitoring framework for maternal morbidity—a harbinger of problems that, if left unchecked, could lead to maternal mortality—exists and has been validated, no similar measure of severe maternal mental health morbidity exists to help identify and target those most at risk for suicide or overdose in the peripartum period.

As noted, indirect causes of maternal mortality are important contributors, so studies that focus on the social and structural determinants of health and their effect on maternal outcomes are needed (Crear-Perry et al., 2021). Gaps also remain in understanding provider access, availability, knowledge, and potential for bias in care around maternal mortality, particularly for acute health events (Howell, 2018; NASEM, 2021; Slaughter-Acey et al., 2023).

RPL

The definition of RPL differs across professional societies.[10] Based on these varying definitions, 1–5 percent of individuals attempting pregnancy will experience it, and fewer than 1 percent will experience three or more consecutive first-trimester pregnancy losses (ACOG, 2024; Practice Committee of the American Society for Reproductive Medicine, 2012; Regan et al., 2023).

While embryonic aneuploidy, or abnormal chromosome number, is the most common cause of any one pregnancy loss, its contribution decreases as consecutive pregnancy losses increase. Other potential explanations include uterine anomalies, endocrine disorders, immune disorders, and thrombophilias, which are genetic or acquired blood clotting disorders (Ford and Schust, 2009; Regan et al., 2023). RPL confers significant mental, emotional, and financial burdens that affect health care costs, personal and family stress, and work productivity (Laijawala, 2024; Quenby et al., 2021). Despite these burdens, it remains unexplained in 50 percent of cases (ACOG, 2024; Ford and Schust, 2009). Furthermore, no treatments have consistently demonstrated effectiveness in maintaining pregnancies afterward. This is true even for interventions, including uterine septum resection and PG supplementation, aimed at specific relevant etiologies (Ford and Schust, 2009; Regan et al., 2023).

---

[10] The American College of Obstetricians and Gynecologists, for example, defines RPL as having two or more miscarriages, while the American Society of Reproductive Medicine defines it as the loss of two or more clinical and consecutive pregnancies with either ultrasound or histopathological documentation, excluding ectopic and molar pregnancies, and the Royal College of Obstetricians and Gynecologists defines it as three or more consecutive first trimester miscarriages (ACOG, 2024; Practice Committee of the American Society for Reproductive Medicine, 2013; Regan et al., 2023).

Recent early trials for subsets of the RPL population have shown some promise. For example, intravenous immunoglobulin IVIG for individuals who have experienced more than four losses and PG supplementation for individuals with more than three losses and vaginal bleeding in the first trimester of a subsequent pregnancy may show promise for these small subsets, but their evidence base and effectiveness in practice remains under investigation given the lack of large-scale, randomized controlled trials and conclusive evidence (ACOG, 2021; Banjar et al., 2023; Coomarasamy et al., 2019, 2020; D'Mello et al., 2021; Habets et al., 2022; Shi et al., 2022; Yamada et al., 2022).

The failure of many proposed treatment strategies is likely due to several heterogenous disease processes that result in a similar clinical phenotype of RPL. Therefore, the entire relevant translational research spectrum would benefit from increased attention; it serves as a clear example of gaps in basic science knowledge. Understanding is limited of the processes that support appropriate implantation and permit early pregnancies to progress when the embryo has normal genes. This inadequate understanding of pathophysiology across both identified and yet-to-be-identified causes of RPL has generally hampered progress toward interventions that could mitigate the substantial emotional, financial, and potential long-term health burdens (Laijawala, 2024; Quenby et al., 2021).

Preeclampsia

Preeclampsia is on a spectrum of hypertensive diseases in pregnancy and affects 2–8 percent of all pregnant people globally (ACOG, n.d.). Classically, pregnant people are diagnosed when they exhibit new-onset elevated blood pressures and proteinuria, or elevated protein in the urine, beyond 20 weeks of pregnancy. More severe forms manifest with pulmonary edema, cardiomyopathy, seizures, uncontrolled headaches, or end-organ damage, such as acute liver or kidney injury. Preeclampsia and other related hypertensive disorders of pregnancy significantly affect maternal and fetal health, with more than 7 percent of maternal deaths stemming from preeclampsia and its complications (CDC, 2022).

In addition, preeclampsia drives a significant proportion of preterm births (PTBs) resulting from the need to induce birth early for maternal safety and from small for gestational age neonates due to associated poor placental function. Black and African American pregnant people in the United States have a moderately increased risk of preeclampsia compared to White individuals and a higher likelihood of related morbidity and mortality, suggesting differences in treatment and care access (MacDorman et al., 2021; Zhang et al., 2020b). Preeclampsia confers lifelong increased cardiovascular risks that compound its health effects and underscore the urgency of understanding, treating, and preventing it and its long-term consequences.

The origins of preeclampsia are not fully understood but likely begin with impaired placental implantation (Dimitriadis et al., 2023; Huppertz, 2008; Kalafat and Thilaganathan, 2017; Kornacki et al., 2023). Advances in understanding the roles of serum markers that indicate dysfunction within the lining of small blood vessels and markers of immune system dysfunction have not yet translated into improved diagnostic or therapeutic options (Amaral et al., 2017; Dimitriadis et al., 2023; Jung et al., 2022). Preeclampsia remains a clinical diagnosis based on symptoms and signs consistent with it; diagnosis is challenging when other comorbidities exist that mimic these, such as chronic hypertension and autoimmune disease (Jung et al., 2022; Staff, 2019). The lack of a definitive diagnostic disease marker increases the potential for bias in interpreting the signs and symptoms by race, ethnicity, or other demographics, thereby increasing the possibility of inequitable outcomes (Dimitriadis et al., 2023; Johnson and Louis, 2022).

No treatments aside from delivery can slow, mitigate, or reverse the effects of preeclampsia (Bokuda and Ichihara, 2023; Dimitriadis et al., 2023; Magee et al., 2023; Staff, 2019). Despite promising results in animal models, trials of phosphodiesterase inhibitors and statins have failed to demonstrate effectiveness in humans; statins may reduce preterm, but not term, preeclampsia (Bokuda and Ichihara, 2023; Dimitriadis et al., 2023; Larré et al., 2018). A daily low-dose aspirin can decrease the likelihood of preeclampsia in individuals at risk, but clinicians continue to lack clarity around why it works, which dosage is most effective, or which population might benefit most (Dimitriadis et al., 2023). The lack of effective preventive and treatment options demonstrates the difficulty in bridging the wide chasm of clinical translation between basic science understanding and clinically meaningful diagnostic, preventive, and therapeutic outcomes. Given the broad effects, including the increased risk of serious conditions later in life, such as chronic hypertension, stroke, heart failure, heart attack, peripheral vascular disease, and kidney disease, and the role preeclampsia plays in inequities in maternal morbidity and mortality, a lagging understanding of diagnosis and treatment places pregnant people and their offspring at significant risk (Bokuda and Ichihara, 2023; Dimitriadis et al., 2023; Howell, 2018).

Gestational Diabetes (GD)

GD results from an inappropriate or dysregulated response to pregnancy-related decreases in insulin sensitivity. An imbalance in glucose intolerance and insulin production can lead to GD, but it remains unclear how the imbalance occurs or what hormones mediate the development of this disorder (Rassie et al., 2022).

Each year, 5–9 percent of U.S. pregnant individuals will develop GD, with an estimated annual cost of $1.6 billion related to additional antenatal surveillance, such as ultrasounds and non-stress tests, and increased maternal, obstetric, and neonatal adverse outcomes (Bolduc et al., 2024; CDC, 2024a; Dall et al., 2019; Sweeting et al., 2024). It disproportionately affects Latina/Latine/Hispanic, NHPI, AIAN, and Asian (notably Asian Indian) people, contributing to an excess burden of perinatal morbidity (Greco et al., 2024; Gregory and Ely, 2022; Shah et al., 2021; Ye et al., 2022). In addition to increased rates, there are also gaps in glycemic control and disease outcomes among pregnant people of color, which might be attributable to lack of access to high-quality care, lack of culturally responsive treatments, and other structural barriers (Bower et al., 2019; CDC, 2023; Erbetta et al., 2022; Palatnik et al., 2022; Shah et al., 2021).

Approximately 20–60 percent of individuals diagnosed with GD will develop Type 2 diabetes in the next 10 years; for some, this results in a young age of onset, with a lifetime of managing a chronic illness and significant potential for cardiovascular, renal, neurologic, and cerebrovascular disease (Buchanan et al., 2012; Li et al., 2022). For individuals who develop Type 2 diabetes later in life, it remains unclear whether GD represents a manifestation of baseline risk for diabetes given the physiologic and hormonal challenges of pregnancy or itself somehow contributes to lifelong increased risk by permanently altering physiology. Recent genome-wide association studies have demonstrated some overlap between genes that increase susceptibility to Type 2 and GD, which provides some early insight into disease pathophysiology but cannot clarify the chronology of these events (Dalfrà et al., 2020).

GD is also associated with increases in adverse perinatal outcomes for birthing parent, fetus, and neonate, including cesarean birth; preeclampsia; shoulder dystocia, a condition where one or both shoulders of the baby become stuck during labor; fetal growth abnormalities, particularly macrosomia, or being oversized; neonatal hypoglycemia; stillbirth; and neonatal intensive care unit admission. Two large randomized controlled trials demonstrated that treating it results in reduced adverse perinatal outcomes, confirming observational studies suggesting that glycemic control reduces the risk of adverse outcomes (Crowther et al., 2005).

Research gaps in GD include understanding the hormonal physiology that contributes to both it and Type 2 diabetes risk and identifying the most effective screening windows, serum glucose thresholds for diagnostic tests, and implementation approaches to ensure all groups have access to high-quality and culturally responsive counseling and treatment.

Spontaneous PTB

PTB, or the birth of a live or stillborn infant before 37 weeks gestation, affects up 10 percent of U.S. pregnant people (CDC, 2024b; March of Dimes, n.d.). The majority occurs at 32–36 weeks of pregnancy, and 70–80 percent of these are spontaneous and not as a result of medical intervention to induce birth (Goldenberg et al., 2008; March of Dimes, n.d.). The causes include spontaneous preterm labor (40–45 percent), premature rupture of membranes that cause amniotic fluid leaking before the onset of labor (25–30 percent), and, more rarely, premature dilation of the cervix (also known as "cervical insufficiency") or placental abruption (premature separation of the placenta from the wall of the uterus) (Goldenberg et al., 2008). Approximately 20–30 percent of PTBs occur when clinicians decide to induce (medically or surgically) given a fetal or maternal complication that substantially increases the risk of ongoing pregnancy to the mother or fetus (Goldenberg et al., 2008; IOM, 2007). However, clinicians and investigators often cannot provide parents with clear reasons for their PTB experience, and many pregnant people feel responsible for the outcome, with associated feelings of guilt and shame.

The underlying processes that can prematurely trigger the labor cascade, resulting in spontaneous PTB, remain unclear (Goldenberg et al., 2008). This is a result, at least in part, to a poor understanding of the labor cascade itself; interventions for slowing or stopping the process in preterm, pathological situations have proven unsuccessful (Goldenberg et al., 2008; Iams et al., 2008; March of Dimes, 2020; Mayo Clinic, 2022).

Studies have demonstrated that inflammation, whether from microbial infection or an endogenous cause, plays a role in PTB (Goldenberg et al., 2008). However, how these abnormal inflammatory states begin—how maternal immune system tolerance for the fetus and vice versa becomes disrupted or dysfunctional—how and why infection may ascend into the uterus, and how the inflammatory milieu can trigger labor remains an area of investigation. In addition, multiple clinical and environmental factors, such as multifetal gestation, air pollution and heat exposure, stress, and others, have an association with PTB (Bekkar et al., 2020; Etzel, 2020; Goldenberg et al., 2008).

Preterm birth is a leading cause of neonatal morbidity and mortality worldwide, and inequities by race persist. Black and AIAN pregnant people's risk of PTB exceeds that of White individuals by about 50 percent (Barreto et al., 2024; Raglan et al., 2016). It is also critical to consider the heterogeneity within racial and ethnic groups when addressing health equity (NASEM, 2023). Birth outcomes among Latino/a/x/e individuals are a salient example; although these outcomes are on average worse than for White pregnant patients, there is considerable variation. For example, in one study that included predominately Puerto Rican individuals, who have some of the highest rates of adverse outcomes, acculturation (measured by language preference and generation in the United States) was associated with higher gestational age and birthweight (Barcelona de Mendoza et al., 2016).

In addition to the immediate neonatal consequences, PTB also exposes mothers to increased cardiovascular complications and earlier all-cause mortality compared to individuals without a history of PTB (Crump et al., 2020; Wu et al., 2018).

Abortion

Even before the Supreme Court decision in *Dobbs v. Jackson Women's Health Organization*,[11] which overturned the federal right to abortion and protections for abortion access, data gaps surrounding abortion made it difficult to study. Reasons for data collection difficulty include the early gestation at which most abortions occur, concerns about criminalization of providers and patients, stigma, and the decentralized and siloed environments in which most abortion care takes place, with abortion clinics typically separated to greater or lesser degree from other health care institutions (NASEM, 2024d). As of August 2024, 14 states have banned abortion with limited and difficult to access exceptions, and an additional six states have limited it to early in pregnancy, often before people even know they are pregnant (KFF, 2024). The Guttmacher Institute estimates there were 1,037,000 abortions in the formal health care system in 2023, the first full year after the Supreme Court overturned *Roe v. Wade* (Maddow-Zimet and Gibson, 2024). This estimate does not include self-managed abortion, which has likely increased but presents even greater barriers to accurate measurement.

Despite the commonality of pregnancy termination, multiple data gaps exist (Gomez et al., 2024; NASEM, 2024d). These include the difficulty identifying which patients or communities might need abortion care but cannot access it, differences in health outcomes caused by delays in care, increased difficulties created by crossing state lines or accessing self-managed abortion resources, and a better understanding of the health implications of self-managed abortions in the present context of broader availability of mifepristone. There are also gaps in documenting changes in abortion access and delivery, understanding short- and long-term ramifications for restrictions, and implications for the workforce (Dennis, 2024).

There are numerous federal policy barriers and challenges to collecting abortion data and undertaking abortion-related research (NIH, n.d.-b,c; Schott et al., 2023). However, given the potential for significant effects of denied abortion and delays in miscarriage management interventions on maternal morbidity and mortality, and other important concerns affecting women's health and well-being, abortion-related research is needed to protect women's health and inform policy. In addition, post-*Roe v. Wade*

---

[11] Dobbs v. Jackson Women's Health Organization, 597 U.S. 215 (2022).

abortion bans have resulted in fewer medical residency applicants choosing to train in abortion-restrictive states; this could directly lead to worsening maternity care access and a negative impact on maternal health outcomes in those states (Orgera and Grover, 2024; Weiner, 2022).

Structural Barriers to Advancing Pregnancy Research

A chief barrier to pregnancy-related research is the prior designation of pregnant individuals as a vulnerable population for research safety. Vulnerable populations have social or medical circumstances that increase their susceptibility to coercion or inability to provide voluntary consent to research. Though pregnancy itself does not render people incapable of providing informed consent, the fetus was felt to be a third party who could not consent. Because of this designation, ethics boards most often required research procedures to have demonstrable *direct* benefit to both the pregnant person and fetus or direct benefit to the pregnant person and no more than minimal risk to the fetus. As discussed in Chapter 2, such barriers resulted in excluding pregnant and lactating individuals from nearly all protocols related to non-obstetric conditions or drug trials. Furthermore, the designation created a particularly high bar for risk tolerance in obstetric research. This has resulted in numerous fundamental questions remaining unanswered, such as the efficacy of certain drugs during pregnancy, safety of medication during lactation, or the pathophysiology of disorders in pregnancy (NASEM, 2024a).

While pregnant people received a new special populations designation by FDA in 2018, which removed some of the most restrictive rules, the significant knowledge gaps created by decades of treatment as a vulnerable population will take dedicated effort and funding to close. Furthermore, these rule changes have not sparked a dramatic increase in including pregnant and lactating individuals in trials (NASEM, 2024a). This has left them and their health care providers faced with the challenging task of determining which medications and vaccines are safe and effective and will affect their own health or that of their fetus or child. Conversely, some may choose to use these and face an unpredictable risk of harm and uncertain potential benefits. A 2024 National Academies report, *Advancing Clinical Research with Pregnant and Lactating Populations: Overcoming Real and Perceived Liability Risks*, recommends ways to improve the safe and ethical inclusion of pregnant and lactating people in clinical research, including recommending that NIH develop a plan to prioritize research with these populations across its ICs (NASEM, 2024a).

The structure and funding of NIH ICs also creates limitations for pregnancy-related research. The *Eunice Kennedy Shriver* National Institute for Child Health and Development (NICHD) is the only IC that specifically includes pregnancy within its charge. However, it enters the NICHD purview largely as a driver of neonatal and infant health rather than an opportunity to understand either pregnancy itself or any maternal effects in the short and long terms. This results in researchers focusing questions and hypotheses from the frame of fetal and neonatal outcomes, leaving important maternal health–related questions understudied or unaddressed because of a lack of alignment with funding opportunities. The risk of becoming pregnant and the immediate and downstream consequences of pregnancy, labor, and birth on the body are unique. However, no permanent NIH infrastructure supports the research needed to advance scientific understanding of pregnancy and postpartum conditions to improve the health and well-being of people who are or capable of becoming pregnant and their families and address prevention (including contraception) to avoid pregnancies that are not desired or mistimed.

Summary of Maternal Disorders/Pregnancy-Related Complications

As demonstrated, researchers and clinicians have only the merest grasp of physiology, pathophysiology, and effective clinical treatments related to pregnancy and pregnancy-related disorders, a unifying thread within this research. In addition, data gaps hamper population health interventions and evidence-based policy making to prevent adverse pregnancy outcomes and close gaps by race, ethnicity, geography, or income. This situation stems from a lack of investment in research at the maternal–fetal interface and lack of research understanding and intervening on structural and policy barriers that have impeded progress.

DIFFERENTIAL EFFECT BY SEX AND INCREASED FEMALE DALYS RESULTING FROM DISABLING CONDITIONS

Mood Disorders (Depressive and Anxiety Disorders)

Depression affects women throughout their life course and includes conditions such as premenstrual dysphoric disorder, perinatal depression, and depression related to the menopause transition. Multiple studies have illustrated that depression is higher among women compared to men and among women of younger compared to older age (NASEM, 2024b). The prevalence of depression from 2015 to 2020 reported within the past year increased in both adolescent and adult women and men but was almost two times higher in women compared to men, at 11.8 percent versus 6.4 percent in 2020 (Goodwin et al., 2022). Although racially and ethnically minoritized women report a lower prevalence of depression, they report exhibiting distinct differences in presentation; for example, Black and Latina women experience greater somatic symptoms compared to White women (Phimphasone-Brady et al., 2023). Postpartum depression, defined as symptoms occurring during pregnancy or in 4 weeks after birth, is 3.0–25.2 percent and higher among AIAN, Asian American and Pacific Islander, and non-Hispanic Black women compared to non-Hispanic White women (Bauman et al., 2020; NASEM, 2024b).

A 2024 National Academies report identified research gaps related to depression in women, such as the mechanisms that underlie sex differences (NASEM, 2024b). Additional models are also needed to better understand the molecular basis of hormonally driven vulnerability to depression. Research on sex hormone and gene interactions and how sex chromosome effects are involved in the pathophysiology of depression in women are also critical (NASEM, 2024b). The report also describes the gaps in research on inflammatory triggers for depression in women, such as trauma, adverse childhood experiences, and stress, that can inform therapy development. More studies on the bidirectional influences of depression and other chronic conditions and how depression manifests across the life course will help to address research gaps. A better understanding of environmental influences in the development of depression in women is also needed (NASEM, 2024b).

Research on factors that may make women more susceptible to depression and biopsychosocial factors, such as nutrition/nutrients, microbiome, lifestyle, that may counter it is needed. Other gaps include developing screening tools that delineate the diagnostic features of perinatal depression, postpartum depression, and major depressive disorder to better identify women at risk along with research to incorporate racial, ethnic, and cultural considerations into clinical trials to treat depression in women at all stages of the life cycle (NASEM, 2024b).

Anxiety disorders are reported to be more prevalent in women compared to men based on national data. They contributed to greater global DALYs in women compared to men both before and during the COVID-19 pandemic and led to an additional 9.05 million DALYs resulting from the pandemic, of which 6.11 million were attributed to women and 2.94 million to men (COVID-19 Mental Disorders Collaborators, 2021). In 2019, 19.0 percent of women compared to 11.9 percent of men in the United States experienced anxiety symptoms within the past 2 weeks (Terlizzi and Villarroel, 2020).

An analysis of pooled studies have found that the prevalence of anxiety disorders during pregnancy or postpartum was 20.7 percent (Fawcett et al., 2019). Sex differences are attributed to both biological and social factors, including experiencing greater stressors, such as childhood abuse and trauma, and the presence and interaction of the central nervous system with hormonal fluctuations during puberty, the menstrual cycle, pregnancy, and the menopause transition (Hantsoo and Epperson, 2017).

In general, research on anxiety disorders in women is lacking (Hantsoo and Epperson, 2017). Further research on improving screening across the life-span is needed, given the clear differences in presentation of anxiety between women and men, and to further understand the exact sex-specific and hormonal mechanisms for treatment considerations and development of pharmacological therapies (Hantsoo and Epperson, 2017; Li and Graham, 2017). Given significant unmet needs for mental health services specifically among Indigenous and Black women, strategies to mitigate disparities in treatment and outcomes are needed (Taiwo et al., 2024). The factors associated with anxiety in racially and ethnically minoritized women, especially during the menopause transition, are less understood. A recent scoping review identified that approaches to address treatment considerations through the use of health care services, intervention, and implementation science are needed (Lewis Johnson et al., 2024)

Osteoarthritis (OA)

Musculoskeletal disorders are among the conditions with highest DALY burden, especially among women. OA is discussed here; see Chapters 2 and 5 for information on osteoporosis, which is also more prevalent among women and, due to the fractures it causes via loss of bone mass, is associated with disability and mortality. OA is generally not present until after the age of 50. Knee OA (KOA) is one of the most disabling diseases among older people and more prevalent in females. During the menopause transition, when serum estrogen levels decline (and then stabilize at a lower level in postmenopause), females have nearly twice the odds of KOA, have higher prevalence after age 55, and are more likely to experience pain and disability compared with males of the same age (Silverwood et al., 2015; Srikanth et al., 2005). Despite the increasing evidence pointing toward a higher risk of KOA in females, sex is often used only as an adjustment factor, and studies rarely report sex-specific estimates.

Hand OA, which often becomes clinically active around the menopause transition and tends to be hereditary, affects females at nearly three times the rate of males. A recent study of 3,588 participants in the Osteoarthritis Initiative found complex differences by age, sex, and race, with increasing prevalence rates with older age in both females and males but rates of incident disease peaking in females at ages 55–64, whereas for males the increase is more gradual and peaks later in life (Eaton et al., 2022). Hip osteoarthritis (HOA) is also prevalent among older adults, and females report a greater prevalence of symptomatic HOA than males (Nelson et al., 2022). A population-based cohort study found that females were more likely than males to report hip symptoms (40 vs. 32 percent) at baseline and to have symptomatic radiographic HOA (16 versus 12 percent) at the fourth follow-up (Nelson et al., 2022).

The etiology of sex differences in KOA, hand OA, and other sites of OA have not been thoroughly studied (Szilagyi et al., 2023). Certain risk factors, including body mass index, have been well documented in the literature, but more longitudinal studies are needed to examine sex differences in risk factors, including lifestyle, occupational, comorbidity, and environmental factors (Szilagyi et al., 2023). The role of estrogen and other hormonal deficiencies associated with the menopause transition and aging in contributing to these sex differences are also not understood. Identifying the risk factors and understanding the physiological differences that affect women more prominently could lead to better sex-specific preventive and treatment strategies (Segal et al., 2024). Furthermore, characterizing the burden of OA in racially and ethnically minoritized populations has been a challenge, with a need to standardize assessments of OA in these populations and provide estimates separately by sex (Nelson et al., 2022).

DIFFERENTIAL EFFECT BY SEX AND INCREASED FEMALE DALYS RESULTING FROM EARLY MORTALITY

Cardiometabolic Disease

Cardiometabolic diseases include conditions such as heart disease, heart failure, stroke, diabetes, and hypertension and contribute to significant morbidity and mortality in women. CVD was the leading cause of death among women in 2021, contributing to 439,729 deaths. In addition, heart disease was a significant cause of death, with 310,656 deaths reported in the same year (Martin et al., 2024). Stroke alone represented the fifth-leading cause of death in women and contributed to 92,038 deaths in 2021 (Martin et al., 2024). The lifetime risk of stroke is reported to be greater in women compared to men (Tsao et al., 2023). Premature deaths due to cardiometabolic disease have increased for women from 1999 to 2018, specifically for diabetes and cerebrovascular disease (Shah et al., 2020). Premature mortality disproportionately affects Black women; 27.4, 21.1, and 33.0 percent of deaths in 2018 were premature due to heart disease, cerebrovascular disease, and diabetes, respectively (Shah et al., 2020). The prevalence of CVD from 2017–2020 was highest in non-Hispanic Black women at 59 percent compared to 44.6 percent in non-Hispanic White, 37.3 percent in Hispanic, and 38.5 in non-Hispanic Asian women (Martin et al., 2024). CVD contributes to significant disparities in health outcomes, which are associated with diagnosing and treating CVD in women (Nguyen et al., 2024; Vogel et al., 2021).

The 2024 National Academies report *Advancing Research on Chronic Conditions in Women* identified research gaps related to cardiometabolic conditions in women (NASEM, 2024b). Specifically, the report calls for a better understanding of the molecular basis for the female-biased propensity to store fat, including through preclinical models. Additional research on gonadal hormone ablation in preclinical models throughout the life-span was also identified as necessary. The report also describes the need for human studies of new diabetes and obesity drugs and sodium glucose cotransporter 2 inhibitors on weight loss and long-term outcomes by sex and gender. Additional tools to support early and accurate diagnosis of CVD in women are also important to fill gaps in knowledge (NASEM, 2024b).

The report also discussed the need for standard diagnostic criteria for ischemia with no obstructive coronary artery disease and research to clarify mechanisms leading to both it and myocardial infarction with no obstructive coronary artery disease in women. No guidelines are available on the evaluation and treatment for spontaneous coronary artery dissection. Finally, disaggregated data on CVD in Hispanic/Latina, Asian American, and NHPI women are needed (NASEM, 2024b).

As noted, depression and anxiety are more common among women than men and are risk factors for developing cardiometabolic disorders, such as hypertension, diabetes, and hyperlipidemia, and adverse cardiometabolic events (Civieri et al., 2024; Mattina et al., 2019; Rome et al., 2022). A 2024 retrospective cohort study of more than 71,000 participants found that those with anxiety and/or depression were at significantly higher risk of developing new cardiometabolic risk factors within a shorter time even after adjustment for demographics and health behaviors; the greatest effect was among young women, potentially mediated by neuroimmune pathways related to stress, such as systemic, chronic inflammation and autonomic nervous system dysfunction (Civieri et al., 2024). In addition, a variety of sex-specific risk factors related to hormonal life course changes in menarche, fertility, pregnancy, breastfeeding, and the menopause transition alter women's risk for cardiometabolic diseases (O'Kelly et al., 2022; Parikh et al., 2021). For example, a history of common adverse pregnancy outcomes, such as PTB, GD, and hypertensive disorders of pregnancy, increase a woman's lifetime risk of cardiometabolic diseases, while lactation and breastfeeding decrease it. Although the American Heart Association recommended screening for adverse birth outcomes as a universal aspect of cardiometabolic risk assessment for women in their 2011 update, improvements in risk prediction have not followed (Bahr, 2016; Gladstone et al., 2019; Mosca et al., 2011). On the other hand, breastfeeding has been considered a protective factor for cardiometabolic health, for women both with and without hypertensive disorders of pregnancy (Magnus et al., 2023).

More research is needed to understand the mechanisms and pathways linking these sex-specific risk and protective factors for identification, prevention, and treatment of later cardiometabolic diseases related to reproductive health (O'Kelly et al., 2022).

DIFFERENTIAL EFFECT BY SEX AND INCREASED FEMALE DALYS RESULTING FROM DISABLING CONDITIONS AND EARLY MORTALITY

Autoimmune Disorders

Autoimmune disorders constitute 80–150 different conditions, and their overall prevalence is difficult to measure, given the lack of consensus in number (NASEM, 2022). The last comprehensive study of U.S. prevalence was in 2009, producing an estimate of 7.6–9.4 percent of the population; however, it only included 29 conditions, and the prevalence is likely underreported (Cooper et al., 2009; NASEM, 2022). A recent U.K. population-based cohort study of 19 autoimmune disorders found that 1 in 10 individuals had an autoimmune disorder, with almost two-thirds of those female and one-third male (Conrad et al., 2023). In the 2022 NASEM report *Enhancing NIH Research on Autoimmune Disease,* the committee points out that several autoimmune disorders are overrepresented in female patients, including Sjögren's Disease, systemic lupus erythematosus, rheumatoid arthritis, multiple sclerosis (MS), celiac disease, and inflammatory bowel disease. The incidence and prevalence of some autoimmune disorders have increased and are associated with the co-occurrence of other chronic conditions.

National Academies reports issued in 2022 and 2024 outlined research gaps related to autoimmune disorders in women (NASEM, 2022, 2024b). The 2024 report, for example, identified the need for more research to understand how inflammatory and immune system pathways affect the development of chronic conditions in women (NASEM, 2024b). Research on MS, which primarily affects women, needs to examine how hormonal and sex chromosome mechanisms intersect. Research is also needed to understand how factors, particularly Epstein-Barr viral infection, body weight, and others may contribute to the development of MS (NASEM, 2024b).

The 2022 National Academies report identified additional research gaps, including the need for population-based surveillance and epidemiological data on autoimmune diseases and measures of autoimmunity. Data are needed on autoantibodies that can predict and diagnose autoimmune diseases; common mechanisms in inflammation; gene–environment interactions within and across these diseases; the role of environmental exposures; and the effect of interventions to address the impact of comorbidities and complications for patients (NASEM, 2022). The report also identified the need for clinical and basic research to understand heterogeneity across and within autoimmune diseases and examine rare ones (NASEM, 2022).

Neurodegenerative Diseases, AD, and Dementias— Cognition Across the Life Course

Both sex and gender affect the etiology, presentation, and treatment outcomes of many neurological disorders. Ongoing research aims to examine the role of sex and gender on cognition in specific neurodegenerative conditions, such as Parkinson's disease, Huntington's disease (HD), frontotemporal disease, and AD.

Sex Differences in Non-AD Neurodegenerative Disorders

The literature from epidemiological and clinic-based studies have generally supported the finding of a greater prevalence and earlier age of onset of Parkinson's disease in men compared to women (Elbaz et al., 2002). Research has also reported sex-specific patterns regarding cognitive function, with female patients generally reporting less cognitive impairment in some but not all studies (Bakeberg et al., 2021; Chen et al., 2021; Reekes et al., 2020); studies have found that female patients had better frontal executive memory, visual perception, and verbal memory performance (Curtis et al., 2019; Liu et al., 2015) and that the apolipoprotein (*APOE*) e4 genotype conferred poorer cognitive performance that was more pronounced in men (Tipton et al., 2021). However, another study found that lower baseline semantic fluency scores were associated with a faster decline in women but not men (Cholerton et al., 2018).

Although the literature does not typically report sex differences in HD, studies have shown sex differences in clinical expression, with female disease gene carriers presenting with worse motor, cognitive, and depressive symptoms compared to male carriers (Hentosh et al., 2021). Female patients, for example, performed worse on verbal fluency, the symbol digits modality test, and the Stroop Interference test compared to men.

Studies in patients with frontotemporal disorders, characterized by changes in the frontal and temporal lobes that often present with significant emotional, language, and behavioral disturbances, reported that sex differences influenced clinical presentation and cognitive function. Some studies have noted the behavioral variant to be more common in male patients, whereas female patients may present with primary progressive aphasia.

In the behavioral variant, female patients outperformed male patients in measures of executive function and had less neurobehavioral changes despite a higher level of frontal atrophy. Consistent with other neurodegenerative conditions, female patients with the behavioral variant have higher behavioral and executive reserve (Illán-Gala et al., 2021).

AD and AD-Related Dementias

AD causes one of the most common types of dementia in older adults, accounting for 60–80 percent of cases. It was the fifth leading cause of death among those 65 and older in 2021 in the United States, and of the 6.9 million affected, 4.2 million are women and 73 percent are 75 years or older (Alzheimer's Association, 2024; Hebert et al., 2001). An additional 5–7 million people age 65 and older are thought to have mild cognitive impairment resulting from AD (Alzheimer's Association, 2024). The number of individuals with AD is expected to increase more in women than men over the coming years, reflecting biological factors and the increased longevity for women (Alzheimer's Association, 2024; Hebert et al., 2013).

Recent evidence does not fully support previous reports that the risk of developing AD or other dementias differs between men and women of the same age (Shaw et al., 2021). This suggests that risk differences could have resulted from survival or selection bias, with projected average survival rates varying between 1.1 and 8.5 years across studies and affected by multiple factors, including age at diagnosis, sex, behavioral features, dementia subtype, motor system involvement, and medical comorbidities (Brodaty et al., 2012).

Biological factors

The strongest genetic risk factor for late-onset AD remains the *APOE* genotype. *APOE* encodes the brain's major cholesterol transporter and has three common alleles: e2, e3 and e4. *APOE* e4 is associated with an increased risk of developing AD compared to e2 and e3 genotypes (Liu et al., 2013), and each *APOE* e4 allele reduces the average age of symptom onset by a decade. Female carriers of *APOE* e4 are at a greater risk of developing AD than male carriers, particularly those aged 65–75 (Neu et al., 2017). One study found for people in their 60s and 70s, females with *APOE* e4 +/+ genotype had less functional decline in an immediate recall memory test with increasing age than females with other genotypes (*APOE* e4 +/- and *APOE* e4 -/-), whereas males with the *APOE* e4 +/+ genotype had the most memory decline than other genotypes (Anstey et al., 2021a,b). The reason for these sex differences remains unclear and warrants further investigation.

The risk of developing AD and related forms of dementia increases in patients with vascular risk factors (Barnes and Yaffe, 2011; Ritchie et al., 2015). The data regarding potential sex differences related to cardio-vascular risk factors and cognitive decline and dementia are inconsistent. For example, males have a higher prevalence of vascular risk factors and conditions up to about the age of 80, although a recent study suggested that despite the higher prevalence of these conditions in midlife, female individuals with vascular risk factors were at the greatest risk of cognitive decline (Huo et al., 2022). This area warrants investigation.

Neuroimaging markers have also been reported to show sex differences, with the increased occurrence of white matter hyperintensities increasing with advanced age in females postmenopause compared to males or pre-menopausal females (Ossenkoppele et al., 2020). It is unclear what specific physiological aspect of menopause might be contributing to this observation, in part because of a lack of quality data collected around the menopausal transition. In addition, the potential psychosocial stressors associated with the menopause transition, which could differ based on age, race, ethnicity, or age of onset, are still not fully examined as potential mediators to changes in physical or cognitive function in many of these research investigations (Faleschini et al., 2022).

Non-biological factors

Multiple lifestyle, psychological, behavioral, and environmental factors have been associated with AD, and the relationships between many of these and dementia vary by sex and gender (Baumgart et al., 2015), though the mechanism by which they contribute to differences in AD risk remain elusive. Multiple studies suggest that sex modifies the association between physical activity and cognition. Older females undergoing aerobic training showed greater cognitive gains than older males (Barha et al., 2017a,b), and physical activity maintenance over 10 years predicted fewer declines in multiple cognitive domains among females compared to males (Barha et al., 2020). Another study showed a positive correlation between physical activity and cognitive processing speed for females but not males, and the *APOE* e4 genotype once again moderated these relationships only in females (Sundermann et al., 2016).

Sex differences in sleep disturbances are commonly seen with neuropsychiatric behavior symptoms (Sateia, 2014) and linked to late-life cognitive decline and AD (Bombois et al., 2010; Ju et al., 2014; Yaffe et al., 2011). Females are especially vulnerable to sleep disruption at or around the menopause transition, with many experiencing symptoms that fit the diagnosis of insomnia (Joffe et al., 2010). Postmenopausal females are three times more likely to experience obstructive sleep apnea than premenopausal women, but whether these sex differences in sleep disruption affect AD risk is still an area of active investigation (Bixler et al., 2001; Ju et al., 2017; Rumble et al., 2023).

Psychological stressors, such as gender- and race-based discrimination, harassment, poverty, and caregiving, may contribute to gender differences in late-life cognitive health, but research has not elucidated the mechanisms by which they may affect cognitive function and decline differentially by sex (Aartsen et al., 2004; Norton et al., 2010; Vitaliano, 2010). For instance, researchers have hypothesized an intersectional relationship between caregiving and cognitive health. Factors such as poor overall health; mental health conditions, such as depression and anxiety; social isolation; and chronic stress from economic hardships—stemming from unpaid caregiving and changes in employment—may interact in a way that negatively impacts a caregiver's brain and cognitive function. This interaction could lead to pathways involving inflammation and excessive cortisol, further diminishing cognitive health (Alzheimer's Association, 2024; Norton et al., 2010; Vitaliano, 2010). Life course research demonstrates that childhood socioeconomic position is more strongly associated with the rate of later-life cognitive decline in women than in men and that formal education was the strong mediator of that relationship (Wolfova et al., 2021).

Collectively, these social factors can affect medical treatment and access to care and the patient's experience of care. Further research is warranted to understand sex-specific responses to early-life socioeconomic stressors and their impact on biological and other pathways that underlie them, setting the stage for differences in cognitive reserve later in life. This research investment will lead to interventions that beneficially affect long-term cognitive outcomes for men and women (Hidalgo et al., 2019).

Implications of Sex Differences in Cognitive Assessment Tools and Biomarkers

Studies are limited regarding sex-specific norms for neurocognitive impairment. Studies have shown that when compared with men, women across the life-span have stronger performance in most cognitive domains. Thus, continued failure to account for sex and gender differences can lead to underdetection of cognitive impairment in women, which can delay diagnosis and compromise access to early interventions.

Researchers are investigating using neuroimaging and blood-based markers to predict risk for decline or dementia. Some neuroimaging studies report that female patients have higher levels of brain glucose metabolism and greater cortical thickness compared to male patients, while other studies of AD biomarkers in blood and cerebrospinal fluid note higher cerebrospinal fluid levels of total tau protein in female patients (Buckley et al., 2019; Mielke, 2020; Ossenkoppele et al., 2020;

Sundermann et al., 2016, 2020). More research is needed to assess sex differences among these biomarkers and examine the properties of these biomarkers in older, racially diverse populations.

CONCLUDING OBSERVATIONS

Many women's health conditions and approaches are not detailed in this chapter—for example, complementary health and naturopathic approaches, such as those the NIH National Center for Complementary and Integrative Health supports to address conditions such as perinatal depression, opioid use disorder, anxiety, and pain management (NCCIH, 2021). However, based on the conditions and factors that were reviewed in Chapters 2, 5, 6, and 7, the committee identified significant gaps for WHR across the life course. These include a lack of understanding of basic female physiology, insufficient study of specific conditions, inattention to SDOH and health inequities on specific health outcomes that focus on women, and the need for research on the interaction of these factors. Addressing these gaps requires a concerted and coordinated effort to include more women in clinical trials, increase funding for WHR, and focus on both biological and social determinants of health. This research is vital to ensure that all women receive the care and treatment they need.

REFERENCES

AACR (American Association for Cancer Research). 2024. *AACR cancer disparities progress report 2024*. Philadelphia, PA: American Association for Cancer Research.

Aartsen, M. J., M. Martin, and D. Zimprich. 2004. Gender differences in level and change in cognitive functioning. Results from the Longitudinal Aging Study Amsterdam. *Gerontology* 50(1):35–38.

Aboseif, C., and P. Liu. 2022. Pelvic organ prolapse. In *Statpearls*. Treasure Island, FL: StatPearls Publishing.

ACOG (American College of Obstetricians and Gynecologists). n.d. *Gestational Hypertension and Preeclampsia*. https://www.acog.org/clinical/clinical-guidance/practice-bulletin/articles/2020/06/gestational-hypertension-and-preeclampsia (accessed August 15, 2024).

ACOG. 2021. *Practice bulletin 200: Early pregnancy loss*. Washington, DC: Committee on Practice Bulletins—Gynecology, American College of Obstetricians and Gynecologists.

ACOG. 2024. *FAQs: Repeated Miscarriages*. https://www.acog.org/womens-health/faqs/repeated-miscarriages (accessed October 14, 2024).

Akre, S., K. Sharma, S. Chakole, and M. B. Wanjari. 2022. Recent advances in the management of polycystic ovary syndrome: A review article. *Cureus* 14(8):e27689.

Al-Hawary, S. I. S., E. A. M. Saleh, N. A. Mamajanov, N. S. Gilmanova, H. O. Alsaab, A. Alghamdi, S. A. Ansari, A. H. R. Alawady, A. H. Alsaalamy, and A. J. Ibrahim. 2023. Breast cancer vaccines; a comprehensive and updated review. *Pathology—Research and Practice* 249:154735.

Al Harbi, R., I. A. McNeish, and M. El-Bahrawy. 2021. Ovarian sex cord-stromal tumors: An update on clinical features, molecular changes, and management. *International Journal of Gynecologic Cancer* 31(2):161–168.

Alblooshi, S., M. Taylor, and N. Gill. 2023. Does menopause elevate the risk for developing depression and anxiety? Results from a systematic review. *Australasian Psychiatry* 31(2):165–173.

Allen, L. A., N. Shrikrishnapalasuriyar, and D. A. Rees. 2022. Long-term health outcomes in young women with polycystic ovary syndrome: A narrative review. *Clinical Endocrinology* 97(2):187–198.

Alzheimer's Association. 2024. *2024 Alzheimer's disease facts and figures. Special report: Mapping a better future for dementia care navigation.* Chicago, IL: Alzheimer's Association.

Amaral, L. M., K. Wallace, M. Owens, and B. LaMarca. 2017. Pathophysiology and current clinical management of preeclampsia. *Current Hypertension Reports* 19(8):61.

American Cancer Society. 2024a. *Cancer facts & figures 2024.* Atlanta, GA: American Cancer Society.

American Cancer Society. 2024b. *Key Statistics for Breast Cancer.* https://www.cancer.org/cancer/types/breast-cancer/about/how-common-is-breast-cancer.html (accessed August 14, 2024).

ANSIRH (Advancing New Standards in Reproductive Health). n.d. *The Turnaway Study.* https://www.ansirh.org/research/ongoing/turnaway-study (accessed August 15, 2024).

Anstey, K. J., L. Ehrenfeld, M. E. Mortby, N. Cherbuin, R. Peters, K. M. Kiely, R. Eramudugolla, and M. H. Huque. 2021a. Gender differences in cognitive development in cohorts of young, middle, and older adulthood over 12 years. *Developmental Psychology* 57(8):1403–1410.

Anstey, K. J., R. Peters, M. E. Mortby, K. M. Kiely, R. Eramudugolla, N. Cherbuin, M. H. Huque, and R. A. Dixon. 2021b. Association of sex differences in dementia risk factors with sex differences in memory decline in a population-based cohort spanning 20–76 years. *Scientific Reports* 11(1):7710.

Augustovski, F., L. D. Colantonio, J. Galante, A. Bardach, J. E. Caporale, V. Zárate, L. H. Chuang, A. Pichon-Riviere, and P. Kind. 2018. Measuring the benefits of healthcare: DALYs and QALYs—does the choice of measure matter? A case study of two preventive interventions. *International Journal of Health Policy and Management* 7(2):120–136.

Bae-Jump, V. 2024. *Obesity-Driven Endometrial Cancer: Gaps and Barriers to Improving Outcomes. Presentation to the NASEM Committee on the Assessment of NIH Research on Women's Health, Meeting 3 (March 7, 2024).* https://www.nationalacademies.org/event/docs/D1E982F058D7054AE8307F645CDE60D49C6215FC49F6?noSaveAs=1 (accessed October 21, 2024).

Bahr, R. 2016. Why screening tests to predict injury do not work—and probably never will. . . : A critical review. *British Journal of Sports Medicine* 50(13):776–780.

Bakeberg, M. C., A. M. Gorecki, J. E. Kenna, A. Jefferson, M. Byrnes, S. Ghosh, M. K. Horne, S. McGregor, R. Stell, S. Walters, P. Chivers, S. J. Winter, F. L. Mastaglia, and R. S. Anderton. 2021. Differential effects of sex on longitudinal patterns of cognitive decline in Parkinson's disease. *Journal Neurology* 268(5):1903–1912.

Banjar, S., E. Kadour, R. Khoudja, S. Ton-leclerc, C. Beauchamp, M. Beltempo, M. H. Dahan, P. Gold, I. Jacques Kadoch, W. Jamal, C. Laskin, N. Mahutte, S. L. Reinblatt, C. Sylvestre, W. Buckett, and G. Genest. 2023. Intravenous immunoglobulin use in patients with unexplained recurrent pregnancy loss. *American Journal of Reproductive Immunology* 90(2):e13737.

Barcelona de Mendoza, V., E. Harville, K. Theall, P. Buekens, and L. Chasan-Taber. 2016. Acculturation and adverse birth outcomes in a predominantly Puerto Rican population. *Maternal and Child Health Journal* 20(6):1151–1160.

Barha, C. K., J. C. Davis, R. S. Falck, L. S. Nagamatsu, and T. Liu-Ambrose. 2017a. Sex differences in exercise efficacy to improve cognition: A systematic review and meta-analysis of randomized controlled trials in older humans. *Frontiers in Neuroendocrinology* 46:71–85.

Barha, C. K., G. R. Hsiung, J. R. Best, J. C. Davis, J. J. Eng, C. Jacova, P. E. Lee, M. Munkacsy, W. Cheung, and T. Liu-Ambrose. 2017b. Sex difference in aerobic exercise efficacy to improve cognition in older adults with vascular cognitive impairment: Secondary analysis of a randomized controlled trial. *Journal of Alzheimer's Disease* 60(4):1397–1410.

Barha, C. K., J. R. Best, C. Rosano, K. Yaffe, J. M. Catov, and T. Liu-Ambrose. 2020. Sex-specific relationship between long-term maintenance of physical activity and cognition in the Health ABC study: Potential role of hippocampal and dorsolateral prefrontal cortex volume. *Journals of Gerontology, Series A* 75(4):764–770.

Barnard, M. E., L. V. Farland, B. Yan, J. Wang, B. Trabert, J. A. Doherty, H. D. Meeks, M. Madsen, E. Guinto, L. J. Collin, K. A. Maurer, J. M. Page, A. C. Kiser, M. W. Varner, K. Allen-Brady, A. Z. Pollack, K. R. Peterson, C. M. Peterson, and K. C. Schliep. 2024. Endometriosis typology and ovarian cancer risk. *JAMA* 332(6):482–489.

Barnes, D. E., and K. Yaffe. 2011. The projected effect of risk factor reduction on Alzheimer's disease prevalence. *Lancet Neurology* 10(9):819–828.

Barreto, A., B. Formanowski, M.-M. Peña, E. G. Salazar, S. C. Handley, H. H. Burris, R. Ortiz, S. A. Lorch, and D. Montoya-Williams. 2024. Preterm birth risk and maternal nativity, ethnicity, and race. *JAMA Network Open* 7(3):e243194.

Bauman, B. L., J. Y. Ko, S. Cox, D. V. D'Angelo Mph, L. Warner, S. Folger, H. D. Tevendale, K. C. Coy, L. Harrison, and W. D. Barfield. 2020. Vital signs: Postpartum depressive symptoms and provider discussions about perinatal depression—United States, 2018. *MMWR* 69(19):575–581.

Baumgart, M., H. M. Snyder, M. C. Carrillo, S. Fazio, H. Kim, and H. Johns. 2015. Summary of the evidence on modifiable risk factors for cognitive decline and dementia: A population-based perspective. *Alzheimer's & Dementia* 11(6):718–726.

Bekkar, B., S. Pacheco, R. Basu, and N. DeNicola. 2020. Association of air pollution and heat exposure with preterm birth, low birth weight, and stillbirth in the U.S.: A systematic review. *JAMA Network Open* 3(6):e208243.

Berek, J. S., M. Renz, S. Kehoe, L. Kumar, and M. Friedlander. 2021. Cancer of the ovary, fallopian tube, and peritoneum: 2021 update. *International Journal of Gynecology & Obstetrics* 155(S1):61–85.

Bixler, E. O., A. N. Vgontzas, H. M. Lin, T. Ten Have, J. Rein, A. Vela-Bueno, and A. Kales. 2001. Prevalence of sleep-disordered breathing in women: Effects of gender. *American Journal of Respiratory and Critical Care Medicine* 163(3 Pt 1):608–613.

Bokuda, K., and A. Ichihara. 2023. Preeclampsia up to date—what's going on? *Hypertension Research* 46(8):1900–1907.

Bolduc, M. L. F., C. I. Mercado, Y. Zhang, E. A. Lundeen, N. D. Ford, K. M. Bullard, and D. C. Carty. 2024. Gestational diabetes prevalence estimates from three data sources, 2018. *Maternal and Child Health Journal* 28(8):1308–1314.

Bombois, S., P. Derambure, F. Pasquier, and C. Monaca. 2010. Sleep disorders in aging and dementia. *Journal of Nutrition, Health and Aging* 14(3):212–217.

Bower, J. K., B. N. Butler, S. Bose-Brill, J. Kue, and C. L. Wassel. 2019. Racial/ethnic differences in diabetes screening and hyperglycemia among U.S. women after gestational diabetes. *Preventing Chronic Disease* 16:E145.

Bozdag, G., S. Mumusoglu, D. Zengin, E. Karabulut, and B. O. Yildiz. 2016. The prevalence and phenotypic features of polycystic ovary syndrome: A systematic review and meta-analysis. *Human Reproduction* 31(12):2841–2855.

Brodaty, H., K. Seeher, and L. Gibson. 2012. Dementia time to death: A systematic literature review on survival time and years of life lost in people with dementia. *International Psychogeriatrics* 24(7):1034–1045.

Bromberger, J. T., and C. N. Epperson. 2018. Depression during and after the perimenopause: Impact of hormones, genetics, and environmental determinants of disease. *Obstetrics and Gynecology Clinics of North America* 45(4):663–678.

Buchanan, T. A., A. H. Xiang, and K. A. Page. 2012. Gestational diabetes mellitus: Risks and management during and after pregnancy. *Nature Reviews Endocrinology* 8(11):639–649.

Buck Louis, G. M., M. L. Hediger, C. M. Peterson, M. Croughan, R. Sundaram, J. Stanford, Z. Chen, V. Y. Fujimoto, M. W. Varner, A. Trumble, and L. C. Giudice. 2011. Incidence of endometriosis by study population and diagnostic method: The Endo study. *Fertility and Sterility* 96(2):360–365.

Buckley, R. F., E. C. Mormino, J. S. Rabin, T. J. Hohman, S. Landau, B. J. Hanseeuw, H. I. L. Jacobs, K. V. Papp, R. E. Amariglio, M. J. Properzi, A. P. Schultz, D. Kirn, M. R. Scott, T. Hedden, M. Farrell, J. Price, J. Chhatwal, D. M. Rentz, V. L. Villemagne, K. A. Johnson, and R. A. Sperling. 2019. Sex differences in the association of global amyloid and regional tau deposition measured by positron emission tomography in clinically normal older adults. *JAMA Neurology* 76(5):542–551.

Bulun, S. 2016. Physiology and pathology of the female reproductive axis. In *Williams Textbook of Endocrinology*, 13th ed., edited by S. Melmed, K. S. Polonsky, P. R. Larsen, and H. M. Kronenberg. Philadelphia, PA: Elsevier Health Sciences. Pp. 589–663.

Buys, S. S., E. Partridge, A. Black, C. C. Johnson, L. Lamerato, C. Isaacs, D. J. Reding, R. T. Greenlee, L. A. Yokochi, B. Kessel, E. D. Crawford, T. R. Church, G. L. Andriole, J. L. Weissfeld, M. N. Fouad, D. Chia, B. O'Brien, L. R. Ragard, J. D. Clapp, J. M. Rathmell, T. L. Riley, P. Hartge, P. F. Pinsky, C. S. Zhu, G. Izmirlian, B. S. Kramer, A. B. Miller, J.-L. Xu, P. C. Prorok, J. K. Gohagan, and C. D. Berg, for the PLCO Project Team. 2011. Effect of screening on ovarian cancer mortality: The Prostate, Lung, Colorectal and Ovarian (PLCO) cancer screening randomized controlled trial. *JAMA* 305(22):2295–2303.

Byatt, N., T. A. Simas, R. S. Lundquist, J. V. Johnson, and D. M. Ziedonis. 2012. Strategies for improving perinatal depression treatment in North American outpatient obstetric settings. *Journal of Psychosomatic Obstetrics and Gynecology* 33(4):143–161.

CDC (Centers for Disease Control and Prevention). n.d.-a. *Maternal Deaths and Mortality Rates: Each State, the District of Columbia, United States, 2018–2022.* https://www.cdc.gov/nchs/maternal-mortality/mmr-2018–2022-state-data.pdf (accessed August 26, 2024).

CDC. n.d.-b. *Pregnancy Mortality Surveillance System.* https://www.cdc.gov/maternal-mortality/php/pregnancy-mortality-surveillance/index.html (accessed August 14, 2024).

CDC. n.d.-c. *Working Together to Reduce Black Maternal Mortality.* https://www.cdc.gov/womens-health/features/maternal-mortality (accessed August 14, 2024).

CDC. 2022. *Four in 5 Pregnancy-Related Deaths in the U.S. Are Preventable.* https://www.cdc.gov/media/releases/2022/p0919-pregnancy-related-deaths.html (accessed August 16, 2024).

CDC. 2023. Quickstats: Percentage of mothers with gestational diabetes, by maternal age—National Vital Statistics System, United States, 2016 and 2021. *MMWR* 72(16).

CDC. 2024a. *About Gestational Diabetes.* https://www.cdc.gov/diabetes/about/gestational-diabetes.html (accessed October 20, 2024).

CDC. 2024b. *Preterm Birth.* https://www.cdc.gov/maternal-infant-health/preterm-birth/index.html (accessed October 22, 2024).

CDMRP. 2024. *Ovarian Cancer.* https://cdmrp.health.mil/ocrp/ (accessed August 16, 2024).

CDMRP. n.d. *Ovarian Cancer Research Program: Strategic Plan.* Fort Detrick, MD: Congressionally Directed Medical Research Porgrams.

Cetin, E., A. Al-Hendy, and M. Ciebiera. 2020. Non-hormonal mediators of uterine fibroid growth. *Current Opinions in Obstetrics and Gynecology* 32(5):361–370.

Che, Y., J. Yu, Y. S. Li, Y. C. Zhu, and T. Tao. 2023. Polycystic ovary syndrome: Challenges and possible solutions. *Journal of Clinical Medicine* 12(4).

Chen, M.-L., C.-H. Tan, H.-C. Su, P.-S. Sung, C.-Y. Chien, and R.-L. Yu. 2021. The impact of sex on the neurocognitive functions of patients with Parkinson's disease. *Brain Sciences* 11(10):1331.

Chin, K., A. Wendt, I. M. Bennett, and A. Bhat. 2022. Suicide and maternal mortality. *Current Psychiatry Reports* 24(4):239–275.

Cholerton, B., C. O. Johnson, B. Fish, J. F. Quinn, K. A. Chung, A. L. Peterson-Hiller, L. S. Rosenthal, T. M. Dawson, M. S. Albert, S. C. Hu, I. F. Mata, J. B. Leverenz, K. L. Poston, T. J. Montine, C. P. Zabetian, and K. L. Edwards. 2018. Sex differences in progression to mild cognitive impairment and dementia in Parkinson's disease. *Parkinsonism & Related Disorders* 50:29–36.

Christ, J. P., and M. I. Cedars. 2023. Current guidelines for diagnosing PCOS. *Diagnostics* 13(6).

Civieri, G., S. Abohashem, S. S. Grewal, W. Aldosoky, I. Qamar, E. Hanlon, K. W. Choi, L. M. Shin, R. P. Rosovsky, S. C. Bollepalli, H. C. Lau, A. Armoundas, A. V. Seligowski, S. M. Turgeon, R. K. Pitman, F. Tona, J. H. Wasfy, J. W. Smoller, S. Iliceto, J. Goldstein, C. Gebhard, M. T. Osborne, and A. Tawakol. 2024. Anxiety and depression associated with increased cardiovascular disease risk through accelerated development of risk factors. *JACC Advances* 3(9):101208.

Clarke, M. A., S. S. Devesa, S. V. Harvey, and N. Wentzensen. 2019. Hysterectomy-corrected uterine corpus cancer incidence trends and differences in relative survival reveal racial disparities and rising rates of nonendometrioid cancers. *Journal of Clinical Oncology* 37(22):1895–1908.

Coleman, R. L., A. M. Oza, D. Lorusso, C. Aghajanian, A. Oaknin, A. Dean, N. Colombo, J. I. Weberpals, A. Clamp, G. Scambia, A. Leary, R. W. Holloway, M. A. Gancedo, P. C. Fong, J. C. Goh, D. M. O'Malley, D. K. Armstrong, J. Garcia-Donas, E. M. Swisher, A. Floquet, G. E. Konecny, I. A. McNeish, C. L. Scott, T. Cameron, L. Maloney, J. Isaacson, S. Goble, C. Grace, T. C. Harding, M. Raponi, J. Sun, K. K. Lin, H. Giordano, and J. A. Ledermann. 2017. Rucaparib maintenance treatment for recurrent ovarian carcinoma after response to platinum therapy (ARIEL3): A randomised, double-blind, placebo-controlled, Phase 3 trial. *Lancet* 390(10106):1949–1961.

Coleman, R. L., G. F. Fleming, M. F. Brady, E. M. Swisher, K. D. Steffensen, M. Friedlander, A. Okamoto, K. N. Moore, N. E. Ben-Baruch, T. L. Werner, N. G. Cloven, A. Oaknin, P. A. DiSilvestro, M. A. Morgan, J.-H. Nam, C. A. Leath, S. Nicum, A. R. Hagemann, R. D. Littell, D. Cella, S. Baron-Hay, J. Garcia-Donas, M. Mizuno, K. Bell-McGuinn, D. M. Sullivan, B. A. Bach, S. Bhattacharya, C. K. Ratajczak, P. J. Ansell, M. H. Dinh, C. Aghajanian, and M. A. Bookman. 2019. Veliparib with first-line chemotherapy and as maintenance therapy in ovarian cancer. *New England Journal of Medicine* 381(25):2403–2415.

Collier, A. Y., and R. L. Molina. 2019. Maternal mortality in the United States: Updates on trends, causes, and solutions. *NeoReviews* 20(10):e561–e574.

Conrad, N., S. Misra, J. Y. Verbakel, G. Verbeke, G. Molenberghs, P. N. Taylor, J. Mason, N. Sattar, J. J. V. McMurray, I. B. McInnes, K. Khunti, and G. Cambridge. 2023. Incidence, prevalence, and co-occurrence of autoimmune disorders over time and by age, sex, and socioeconomic status: A population-based cohort study of 22 million individuals in the U.K. *Lancet* 401(10391):1878–1890.

Coomarasamy, A., A. J. Devall, V. Cheed, H. Harb, L. J. Middleton, I. D. Gallos, H. Williams, A. K. Eapen, T. Roberts, C. C. Ogwulu, I. Goranitis, J. P. Daniels, A. Ahmed, R. Bender-Atik, K. Bhatia, C. Bottomley, J. Brewin, M. Choudhary, F. Crosfill, S. Deb, W. C. Duncan, A. Ewer, K. Hinshaw, T. Holland, F. Izzat, J. Johns, K. Kriedt, M. A. Lumsden, P. Manda, J. E. Norman, N. Nunes, C. E. Overton, S. Quenby, S. Rao, J. Ross, A. Shahid, M. Underwood, N. Vaithilingam, L. Watkins, C. Wykes, A. Horne, and D. Jurkovic. 2019. A randomized trial of progesterone in women with bleeding in early pregnancy. *New England Journal of Medicine* 380(19):1815–1824.

Coomarasamy, A., A. J. Devall, J. J. Brosens, S. Quenby, M. D. Stephenson, S. Sierra, O. B. Christiansen, R. Small, J. Brewin, T. E. Roberts, R. Dhillon-Smith, H. Harb, H. Noordali,

A. Papadopoulou, A. Eapen, M. Prior, G. C. Di Renzo, K. Hinshaw, B. W. Mol, M. A. Lumsden, Y. Khalaf, A. Shennan, M. Goddijn, M. van Wely, M. Al-Memar, P. Bennett, T. Bourne, R. Rai, L. Regan, and I. D. Gallos. 2020. Micronized vaginal progesterone to prevent miscarriage: A critical evaluation of randomized evidence. *American Journal of Obstetrics and Gynecology* 223(2):167–176.

Cooper, G. S., M. L. Bynum, and E. C. Somers. 2009. Recent insights in the epidemiology of autoimmune diseases: Improved prevalence estimates and understanding of clustering of diseases. *Journal of Autoimmunity* 33(3–4):197–207.

COVID-19 Mental Disorders Collaborators. 2021. Global prevalence and burden of depressive and anxiety disorders in 204 countries and territories in 2020 due to the COVID-19 pandemic. *Lancet* 398(10312):1700–1712.

Cox, E. Q., N. A. Sowa, S. E. Meltzer-Brody, and B. N. Gaynes. 2016. The perinatal depression treatment cascade: Baby steps toward improving outcomes. *Journal of Clinical Psychiatry* 77(9):1189–1200.

Crear-Perry, J., R. Correa-de-Araujo, T. Lewis Johnson, M. R. McLemore, E. Neilson, and M. Wallace. 2021. Social and structural determinants of health inequities in maternal health. *Journal of Women's Health* 30(2):230–235.

Cronin, K. A., S. Scott, A. U. Firth, H. Sung, S. J. Henley, R. L. Sherman, R. L. Siegel, R. N. Anderson, B. A. Kohler, V. B. Benard, S. Negoita, C. Wiggins, W. G. Cance, and A. Jemal. 2022. Annual report to the nation on the status of cancer, part 1: National cancer statistics. *Cancer* 128(24):4251–4284.

Crowther, C. A., J. E. Hiller, J. R. Moss, A. J. McPhee, W. S. Jeffries, and J. S. Robinson. 2005. Effect of treatment of gestational diabetes mellitus on pregnancy outcomes. *New England Journal of Medicine* 352(24):2477–2486.

Crump, C., J. Sundquist, and K. Sundquist. 2020. Preterm delivery and long term mortality in women: National cohort and co-sibling study. *BMJ* 370:m2533.

Cuijpers, P., and E. Karyotaki. 2021. The effects of psychological treatment of perinatal depression: An overview. *Archives of Women's Mental Health* 24(5):801–806.

Curtis, A. F., M. Masellis, R. Camicioli, H. Davidson, and M. C. Tierney. 2019. Cognitive profile of non-demented Parkinson's disease: Meta-analysis of domain and sex-specific deficits. *Parkinsonism & Related Disorders* 60:32–42.

D'Mello, R. J., C.-D. Hsu, P. Chaiworapongsa, and T. Chaiworapongsa. 2021. Update on the use of intravenous immunoglobulin in pregnancy. *NeoReviews* 22(1):e7–e24.

Dagher, R. K., H. E. Bruckheim, L. J. Colpe, E. Edwards, and D. B. White. 2021. Perinatal depression: Challenges and opportunities. *Journal of Women's Health* 30(2):154–159.

Dalfrà, M. G., S. Burlina, G. G. Del Vescovo, and A. Lapolla. 2020. Genetics and epigenetics: New insight on gestational diabetes mellitus. *Frontiers in Endocrinology* 11:602477.

Dall, T. M., W. Yang, K. Gillespie, M. Mocarski, E. Byrne, I. Cintina, K. Beronja, A. P. Semilla, W. Iacobucci, and P. F. Hogan. 2019. The economic burden of elevated blood glucose levels in 2017: Diagnosed and undiagnosed diabetes, gestational diabetes mellitus, and prediabetes. *Diabetes Care* 42(9):1661–1668.

de Wit, A. E., E. J. Giltay, M. K. de Boer, M. Nathan, A. Wiley, S. Crawford, and H. Joffe. 2021. Predictors of irritability symptoms in mildly depressed perimenopausal women. *Psychoneuroendocrinology* 126:105128.

Deligiannidis, K. M. 2024. *Research Gaps in Perinatal Mental Health Disorders: Perinatal Depression. Presentation to the NASEM Committee on the Assessment of NIH Research on Women's Health, Meeting 3 (March 7, 2024).* https://www.nationalacademies.org/event/docs/D6302B045662CDB06C85FC9E9EADAE8BFCB02A394EC5?noSaveAs=1 (accessed October 21, 2024).

Dennett, C. C., and J. Simon. 2015. The role of polycystic ovary syndrome in reproductive and metabolic health: Overview and approaches for treatment. *Diabetes Spectrum* 28(2):116–120.

Dennis, A. 2024. *Research Gaps in Family Planning. Presentation to the NASEM Committee on the Assessment of NIH Research on Women's Health, Meeting 2 (March 7, 2024).* https://www.nationalacademies.org/documents/embed/link/LF2255DA3DD1C 41C0A42D3BEF0989ACAECE3053A6A9B/file/D34E83DA13AE295302AE8CB1F2E5 AD52868CFD491120?noSaveAs=1 (accessed August 16, 2024).

Dimitriadis, E., D. L. Rolnik, W. Zhou, G. Estrada-Gutierrez, K. Koga, R. P. V. Francisco, C. Whitehead, J. Hyett, F. da Silva Costa, K. Nicolaides, and E. Menkhorst. 2023. Pre-eclampsia. *Nature Reviews Disease Primers* 9(1):8.

Early Breast Cancer Trialists' Collaborative Group. 2015. Aromatase inhibitors versus tamoxifen in early breast cancer: Patient-level meta-analysis of the randomised trials. *Lancet* 386(10001):1341–1352.

Eaton, C. B., L. F. Schaefer, J. Duryea, J. B. Driban, G. H. Lo, M. B. Roberts, I. K. Haugen, B. Lu, M. C. Nevitt, M. C. Hochberg, R. D. Jackson, C. K. Kwoh, and T. McAlindon. 2022. Prevalence, incidence, and progression of radiographic and symptomatic hand osteoarthritis: The Osteoarthritis Initiative. *Arthritis & Rheumatology* 74(6):992–1000.

Elbaz, A., J. H. Bower, D. M. Maraganore, S. K. McDonnell, B. J. Peterson, J. E. Ahlskog, D. J. Schaid, and W. A. Rocca. 2002. Risk tables for Parkinsonism and Parkinson's disease. *Journal of Clinical Epidemiology* 55(1):25–31.

Ellis, K., D. Munro, and J. Clarke. 2022. Endometriosis is undervalued: A call to action. *Frontiers in Global Women's Health* 3:902371.

Eltoukhi, H. M., M. N. Modi, M. Weston, A. Y. Armstrong, and E. A. Stewart. 2014. The health disparities of uterine fibroid tumors for African American women: A public health issue. *American Journal of Obstetrics and Gynecology* 210(3):194–199.

Erbetta, K., J. Almeida, and M. R. Waldman. 2022. Racial, ethnic and nativity inequalities in gestational diabetes mellitus: The role of racial discrimination. *SSM Population Health* 19:101176.

Etzel, R. A. 2020. Is the environment associated with preterm birth? *JAMA Network Open* 3(4):e202239.

Faleschini, S., H. Tiemeier, S. L. Rifas-Shiman, J. Rich-Edwards, H. Joffe, W. Perng, J. Shifren, J. E. Chavarro, M. F. Hivert, and E. Oken. 2022. Longitudinal associations of psychosocial stressors with menopausal symptoms and well-being among women in midlife. *Menopause* 29(11):1247–1253.

Fawcett, E. J., N. Fairbrother, M. L. Cox, I. R. White, and J. M. Fawcett. 2019. The prevalence of anxiety disorders during pregnancy and the postpartum period: A multivariate Bayesian meta-analysis. *Journal of Clinical Psychiatry* 80(4).

FDA (Food and Drug Administration). 2016. *FDA Grants Accelerated Approval to New Treatment for Advanced Ovarian Cancer.* https://www.fda.gov/news-events/press-announcements/fda-grants-accelerated-approval-new-treatment-advanced-ovarian-cancer (accessed August 26, 2024).

Ford, H. B., and D. J. Schust. 2009. Recurrent pregnancy loss: Etiology, diagnosis, and therapy. *Reviews in Obstetrics and Gynecology* 2(2):76–83.

GBD 2021 Diseases and Injuries Collaborators. 2024. Global incidence, prevalence, years lived with disability (YLDs), disability-adjusted life-years (DALYs), and healthy life expectancy (HALE) for 371 diseases and injuries in 204 countries and territories and 811 subnational locations, 1990–2021: A systematic analysis for the Global Burden of Disease study 2021. *Lancet* 403(10440):2133–2161.

Gerdts, C., L. Dobkin, D. G. Foster, and E. B. Schwarz. 2016. Side effects, physical health consequences, and mortality associated with abortion and birth after an unwanted pregnancy. *Women's Health Issues* 26(1):55–59.

Gladstone, R. A., J. Pudwell, K. A. Nerenberg, S. A. Grover, and G. N. Smith. 2019. Cardiovascular risk assessment and follow-up of women after hypertensive disorders of pregnancy: A prospective cohort study. *Journal of Obstetrics and Gynaecology Canada* 41(8):1157–1167.e1151.

Gnanasegar, R., W. Wolfman, L. H. Galan, A. Cullimore, and A. K. Shea. 2024. Does menopause hormone therapy improve symptoms of depression? Findings from a specialized menopause clinic. *Menopause* 31(4):320–325.

Goldenberg, R. L., J. F. Culhane, J. D. Iams, and R. Romero. 2008. Epidemiology and causes of preterm birth. *Lancet* 371(9606):75–84.

Gomez, I., K. Diep, B. Frederiksen, U. Ranji, and A. Salganicoff. 2024. *Abortion Experiences, Knowledge, and Attitudes Among Women in the U.S.: Findings from the 2024 KFF Women's Health Survey*. https://www.kff.org/womens-health-policy/issue-brief/abortion-experiences-knowledge-attitudes-among-u-s-women-2024-womens-health-survey/ (accessed August 16, 2024).

González-Martín, A., B. Pothuri, I. Vergote, R. D. Christensen, W. Graybill, M. R. Mirza, C. McCormick, D. Lorusso, P. Hoskins, G. Freyer, K. Baumann, K. Jardon, A. Redondo, R. G. Moore, C. Vulsteke, R. E. O'Cearbhaill, B. Lund, F. Backes, P. Barretina-Ginesta, A. F. Haggerty, M. J. Rubio-Pérez, M. S. Shahin, G. Mangili, W. H. Bradley, I. Bruchim, K. Sun, I. A. Malinowska, Y. Li, D. Gupta, and B. J. Monk. 2019. Niraparib in patients with newly diagnosed advanced ovarian cancer. *New England Journal of Medicine* 381(25):2391–2402.

Goodman, J. H. 2009. Women's attitudes, preferences, and perceived barriers to treatment for perinatal depression. *Birth* 36(1):60–69.

Goodwin, R. D., L. C. Dierker, M. Wu, S. Galea, C. W. Hoven, and A. H. Weinberger. 2022. Trends in U.S. depression prevalence from 2015 to 2020: The widening treatment gap. *American Journal of Preventive Medicine* 63(5):726–733.

Greco, E., M. Calanducci, K. H. Nicolaides, E. V. H. Barry, M. S. B. Huda, and S. Iliodromiti. 2024. Gestational diabetes mellitus and adverse maternal and perinatal outcomes in twin and singleton pregnancies: A systematic review and meta-analysis. *American Journal of Obstetrics and Gynecology* 230(2):213–225.

Greenberg, P. E., A.-A. Fournier, T. Sisitsky, M. Simes, R. Berman, S. H. Koenigsberg, and R. C. Kessler. 2021. The economic burden of adults with major depressive disorder in the United States (2010 and 2018). *PharmacoEconomics* 39(6):653–665.

Gregory, E. C., and D. M. Ely. 2022. Trends and characteristics in gestational diabetes: United States, 2016–2020. *National Vital Statistics Report* 71(3):1–15.

Grossman, D., C. Joffe, S. Kaller, K. Kimport, E. Kinsey, K. Lerma, N. Morris, and K. White. 2023. *Care post-Roe: Documenting cases of poor-quality care since the Dobbs decision.* San Francisco, CA: Advancing New Standards in Reproductive Health.

Guevara, L. Z., E. Myers, R. Spencer, L. Havrilesky, and H. Moss. 2023. Disparities in allocation of research funding for female reproductive cancers based on race-specific disease burden (015). *Gynecologic Oncology* 176:S12.

Gunja, M. Z., E. D. Gumas, R. Masitha, and L. C. Zephyrin. 2024. *Insights into the U.S. maternal mortality crisis: An international comparison.* New York: The Commonwealth Fund.

Habets, D. H. J., K. Pelzner, L. Wieten, M. E. A. Spaanderman, E. Villamor, and S. Al-Nasiry. 2022. Intravenous immunoglobulins improve live birth rate among women with underlying immune conditions and recurrent pregnancy loss: A systematic review and meta-analysis. *Allergy, Asthma & Clinical Immunology* 18(1):23.

Han, B., W. M. Compton, E. B. Einstein, E. Elder, and N. D. Volkow. 2024. Pregnancy and postpartum drug overdose deaths in the U.S. before and during the COVID-19 pandemic. *JAMA Psychiatry* 81(3):270–283.

Hantsoo, L., and C. N. Epperson. 2017. Anxiety disorders among women: A female lifespan approach. *Focus* 15(2):162–172.

Hebert, L. E., P. A. Scherr, J. J. McCann, L. A. Beckett, and D. A. Evans. 2001. Is the risk of developing Alzheimer's disease greater for women than for men? *American Journal of Epidemiology* 153(2):132–136.

Hebert, L. E., J. Weuve, P. A. Scherr, and D. A. Evans. 2013. Alzheimer disease in the United States (2010–2050) estimated using the 2010 census. *Neurology* 80(19):1778–1783.

Hellberg, S. N., L. Lundegard, T. A. Hopkins, K. A. Thompson, M. Kang, T. Morris, and C. E. Schiller. 2023. Psychological distress and treatment preferences among parents amidst the COVID-19 pandemic. *Psychiatry Research Communications* 3(2):100109.

Hentosh, S., L. Zhu, J. Patino, J. W. Furr, N. P. Rocha, and E. Furr Stimming. 2021. Sex differences in Huntington's disease: Evaluating the Enroll-HD database. *Movement Disorders Clinical Practice* 8(3):420–426.

Hidalgo, V., M. M. Pulopulos, and A. Salvador. 2019. Acute psychosocial stress effects on memory performance: Relevance of age and sex. *Neurobiology of Learning and Memory* 157:48–60.

Hill, L., S. Artiga, and U. Ranji. 2022. *Racial disparities in maternal and infant health: Current status and efforts to address them.* San Francisco, CA: KFF.

Hinchcliff, E. M., E. M. Bednar, K. H. Lu, and J. A. Rauh-Hain. 2019. Disparities in gynecologic cancer genetics evaluation. *Gynecologic Oncology* 153(1):184–191.

Howell, E. A. 2018. Reducing disparities in severe maternal morbidity and mortality. *Clinical Obstetrics and Gynecology* 61(2):387–399.

Hoyert, D. 2024. *Maternal Mortality Rates in the United States, 2022.* https://www.cdc.gov/nchs/data/hestat/maternal-mortality/2022/maternal-mortality-rates-2022.htm (accessed August 14, 2024).

Huddleston, H. G., E. G. Jaswa, K. B. Casaletto, J. Neuhaus, C. Kim, M. Wellons, L. J. Launer, and K. Yaffe. 2024. Associations of polycystic ovary syndrome with indicators of brain health at midlife in the CARDIA cohort. *Neurology* 102(4):e208104.

Huo, N., P. Vemuri, J. Graff-Radford, J. Syrjanen, M. Machulda, D. S. Knopman, C. R. Jack, Jr., R. Petersen, and M. M. Mielke. 2022. Sex differences in the association between midlife cardiovascular conditions or risk factors with midlife cognitive decline. *Neurology* 98(6):e623–e632.

Huppertz, B. 2008. Placental origins of preeclampsia: Challenging the current hypothesis. *Hypertension* 51(4):970–975.

Iams, J. D., R. Romero, J. F. Culhane, and R. L. Goldenberg. 2008. Primary, secondary, and tertiary interventions to reduce the morbidity and mortality of preterm birth. *Lancet* 371(9607):164–175.

IHME (Institute for Health Metrics and Evaluation). n.d.-a. *GBD Results.* https://vizhub.healthdata.org/gbd-results/ (accessed August 13, 2024).

IHME. n.d.-b. *Global Burden of Disease 2021 Disease Injury, and Impairment Factsheets.* https://www.healthdata.org/research-analysis/diseases-injuries/factsheets-overview/about-disease-injury-impairment (accessed October 18, 2024).

IHME. n.d.-c. *Global Burden of Disease Study 2021 (GBD 2021) Disability Weights.* https://ghdx.healthdata.org/record/ihme-data/gbd-2021-disability-weights (accessed August 28, 2024).

Illán-Gala, I., K. B. Casaletto, S. Borrego-Écija, E. M. Arenaza-Urquijo, A. Wolf, Y. Cobigo, S. Y. M. Goh, A. M. Staffaroni, D. Alcolea, J. Fortea, R. Blesa, J. Clarimon, M. F. Iulita, A. Brugulat-Serrat, A. Lladó, L. T. Grinberg, K. Possin, K. P. Rankin, J. H. Kramer, G. D. Rabinovici, A. Boxer, W. W. Seeley, V. E. Sturm, M. L. Gorno-Tempini, B. L. Miller, R. Sánchez-Valle, D. C. Perry, A. Lleó, and H. J. Rosen. 2021. Sex differences in the behavioral variant of frontotemporal dementia: A new window to executive and behavioral reserve. *Alzheimer's & Dementia Journal* 17(8):1329–1341.

IOM (Institute of Medicine). 2007. *Preterm birth: Causes, consequences, and prevention.* Washington DC: The National Academies Press.

Jagsi, R. 2024. *Lessons from Breast Cancer Research and Remaining Gaps. Presentation to the NASEM Committee on the Assessement of NIH Research on Women's Health, Meeting 3 (March 7, 2024).* https://www.nationalacademies.org/event/docs/D44D1CC8D876137F76CCDC62F785C004079114963A63?noSaveAs=1 (accessed October 21, 2024).

Jagsi, R., S. T. Hawley, K. A. Griffith, N. K. Janz, A. W. Kurian, K. C. Ward, A. S. Hamilton, M. Morrow, and S. J. Katz. 2017. Contralateral prophylactic mastectomy decisions in a population-based sample of patients with early-stage breast cancer. *JAMA Surgery* 152(3):274–282.

Joffe, H., A. Massler, and K. M. Sharkey. 2010. Evaluation and management of sleep disturbance during the menopause transition. *Seminars in Reproductive Medicine* 28(5):404–421.

Johnson, J. D., and J. M. Louis. 2022. Does race or ethnicity play a role in the origin, pathophysiology, and outcomes of preeclampsia? An expert review of the literature. *American Journal of Obstetrics & Gynecology* 226(2):S876–S885.

Joseph, K. S., S. Lisonkova, A. Boutin, G. M. Muraca, N. Razaz, S. John, Y. Sabr, W.-S. Chan, A. Mehrabadi, J. S. Brandt, E. F. Schisterman, and C. V. Ananth. 2024. Maternal mortality in the United States: Are the high and rising rates due to changes in obstetrical factors, maternal medical conditions, or maternal mortality surveillance? *American Journal of Obstetrics & Gynecology* 230(4):440.e441–440.e413.

Ju, Y.-E. S., B. P. Lucey, and D. M. Holtzman. 2014. Sleep and Alzheimer disease pathology—a bidirectional relationship. *Nature Reviews Neurology* 10(2):115–119.

Ju, Y.-E. S., S. J. Ooms, C. Sutphen, S. L. Macauley, M. A. Zangrilli, G. Jerome, A. M. Fagan, E. Mignot, J. M. Zempel, J. A. H. R. Claassen, and D. M. Holtzman. 2017. Slow wave sleep disruption increases cerebrospinal fluid amyloid-β levels. *Brain* 140(8):2104–2111.

Jung, E., R. Romero, L. Yeo, N. Gomez-Lopez, P. Chaemsaithong, A. Jaovisidha, F. Gotsch, and O. Erez. 2022. The etiology of preeclampsia. *American Journal of Obstetrics and Gynecology* 226(2, Supplement):S844–S866.

Kalafat, E., and B. Thilaganathan. 2017. Cardiovascular origins of preeclampsia. *Current Opinion in Obstetrics and Gynecology* 29(6):383–389.

Karlan, B. Y. 2024. *Ovarian Cancer 2024: Knowledge Gaps and Barriers to Improving Outcomes. Presentation to the NASEM Committee on the Assessment of NIH Research on Women's Health, Meeting 3 (March 7, 2024).* https://www.nationalacademies.org/event/docs/DC0C4FBDCA3CD136898AEE4C97B2D38780CE6060245B?noSaveAs=1 (accessed October 21, 2024).

KFF. 2024. *Abortion in the United States Dashboard.* https://www.kff.org/womens-health-policy/dashboard/abortion-in-the-u-s-dashboard/ (accessed August 15, 2024).

Kornacki, J., O. Olejniczak, R. Sibiak, P. Gutaj, and E. Wender-Ożegowska. 2023. Pathophysiology of pre-eclampsia—two theories of the development of the disease. *International Journal of Molecular Sciences* 25(1).

Laijawala, R. A. 2024. Recurrent pregnancy loss: Immunological aetiologies and associations with mental health. *Brain, Behavior, & Immunity—Health* 41:100868.

Larré, A. B., F. Sontag, D. M. Pasin, N. Paludo, R. R. do Amaral, B. E. P. da Costa, and C. E. Poli-de-Figueiredo. 2018. Phosphodiesterase inhibition in the treatment of preeclampsia: What is new? *Current Hypertension Reports* 20(10):83.

Lewis Johnson, T., L. M. Rowland, M. S. Ashraf, C. T. Clark, V. M. Dotson, A. A. Livinski, and M. Simon. 2024. Key findings from mental health research during the menopause transition for racially and ethnically minoritized women living in the United States: A scoping review. *Journal of Women's Health* 33(2):113–131.

Li, L., J. Ji, Y. Li, Y. Huang, J. Y. Moon, and K. R.S. 2022. Gestational diabetes, subsequent Type 2 diabetes, and food security status: National Health and Nutrition Examination Survey, 2007–2018. *Preventing Chronic Disease* 19.

Li, S. H., and B. M. Graham. 2017. Why are women so vulnerable to anxiety, trauma-related and stress-related disorders? The potential role of sex hormones. *Lancet Psychiatry* 4(1):73–82.

Liu, C.-C., T. Kanekiyo, H. Xu, and G. Bu. 2013. Apolipoprotein E and Alzheimer disease: Risk, mechanisms and therapy. *Nature Reviews Neurology* 9(2):106–118.

Liu, R., D. M. Umbach, S. D. Peddada, Z. Xu, A. I. Tröster, X. Huang, and H. Chen. 2015. Potential sex differences in nonmotor symptoms in early drug-naive Parkinson disease. *Neurology* 84(21):2107–2115.

MacDorman, M. F., and E. Declercq. 2018. The failure of United States maternal mortality reporting and its impact on women's lives. *Birth* 45(2):105–108.

MacDorman, M. F., M. Thoma, E. Declcerq, and E. A. Howell. 2021. Racial and ethnic dispari-
ties in maternal mortality in the United States using enhanced vital records, 2016–2017.
American Journal of Public Health 111(9):1673–1681.
Maddow-Zimet, I., and C. Gibson. 2024. *Despite Bans, Number of Abortions in the United
States Increased in 2023*. https://www.guttmacher.org/2024/03/despite-bans-number-
abortions-united-states-increased-2023 (accessed August 15, 2024).
Magee, L. A., D. Wright, A. Syngelaki, P. von Dadelszen, R. Akolekar, A. Wright, and K.
H. Nicolaides. 2023. Preeclampsia prevention by timed birth at term. *Hypertension*
80(5):969–978.
Magnus, M. C., M. K. Wallace, J. R. Demirci, J. M. Catov, M. J. Schmella, and A. Fraser. 2023.
Breastfeeding and later-life cardiometabolic health in women with and without hyperten-
sive disorders of pregnancy. *Journal of the American Heart Association* 12(5):e026696.
Maki, P. M., S. G. Kornstein, H. Joffe, J. T. Bromberger, E. W. Freeman, G. Athappilly, W. V.
Bobo, L. H. Rubin, H. K. Koleva, L. S. Cohen, and C. N. Soares. 2019. Guidelines for the
evaluation and treatment of perimenopausal depression: Summary and recommendations.
Journal of Women's Health 28(2):117–134.
March of Dimes. n.d. *A Profile of Prematurity in the United States*. https://www.marchofdimes.
org/peristats/reports/united-states/prematurity-profile (accessed October 22, 2024).
March of Dimes. 2020. *Treatments for Preterm Labor*. https://www.marchofdimes.org/find-
support/topics/birth/treatments-preterm-labor (accessed October 22, 2024).
Marsh, E. E., G. Wegienka, and D. R. Williams. 2024. Uterine fibroids. *JAMA* 331(17):1492–1493.
Martin, S. S., A. W. Aday, Z. I. Almarzooq, C. A. M. Anderson, P. Arora, C. L. Avery, C. M.
Baker-Smith, B. Barone Gibbs, A. Z. Beaton, A. K. Boehme, Y. Commodore-Mensah, M.
E. Currie, M. S. V. Elkind, K. R. Evenson, G. Generoso, D. G. Heard, S. Hiremath, M.
C. Johansen, R. Kalani, D. S. Kazi, D. Ko, J. Liu, J. W. Magnani, E. D. Michos, M. E.
Mussolino, S. D. Navaneethan, N. I. Parikh, S. M. Perman, R. Poudel, M. Rezk-Hanna, G.
A. Roth, N. S. Shah, M.-P. St-Onge, E. L. Thacker, C. W. Tsao, M. W. Urbut, H. G. C. Van
Spall, J. H. Voeks, N.-Y. Wang, N. D. Wong, S. S. Wong, K. Yaffe, and L. P. Palaniappan,
on behalf of the American Heart Association Council on Epidemiology and Prevention
Statistics Committee and Stroke Statistics Subcommittee. 2024. 2024 heart disease and
stroke statistics: A report of U.S. and global data from the American Heart Association.
Circulation 149(8):e347–e913.
Mattina, G. F., R. J. Van Lieshout, and M. Steiner. 2019. Inflammation, depression and cardio-
vascular disease in women: The role of the immune system across critical reproductive
events. *Therapeutic Advances in Cardiovascular Disease* 13:1753944719851950.
Mayo Clinic. 2022. *Preterm Labor*. https://www.mayoclinic.org/diseases-conditions/preterm-
labor/diagnosis-treatment/drc-20376848 (accessed October 22, 2024).
Meltzer-Brody, S., H. Colquhoun, R. Riesenberg, C. N. Epperson, K. M. Deligiannidis, D. R.
Rubinow, H. Li, A. J. Sankoh, C. Clemson, A. Schacterle, J. Jonas, and S. Kanes. 2018.
Brexanolone injection in post-partum depression: Two multicentre, double-blind, ran-
domised, placebo-controlled, phase 3 trials. *Lancet* 392(10152):1058–1070.
Menon, U., A. Gentry-Maharaj, M. Burnell, N. Singh, A. Ryan, C. Karpinskyj, G. Carlino, J.
Taylor, S. K. Massingham, M. Raikou, J. K. Kalsi, R. Woolas, R. Manchanda, R. Arora, L.
Casey, A. Dawnay, S. Dobbs, S. Leeson, T. Mould, M. W. Seif, A. Sharma, K. Williamson,
Y. Liu, L. Fallowfield, A. J. McGuire, S. Campbell, S. J. Skates, I. J. Jacobs, and M. Parmar.
2021. Ovarian cancer population screening and mortality after long-term follow-up in
the U.K. Collaborative Trial of Ovarian Cancer Screening (UKCTOCS): A randomised
controlled trial. *Lancet* 397(10290):2182–2193.
Mielke, M. M. 2020. Consideration of sex differences in the measurement and interpretation
of Alzheimer disease-related biofluid-based biomarkers. *Journal of Applied Laboratory
Medicine* 5(1):158–169.

Moore, K., N. Colombo, G. Scambia, B.-G. Kim, A. Oaknin, M. Friedlander, A. Lisyanskaya, A. Floquet, A. Leary, G. S. Sonke, C. Gourley, S. Banerjee, A. Oza, A. González-Martín, C. Aghajanian, W. Bradley, C. Mathews, J. Liu, E. S. Lowe, R. Bloomfield, and P. DiSilvestro. 2018. Maintenance olaparib in patients with newly diagnosed advanced ovarian cancer. *New England Journal of Medicine* 379(26):2495–2505.

Morrison, L., S. Loibl, and N. C. Turner. 2024. The CDK4/6 inhibitor revolution—a game-changing era for breast cancer treatment. *Nature Reviews Clinical Oncology* 21(2):89–105.

Mosca, L., E. J. Benjamin, K. Berra, J. L. Bezanson, R. J. Dolor, D. M. Lloyd-Jones, L. K. Newby, I. L. Piña, V. L. Roger, L. J. Shaw, D. Zhao, T. M. Beckie, C. Bushnell, J. D'Armiento, P. M. Kris-Etherton, J. Fang, T. G. Ganiats, A. S. Gomes, C. R. Gracia, C. K. Haan, E. A. Jackson, D. R. Judelson, E. Kelepouris, C. J. Lavie, A. Moore, N. A. Nussmeier, E. Ofili, S. Oparil, P. Ouyang, V. W. Pinn, K. Sherif, S. C. Smith, Jr., G. Sopko, N. Chandra-Strobos, E. M. Urbina, V. Vaccarino, and N. K. Wenger. 2011. Effectiveness-based guidelines for the prevention of cardiovascular disease in women—2011 update: A guideline from the American Heart Association. *Circulation* 123(11):1243–1262.

Nabi, M. Y., S. Nauhria, M. Reel, S. Londono, A. Vasireddi, M. Elmiry, and P. Ramdass. 2022. Endometriosis and irritable bowel syndrome: A systematic review and meta-analyses. *Frontiers in Medicine* 9:914356.

NASEM (National Academies of Sciences, Engineering, and Medicine). 2019. *Vibrant and healthy kids: Aligning science, practice, and policy to advance health equity.* Washington, DC: The National Academies Press.

NASEM. 2020. *Birth settings in America: Outcomes, quality, access, and choice.* Washington, DC: The National Academies Press.

NASEM. 2021. *Advancing maternal health equity and reducing maternal morbidity and mortality: Proceedings of a workshop.* Washington, DC: The National Academies Press.

NASEM. 2022. *Enhancing NIH research on autoimmune disease.* Washington, DC: The National Academies Press.

NASEM. 2023. *Federal policy to advance racial, ethnic, and tribal health equity.* Washington, DC: The National Academies Press.

NASEM. 2024a. *Advancing clinical research with pregnant and lactating populations: Overcoming real and perceived liability risks.* Washington, DC: The National Academies Press.

NASEM. 2024b. *Advancing research on chronic conditions in women.* Washington, DC: The National Academies Press.

NASEM. 2024c. *Overview of research gaps for selected conditions in women's health research at the National Institutes of Health: Proceedings of a workshop—in brief.* Washington, DC: The National Academies Press.

NASEM. 2024d. *Reproductive health, equity, and society: Exploring data challenges and needs in the wake of the Dobbs v. Jackson women's health organization decision: Proceedings of a workshop—in brief.* Washington, DC: The National Academies Press.

NCCID (National Collaborating Centre for Infectious Diseases). 2015. *Understanding Summary Measures Used to Estimate the Burden of Disease: All About HALYs, DALYs and QALYs.* https://nccid.ca/publications/understanding-summary-measures-used-to-estimate-the-burden-of-disease/ (accessed August 8, 2024).

NCCIH (National Center for Complementary and Integrative Health). 2021. *NCCIH strategic plan FY 2021–2025: Mapping a pathway to research on whole person health.* Bethesda, MD: National Center for Complementary and Integrative Health.

NCCN (National Comprehensive Cancer Network). 2024. *NCCN guidelines for patients: Ovarian cancer.* Plymouth Meeting, PA: National Comprehensive Cancer Network.

NCI (National Cancer Institute). n.d.-a. *NCI Cervical Cancer "Last Mile" Initiative*. https:// prevention.cancer.gov/major-programs/nci-cervical-cancer-last-mile-initiative (accessed August 14, 2024).

NCI. n.d.-b. *SEER Cancer Stat Facts: Cervical Cancer*. https://seer.cancer.gov/statfacts/html/ cervix.html (accessed October 20, 2024).

NCI. n.d.-c. *SEER Cancer Stat Facts: Ovarian Cancer*. https://seer.cancer.gov/statfacts/html/ ovary.html (accessed October 20, 2024).

NCI. n.d.-d. *SEER Cancer Stat Facts: Uterine Cancer*. https://seer.cancer.gov/statfacts/html/ corp.html (accessed July 15, 2024).

NCI. 2020. *With Two FDA Approvals, Prostate Cancer Treatment Enters the PARP Era*. https://www.cancer.gov/news-events/cancer-currents-blog/2020/fda-olaparib-rucaparib-prostate-cancer (accessed October 20, 2024).

NCI. 2024a. *All Cancer Sites Combined: Recent Trends in SEER age-Adjusted Incidence Rates, 2000–2021*. https://seer.cancer.gov/statistics-Network/explorer/application.html? site=1&data_type=1&graph_type=2&compareBy=sex&chk_sex_3=3&chk_sex_2=2& rate_type=2&race=1&age_range=1&hdn_stage=101&advopt_precision=1&advopt_ show_ci=on&hdn_view=0&advopt_show_apc=on&advopt_display=2#resultsRegion0 (accessed August 21, 2024).

NCI. 2024b. *Breast: Recent Trends in SEER Relative Survival Rates, 2000–2021: By Race/ Ethnicity, 3-year Relative Survival, Female, All Ages, All Stages*. https://seer.cancer. gov/statistics-network/explorer/application.html?site=55&data_type=4&graph_ type=2&compareBy=race&chk_race_1=1&chk_race_3=3&chk_race_2=2&relative_ survival_interval=3&sex=3&age_range=1&stage=101&advopt_precision=1&advopt_ show_ci=on&hdn_view=0&advopt_show_apc=on&advopt_display=1#resultsRegion0 (accessed October 20, 2024).

NCI. 2024c. *Cervix Uteri: Recent Trends in SEER Relative Survival Rates, 2000–2021: Female by Race/Ethnicity, 3-Year Relative Survival, All Ages, All Stages*. https://seer. cancer.gov/statistics-network/explorer/application.html?site=57&data_type=4&graph_ type=2&compareBy=race&chk_race_1=1&chk_race_3=3&chk_race_2=2&relative_sur- vival_interval=3&hdn_sex=3&age_range=1&stage=101&advopt_precision=1&advopt_ show_ci=on&hdn_view=0&advopt_show_apc=on&advopt_display=1#resultsRegion0 (accessed October 20, 2024).

NCI. 2024d. *Corpus and Uterus, Nos: Recent Trends in SEER Relative Survival Rates, 2000– 2021: Female by Race/Ethnicty, 3-Year Relative Survival, All Ages, All Stages*. https://seer. cancer.gov/statistics-network/explorer/application.html?site=58&data_type=4&graph_ type=2&compareBy=race&chk_race_1=1&chk_race_3=3&chk_race_2=2&relative_ survival_interval=3&hdn_sex=3&age_range=1&stage=101&advopt_precision= 1&advopt_show_ci=on&hdn_view=0&advopt_show_apc=on&advopt_display=2# resultsRegion0 (accessed October 20, 2024).

NCI. 2024e. *Funding for Research Areas*. https://www.cancer.gov/about-nci/budget/fact-book/ data/research-funding (accessed August 14, 2024).

NCI. 2024f. *Ovary: Recent Trends in SEER Relative Survival Rates, 2000–2021: Female by Race/Ethnicity, 3-Year Relative Survival, All Ages, All Stages*. https://seer.cancer. gov/statistics-network/explorer/application.html?site=61&data_type=4&graph_ type=2&compareBy=race&chk_race_3=3&chk_race_2=2&relative_survival_ interval=3&hdn_sex=3&age_range=1&stage=101&advopt_precision=1&advopt_ show_ci=on&hdn_view=0&advopt_show_apc=on&advopt_display=2#resultsRegion0 (accessed August 21, 2024).

Nelson, A. E., D. Hu, L. Arbeeva, C. Alvarez, R. J. Cleveland, T. A. Schwartz, L. B. Murphy, C. G. Helmick, L. F. Callahan, J. B. Renner, J. M. Jordan, and Y. M. Golightly. 2022. Point preva- lence of hip symptoms, radiographic, and symptomatic OA at five time points: The Johnston County Osteoarthritis Project, 1991–2018. *Osteoarthritis and Cartilage Open* 4(2).

Neu, S. C., J. Pa, W. Kukull, D. Beekly, A. Kuzma, P. Gangadharan, L. S. Wang, K. Romero, S. P. Arneric, A. Redolfi, D. Orlandi, G. B. Frisoni, R. Au, S. Devine, S. Auerbach, A. Espinosa, M. Boada, A. Ruiz, S. C. Johnson, R. Koscik, J. J. Wang, W. C. Hsu, Y. L. Chen, and A. W. Toga. 2017. Apolipoprotein E genotype and sex risk factors for Alzheimer disease: A meta-analysis. *JAMA Neurology* 74(10):1178–1189.

Nguyen, A. H., M. Hurwitz, S. A. Sullivan, A. Saad, J. L. W. Kennedy, and G. Sharma. 2024. Update on sex specific risk factors in cardiovascular disease. *Frontiers in Cardiovascular Medicine* 11:1352675.

NIA (National Institute on Aging). 2022. *Research Highlights: Research Explores the Impact of Menopause on Women's Health and Aging.* https://www.nia.nih.gov/news/research-explores-impact-menopause-womens-health-and-aging (accessed October 21, 2024).

NIH (National Institutes of Health). n.d.-a. *Improving Health: Cancer.* https://www.nih.gov/about-nih/what-we-do/impact-nih-research/improving-health/cancer (accessed August 14, 2024).

NIH. n.d.-b. *NIH Grants Policy Statement: 4.1.14 Human Fetal Tissue Research.* https://grants.nih.gov/grants/policy/nihgps/html5/section_4/4.1.14_human_fetal_tissue_research.htm (accessed August 21, 2024).

NIH. n.d.-c. *NIH Grants Policy Statement: 4.2.7 Restriction on Abortion Funding.* https://grants.nih.gov/grants/policy/nihgps/HTML5/section_4/4.2.7_restriction_on_abortion_funding.htm (accessed August 21, 2024).

NIH. 2013. *Understanding Breast Cancer: Early Detection, Improved Treatments Save Lives.* https://newsinhealth.nih.gov/sites/newsinhealth/files/2013/October/NIHNiHOct2013.pdf (accessed August 14, 2024).

Nordin, M. L., A. K. Azemi, A. H. Nordin, W. Nabgan, P. Y. Ng, K. Yusoff, N. Abu, K. P. Lim, Z. A. Zakaria, N. Ismail, and F. Azmi. 2023. Peptide-based vaccine against breast cancer: Recent advances and prospects. *Pharmaceuticals* 16(7).

Norton, M. C., K. R. Smith, T. Østbye, J. T. Tschanz, C. Corcoran, S. Schwartz, K. W. Piercy, P. V. Rabins, D. C. Steffens, I. Skoog, J. C. Breitner, and K. A. Welsh-Bohmer. 2010. Greater risk of dementia when spouse has dementia? The Cache County study. *Journal of the American Geriatric Society* 58(5):895–900.

O'Kelly, A. C., E. D. Michos, C. L. Shufelt, J. V. Vermunt, M. B. Minissian, O. Quesada, G. N. Smith, J. W. Rich-Edwards, V. D. Garovic, S. R. El Khoudary, and M. C. Honigberg. 2022. Pregnancy and reproductive risk factors for cardiovascular disease in women. *Circulation Research* 130(4):652–672.

Orgera, K., and A. Grover. 2024. *States with Abortion Bans See Continued Decrease in U.S. MD Senior Residency Applicants.* https://www.aamcresearchinstitute.org/our-work/data-snapshot/post-dobbs-2024 (accessed August 19, 2024).

Ossenkoppele, R., C. H. Lyoo, J. Jester-Broms, C. H. Sudre, H. Cho, Y. H. Ryu, J. Y. Choi, R. Smith, O. Strandberg, S. Palmqvist, J. Kramer, A. L. Boxer, M. L. Gorno-Tempini, B. L. Miller, R. La Joie, G. D. Rabinovici, and O. Hansson. 2020. Assessment of demographic, genetic, and imaging variables associated with brain resilience and cognitive resilience to pathological tau in patients with Alzheimer disease. *JAMA Neurology* 77(5):632–642.

Palatnik, A., R. K. Harrison, R. J. Walker, M. Y. Thakkar, and L. E. Egede. 2022. Maternal racial and ethnic disparities in glycemic threshold for pharmacotherapy initiation for gestational diabetes. *Journal of Maternal-Fetal & Neonatal Medicine* 35(1):58–65.

Pallerla, S., A. Abdul, J. Comeau, and S. Jois. 2021. Cancer vaccines, treatment of the future: With emphasis on HER2-positive breast cancer. *International Journal of Molecular Sciences* 22(2).

Parikh, N. I., J. M. Gonzalez, C. A. M. Anderson, S. E. Judd, K. M. Rexrode, M. A. Hlatky, E. P. Gunderson, J. J. Stuart, and D. Vaidya, on behalf of the American Heart Association Council on Epidemiology and Prevention; Council on Arteriosclerosis, Thrombosis, and Vascular Biology; Council on Cardiovascular and Stroke Nursing; and the Stroke

Council. 2021. Adverse pregnancy outcomes and cardiovascular disease risk: Unique opportunities for cardiovascular disease prevention in women: A scientific statement from the American Heart Association. *Circulation* 143(18):e902–e916.

Patterson, R., I. Balan, A. L. Morrow, and S. Meltzer-Brody. 2024. Novel neurosteroid therapeutics for post-partum depression: Perspectives on clinical trials, program development, active research, and future directions. *Neuropsychopharmacology* 49(1):67–72.

Payne, J. L., and J. Maguire. 2019. Pathophysiological mechanisms implicated in postpartum depression. *Frontiers in Neuroendocrinology* 52:165–180.

Peacock, K., K. Carlson, and K. M. Ketvertis. 2023. Menopause. In *Statpearls*. Treasure Island, FL: StatPearls Publishing.

Petersen, E. E., N. L. Davis, D. Goodman, S. Cox, C. Syverson, K. Seed, C. Shapiro-Mendoza, W. M. Callaghan, and W. Barfield. 2019. Racial/ethnic disparities in pregnancy-related deaths—United States, 2007–2016. *MMWR* 68(35):762–765.

Phimphasone-Brady, P., C. E. Page, D. A. Ali, H. C. Haller, and K. A. Duffy. 2023. Racial and ethnic disparities in women's mental health: A narrative synthesis of systematic reviews and meta-analyses of the U.S.-based samples. *Fertility and Sterility* 119(3):364–374.

Pinna, G. 2020. Allopregnanolone, the neuromodulator turned therapeutic agent: Thank you, next? *Frontiers in Endocrinology* 11:236.

Practice Committee of the American Society for Reproductive Medicine. 2012. Evaluation and treatment of recurrent pregnancy loss: A committee opinion. *Fertility and Sterility* 98(5):1103–1111.

Practice Committee of the American Society for Reproductive Medicine. 2013. Definitions of infertility and recurrent pregnancy loss: A committee opinion. *Fertility and Sterility* 99(1):63.

Quenby, S., I. D. Gallos, R. K. Dhillon-Smith, M. Podesek, M. D. Stephenson, J. Fisher, J. J. Brosens, J. Brewin, R. Ramhorst, E. S. Lucas, R. C. McCoy, R. Anderson, S. Daher, L. Regan, M. Al-Memar, T. Bourne, D. A. MacIntyre, R. Rai, O. B. Christiansen, M. Sugiura-Ogasawara, J. Odendaal, A. J. Devall, P. R. Bennett, S. Petrou, and A. Coomarasamy. 2021. Miscarriage matters: The epidemiological, physical, psychological, and economic costs of early pregnancy loss. *Lancet* 397(10285):1658–1667.

Raglan, G. B., S. M. Lannon, K. M. Jones, and J. Schulkin. 2016. Racial and ethnic disparities in preterm birth among American Indian and Alaska Native women. *Maternal and Child Health Journal* 20(1):16–24.

Ralph, L. J., E. B. Schwarz, D. Grossman, and D. G. Foster. 2019. Self-reported physical health of women who did and did not terminate pregnancy after seeking abortion services. *Annals of Internal Medicine* 171(4):238–247.

Rassie, K., R. Giri, A. E. Joham, H. Teede, and A. Mousa. 2022. Human placental lactogen in relation to maternal metabolic health and fetal outcomes: A systematic review and meta-analysis. *International Journal of Molecular Sciences* 23(24).

Reddy, D. S., R. H. Mbilinyi, and E. Estes. 2023. Preclinical and clinical pharmacology of brexanolone (allopregnanolone) for postpartum depression: A landmark journey from concept to clinic in neurosteroid replacement therapy. *Psychopharmacology* 240(9): 1841–1863.

Reekes, T. H., C. I. Higginson, C. R. Ledbetter, N. Sathivadivel, R. M. Zweig, and E. A. Disbrow. 2020. Sex specific cognitive differences in parkinson disease. *NPJ Parkinson's Disease* 6(1):7.

Regan, L., R. Rai, S. Saravelos, and T.-C. Li on behalf of the Royal College of Obstetricians and Gynaecologists. 2023. Recurrent miscarriage: Green-top guideline no. 17. *BJOG* 130(12):e9–e39.

Reis, F. M., E. Bloise, and T. M. Ortiga-Carvalho. 2016. Hormones and pathogenesis of uterine fibroids. *Best Practice and Research Clinical Obstetrics and Gynecology* 34:13–24.

Rimel, B. J., C. A. Kunos, N. Macioce, and S. M. Temkin. 2022. Current gaps and opportunities in screening, prevention, and treatment of cervical cancer. *Cancer* 128(23):4063–4073.

Ritchie, K., C. W. Ritchie, K. Yaffe, I. Skoog, and N. Scarmeas. 2015. Is late-onset Alzheimer's disease really a disease of midlife? *Alzheimer's & Dementia* 1(2):122–130.

Rome, D., A. Sales, R. Leeds, J. Usseglio, T. Cornelius, C. Monk, K. G. Smolderen, and N. Moise. 2022. A narrative review of the association between depression and heart disease among women: Prevalence, mechanisms of action, and treatment. *Current Atherosclerosis Reports* 24(9):709–720.

Rossen, L. M., B. E. Hamilton, J. C. Abma, E. C. W. Gregory, V. Beresovsky, A. V. Resendez, A. Chandra, and J. A. Martin. 2023. *Updated methodology to estimate overall and unintended pregnancy rates in the United States: Data evaluation and methods research.* Hyattsville, MD: National Center for Health Statistics, Centers for Disease Control and Prevention.

Rössler, W., V. Ajdacic-Gross, A. Riecher-Rössler, J. Angst, and M. P. Hengartner. 2016. Does menopausal transition really influence mental health? Findings from the prospective long-term Zurich study. *World Psychiatry* 15(2):146–154.

Rumble, M. E., P. Okoyeh, and R. M. Benca. 2023. Sleep and women's mental health. *Psychiatric Clinics of North America* 46(3):527–537.

Salomon, J. A., T. Vos, D. R. Hogan, M. Gagnon, M. Naghavi, A. Mokdad, N. Begum, R. Shah, M. Karyana, S. Kosen, M. R. Farje, G. Moncada, A. Dutta, S. Sazawal, A. Dyer, J. Seiler, V. Aboyans, L. Baker, A. Baxter, E. J. Benjamin, K. Bhalla, A. Bin Abdulhak, F. Blyth, R. Bourne, T. Braithwaite, P. Brooks, T. S. Brugha, C. Bryan-Hancock, R. Buchbinder, P. Burney, B. Calabria, H. Chen, S. S. Chugh, R. Cooley, M. H. Criqui, M. Cross, K. C. Dabhadkar, N. Dahodwala, A. Davis, L. Degenhardt, C. Díaz-Torné, E. R. Dorsey, T. Driscoll, K. Edmond, A. Elbaz, M. Ezzati, V. Feigin, C. P. Ferri, A. D. Flaxman, L. Flood, M. Fransen, K. Fuse, B. J. Gabbe, R. F. Gillum, J. Haagsma, J. E. Harrison, R. Havmoeller, R. J. Hay, A. Hel-Baqui, H. W. Hoek, H. Hoffman, E. Hogeland, D. Hoy, D. Jarvis, G. Karthikeyan, L. M. Knowlton, T. Lathlean, J. L. Leasher, S. S. Lim, S. E. Lipshultz, A. D. Lopez, R. Lozano, R. Lyons, R. Malekzadeh, W. Marcenes, L. March, D. J. Margolis, N. McGill, J. McGrath, G. A. Mensah, A. C. Meyer, C. Michaud, A. Moran, R. Mori, M. E. Murdoch, L. Naldi, C. R. Newton, R. Norman, S. B. Omer, R. Osborne, N. Pearce, F. Perez-Ruiz, N. Perico, K. Pesudovs, D. Phillips, F. Pourmalek, M. Prince, J. T. Rehm, G. Remuzzi, K. Richardson, R. Room, S. Saha, U. Sampson, L. Sanchez-Riera, M. Segui-Gomez, S. Shahraz, K. Shibuya, D. Singh, K. Sliwa, E. Smith, I. Soerjomataram, T. Steiner, W. A. Stolk, L. J. Stovner, C. Sudfeld, H. R. Taylor, I. M. Tleyjeh, M. J. van der Werf, W. L. Watson, D. J. Weatherall, R. Weintraub, M. G. Weisskopf, H. Whiteford, J. D. Wilkinson, A. D. Woolf, Z. J. Zheng, C. J. Murray, and J. B. Jonas. 2012. Common values in assessing health outcomes from disease and injury: Disability weights measurement study for the Global Burden of Disease study 2010. *Lancet* 380(9859):2129–2143.

Salomon, J. A., J. A. Haagsma, A. Davis, C. M. de Noordhout, S. Polinder, A. H. Havelaar, A. Cassini, B. Devleesschauwer, M. Kretzschmar, N. Speybroeck, C. J. L. Murray, and T. Vos. 2015. Disability weights for the Global Burden of Disease 2013 study. *Lancet Global Health* 3(11):e712–e723.

Santen, R. J., H. Brodie, E. R. Simpson, P. K. Siiteri, and A. Brodie. 2009. History of aromatase: Saga of an important biological mediator and therapeutic target. *Endocrine Reviews* 30(4):343–375.

Sassi, F. 2006. Calculating QALYs, comparing QALY and DALY calculations. *Health Policy Plan* 21(5):402–408.

Sateia, M. J. 2014. International classification of sleep disorders-third edition. *Chest* 146(5):1387–1394.

Sayres Van Niel, M., and J. L. Payne. 2020. Perinatal depression: A review. *Cleveland Clinic Journal of Medicine* 87(5):273–277.

Scalici, J., M. A. Finan, J. Black, M. D. Harmon, W. Nicolson, H. A. Lankes, W. E. Brady, and R. P. Rocconi. 2015. Minority participation in gynecologic oncology group (GOG) studies. *Gynecologic Oncology* 138(2):441–444.

Schmidt, P. J., N. Haq, and D. R. Rubinow. 2004. A longitudinal evaluation of the relationship between reproductive status and mood in perimenopausal women. *American Journal of Psychiatry* 161(12):2238–2244.

Schoenbaum, M., J. M. Sutherland, A. Chappel, S. Azrin, A. B. Goldstein, A. Rupp, and R. K. Heinssen. 2017. Twelve-month health care use and mortality in commercially insured young people with incident psychosis in the United States. *Schizophrenia Bulletin* 43(6):1262–1272.

Schott, S. L., A. Adams, R. J. Dougherty, T. Montgomery, F. C. Lapite, and F. E. Fletcher. 2023. Renewed calls for abortion-related research in the post-Roe era. *Frontiers Public Health* 11:1322299.

Sefah, N., S. Ndebele, L. Prince, E. Korasare, M. Agbleke, A. Nkansah, H. Thompson, A. Al-Hendy, and A. A. Agbleke. 2022. Uterine fibroids—causes, impact, treatment, and lens to the African perspective. *Frontiers in Pharmacology* 13:1045783.

Segal, N. A., J. M. Nilges, and W. M. Oo. 2024. Sex differences in osteoarthritis prevalence, pain perception, physical function and therapeutics. *Osteoarthritis Cartilage* 32(9):1045–1053.

Seritan, A. L., A.-M. Iosif, J. H. Park, D. DeatherageHand, R. L. Sweet, and E. B. Gold. 2010. Self-reported anxiety, depressive, and vasomotor symptoms: A study of perimenopausal women presenting to a specialized midlife assessment center. *Menopause* 17(2):410–415.

Shah, N. S., D. M. Lloyd-Jones, N. R. Kandula, M. D. Huffman, S. Capewell, M. O'Flaherty, K. N. Kershaw, M. R. Carnethon, and S. S. Khan. 2020. Adverse trends in premature cardiometabolic mortality in the United States, 1999 to 2018. *Journal of the American Heart Association* 9(23):e018213.

Shah, N. S., M. C. Wang, P. M. Freaney, A. M. Perak, M. R. Carnethon, N. R. Kandula, E. P. Gunderson, K. M. Bullard, W. A. Grobman, M. J. O'Brien, and S. S. Khan. 2021. Trends in gestational diabetes at first live birth by race and ethnicity in the U.S., 2011–2019. *JAMA* 326(7):660–669.

Shaw, C., E. Hayes-Larson, M. M. Glymour, C. Dufouil, T. J. Hohman, R. A. Whitmer, L. C. Kobayashi, R. Brookmeyer, and E. R. Mayeda. 2021. Evaluation of selective survival and sex/gender differences in dementia incidence using a simulation model. *JAMA Network Open* 4(3):e211001.

Shi, Y., D. Tan, B. Hao, X. Zhang, W. Geng, Y. Wang, J. Sun, and Y. Zhao. 2022. Efficacy of intravenous immunoglobulin in the treatment of recurrent spontaneous abortion: A systematic review and meta-analysis. *American Journal of Reproductive Immunology* 88(5):e13615.

Siegel, R. L., A. N. Giaquinto, and A. Jemal. 2024. Cancer statistics, 2024. *CA* 74(1):12–49.

Silverwood, V., M. Blagojevic-Bucknall, C. Jinks, J. L. Jordan, J. Protheroe, and K. P. Jordan. 2015. Current evidence on risk factors for knee osteoarthritis in older adults: A systematic review and meta-analysis. *Osteoarthritis and Cartilage* 23(4):507–515.

Slaughter-Acey, J., K. Behrens, A. Claussen, T. Usset, C. Neerland, S. Bilal-Roby, H. Bashir, A. Westby, B. Wagner, M. Dixon, M. Xiao, and M. Butler. 2023. *Social and structural determinants of maternal morbidity and mortality: An evidence map.* Rockville, MD: Agency for Healthcare Research and Quality.

Spencer, R. J., L. W. Rice, C. Ye, K. Woo, and S. Uppal. 2019. Disparities in the allocation of research funding to gynecologic cancers by funding to lethality scores. *Gynecologic Oncology* 152(1):106–111.

Srikanth, V. K., J. L. Fryer, G. Zhai, T. M. Winzenberg, D. Hosmer, and G. Jones. 2005. A meta-analysis of sex differences prevalence, incidence and severity of osteoarthritis. *Osteoarthritis and Cartilage* 13(9):769–781.

St. Pierre, A., J. Zaharatos, D. Goodman, and W. M. Callaghan. 2018. Challenges and opportunities in identifying, reviewing, and preventing maternal deaths. *Obstetrics and Gynecology* 131(1):138–142.

Staff, A. C. 2019. The two-stage placental model of preeclampsia: An update. *Journal of Reproductive Immunology* 134–135:1–10.

Statista. 2023. *Resident Population of the United States by Sex and Age as of July 1, 2022.* https://www.statista.com/statistics/241488/population-of-the-us-by-sex-and-age/ (accessed 7/12/2024, 2024).

Stevenson, A. J., and L. Root. 2024. Trends in maternal death post-Dobbs v Jackson Women's Health. *JAMA Network Open* 7(8):e2430035.

Stewart, S. L., N. Lakhani, P. M. Brown, O. A. Larkin, A. R. Moore, and N. S. Hayes. 2013. Gynecologic cancer prevention and control in the National Comprehensive Cancer Control Program: Progress, current activities, and future directions. *Jounal of Women's Health* 22(8):651–657.

Sundermann, E. E., P. M. Maki, L. H. Rubin, R. B. Lipton, S. Landau, and A. Biegon. 2016. Female advantage in verbal memory: Evidence of sex-specific cognitive reserve. *Neurology* 87(18):1916–1924.

Sundermann, E. E., M. S. Panizzon, X. Chen, M. Andrews, D. Galasko, and S. J. Banks, for the Alzheimer's Disease Neuroimaging Initiative. 2020. Sex differences in Alzheimer's-related Tau biomarkers and a mediating effect of testosterone. *Biology of Sex Differences* 11(1):33.

Surana, K. 2024a. *Abortion Bans Have Delayed Emergency Medical Care. In Georgia, Experts Say This Mother's Death Was Preventable.* https://www.propublica.org/article/georgia-abortion-ban-amber-thurman-death (accessed October 10, 2024).

Surana, K. 2024b. *Afraid to Seek Care Amid Georgia's Abortion Ban, She Stayed Home and Died.* https://www.propublica.org/article/candi-miller-abortion-ban-death-georgia (accessed October 10, 2024).

Sweeting, A., W. Hannah, H. Backman, P. Catalano, M. Feghali, W. H. Herman, M.-F. Hivert, J. Immanuel, C. Meek, M. L. Oppermann, C. J. Nolan, U. Ram, M. I. Schmidt, D. Simmons, T. Chivese, and K. Benhalima. 2024. Epidemiology and management of gestational diabetes. *Lancet* 404(10448):175–192.

Swenson, C. 2024. *Research on Pelvic Floor Disorders.* https://www.nationalacademies.org/documents/embed/link/LF2255DA3DD1C41C0A42D3BEF0989ACAECE3053A6A9B/file/DDCEB46107AB492040A1FCD09695BB1812A6FF641CBB?noSaveAs=1 (accessed July 18, 2024).

Szilagyi, I. A., J. H. Waarsing, J. B. J. van Meurs, S. M. A. Bierma-Zeinstra, and D. Schiphof. 2023. A systematic review of the sex differences in risk factors for knee osteoarthritis. *Rheumatology* 62(6):2037–2047.

Taiwo, T. K., K. Goode, P. M. Niles, K. Stoll, N. Malhotra, and S. Vedam. 2024. Perinatal mood and anxiety disorder and reproductive justice: Examining unmet needs for mental health and social services in a national cohort. *Health Equity* 8(1):3–13.

Terlizzi, E. P., and M. A. Villarroel. 2020. Symptoms of generalized anxiety disorder among adults: United States, 2019. *NCHS Data Brief* (378):1–8.

Tillmanns, T., A. Masri, C. Stewart, D. Chase, A. Karnezis, L.-m. Chen, and R. Urban. 2024. Advanced endometrial cancer—the next generation of treatment: A Society of Gynecologic Oncology Journal Club clinical commentary. *Gynecologic Oncology Reports* 55:101462.

Tipton, P., N. Bülbül, J. Crook, Z. Quicksall, O. Ross, R. Uitti, Z. Wszolek, and N. Ertekin-Taner. 2021. Effects of sex and APOE on Parkinson's disease-related cognitive decline. *Neurologia i Neurochirurgia Polska* 55(6):559–566.

Towner, M., J. J. Kim, M. A. Simon, D. Matei, and D. Roque. 2022. Disparities in gynecologic cancer incidence, treatment, and survival: A narrative review of outcomes among Black and White women in the United States. *International Journal of Gynecological Cancer* 32(7):931–938.

Trost, S., J. Beauregard, G. Chandra, F. Njie, J. Berry, A. Harvey, and D. A. Goodman. 2022. *Pregnancy-related deaths: Data from maternal mortality review committees in 36 U.S. states, 2017–2019.* Atlanta, GA: Centers for Disease Control and Prevention.

Tsao, C. W., A. W. Aday, Z. I. Almarzooq, C. A. M. Anderson, P. Arora, C. L. Avery, C. M. Baker-Smith, A. Z. Beaton, A. K. Boehme, A. E. Buxton, Y. Commodore-Mensah, M. S. V. Elkind, K. R. Evenson, C. Eze-Nliam, S. Fugar, G. Generoso, D. G. Heard, S. Hiremath, J. E. Ho, R. Kalani, D. S. Kazi, D. Ko, D. A. Levine, J. Liu, J. Ma, J. W. Magnani, E. D. Michos, M. E. Mussolino, S. D. Navaneethan, N. I. Parikh, R. Poudel, M. Rezk-Hanna, G. A. Roth, N. S. Shah, M. P. St-Onge, E. L. Thacker, S. S. Virani, J. H. Voeks, N. Y. Wang, N. D. Wong, S. S. Wong, K. Yaffe, and S. S. Martin. 2023. Heart disease and stroke statistics—2023 update: A report from the American Heart Association. *Circulation* 147(8):e93–e621.

U.K. Health Security Agency. 2015. *GBD Compare: A New Data Tool for Professionals.* https://ukhsa.blog.gov.uk/2015/09/15/gbd-compare-a-new-data-tool-for-professionals/ (accessed August 13, 2024).

Ulm, M., A. V. Ramesh, K. M. McNamara, S. Ponnusamy, H. Sasano, and R. Narayanan. 2019. Therapeutic advances in hormone-dependent cancers: Focus on prostate, breast and ovarian cancers. *Endocrine Connections* 8(2):R10–R26.

USPSTF (U.S. Preventive Services Task Force). 2024. Screening for breast cancer: U.S. Preventive Services Task Force recommendation statement. *JAMA* 331(22):1918–1930.

van den Akker, T., M. Nair, M. Goedhart, J. Schutte, T. Schaap, and M. Knight. 2017. Maternal mortality: Direct or indirect has become irrelevant. *Lancet Global Health* 5(12):e1181.

Vigo, D., L. Jones, R. Atun, and G. Thornicroft. 2022. The true global disease burden of mental illness: Still elusive. *Lancet Psychiatry* 9(2):98–100.

Vilda, D., M. E. Wallace, C. Daniel, M. G. Evans, C. Stoecker, and K. P. Theall. 2021. State abortion policies and maternal death in the United States, 2015–2018. *American Journal of Public Health* 111(9):1696–1704.

Vitaliano, P. P. 2010. An ironic tragedy: Are spouses of persons with dementia at higher risk for dementia than spouses of persons without dementia? *Journal of the American Geriatrics Society* 58(5):976–978.

Vogel, B., M. Acevedo, Y. Appelman, C. N. Bairey Merz, A. Chieffo, G. A. Figtree, M. Guerrero, V. Kunadian, C. S. P. Lam, A. Maas, A. S. Mihailidou, A. Olszanecka, J. E. Poole, C. Saldarriaga, J. Saw, L. Zühlke, and R. Mehran. 2021. The Lancet Women and Cardiovascular Disease Commission: Reducing the global burden by 2030. *Lancet* 397(10292):2385–2438.

Wariso, B. A., G. M. Guerrieri, K. Thompson, D. E. Koziol, N. Haq, P. E. Martinez, D. R. Rubinow, and P. J. Schmidt. 2017. Depression during the menopause transition: Impact on quality of life, social adjustment, and disability. *Archive of Women's Mental Health* 20(2):273–282.

Weiner, S. 2022. *How the Repeal of Roe v. Wade Will Affect Training in Abortion and Reproductive Health.* https://www.aamc.org/news/how-repeal-roe-v-wade-will-affect-training-abortion-and-reproductive-health (accessed August 15, 2024).

Whetstone, S., W. Burke, S. S. Sheth, R. Brooks, A. Cavens, K. Huber-Keener, D. M. Scott, B. Worly, and D. Chelmow. 2022. Health disparities in uterine cancer: Report from the Uterine Cancer Evidence Review Conference. *Obstetrics & Gynecology* 139(4):645–659.

Whiteley, J., M. DiBonaventura, J. S. Wagner, J. Alvir, and S. Shah. 2013. The impact of menopausal symptoms on quality of life, productivity, and economic outcomes. *Journal of Women's Health* 22(11):983–990.

WHO (World Health Organization). n.d. *Maternal Deaths.* https://www.who.int/data/gho/indicator-metadata-registry/imr-details/ (accessed August 14, 2024).

Wolfova, K., Z. Csajbok, A. Kagstrom, I. Kåreholt, and P. Cermakova. 2021. Role of sex in the association between childhood socioeconomic position and cognitive ageing in later life. *Scientific Reports* 11(1):4647.

Woods, N. F., and E. S. Mitchell. 2005. Symptoms during the perimenopause: Prevalence, severity, trajectory, and significance in women's lives. *American Journal of Medicine* 118(12, Suppl 2):14–24.

Wu, P., M. Gulati, C. S. Kwok, C. W. Wong, A. Narain, S. O'Brien, C. A. Chew-Graham, G. Verma, U. T. Kadam, and M. A. Mamas. 2018. Preterm delivery and future risk of maternal cardiovascular disease: A systematic review and meta-analysis. *Journal of the American Heart Association* 7(2).

Yaffe, K., A. M. Laffan, S. L. Harrison, S. Redline, A. P. Spira, K. E. Ensrud, S. Ancoli-Israel, and K. L. Stone. 2011. Sleep-disordered breathing, hypoxia, and risk of mild cognitive impairment and dementia in older women. *JAMA* 306(6):613–619.

Yamada, H., M. Deguchi, S. Saito, T. Takeshita, M. Mitsui, T. Saito, T. Nagamatsu, K. Takakuwa, M. Nakatsuka, S. Yoneda, K. Egashira, M. Tachibana, K. Matsubara, R. Honda, A. Fukui, K. Tanaka, K. Sengoku, T. Endo, and H. Yata. 2022. Intravenous immunoglobulin treatment in women with four or more recurrent pregnancy losses: A double-blind, randomised, placebo-controlled trial. *eClinicalMedicine* 50.

Ye, W., C. Luo, J. Huang, C. Li, Z. Liu, and F. Liu. 2022. Gestational diabetes mellitus and adverse pregnancy outcomes: Systematic review and meta-analysis. *BMJ* 377:e067946.

Young, S. 2024. *Endometriosis Research: Barriers to Progress. Presentation to the NASEM Committee on the Assessment of NIH Research on Women's Health, Meeting 2 (March 7, 2024).* https://www.nationalacademies.org/documents/embed/link/LF2255DA3DD1C 41C0A42D3BEF0989ACAECE3053A6A9B/file/D88A63BB015C48DB61FD1575954A5 9AE902C6A858D9C?noSaveAs=1 (accessed August 14, 2024).

Zhang, C., C. Zhang, Q. Wang, Z. Li, J. Lin, and H. Wang. 2020a. Differences in stage of cancer at diagnosis, treatment, and survival by race and ethnicity among leading cancer types. *JAMA Network Open* 3(4):e202950.

Zhang, M., P. Wan, K. Ng, K. Singh, T. H. Cheng, I. Velickovic, M. Dalloul, and D. Wlody. 2020b. Preeclampsia among African American pregnant women: An update on prevalence, complications, etiology, and biomarkers. *Obstetrical & Gynecological Survey* 75(2):111–120.

8

A Workforce to Advance
Women's Health Research

The committee's charge included providing recommendations to improve training and education efforts to build, support, and maintain a robust women's health research (WHR) workforce (i.e., researchers who undertake such research, not only women researchers) at the National Institutes of Health (NIH) and recommendations to achieve an NIH-wide workforce to effectively solicit, review, and support WHR. The committee was asked to look broadly at NIH's structure (extra- and intramural) systems and review processes within all domains, including workforce. The NIH intra- and extramural workforce is essential—without a properly trained and supported workforce, the nation cannot address the research needs and gaps highlighted in Chapters 2, 4, 5, 6 and 7. This chapter reviews some of NIH's programs, grants, and processes that affect the WHR workforce. For this report, the "workforce" includes extramural researchers who could or have applied for NIH funding and intramural staff at NIH: scientists and researchers who are part of the NIH Intramural Research Program (IRP), NIH program staff who oversee grants and programs, and other NIH staff, such as in the Center for Scientific Review, who organize, review, and administer peer review. The committee focused on the extramural research workforce and needed support, as that is where NIH spends the majority of its research dollars and where data are available to assess. However, the committee recognizes that the entire NIH workforce has a critical role in shaping the WHR workforce nationally.

EXTRAMURAL WORKFORCE

To ensure a diverse workforce, including those with expertise in women's health and sex differences research, workforce development grants are essential to support researchers' development and ability to continue to progress in their research in a given field (see Figure 8-1 for trends of funded career development grants). The role of NIH in workforce development is crucial as the primary funder of biomedical research in the United States; it is essential to ensure these funds are allocated to maximize their effect on research discoveries and researchers have the needed experiences, training, and expertise from high school forward.

NIH provides a range of grants to extramural researchers that vary by career stage, focus, length, funding level, and mechanism. Not all NIH Institutes and Centers (ICs) offer all grant types, and the number they award varies over time (see Table 8-1 for types of workforce support/development grants). When looking at all grants, including for career development, NIH awards over 58,000 extramural grants each year, representing nearly 83 percent of its budget, that directly support more than 300,000

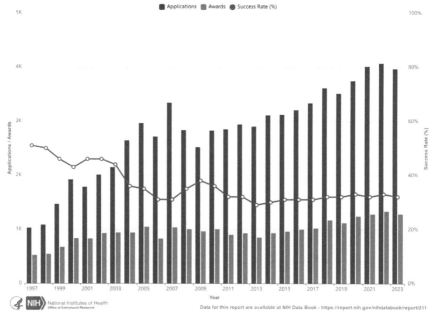

FIGURE 8-1 Research career development awards: Competing applications, awards, and success rates.
SOURCE: NIH, 2024i.

TABLE 8–1 Categories for Fellowship, Training, and Training Center Grants

Types of NIH Grants		
Activity Code	Purpose	
Fellowships, Training, Training Centers		
F	Fellowship Programs	Fellowships provide individual research training opportunities (including international) for those at the undergraduate, graduate, and postdoctoral levels.
K	Research Career Development Programs	Research Career Development awards provide individual and institutional research training opportunities (including international) to those at the undergraduate, graduate, and postdoctoral levels.
T	Institutional Training Programs	Institutional Training awards enable institutions to provide individual research training opportunities (including international) for those at the undergraduate, graduate, and postdoctoral levels.

SOURCES: Data from NIH, 2017a,b,c.
NOTES: Specific grant awards and programs in other grant mechanisms also support workforce development, such as some D (Institutional Training and Director Program Projects), R (Research Projects), and supplemental grant awards. More information on these grants is available at https://researchtraining.nih.gov/ (accessed August 5, 2024).

researchers at more than 2,700 different institutions (Lauer, 2024; NIH, 2023a, 2024a). Who can obtain these grants depends heavily on their understanding of the NIH application process, expertise in research, support offered by their home institution, and time available to apply. Whom NIH funds also depends on the priorities of the IC to which the researcher is applying—topics that do not align with an IC's priorities or purview are less likely to be funded by it. As previous chapters noted, this is problematic because many women's health conditions do not align with the purview or priorities of ICs, leaving such researchers with fewer funding opportunities.

Based on the committee's funding analysis (see Chapter 4 and Appendix A), from 2013 to 2023, extramural funding on WHR was predominantly research project grants (R series). Workforce training and development grants that focused on WHR had a low level of funding. Across ICs 2013–2023, $1.01 billion (3.05 percent) was spent on career development (K series), $0.16 billion (0.49 percent) on fellowships (F series), and $0.12 billion (0.37 percent) on training grants for WHR; the *Eunice Kennedy Shriver* National Institute of Child Health and Human Development (NICHD) invested the most on career development grants, followed by the National Cancer Institute (NCI) and the Office of the Director (OD). For training grants, NICHD invested the most, followed by NCI and the

National Institute of Allergy and Infectious Diseases (NIAID). NCI invested the most in fellowships, followed by NICHD and the National Institute on Mental Health (NIMH).

Whom Does NIH Fund?

This section briefly summarizes the makeup of the NIH extramural workforce by sex, race, and ethnicity as reported by NIH (see later in this chapter for an overview of the intramural workforce). Trends of NIH grant funding can serve as one indicator of the level of support for WHR, including support of investigators from minoritized populations. Ensuring a diverse pool of funded researchers across sex, race, ethnicity, and other demographic characteristics can lead to a broader range of perspectives and innovative approaches in research, including for WHR. When available, data at the intersection of gender/sex and race and ethnicity are reported.

Distribution of Grantees by Sex

NIH tracks the sex but not the gender identity of extramural research-ers receiving grants. For fiscal year (FY) 2016–2022, female principal inves-tigators (PIs) supported by R01-equivalent grants[1] increased from 29.4 to 34.0 percent. This represents an average annual increase of about 0.8 per-centage points (see Figure 8-2) (ORWH, 2023).

For all research project grants (RPGs), the proportion of female PIs grew from 30.8 percent in 2016 to 36.2 percent in 2022, with an average annual increase of 0.9 percentage points (ORWH, 2023), and the percent-age of female PIs on R01-equivalent grants who identified as non-Hispanic White decreased from 70.6 percent to 63.0 percent, with a rise in the percentage of female PIs from Asian, Hispanic, Black, and other racial and ethnic groups. The NIH Office of Research on Women's Health (ORWH) reported that during that FY 2016–FY 2022 period, 32 percent of PIs sup-ported on research career, other research, and RPG awards were female and 31 percent or fewer were supported by center grants, Small Business Innovation Research grants, and Small Business Technology Transfer awards (ORWH, 2023). In FY 2021, women made up 60 percent of the postdoc-toral institutional trainees, up from 56 percent in FY 2020 and 2022. Female postdoctoral fellows increased from 50 percent in FY 2020 to 57 percent in FY 2021 but then dropped slightly to 55 percent in FY 2022. Female predoctoral trainees decreased from 58 percent in FY 2020 to 53 percent in FY 2021 before rising again to 61 percent in FY 2022 (ORWH, 2023).

---

[1] The Research Project (R01) grant is an award to support a discrete, specified, circumscribed project to be performed by the investigator(s) in an area representing their specific interest and competencies, based on NIH's mission.

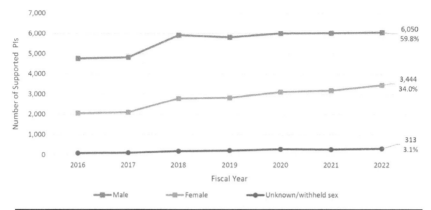

Year	Female	Male	Unknown/withheld sex
2016	2057	4765	93
2017	2097	4818	109
2018	2789	5913	189
2019	2825	5811	222
2020	3112	6007	288
2021	3180	6021	278
2022	3444	6050	313

FIGURE 8-2 Supported principal investigators (PIs) on R01 equivalent grants by sex and fiscal year.
NOTES: Data were drawn from the frozen Success Rate Demographic file on February 14, 2023. Data were produced by the Division of Statistical Analysis and Reporting within the National Institutes of Health (NIH) Office of Extramural Research's Office of Research Reporting and Analysis. Percentages do not add up to 100 percent because of rounding. R0-1-equivelent grants are defined in Annex B of the original source. Data on sex profiles are maintained by the investigator in the NIH Electronic Research Administration (eRA) system and are subject to change. Data include direct budget authority only and include all competing applications.
SOURCE: ORWH, 2023.

Since FY 2016, female PIs accounted for 50 percent or more of those receiving research career and training awards, and in FY 2022, they had funding rates comparable to male PIs (see Figure 8-3). However, for R01-equivalent grants between FY 2016 and FY 2022, female PIs represented 31–34 percent of applicants and 29–34 percent of recipients. In FY 2022, female PIs constituted 48 percent of early-stage R01-equivalent grant recipients (ORWH, 2023) and received about the same or higher funding amounts for R01-equivalents 2016 to 2022. Male PIs generally receive higher average funding overall than their female counterparts and are more likely to receive certain types of grants, such as center grants. While funding rates for female PIs from minoritized backgrounds have improved since FY 2016, these populations are still funded at lower rates than non-Hispanic White female PIs (ORWH, 2023).

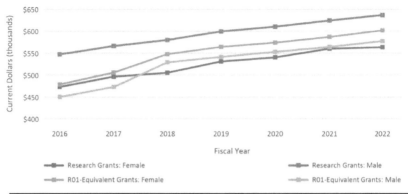

Year	Research Grants: Female	Research Grants: Male	R01 Equivalent Grants: Female	R01 Equivalent Grants: Male
2016	$472,889	$547,136	$478,624	$450,130
2017	$496,360	$566,037	$505,649	$472,930
2018	$505,271	$579,673	$547,492	$528,776
2019	$530,694	$599,511	$564,094	$541,184
2020	$540,256	$610,479	$573,752	$552,810
2021	$560,238	$624,339	$586,746	$564,186
2022	$563,386	$636,889	$601,771	$577,139

FIGURE 8-3 National Institutes of Health (NIH) research grants and R01-equivalent grants: Average funding in current dollars by sex of the supported principal investigator and fiscal year.
NOTES: Data from NIH IMPAC Pub File. Data were produced by the Division of Statistical Analysis and Reporting within the NIH Office of Extramural Research's Office of Research Reporting and Analysis and drawn on December 16, 2022. Each data point reflects only current dollars and is not adjusted for inflation. R01-equivelent grants are defined in Annex B of the original source. Research grants are defined as extramural awards made for research centers, research projects, Small Business Innovation Research/Small Business Technology Transfer program grants, and other research grants. Research grants are defines by the following activity codes: R, P, M, S, K, U (excluding UC6), DP1, DP2, DP3, DP4, DP5, DP42, and G12. Analysis is restricted to Principle Investigators who reported their sex. Data on sex profiles are maintained by the investigator in the NIH eRA system and are subject to change.
SOURCE: ORWH, 2023.

Race and Ethnicity

A 2011 review of grants awarded over a 7-year period revealed that, for independent research grants, applications from White PIs were 1.7 times more likely to be funded than those from Black PIs (Ginther et al., 2011). A 2019 follow-up study showed no change (Hoppe et al., 2019) and that the decision to discuss applications at a study section and the impact score combined accounted for 42 percent of gap in funding, with the proposed research topic accounting for 20 percent. A 2018 analysis found that factors related to higher success rates in general, such as being a full professor or

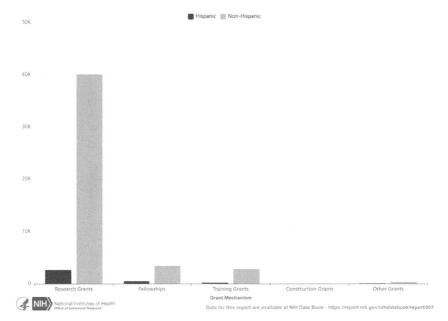

FIGURE 8-4 Number of National Institutes of Health (NIH) principal investigators funded by grant mechanism and ethnicity, 2023.
SOURCE: NIH, 2024e.

publishing with coauthors who publish in the upper quartile of their fields, did not close the funding gap (Ginther et al., 2018). See Figures 8-4 and 8-5 for funding by race and ethnicity for NIH grants.

A 2018 Government Accountability Office (GAO) study also found disparities for underrepresented racial and ethnic groups and female investigators from 2013 through 2017 (GAO, 2018). In 2017, about 17 percent of Black, American Indian and Alaska Native (AIAN), and Native Hawaiian and Pacific Islander (NHPI) applicants combined for large grants received them, compared to approximately 24 percent of Hispanic or Latino, 24 percent of Asian, and 27 percent of White applicants. The GAO report concluded that "NIH has taken positive steps such as establishing the position of Chief Officer of Scientific Workforce Diversity, who in turn created a strategic workforce diversity plan, which applies to both extramural and intramural investigators. The plan includes five broad goals for expanding and supporting these investigators. However, NIH has not developed quantitative metrics, evaluation details, or specific time frames by which it could measure the agency's progress against these goals" (GAO, 2018).

NIH has developed programs and initiatives to close these gaps and is making some progress (NIH, 2022b, 2024b, n.d.-d). In July 2024, NIH published a report on mentored career development application (K award)

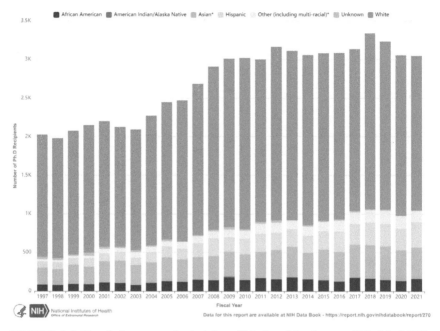

FIGURE 8-5 Trends in race and ethnicity of National Institutes of Health (NIH)-supported Ph.D. recipients, 1997–2021.
NOTES: From 1982 to 2000, the racial categories used in the Survey of Earned Doctorates included "Asian and Pacific Islander." In 2001, the survey was revised, and "Asian" and "Native Hawaiian or other Pacific Islander" became separate categories. For the purposes of reporting, Native Hawaiians are included in the "Other" category.
SOURCE: NIH, 2023c.

funding rates[2] (Figures 8-6 and 8-7) (Lauer and Roychowdhury, 2024). For scientists designated as a PI on at least one K application submitted in FY 2011 and FY 2023, Black applicants in FY 2023 were more likely to submit a K01 application and less likely to submit K08 or K23 applications compared to White applicants. Black applicants were more likely to submit proposals including human participants and less likely to submit proposals including animal models (Lauer and Roychowdhury, 2024).[3] This analysis

---

[2] Data include K01, K08, K23, K25, and K99 career development awards. Some ICs use the K01 mechanism to enhance workforce diversity.

[3] A separate analysis by NIH showed that Black applicants were more likely to be associated with topics such as health disparities, disease prevention and intervention, socioeconomic factors, health care, lifestyle, psychosocial, adolescent, and risk and that, in general, applications using those terms were less likely to be funded than topics such as neuron, corneal, cell, and iron (Hoppe et al., 2019).

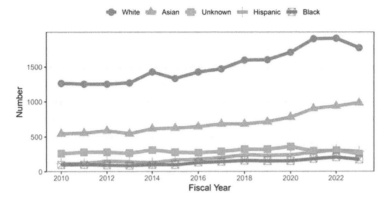

FIGURE 8-6 K applicants according to race and ethnicity by fiscal year.
SOURCE: Lauer and Roychowdhury, 2024.

did not include data on NHPI and AIAN researchers, likely the result of the larger problem of AIAN and NHPI researchers being underrepresented in NIH grants.

These data show applicants and funding rates from underrepresented groups trending upward. However, AIAN and NHPI researchers are not visible in NIH data reporting of grant funding for almost all years (NIH, 2022c). This is also the case when looking at the funding mechanisms and who is funded by race and ethnicity, including research grants, training grants, and fellowships. Overall, while the race and ethnicity gaps in funding are beginning to narrow, significant gaps for certain groups persist.

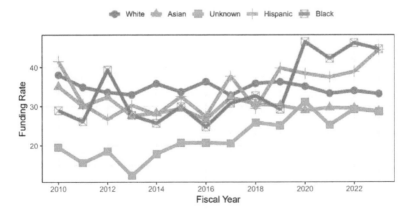

FIGURE 8-7 Funding rates for K applicants according to race and ethnicity by fiscal year.
SOURCE: Lauer and Roychowdhury, 2024.

Summary of Whom NIH Funds

Unfortunately, data on racial and ethnic trends in funding among women are not readily available on the NIH dashboard. Such data would indicate whether there are multiplicative effects of being a woman and racially minoritized in the NIH workforce. However, given research on the scientific workforce and trends in the general workforce, it would be expected that AIAN and Black women in particular are funded at lower rates than White women (Kaiser, 2023; Malcom et al., 1976; Nguyen et al., 2023). Furthermore, the data do not indicate any information on transgender or nonbinary identities among investigators, and the measurement of sex is inadequate to assess gender.

NIH EXTRAMURAL GRANTS TO DEVELOP AND SUPPORT WHR WORKFORCE

In this section, the committee reviews some career development grants awarded by NIH and how they affect the initiation and sustainability of research careers. This section also reviews workforce development and support programs for the NIH extramural workforce that specifically focus on women or on sex differences (see Table 8-2). It was beyond the scope of this report to review all NIH programs that could potentially impact the WHR workforce.

TABLE 8-2 National Institutes of Health (NIH) Extramural Workforce Programs Focusing on Women's and/or Sex Differences Research Reviewed

Program	Target Population	Type of Award	Duration*
Building Interdisciplinary Research Careers in Women's Health (BIRCWH)	Early-career faculty who have recently completed clinical training or postdoctoral fellowship and plan to conduct interdisciplinary basic, translational, behavioral, clinical, and/or health-services research relevant to women's health	K12, Internal K	Up to 5 years
Women's Reproductive Health Research (WRHR)	Obstetrician-gynecologists who recently completed postgraduate clinical instruction	K12	5 years
Reproductive Scientist Development Program (RSDP)	Early-career physician-scientists	K12	Up to 5 years
Specialized Centers of Research Excellence (SCORE) on Sex Differences	Any individual(s) with the skills, knowledge, and resources necessary to carry out the research	U54	5 years

NOTE: * Duration based on the most recent NIH Request for Proposal for each program.
SOURCES: Data from HHS, 2018; NICHD, 2023b; NIH, 2022d,e, 2024f,g.

Research Career Development Awards (K)

I am fortunate to have experienced over a decade some kind of support from the NIH and it would not have been possible without a K award. I see far too many capable junior researchers fall away because of the lack of time to really pursue important research questions and because the clinical mission is what is emphasized.
—Participant at committee information-gathering meeting

External Research Career Development Program K awards are available to early-career researchers to apply for mentored research projects. They support and protect time for faculty to develop research skills and ultimately ensure a pool of highly trained research scientists and enable scientists with diverse backgrounds to enhance their careers in biomedical research and provide support for senior postdoctoral fellows or faculty-level candidates. Individual ICs fund K awards for up to 5 years, and the specific terms vary, particularly regarding salary limitations. K awards fall into three categories (see Appendix B for examples):

1. Mentored awards to individuals are intended primarily for researchers at the beginning of their careers and provide a transition to full independent research awards.
2. Independent or nonmentored awards provide protected research time for midcareer or even senior faculty to enhance their research potential.
3. Institutional awards provide mentored experiences for multiple individuals.

The objective of K awards is to provide candidates with the experience and support needed to be able to conduct their research independently and be ready to compete for major grant support. These are traditional mentored research awards, and applicants are judged on their ability to perform research and publish, the mentor's ability to advance the careers of their mentees, and their institutional support. External K awards are the mechanism for most Building Interdisciplinary Research Careers in Women's Health (BIRCWH) awardees (see later in the chapter for more information) to progress in developing into independent researchers. However, not all K awardees continue to conduct research after their award ends (Jagsi et al., 2017). The reasons for this attrition for M.D.s and Ph.D.s are multifaceted but center around the need for higher income for researchers to pay off large training debts, lack of a tenure or other funded position at their home or other research institutions, inability to become independent from their mentors (e.g., acquisition of R01 or R01 equivalent), and caregiving responsibilities (Bates et al., 2023; Jagsi et al., 2017). This is an especially salient issue in women's health and sex differences research. However, some WHR-focused workforce programs demonstrated greater success in retaining clinician-researchers (see later in this chapter for more information).

A shortcoming of the mentored K awards is that there is no direct financial support for the mentor, limiting their ability to guide their mentees. In addition, support for K awardee salaries is capped at $100,000 per year, which is often not sufficient for physicians to juggle debt repayment and the cost of living near most academic medical centers (NIH, 2019, 2024j). After 5 years of K funding, some awardees may not be ready to launch an independent research program with R awards, with no clear mechanisms to obtain supplemental funding to extend the mentored training period to achieve independent funding.

This section discusses three K award workforce development programs that support WHR. All are either administered by or offered in coordination with ORWH.

BIRCWH

Through a partnership among ORWH and other Institutes, Centers, and Offices (ICOs), the BIRCWH career development K12 program was established in 2000 (ORWH, n.d.-a). It focuses on training early-career faculty, the BIRCWH scholars, and provides them with the opportunity to develop research skills to investigate women's health and sex differences. The main goal is to provide early-career faculty with protected time to conduct research, write manuscripts, and obtain peer-reviewed funding to advance the understanding of this research (ORWH, n.d.-a). The program has played a significant role in launching the current generation of researchers who go on to become tenured professors and lead impactful research on women's health and sex differences nationwide (Berge et al., 2022; Choo et al., 2020; Nagel et al., 2013). In turn, those researchers will acquire the expertise to train new researchers.

A key component of the program is mentorship by senior faculty who share interests in women's health and sex and gender differences and have obtained peer-reviewed funding (NIH R01s or an equivalent). The program supports scholars in interdisciplinary basic, translational, behavioral, clinical, and health services research on these topics. Individuals who have completed clinical training or a postdoctoral fellowship and are within 6 years of their terminal degrees or have not had protected time to research since that degree are eligible; they will plan and conduct relevant research within their discipline.

Since its inception in 2000, over 750 BIRCWH scholars have received career development training (ORWH, n.d.-a). ORWH and its partner ICs provide over $15 million per year to the 19 active BIRCWH programs (see

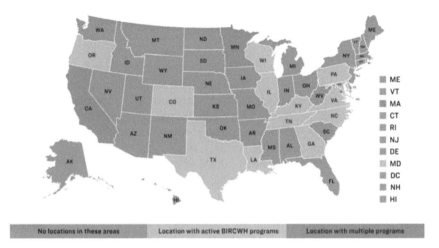

FIGURE 8-8 Locations of the 19 active Building Interdisciplinary Research Careers in Women's Health programs.
SOURCE: ORWH, n.d.-a.

Figure 8-8).[4] For example, the National Institute of Arthritis and Musculo-skeletal and Skin Diseases (NIAMS) and National Institute on Drug Abuse provide grant management for BIRCWH awards (ORWH, n.d.-a).[5]

BIRCWH has focused on supporting early-career faculty, typically newly appointed assistant professors. Initially, it provided support for four scholars at each program site. Over time, the program budget has changed, resulting in a reduction or addition of the number of scholars per site (NIH, 2020). Starting in FY 2023, the program expanded to include a postdoctoral fellow (clinical degree, Ph.D., or comparable degree) or instructor-level faculty for each BIRCWH program for 1 additional year of support to obtain additional methodological training and conduct a mentored research project (HHS, 2024). The April 2024 funding announcement for renewal of the grants includes a budget in direct dollars (not including indirect costs) of $840,000 per program, which will fund up to five scholars each (HHS, 2024) This increase in sponsored scholars per program could have lasting impact on the size of the workforce of women's health researchers with

---

[4] For active 2024 BIRCWH programs, see https://orwh.od.nih.gov/our-work/building-interdisciplinary-research-careers-in-womens-health-bircwh/funded-programs-and-principal-investigators (accessed June 11, 2024).

[5] Past cosponsors include NICHD, NCI, the National Institute on Aging, the National Institute on Alcohol Abuse and Alcoholism, NIAID, the National Institute of Dental and Craniofacial Research (NIDCR), the National Institute of Environmental Health Sciences (NIEHS), NIMH, and the Office of AIDS Research.

the goal of improving women's health and understanding sex differences across the nation.

One unique aspect of this program is mentorship by a senior faculty member with experience in obtaining NIH or equivalent funding and expertise in mentoring early-career researchers. However, a significant shortcoming is that they receive no funds to cover their time and effort. In addition to the primary mentor, the BIRCWH program requires "mentoring teams" who provide career advice, additional research direction, and education about how to navigate early careers at research institutions. It also requires scholars to write career development plans that are reviewed by their mentors at least twice a year to ensure they are progressing and identify challenges that need to be addressed to advance their research and careers. Scholars across the sites are networked and work together through quarterly virtual meetings organized by ORWH and BIRCWH programs on issues related to career advancements. ORWH brings all scholars and program directors to the NIH campus each year for in-person career advancement education and scientific exchanges.

An important benefit of BIRCWH is that it educates researchers on how to integrate sex and gender differences into clinical research and connects scholars to national resources. A 2020 study found that 45 percent of BIRCWH institutions offered education on integration in clinical translational research; of those, 54 percent offered in-person training and 31 percent offered content within existing for-credit courses (Libby et al., 2020).

Individual programs have conducted their own assessments to identify best practices and program outcomes and an overall evaluation of the success of the BIRCWH scholars in obtaining funds or success in academic research. One program conducted an electronic survey and in-person discussions with BIRCWH program leaders and concluded that the programs have been highly successful; the most commonly cited factors associated with success were sufficient time for mentors and scholars to meet and the interdisciplinary and collaborative team mentoring approach (Guise et al., 2012). A 2017 study found that interdisciplinary teams helped BIRCWH scholars strengthen study designs, expand their research topics, and expose them to research areas in which they were not directly trained (Guise et al., 2017). Other benefits noted by scholars include opportunities to meet local and national investigators with whom they subsequently established research collaborations.

A 2017 review of BIRCWH found that mentoring plays a critical role in academic success. Fellows and faculty who are mentored are more likely to report greater job satisfaction, pursue and remain in an academic career, experience improvements in annual performance reviews, are more than two times more likely to be promoted to professor, and are two to three times more likely to become a PI on research grants. These outcomes underscore the importance of mentored grant programs to developing a WHR workforce. One study found that BIRCWH directors identified persistence and resilience and developing community, networks, and other support opportunities as elements of scholar success and noted the critical role of mentors (Choo et al., 2020). A 2022 review evaluated 16 BIRCWH scholars against a comparison group of 17 non-BIRCWH scholars for traditional bibliometric impact (Berge et al., 2022). This review found that BIRCWH scholars had significantly more publications from pre- to post-BIRCWH experience and accelerated network growth, interdisciplinary collaborations, international citations, and policy impact. Specifically, BIRCWH scholars had a 38 percent grant award success rate in comparison to the NIH overall early-stage investigator rate of 29 percent.

Another study reviewed the Minnesota BIRCWH program and showed that a rigorous evaluation plan can increase the effectiveness of a research career development plan (Raymond et al., 2018). This study demonstrated the importance of a formal research career development program and found that 28 of 29 BIRCWH programs incorporated structured evaluations of mentoring and training components.

In summary, the BIRCWH program has successfully trained a workforce of investigators in women's health and sex differences research. It provides protected time to perform research, write, and publish and oversight of scholars' work and career progression by both mentors in their disciplines and program directors. In addition, the annual meeting of scholars from all programs enables them to share research, build collaborations, and gain perspectives on future career directions. The recent increase from two to five scholars for each program is a sufficient size to form a supportive and cohesive group for feedback on grant ideas and career advice.

However, BIRCWH could be strengthened. Although many of the programs function as stepping-stones for scholars to obtain an external K award and give them more time to develop an independent research career, it does prolong training. While the mentors have a history of or current NIH funding, they do not receive salary support for their mentoring, and as most seasoned mentors are keenly aware, it can take over 10 percent effort to train a mentee to become a successful independent researcher. In addition, the institution receives only 8 percent indirect costs for the BIRCWH training grant, which can disincentivize it from adding the needed extra support for administering these grants (HHS, 2024).

To improve the effectiveness of the BIRCWH program to further grow women's health and sex differences research and the WHR workforce, NIH could consider expanding funding to allow mentors to be funded at 10 percent time to allow them time to be more effective and involved (i.e., an increased budget of approximately $100,000 per year for a mentoring component). Extending the term of support to up to 5 years per scholar—some have only 2–3 years—would increase their ability to obtain and analyze data, publish a paper, and have the necessary research portfolio to write and obtain an R01 or equivalent grant. NIH could consider designing a K99/R00 for BIRCWH scholars to allow them to develop an independent research program and stay at the same institution or be able to move to another. This would allow for a two-tier program in which the scholar would be mentored within the institution and then be eligible for a K99/R00 within the same institution and become independent. One additional consideration would be to develop a Request for Application exclusive for BIRCWH graduates for independent funding related to women's health and sex differences. This could be done through the NIH Foundation, which would allow for industry and philanthropy to partner with NIH in areas of women's research and sex differences that are poorly funded and in need of novel interventions. See Chapter 9 for recommendations in this area.

Women's Reproductive Health Research (WRHR) Career Development Program

The WRHR Career Development Program was launched in 1998 by NICHD with support from ORWH. It aims to enhance the research capabilities of newly trained obstetrician-gynecologists (OB/GYNs) (NIH, 1998, n.d.-b). It offers academic opportunities to receive state-of-the-art education and practical experience in women's reproductive health research, spanning basic science, translational, and clinical research (NICHD, 2023b). This includes providing obstetrics and gynecology departments with investigators specializing in women's reproductive health research.

Experienced investigators from well-established research programs offer an intellectual and technical base for mentoring WRHR scholars, addressing a wide range of basic and applied biomedical and biobehavioral sciences in obstetrics, gynecology, and partnering departments. The program sites for 2020–2025 include the University of North Carolina, Chapel Hill, Baylor College of Medicine and Texas Children's Hospital, University of Colorado, Duke University, Johns Hopkins University, Oregon Health & Science University, University of Pennsylvania, Stanford University, Harvard University, University of California, San Diego, University of Utah, Northwestern University, University of California, San Francisco, University of Washington, and Yale University (NICHD, 2023b).

The Gynecologic Health and Disease Branch in NICHD funds WRHR as part of NICHD's K12 Institutional Career Development Program and is co-sponsored by ORWH, which supports local institutions that foster the development of OB/GYNs into independent research investigators (NIH, 2023d). WRHR covers the entire spectrum of obstetrics and gynecology research, including both general and specialized topics. Areas of focus include maternal and fetal medicine, gynecologic oncology, reproductive endocrinology and infertility, and female pelvic medicine and reconstructive surgery, along with related fields, such as perimenopausal management and adolescent gynecology. This is essential because the OB/GYN workforce is small, and even fewer are clinician-scientists (see later in this chapter for more information). Funding is approximately $315,000 in direct costs per center each year for a maximum of 5 years (NIH, 2024l).

In 1998, WRHR started with 12 programs, growing to 20 in 1999, with three scholar slots per program for a total of 60 slots nationally. However, in 2024, there are only 15 programs with two slots per program for a total of 30 slots nationally, as a result of decreased funding. Since its inception, 28 institutions have participated; departmental benefits include developing and expanding research programs and the number of physician investigators (Coutifaris, 2024). Benefits to scholars are dedicated time for research, networking, and exposure to NIH (Coutifaris, 2024). However, there are drawbacks because the investment of time in the program by scholars (75 percent) is more than what is financially covered by the grants. In addition, mentor time is not covered (Coutifaris, 2024).

One group evaluated the WRHR program and found that 40 percent of scholars received additional independent NIH funding. Moreover, the return on investment was substantial, with 25 and 13 percent of scholars receiving at least one R01 or two to five R01 grants, respectively (McCoy et al., 2023). In addition, 81 percent continue to hold an academic position, with 75 percent achieving leadership in departmental or institutional positions, including vice chair (20 percent), chair (9 percent), or dean (3 percent). Fifty-two percent had participated in a NIH study section. The authors concluded that "the infrastructure provided by an institutional K award is an advantageous career development award mechanism for obstetrician-gynecologists," who are predominantly women surgeons and noted that it "may serve as a corrective [program] for the known inequities in NIH funding by gender" (McCoy et al., 2023, p. 425.e1).

There are several opportunities to improve WRHR. For example, NICHD could allow flexibility for the percent of effort K awardees allocate to research (as some ICs do). Since OB/GYN is a surgical specialty that has a multistage certification process and examinations for 3–5 years after training, it is reasonable to consider flexibility in assigning the time dedicated to research effort. In addition, depending on the career path of the scholar (laboratory focused vs. clinical research focused), such flexibility would be advantageous for the overall development of their academic career. For example, developing laboratory researchers who have had no or minimal experience at the bench would likely need 75–100 percent dedicated time for research at the beginning. However, an M.D./Ph.D. starting out their faculty years as laboratory investigators may be equally successful with 50–75 percent time. Allowing such flexibility (50–100 percent protected time for research, with the ability to change the percent during the program) based on the candidates' qualifications, past experience in research, and lines of investigation being pursued could be beneficial for career development of surgeon-scientists.

Because the WRHR career development slots have been decreased by 50 percent since the program's inception, it would be beneficial for the development of the WHR workforce to earmark a certain number of individual K awards for research focused on women's health (with some being specifically earmarked for OB/GYNs).

Reproductive Scientist Development Program (RSDP)

RSDP, launched in 1988, is a national K12 career development program aimed at developing a "cadre of reproductive physician-scientists based in academic departments who could employ cutting-edge cell and molecular technologies to address important problems in the field of obstetrics and gynecology" and training physician-scientists with a particular emphasis on developing basic science skills (NICHD, 2023a). Early-career faculty receive mentored research opportunities to advance as independent physician-scientists.

RSDP is primarily funded by NICHD's Fertility and Infertility Branch, with nongovernmental organizations and corporations offering additional support.[6] It is administered centrally through the PI's home institution and grants individual awards to scholars throughout the United States and Canada (Lo et al., 2023). RSDP scholars study a broad array of reproductive science topics, such as the molecular mechanisms of preeclampsia, transposons and piwi-interacting RNA and their roles in gynecological health and disease, and epigenetics mechanisms involved in the prenatal origins of age-related disease (NICHD, 2023a).

The program historically accepted approximately two to three scholars each year for a 5-year training period (Lo et al., 2023; Schust, 2024). During the first 2–3 years, scholars receive intensive basic science training at a research laboratory while under the supervision of experienced mentors. Scholars then spend an additional 2 years establishing their research programs as early-career faculty in an OB/GYN department, with 75 percent of their time in the laboratory as they return to their sponsoring clinical department duties (Lo et al., 2023; NICHD, 2023a). In 2023, the program

---

[6] American College of Obstetricians and Gynecologists, American Society for Reproductive Medicine, American Board of Obstetrics and Gynecology, Bayer HealthCare, Burroughs Wellcome Fund, March of Dimes Birth Defects Foundation, National Cancer Institute, Ovarian Cancer Research Fund, Inc., and Society for Gynecologic Investigation (NICHD, 2023a).

was reduced from 100 percent protected time during the first 2–3 years and 75 percent for the remainder of the program to 75 percent in both phases (Lo et al., 2023). The overall training program was reduced from 5 to 4 years (Schust, 2024).

The program receives an annual budget of $770,000 a year for seven scholars, with enough funding to cover the salaries of two new scholars for 4 out of 5 years and only one new scholar using NIH funds in 1 of the 4 years of the grant (Schust, 2024). Although the RSDP award states that the scholars will receive $25,000 per year for supplies and travel, no NIH funds in the grant are available to cover these costs (Lo et al., 2023; Schust, 2024). RSDP is meant to be a stepping-stone for a successful career as a physician-scientist and provides a salary and fringe support, research supply costs, protected research time, the ability work with accomplished researchers in biomedical research, potential collaborations for future projects, and continuous scientific and career support (Lo et al., 2023; Schust, 2024).

A 2023 study on RSDP provides data on scholars' academic achievements (Lo et al., 2023).[7] Seventy percent have remained active in academia and span from instructor (4 percent), assistant professor (19 percent), associate professor (21 percent), to full professor (25 percent), with many in leadership roles—academic director (32 percent), medical director (10 percent), department chair or vice chair (15 percent), and dean or associate dean or vice dean (3 percent). The study found that RSDP's unique two-phase structure has affected scholars' career development and highlights how programs like this are critical for maintaining a well-trained workforce of OB/GYN scientists, especially in light of that workforce diminishing and underinvestment in WHR (Lo et al., 2023). For example, compared to K08 and K23 recipients from other medical specialties, and OB/GYN K08 and K23 recipients, RSDP scholars had similar R01 success rates. In addition, the 8-year conversion time from RSDP K12 to an R01 was comparable to published rates for K08 and K23 (6 and 7 years, respectively) (Lo et al., 2023).

The Effect of NICHD K Awards

In addition to the program successes described, several authors have studied the success of K award programs. One group evaluated the outcomes for NICHD career development and training grant awardees from 1999 to 2001 and reported that M.D.s with individual K awards were more successful at achieving independent funding compared to those with institutional K12 support. M.D.s/Ph.D.s had no significant difference in subsequent funding whether they had an individual or institution career

---

[7] A 30-item survey was used to assess the demographics and career details of all current and former RSDP scholars.

development award (Twombly et al., 2018). Both the individual K and institutional K12 awards led to successful development of a cohort of research, with 75.2 percent who remained in academic medicine.

Another group also reported on recipients who received K08, K12, and K23 awards from 1988 to 2015 (Okeigwe et al., 2017). Their findings demonstrated that OB/GYN physician-scientists who received mentored early-career development K programs had a higher likelihood of receiving NIH independent research funding compared to nonrecipients. This study identified 388 K award recipients, including 66 percent women and 82 percent M.D.s. Over 80 percent were K12 awards, while 10 percent and 8 percent were K08 and K23, respectively, with 22 percent succeeding at obtaining an R01 between 1988 and 2009. There did not appear to be significant differences in sex, educational degree, or subspecialty and successful independent funding (Okeigwe et al., 2017).

These studies, along with those discussed regarding the BIRCWH, WRHR, and RSDP programs collectively, reveal the importance of NIH K awards in training a WHR workforce. While individual K awards may lead to higher success in NIH funding, the value of institutional K12 awards indicated high retention of the workforce in academia. NIH could improve these and similar K awards by increasing the duration of appointments to allow flexibility in effort, such as providing more protected time for bench and translational research and clinical and health services research. See later in this chapter for additional opportunities to address barriers to becoming a clinician-researcher.

Other Programs and Awards

Specialized Centers of Research Excellence (SCORE) on Sex Differences

SCORE programs focus on identifying the role of biological sex differences on women's health through research at multifaceted levels. SCORE is the sole NIH Center program dedicated to disease-agnostic research on sex differences (NIH, 2024h). It is a U54 grant mechanism managed by ORWH and a significant initiative aimed at understanding the role of biological sex differences in health outcomes. It serves as a national resource for translational research and promotes integrating sex as a biological variable in biomedical research. It is not limited to specific diseases but rather focuses broadly on sex differences across conditions affecting women (ORWH, n.d.-c).

SCORE was established in 2018, but before that, the Specialized Centers of Research P50 program funded scientists making contributions to sex differences research related to women's health from 2002 to 2017 (NIH, n.d.-w). SCORE established 12 new Centers: Los Angeles, CA (2 Centers), Denver,

CO, Rochester, MN, Atlanta, GA, Augusta, GA, Charleston, SC, Baltimore, MD, New Haven, CT, and Boston, MA (3 Centers), with investigators studying varied topics, such as aging, cardiovascular disease, influenza, microbiome, fatty liver, inflammation, and stress (ORWH, n.d.-c).[8] Each SCORE Center receives $1.5 million a year in funding (NIH, 2022e).

The program implemented SCORE's Career Enhancement Core to train the next generation of sex difference researchers. It consists of financial resources for early-career and senior faculty, educational curricula for graduate and medical students, standards for researching sex differences, and state-of-the-art research methodologies, along with pilot projects and complementary training programs (HHS, 2018). Each SCORE Center acts as a national hub for research on sex and gender, facilitating collaboration among researchers from academia, private industry, and federal settings. This collaborative environment enhances the program's ability to address complex scientific questions.

The program has led to significant contributions in the field of sex differences research, influencing the development of new medical interventions and improving health outcomes for women (ORWH, n.d.-c). In 2023, the *Journal of Women's Health* published a special issue highlighting the program's work. The studies found that it has significantly advanced the field's understanding of how sex differences affect health and disease and highlighted how biological, physiological, and behavioral differences between men and women influence the prevalence, progression, and treatment outcomes of various diseases. The research has employed innovative methodologies to better capture and analyze sex differences, including nuanced experimental designs and analytical techniques that account for gender-specific variables (Agarwal et al., 2023; Bennett et al., 2023; Reue and Arnold, 2023).

SCORE programs allow for studying women's health and sex differences with more focus on individual research areas and for projects to mature to the point they are ready for R01 or equivalent funding. They also provide a community of researchers and trainees within the programs who come together and share their science annually. Their challenge is that they tend to be limited to a research focus that has funding support by individual ICs. Therefore, SCORE programs, like many program project grants, need individual IC support and buy-in while the application is being developed; if it receives a good score, it will be funded. It is likely that many investigators do not know this, limiting the SCORE grants on sex differences and

---

[8] Augusta University, Brigham and Women's Hospital, Cedars-Sinai Medical Center, Emory University, Johns Hopkins University, Massachusetts General Hospital/Harvard Medical School, Mayo Clinic, Medical University of South Carolina, University of California, Los Angeles, University of Colorado, and Yale University have SCORE programs.

women's health to the ICs that want to fund the applications. At this time, few ICs participate in the funding,[9] which constrains the breadth and depth of the research.

R35 Grants

Most programs and grant mechanisms described have focused on early- and midcareer researchers. R35s are one mechanism designed to better support more senior investigators. "The purpose is to promote scientific productivity and innovation by providing long-term support and increased flexibility to experienced [PIs]" and those "whose outstanding record of research demonstrate their ability to make major contributions" to the particular IC's mission (NIH, 2024d). The R35 is intended to support a research program, rather than a research project, by providing the primary source—and most likely the sole source—of funding for an investigator receiving an individual grant award (NIH, 2024d). The advantage over standard R01 grants is the amount and duration. For example, a standard R01 can be funded up to $500,000[10] in direct costs per year without asking permission from the IC. However, these grants are for 5 years at most. In contrast, the R35 provides up to $750,000 per year in direct costs for up to 7 years (length varies by IC), allowing investigators more freedom to perform experiments that might be hypothesis generating and conduct follow-up studies based on data generated in prior research.[11] Only select ICs offer R35s.

Recently, Congress mandated greater funding for Type 1 diabetes research to make breakthroughs in both the biology and treatments to improve the outcomes of this chronic debilitating disease (NIDDK, 2024). The investigators have been allotted $250 million annually. This mechanism could be used as a model to catalyze women's health and sex differences research and allow for rapid discoveries at both the laboratory and the clinic in areas that desperately need funding and attention. Research funded by such a mechanism could, for example, study the changes in activity levels controlled by estrogen in the hypothalamus that may reduce dementia in women. The R35 mechanism could also be used to provide foundation funding for interdisciplinary groups that study the biology and treatments of endometriosis. Since R35s provide 7 years of continuous funding,

---

[9] The following ICs support one or more SCORE programs: NIA (6 centers), National Institute on Alcohol Abuse and Alcoholism (1 center), National Institute of Diabetes and Digestive and Kidney Diseases (1 center), National Institute on Drug Abuse (1 center), National Heart, Lung, and Blood Institute (NHLBI; 2 centers), and NIMH (1 center) (NIH, n.d.-w).

[10] See, for example, https://www.nhlbi.nih.gov/grants-and-training/policies-and-guidelines/applications-with-direct-costs-of-500000-or-more-in-any-one-year (accessed October 22, 2024).

[11] See, for example, https://www.aamc.org/news/nih-funds-more-long-term-grants (accessed October 22, 2024).

investigators can take the time needed to study the underlying mechanisms in depth and translate the findings to the clinic.

A senior NIH-funded investigator can obtain funding for their grants for up to 5 years via other grant mechanisms. Grant renewal efforts need to start after 3 years of funding to allow time for peer review. In addition, only about 20 percent of all R grants are funded (Lauer, 2024), making it a competitive climate. For these reasons, it often takes approximately 3 years for a senior investigator to obtain funding for a new R01 grant. A 7-year grant would allow them to make foundational observations, publish their work, and inform clinicians about both the biology of and best treatments for ailments that affect women or have sex differences in presentation or outcomes. In summary, IC support of R35 grants for specific investigators who are experienced and can undertake research to address important women's health questions could be an effective mechanism to increase and support those studying women's health and sex differences and make significant breakthroughs.

Reentry and Retention of Women's Health Researchers

A large number of trained women's health and sex differences researchers, particularly those who are female, need to leave their field or scale back research because of other demands, both career and external, that prevent them from finishing current projects (NASEM, 2024c). This includes pregnancy and the number and timing of children as a particular point of inflection in women's careers in submitting applications and funding applications. These factors prevent them from being competitive for peer-reviewed funding from NIH or other peer-reviewed grant applications. Lack of policies that support informal caregiving and eldercare also have a negative effect on the physician workforce conducting WHR. A recent study found that among midcareer, full-time medical school faculty aged 55+, 22 percent of women and 17 percent of men were caregivers, and 90 percent of them were experiencing mental or emotional strain from those responsibilities (Skarupski et al., 2021). In another study, women faculty were 2.5 times more likely to be caregivers than men, as were older compared to younger faculty (Rennels et al., 2024). Among physicians who were mothers, those with additional informal caregiving responsibilities experience more burnout and mental health concerns than those without (Yank et al., 2019). Without investment in policies, programs, and resources to support women faculty engaged in informal caregiving, women academicians in WHR and clinical care delivery are at risk of leaving the workforce, further impeding progress in women's health equity. Data on researchers who leave the workforce due to caregiving responsibilities and on reentry are important to collect to assess impact on the careers of the NIH intra- and extramural workforce.

To encourage researchers to re-enter the workforce, ORWH put out a Notice of Special Interest (NOSI) in 2023 titled *Research Supplements to Promote Reentry and Reintegration into Health-Related Research Careers* (NOT-OD-23–170). The Reentry Supplements Program was established in 1992, and since 2012, 24 ICs have participated in this career development program for full- or part-time research. The program has three components: reentry supplements, reintegration, and retraining and retooling. Designed to enhance existing research skills and knowledge in preparation for grantees to apply for a fellowship (F), career development (K) award, a research grant (R), or another type of independent research support, these programs allow administrative supplements to be given to existing NIH research grants for researchers to continue their work after leaving the workforce for family care responsibilities[12] or if they were affected by hostile work environments. The program is also open to those who want to broaden their skill set (ORWH, n.d.-b). Twenty-four ICs have participated, with the NCI and National Institute of General Medical Sciences being the most active (ORWH, n.d.-b).

The reentry program provides mentored research training for at least 1 year. A researcher needs to have at least 6 months of career interruptions arising from qualifying circumstances, such as family responsibilities, and a doctorate or equivalent degree. Some ICs also consider predoctoral students or those enrolled in dual-degree programs (ORWH, n.d.-b). The reintegration program is for pre- and postdoctoral students who have experienced unlawful harassment and helps them find a new work environment that is safe and supportive. The retraining and retooling program, which provides up to $90,000 per year in salary support and $50,000 per year in program-related expenses, is aimed at early- or midcareer researchers and provides new environments to expand skill sets while continuing to support their parent grant; the aim is cross-sectional collaboration and interdisciplinary partnerships to prepare and successfully apply for independent research funding.[13] According to ORWH, 80 percent of the awardees have been women, with 61 percent of applicants receiving awards (ORWH, n.d.-b).

Recommendations from a 2024 National Academies Report

In 2024, the National Academies of Sciences, Engineering, and Medicine released the report *Supporting Family Caregivers in STEMM: A Call to Action* (NASEM, 2024c). It describes how the labor and contributions of caregivers are often invisible and undervalued, with a specific focus on the academic science, technology, engineering, mathematics, and medicine

---

[12] Childrearing is the most cited reason for hiatus among applicants.

[13] See https://grants.nih.gov/grants/guide/notice-files/NOT-OD-23–170.html (accessed August 11, 2024).

(STEMM) ecosystem, including undergraduate and graduate students, postdoctoral scholars, resident physicians and other trainees, tenure-track and non-tenure-track faculty, staff, and researchers. That report made several important recommendations to federal agencies for improvement (see Box 8-1), so this committee focused its recommendations on other areas to improve the women's health and sex differences research workforce.

BOX 8-1
Relevant Recommendations from the 2024 report Supporting Family Caregivers in STEMM: A Call to Action

- Allow and support flexibility in the timing of grant eligibility as well as grant application and delivery deadlines for those with caregiving responsibilities and provide support for coverage while a grantee is on caregiving leave (e.g., decrease and streamline the paperwork and approval processes for grant applications).
- Allow no-cost grant extensions based on caregiving needs.
- Provide flexibility in eligibility timelines when an investigator has taken caregiving leave, such as eligibility deadlines for early-career scholars.
- Consider caregiving leave and acute caregiving demands as valid reasons for acceptance of a late application along the same timelines as other late applications.
- Introduce and allow grant supplements or the redistribution of funding within a grant budget to support coverage for someone to continue scholarly work while the grantee is on caregiving leave.
- Facilitate the leave and reentry processes for those who take a caregiving leave (e.g., provide research supplements to promote reentry following a period of caregiving leave; make supplements available to all types of caregivers, not solely parents; and cover costs associated with restarting a laboratory or research program as well as professional retraining).
- Fund innovative research on family caregiving in academic STEMM by providing competitive grants to institutions to support pilot projects and develop policy innovations.
- Congress should enact legislation to mandate a minimum of 12 weeks of paid, comprehensive caregiving leave. This leave should cover various contexts of caregiving, including childcare, older adult care, spousal care, dependent adult care, extended family care, end-of-life care, and bereavement care.

SOURCE: NASEM, 2024c.

Additional Workforce Support from ORWH

To address in part the inadequate representation of women in biomedical research, the NIH ORWH Working Group on Women in Biomedical Careers released two NOSIs in December 2022 that aim to retain early-career researchers. One, *Administrative Supplements to Promote Research Continuity and Retention of NIH Mentored Career Development (K) Award Recipients and Scholars* (NOT-OD-23-031), supports individuals with K awards during their shift from a mentored career development to independent research. The second, *Administrative Supplement for Continuity of Biomedical and Behavioral Research Among First-Time Recipients of NIH Research Project Grant Awards*, aims to improve the retention of first-time recipients of NIH research project grant awards who are experiencing a critical life event, including high-risk pregnancy, childbirth, adoption, serious personal health issues, or primary caregiving responsibilities for an ailing child, partner, parent, or immediate family (NOT-OD-23-032). During FY 2020 and 2021, the first 2 years of the program, data showed 87 percent of awardees were women and 10 percent were men. The racial breakdown of the participants was 60 percent White, 23 percent Asian, 6 percent African American or Black, and 5 percent more than one race (6 percent did not report). The most common reason for requesting the supplement was childbirth (77 percent) (NIH, n.d.-l).

ORWH is also involved in other mentored career development programs in partnership with ICs, such as the Team Science Leadership Scholars Program launched in 2022 with the NIAMS as a pilot with $2.5 million from ORWH. The program aims to fund four to five applicants with 20–50 percent protected time.

Loan Repayment Programs (LRPs)

Congress established NIH LRPs "to recruit and retain highly qualified health professionals into biomedical or biobehavioral research careers." The programs are designed to address increasing costs of education that are causing scientists to leave research (NIH, n.d.-e). They offer applicants up to $50,000 annually to repay qualified educational debt in return for their commitment to engage in NIH mission-relevant research (NIH, n.d.-e). Specifically, awardees are required to conduct "qualifying research supported by a domestic nonprofit or U. S. government (federal, state, or local) entity" for at least 20 hours per week over a 2-year period (NIH, n.d.-h). There are several basic eligibility requirements, including holding an advanced degree, having qualifying educational debt, conducting qualifying research that represents 50 percent or more of total level of effort, and being a U.S. citizen (NIH, n.d.-h).

The LRPs are available to both researchers not employed by NIH (extramural) and those employed by the agency (intramural) under one of the following subcategories (NIH, n.d.-c):

- **"Clinical Research**: Patient-oriented and conducted with humans.
- **Pediatric Research**: Directly related to diseases, disorders, and other conditions in children.
- **Health Disparities Research**: Focuses on minority and other health disparity populations.
- **Research in Emerging Areas Critical to Human Health**: For researchers pursuing major opportunities or gaps in emerging areas of human health.
- **Clinical Research for Individuals from Disadvantaged Backgrounds**: Available to clinical investigators from disadvantaged backgrounds.
- **Contraception and Infertility Research**: On conditions affecting the ability to conceive and bear young."

LRP awards are intended to support and build a scientist's research career rather than fund research related to these specific topics. New LRP awards are typically offered for 2 years. Repayments for a new award are calculated using the eligible educational debt at the start of the contract (NIH, n.d.-f). Renewal award applicants must have eligible debt of at least $2,000 to apply (NIH, n.d.-f). Payments are made quarterly, starting with the highest-priority loan, with no limit on the number of renewal awards someone can receive. Until their debt is repaid, successful renewal award applicants may continue to apply for, and potentially receive, competitive renewal awards (NIH, n.d.-f).

Each IC convenes external peer reviewers to assess applications to identify those most closely aligned with the IC's mission and priorities. Criteria include the potential to pursue a career in research and the quality of the overall research environment (NIH, n.d.-h).

Extramural LRP Awards and Success Rates

Between 2011 and 2023, $991,946,952 was awarded through the extramural LRP; 33,611 LRP applications were received (new and renewals), with 17,584 awarded—a success rate of 52 percent. The mean award was $56,412 (NIH, n.d.-n). During this same period, 20,270 new applications were received, with 8,460 of these awarded—a success rate of 42 percent. The mean award was $72,079. There were also 13,341 renewal applications; 9,124 of these were awarded, with a success rate of 68 percent. The mean renewal award was $41,885 (NIH, n.d.-n).

While success rates for applications have steadily increased, from 50 percent to 69 percent between 2011 and 2023, applications overall have declined from 3,159 in 2011 to 1,906 in 2023 for reasons that are unclear but could be related to fewer researchers staying in academia (Rothenberg, 2024; Wosen, 2023). Total funding for the program, however, has grown from $72 million in 2011 to $93 million in 2023 (NIH, n.d.-n).

Table 8-3 includes LRP grant success rates by race for all, new, and renewal awards in 2011 and 2023. Success rates have generally increased among all races. Among all awards, Black/African American success rates increased the most (from 37 to 67 percent); however, they continued to lag slightly behind White, Asian, and Other applicants (70, 69, and 68 percent, respectively). This trend is also noted among success rates for new awards,

TABLE 8-3 Loan Repayment Program Grant Success Rates for All, New, and Renewal Awards by Race

Success Rate (All Awards)

Race of Applicants	2011	2023
Asian	52%	69%
Black/African American	37%	67%
White	52%	70%
Other	49%	68%

Success Rate (New Awards)

Race of Applicants	2011	2023
Asian	43%	63%
Black/African American	30%	57%
White	39%	62%
Other	41%	59%

Success Rate (Renewal Awards)

Race of Applicants	2011	2023
Asian	68%	77%
Black/African American	50%	83%
White	70%	82%
Other	64%	83%

SOURCE: Data from NIH, n.d.-g.

while Black/African American and Other race applicants have the highest success rates (83 percent) for renewal awards (see Table 8-3).

In 2023, LRP funding varied significantly by IC, with NHLBI providing $15.67 million, NCI $13.97 million, NICHD $7.53 million, and NIAID $7.41 million being the largest funders by dollar amount (not percentage); the NIH OD, National Institute of Biomedical Imaging and Bioengineering, and National Library of Medicine provide some of the lowest levels at $144,023, $183,694, and $313,818 respectively. NICHD and the OD allocate a higher percentage of their total budgets to LRP, though they have smaller budgets (NIH, n.d.-i).

Intramural LRP Awards and Success Rates

Within the intramural LRP, the overall success rate has increased between 2015 and 2023, while the number of applications and awards has fallen. In 2015, 82 applications were received and 69 funded, for an 84 percent success rate. In 2023, 68 applications were received and 63 funded, for a 93 percent success rate (NIH, n.d.-k).

Regarding funding and awards by IC, in 2023, NCI, NIAID, and NIMH provided the most funding, with NIH Clinical Center and National Human Genome Research Institute (NHGRI) funding the least (see Table 8-4) (NIH, n.d.-k).

Table 8-4 Intramural Loan Repayment Program Awards By Institutes and Centers in 2023

IC	Awards	Funding
CC	1	$92,580
NCI	9	$1,374,374
NHGRI	1	$92,580
NIAID	5	$651,962
NICHD	2	$185,160
NIDCR	1	$231,450
NIMH	5	$511,946
NINDS	2	$266,943
Total	26	$3,406,995

NOTE: CC = Clinical Center; NCI = National Cancer Institute; NHGRI = National Human Genome Research Institute; NIAID = National Institute of Allergy and Infectious Diseases; NICHD = *Eunice Kennedy Shriver* National Institute of Child Health and Human Development; NIDCR = National Institute of Dental and Craniofacial Research; NIMH = National Institute of Mental Health; NINDS = National Institute of Neurological Disorders and Stroke.
SOURCE: Data from NIH, n.d.-k.

NIH LRP Evaluations

Evaluations of the LRP program have been conducted, with varying results, though several studies have noted that it has been helpful in retaining researchers and increasing their productivity. A 2009 evaluation of the extramural LRP noted that it has been effective in recruiting and retaining its physician doctorate target population overall, but has not as effectively retained women Ph.D.s, stating that "the LRPs are selectively losing women awardees." The report further noted it "would be appropriate to examine program design and retention in more detail to determine how the LRP can better serve women PhDs" (National Institutes of Health Loan Repayment Program Evaluation Working Group, 2009). It also commented the LRPs are attracting more African American and Black applicants compared to the demographics of recent M.D. and Ph.D. graduating classes, with no racial or ethnic differences in success rate (National Institutes of Health Loan Repayment Program Evaluation Working Group, 2009).

Another evaluation examined research productivity among LRP participants followed for 10 years after receiving an award between 2003 and 2009 (Lauer, 2019). Results indicated that awardees demonstrated consistently higher levels of "persistence in research," defined as submitting grant or fellowship applications, receiving grant or fellowship awards, and publications (see Figure 8-9). Over time, LRP-funded individuals demonstrated an approximate twofold increase in research productivity, compared to those who did not receive awards, a difference that continued at 14 years after their LRP application (Lauer, 2019).

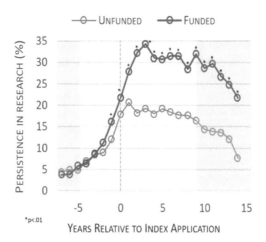

FIGURE 8-9 Assessment of persistence in research among Loan Repayment Program-funded and unfunded researchers.
SOURCE: Lauer, 2019.

In a survey of 1,938 LRP awardees, nearly all discussed benefiting professionally and personally from participating in the program, citing ability to pursue research goals, reduced clinical duties, and added confidence in their research career (Lauer, 2019). Another evaluation followed two cohorts of NHLBI LRP applicants who received awards in 2003 and 2008 over a 10-year period; obtaining the LRP award was strongly associated with increased submission of and success in obtaining grant funding and publications. Furthermore, "the LRP award appears to enhance retention in the biomedical research workforce when measured using metrics of grant application and award rates as well as research publications over a 10-year period" (Kalantari et al., 2021). Similarly, in a 2005 assessment of the intramural LRP, participation was associated with higher rates of both NIH and research retention, including in HIV/AIDS-related and clinical research (Glazerman and Seftor, 2005).

Student Loans and Early-Career Salaries in Academia

The burden of student loans differs significantly between women and men, with women generally facing a heavier financial load. This disparity is influenced by several factors, including the amount of debt taken on, repayment periods, and wage gaps.

Women hold approximately 64 percent of all U.S. student loan debt, totaling some $929 billion (Education Data Initiative, n.d.-b). On average, women graduate with $3,120 more (an average debt of $22,000 compared to $18,880 for men) (AAUW, n.d.-b). Men are less likely to take out loans, though parents of White male students are more likely to take out loans on their behalf or pay out of pocket than they are for female students. This difference in debt is exacerbated by disparities in salaries after graduation, with women earning between 26 and 81 percent of what their male counterparts do, making repayment more challenging (AAUW, n.d.-a; Education Data Initiative, n.d.-b). For women of color, the wage gap is even more pronounced, with Black women earning 64 cents and Latinas earning 51 cents for every dollar paid to White, non-Hispanic men (National Partnership for Women and Families, 2024).

Women in science, technology, engineering, and mathematics fields, including scientists, face unique challenges. Women are more likely to pursue advanced degrees, which increases their overall student debt, and women in these fields often earn less than their male counterparts. This disparity can exacerbate the financial strain of repaying student loans and deter women from pursuing lengthy and costly training programs required for physician-scientist roles (Fry et al., 2021; Hardy et al., 2021). The average debt for medical school alone is approximately $202,453 (Education Data Initiative, n.d.-a).

Having fewer women scientists contributes to gaps in knowledge about women's health, as women are more likely to study relevant diseases and conditions. For example, a study that analyzed the sex of PIs for cardio-vascular clinical trials found that only 18 percent were led by women, but those enrolled more female participants (Yong et al., 2023). Furthermore, a study of 1.5 million papers in the medical literature found that studies authored by women were more likely to include gender and sex analysis (Nielsen et al., 2017). Another study analyzed biomedical research articles from 2002 to 2020; women were more likely to study topics that benefit women (Koning et al., 2021). That study also reviewed biomedical patents and found that female research teams are 35 percent more likely to create treatments for women's conditions than male teams.

Importantly for WHR, 85 percent of OB/GYN medical residents are female (Vassar, 2015). Women are less likely to stay in academic medicine and more at risk of not independently obtaining grants because of the barriers discussed in this chapter. Since OB/GYNs are more likely to conduct research on related topics, failing to support OB/GYN physician-scientist development will continue to widen the gaps in WHR related to these conditions.

LRPs Summary

Women scientists and women's health researchers in general are essential to grow the WHR portfolio at NIH. However, early-career investigators with potential to study women's health and sex differences have a substantial debt burden from training, leading them to exit research because of the need for higher salaries and lack of steady funding to support them as they apply for grants at the start of their career. The LRP program, by relieving debt, might enhance their ability to stay on the research and physician-scientist path. Since women earn less money in research and academic positions, LRP may be an even greater and more urgent need for them. If the goal is to increase such research, retaining and supporting the workforce is key.

OVERVIEW OF THE NIH PROGRAM AND INTRAMURAL WORKFORCE

As of September 2023, the NIH workforce was 19,595 staff (including administrative) working in a wide range of positions in ICOs throughout the agency; over 60 percent were female. The racial and ethnic breakdown of the workforce is as follows (NIH, n.d.-q).

- 5.1 percent (1,006) identify as Hispanic or Latino.
- 51.5 percent (10,097) identify as White.
- 20.6 percent (4,031) identify as Black or African American.

- 20.6 percent (4,027) identify as Asian.
- 0.1 percent (21) identify as Native Hawaiian or Other Pacific Islander.
- 0.7 percent (134) identify as American Indian or Alaska Native.
- 1.4 percent (279) identify as two or more race groups.

The following section summarizes the workforce of Offices with a role in grantmaking or other responsibilities relevant to WHR, such as portfolio analysis. However, because limited information is publicly available detailing the composition of the intramural workforce by function and IC, the committee was constrained in its ability to characterize it. Data on specific expertise related to women's health or sex differences were not readily available.

Center for Scientific Review (CSR)

CSR is the primary Center that assesses grant applications for scientific merit. It organizes peer review groups and study sections to evaluate them. CSR's mission is to ensure that all grant applications receive "fair, independent, expert, and timely scientific reviews—free from inappropriate influences" (CSR, 2022). See Chapter 3 for more information.

According to FY 2023 data, 476 staff worked at CSR, with 61.6 percent (293) females and 38.4 percent (183) males (NIH, n.d.-p). As of 2021, Black and Hispanic individuals accounted for only 18.7 and 6.5 percent of CSR staff, respectively, indicating a lack of diversity among those evaluating grant applications (NIH, n.d.-q). These staff are experts who work with the external reviewers (CSR, 2022). Each CSR scientific division has six scientific review branches, including specific groups with key staff supporting those reviews (CSR, 2022). Staff have expertise in a large range of areas, corresponding to the ICs they support (CSR, 2022). Women's health and sex differences are not listed among the areas of expertise on the CSR website, although individuals within the listed categories could have such expertise.

Given the lack of focus on WHR in general at NIH, staff with expertise in this area may be inadequate. Moreover, if there is an influx of grants on women's health and sex differences research, such as in response to the recommendations of this report (see Chapter 9), the insufficiency will be exacerbated.

ORWH

ORWH has almost 30 staff members with a diverse range of professional and scientific expertise in areas to support and advance the consideration of women's health and sex and gender influences across the entire research continuum to improve women's health (NIH, n.d.-x). Staff have expertise in autoimmune ocular diseases, the role of sex and gender in health and disease, gender and women's studies, community-led HIV research, reproductive justice, applied developmental psychology, children's development, sex and gender differences in autoimmune diseases, orthopedics, obstetrics, gynecologic oncology, obesity, diabetes, aging, and community-based epidemiology, among many others (NIH, n.d.-x).

Division of Program Coordination, Planning, and Strategic Initiatives (DPCPSI)

"DPCPSI plans and coordinates trans-NIH initiatives and research supported by the NIH Common Fund, and develops resources to support portfolio analyses" (NIH, n.d.-o). Twenty staff with a wide range of expertise support the division in the main office and over 500 staff makeup the offices within DPCPSI, including those with backgrounds in biochemistry, biophysics, health science policy, substance use disorder, bioethics, and nutrition, among others (NIH, 2024c, n.d.-o).

DPCPSI's Office of Portfolio Analysis has 34 staff with a wide range of expertise, including molecular biology, systems biology, chemical engineering, computer science, machine learning, electrical engineering, science policy, chemistry, toxicology, biomedical science, molecular genetics, epidemiology, international science policy, data analytics and data science, bioinformatics, and neuroscience (NIH, n.d.-s).

OD's Office of Extramural Research (OER)

OER within the OD supports NIH's framework for research administration, with responsibilities to ensure scientific integrity, public accountability, and stewardship of the agency's extramural research portfolio. OER oversees a range of activities, such as digital platforms, grant compliance, peer review, communications, scientific misconduct, human participant protection, and laboratory animal welfare (NIH, n.d.-a). OER has nine key staff in the immediate Office of the Director (NIH, n.d.-j), with responsibilities including program administration, peer review, and research integrity. OER has over 200 staff whose expertise includes epidemiology, biostatistics, neuroscience, molecular biology, family studies, and genomics.[14]

OER's Office of Research Reporting and Analysis (ORRA)

ORRA provides data and reporting oversight related to NIH grants processing. Its staff have a range of expertise that supports their work

---

[14] The preceding two sections were changed after release of the report to clarify the number of DPCPSI and OER staff in the immediate Office of the Director of NIH and other staff.

in developing policy implementation strategies, and providing guidance, systems, and resources for the publication of funding opportunities to the public and scientific research community (NIH, n.d.-r).

ORRA's Division of Scientific Categorization and Analysis (DSCA)

DSCA is responsible for curating and maintaining the Research, Condition, and Disease Categorization research portfolios for public reporting and analysis. Staff include scientific information analysts, data analysts, and computational linguists (Cebotari and Praskievicz, 2024).

NIH IC Workforce Data

Staff who support the various ICs and Offices, including administrative staff, vary in size from under 100 at the Fogarty International Center and the National Center for Complementary and Integrative Health to over 500 at NICHD, about 900 at NHLBI, and over 3,000 at NCI, with most having at least 50 percent female staff (NIH, n.d.-p). Each has varied expertise aligned with its mission.

Overview of NIH's IRP Workforce

IRP supports basic, translational, and clinical biomedical research throughout NIH and is overseen by the Office of Intramural Research (OIR). OIR is responsible for overseeing and coordinating intramural research within NIH laboratories and clinics embedded in 24 of the ICs. IRP supports about 1,200 PIs who lead research projects involving nearly 6,000 trainees (NIH, 2022a, n.d.-t-u). According to the NIH Triennial report, "the IRP research environment is. . . designed to attract and train a highly talented and diverse cadre of scientists who will lead biomedical research in the 21st century. Its unique funding environment means the IRP can facilitate opportunities to conduct both long-term and high-impact science that would otherwise be difficult to undertake" (NIH, n.d.-u, p. 18). Unlike extramural research, IRP directions and research priorities are not shaped primarily through grant awards but through professional hiring and promotion decisions, external reviews, and the allocation of resources to laboratories and branches. In 2024, the president's Women's Health Initiative directed the IRP at each IC to expand research on understanding, treating, and preventing disorders that disproportionately affect women, recognizing the unique clinical presentations of disorders common to people of both sexes (Harker, 2024).

"IRP in each IC has a promotion and tenure committee that evaluates all recommendations for appointment or promotion. Formal internal reviews are conducted annually for tenured and tenure-track scientists, determining resource allocations and promotions" (NIH, n.d.-u, p. 18).

IRP supports research in various broad scientific areas, including biomedical engineering and biophysics, cancer biology, cell biology, chemical biology, computational biology, developmental biology, epidemiology, genetics and genomics, health disparities, immunology, microbiology and infectious diseases, molecular biology and biochemistry, molecular pharmacology, neuroscience, RNA biology, social and behavioral sciences, stem cell biology, structural biology, systems biology, and virology (NIH, n.d.-v).

Overview of the IRP Workforce

IRP staff are grouped into basic and clinical research tracks. PI data from 2023 show

- 770 senior investigators (27 percent female);
- 232 investigators (tenure-track) (45 percent female);
- 37 senior clinicians (46 percent female);
- 40 senior scientists (30 percent female); and
- 37 assistant clinical investigators (51 percent female).

IRP non-PIs included

- 324 staff clinicians (57 percent female);
- 1,693 staff scientists (39 percent female);
- 261 clinical fellows/senior clinical fellows (50 percent female); and
- 456 research fellows/senior research fellows (47 percent female) (NIH, 2023b).

There were also 163 lab/branch chiefs (31 percent female). IRP PIs focus on various scientific areas, however none is listed as an expert in women's health or sex differences research (NIH, n.d.-v).

OIR runs four NIH-wide early-career faculty recruitment and career development programs, each aimed at a different segment of the intramural research workforce and serving one of the eight strategic aims of NIH's IRP (NIH, n.d.-u). While OIR, and NIH more broadly, has many training and workforce development programs for IRP workforce, none identified by the committee, other than one-off trainings and available seminars, focuses on women's health or sex differences.

Funding of WHR in IRP

Notably, based on the committee's funding analysis, the proportion of intramural funding directed to WHR has been low compared to total intramural funding and within all ICs—only $3.0 billion of the $45.3 billion intramural funding (6.5 percent of the IRP funding) from 2011 to 2023 (see Chapter 4 and Appendix A for more information). NCI, NICHD, NIEHS, and NIAID intramural programs invested the most in WHR.

GAPS IN THE WHR WORKFORCE

To address WHR, it is essential to have a robust and productive trained NIH intramural and extramural research workforce with broad expertise in biomedical research, clinical trials, and implementation science. The committee found that NIH support of the WHR workforce was not sufficient to address the unmet needs of women's health, much less the next generation of researchers studying female-specific ailments and diseases that are more frequent or severe in women. However, there is the sentiment that the workforce of OB/GYNs most likely to address female-specific diseases, such as gynecologic cancers, leiomyoma, endometriosis, vulvodynia, and obstetric-related conditions, is most in jeopardy.

Inadequate Support

Leading experts and respected NIH researchers in women's health are deeply concerned NIH has not sufficiently invested in career development awards (Catherino, 2024; Coutifaris, 2024; NASEM, 2024a,b; Sadovsky et al., 2018; Schust, 2024). There has been a disproportionate decline for procedural clinician-scientists, particularly in obstetrics and gynecology, for reasons that are not completely understood. In part, the lack of funding and support for WHR may have deterred researchers. Moreover, the effect is unknown on gaps in WHR from female researchers having fewer citations in premier journals, less recognition for their scientific scholarship, and repercussions from securing fewer NIH research program and R01 grants in the past compared to men (Heggeness et al., 2016; Nature, 2024). The concern is that fewer trainees, women, and those from underrepresented groups in medicine will be interested in pursuing academic careers focused on WHR. It is a vicious cycle, as an adequate workforce of skilled researchers is imperative to address gaps in WHR, and without a tangible focus and critical investment in women's health and mentorship of investigators in WHR, a cadre of researchers will not pursue a career in it.

Furthermore, potential research talent is discouraged by the lack of institutional support, pressure to be more productive clinically, insufficient protected effort, and a shortage of mature research teams and mentors to direct these efforts within institutions. In addition, developing a research career for surgery-dominant specialties/subspecialties, such as obstetrics and gynecology, is more challenging given the need to maintain a surgical practice. A longer latency period of 5–7 years for the equivalent surgical training with greater flexibility with 50/50 or 60/40 research/clinical care may be beneficial to support early research career development. Non-NIH-supported organizations are attempting to fill the gaps and provide training support to ensure that OB/GYNs have the skills to become competitive and independent researchers. However, without NIH support, these other funding agencies cannot support the number needed to effectively address the gaps in workforce.

Despite NIH programs, OB/GYNs have the lowest number of K08 and K23 awards compared to all other disciplines (Parchem et al., 2022). Early and talented career researchers are often dissuaded from pursuing a career in WHR and turn their attention to other fields as a result of decreased NIH funding. Ultimately, the shortage in physicians and physician-scientists in WHR will lead to a decrease in U.S.-based researchers, applicants, reviewers, mentors, and novel and more effective treatments for often disabling diseases. Therefore, more funding and increased development opportunities are critical to the research training programs described in this chapter, including institutional K12 (such as BIRCWH) and T32 grants[15] across all WHR fields, K01 eligibility for women-specific conditions, K99-R00 awards, and R35 grants. In addition, the requirements for T and F award eligibility could be modified and/or increased to allow OB/GYN physicians to be competitive for such training awards, as could requirements for K99-R00 awards.

It may be important to identify mechanisms for early mentorship for women's health researchers that will not require institutions making significant financial investments. This could be accomplished by increasing funding to women's health and providing additional monetary support to universities to offset costs of protecting clinician time. Increasing NIH's budget for women's health researchers and grant awards to institutions for this express purpose would likely help address this issue. It would be important to have clear guidelines in terms of incorporating early-career faculty and multidisciplinary teams that include members with research doctorates representing complementary fields of expertise to maximize outcomes of this investment.

Bias and Sexism

Another key issue for increasing the focus on WHR is to address the underlying sexism and imbalance of power in the United States. Abundant literature supports the assertion that research on women or females and

---

[15] National Research Service Award Institutional Research Training Grants (T32) provide domestic, nonprofit, and private or public graduate-level academic institutions with funds for training predoctoral and postdoctoral candidates.

conducted by women is less likely to be funded, published, and prioritized than research done by or focusing on men or males (Hamberg, 2008; Mirin, 2021; Nguyen et al., 2023). This is a systemic problem that goes beyond NIH. Nonetheless, addressing it requires women to be equally represented in positions of power at top biomedical journals, Nobel Prize and other important award-bestowing committees, leadership positions at funding agencies and institutes, academic institutions, and councils within NIH and other funding agencies that make recommendations for funding of women's health and sex differences research (see Figure 8-10 for a summary of pres-tigious prizes awarded for research regarding female physiology or women's health versus other topics).

For health equity in terms of the committee's statement of task, research design has two main considerations. Racial and ethnic comparisons with White individuals have been well documented in epidemiologic research, and Black and Native individuals particularly bear a higher burden of

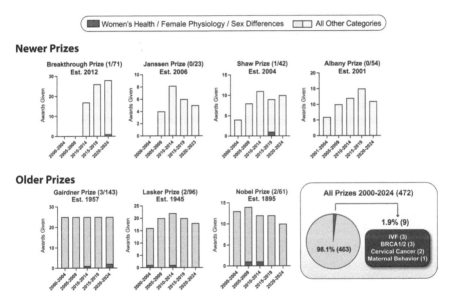

FIGURE 8-10 Major biomedical research prizes recognizing breakthroughs in women's health research compared to all other categories, 2000–2024.

NOTES: Numbers in parentheses after prize name show number of prizes awarded related to women's health, female physiology, or sex differences research of the total number of prizes awarded between 2000 and 2024. BRCA1/2 = BReast CAncer genes 1 and 2; IVF = in vitro fertilization.

SOURCES: Albany Med Health System, n.d.; Albert and Mary Lasker Foundation, n.d.; Dr. Paul Janssen Award, n.d.; Gairdner Foundation, n.d.; The Breakthrough Prize Foundation, n.d.; The Nobel Foundation, 2024; The Shaw Prize, n.d.

morbidity and mortality nearly universally across disease states. Within-group studies are needed given the unique cultural, political, and social exposures as a legacy of structural policies and racism to identify opportunities for study and intervention. This needs to include epistemic justice, where communities most affected by these health disparities are partners in designing, implementing, evaluating and disseminating research findings. Building researcher and reviewer expertise in race, racism, and equity-based research is also imperative for the effective study of the health and disease of women of color.

The top R1 and elite universities receive the bulk of NIH funding (Nietzel, 2024; NIH, n.d.-m). Scientists who are racially and ethnically minoritized are less likely to be hired or tenured at these institutions but more likely to study health equity issues, racism, and socioeconomic factors (Arenson, 2005; Headen, 2024; Hoppe et al., 2019). Women scientists, if hired, are less likely to receive sufficient financial support, mentorship, and tenure at many top universities.

The fallacy that outcomes of the scientific review processes are simply a function of NIH funding "good science" is recognized as bias against WHR; it suggests that WHR is in general not considered innovative or groundbreaking enough to be funded (factors peer reviewers are asked to look for in applications). This was also a clear message relayed by researchers who presented to the committee based on comments they received in the grant review process. This systematic bias results in the huge gaps in knowledge in female physiology and diseases specific to, differentially expressed in, or disproportionately affecting women. For example, a 2018 study showed that female applicants with past grant success rates equivalent to male applicants were given poorer application scores by reviewers, and male applicants with less experience than female applicants were favored and awarded grants at a higher rate (Morgan et al., 2018). A 2023 study found significant gender, racial, and ethnic inequalities in both NIH funding amounts and success rates. For example, Black faculty receive poorer scores and are less likely to be funded after grant resubmission compared to their White counterparts, even after controlling for factors such as training record, prior awards, and publication history (Nguyen et al., 2023). In addition, scientists with multiple NIH grants are overwhelmingly male and White. Women and investigators from underrepresented racial and ethnic groups are less likely to become "super-PIs" with multiple simultaneous research grants (Nguyen et al., 2023). Gender bias in grant reviews may manifest as a greater likelihood of highlighting inadequacies in women's grants (Biernat et al., 2020). Some evidence also suggests that women may be more likely to internalize negative comments from reviewers as personal shortcomings, potentially deterring resubmissions (Biernat et al., 2020; Coffman et al., 2024).

These examples demonstrate that bias and sexism persist in various aspects of the NIH grantmaking process, from the initial application and review stages to funding allocation and awarding multiple grants. NIH has acknowledged these issues and implemented some initiatives to address them, such as UNITE in 2021 to combat systemic racism (NIH, 2024k). However, research suggests that significant disparities remain, and further structural changes may be necessary to achieve equity in the grantmaking process.

Another area to be addressed by NIH is program officer training in women's health and health equity. It is unknown what the gaps are in this area, yet this is a key area to address to improve women's health, as program staff are key to ensuring women's health and sex differences research receives the full attention and funding it warrants.

NIH could, as a report to the Congress, address the workforce required to foster the development of competitive researchers capable of conducting innovative research to address female-specific medical issues. Overarching critical workforce gaps to continually assess include

- baseline information regarding the NIH intramural and extramural research workforce and how WHR is supported in each;
- barriers to attract, develop, and retain successful independent researchers in obstetrics and gynecology and other specialists with a focus in WHR;
- better understanding and elimination of sex- and gender-based bias in research grant awards, citations, and scientific recognition; and
- insufficient IC focus to support grants related to gynecologic conditions.

CONCLUDING OBSERVATIONS

This chapter underscores the need for NIH and other stakeholders to comprehensively prepare a broad-based effort to train a robust research workforce that meets the needs for WHR. Achieving this goal requires a multifaceted, coordinated approach, including substantial support for training and retaining both laboratory-based researchers and physician-scientists specializing in women's health. While the existing programs that focus on WHR workforce development are effective, there are not enough opportunities to build the workforce substantially, and funding is inadequate. Addressing workforce issues throughout the research career continuum is crucial. This includes enhancing educational opportunities for scientists at various stages, such as clinical and doctoral training programs. In addition, it is essential to address the need for protected research time for academic and clinical scientists. Support mechanisms also need to be in place to assist female scientists with childbearing and eldercare responsibilities, ensuring that such duties do not hinder their career progression in research. Furthermore, increased funding and expansion of successful existing programs—BIRCWH, SCORE, WRHR, and RSDP—are vital to support and sustain these efforts. By addressing these critical issues and leveraging proven programs, NIH can help build a robust research workforce capable of addressing the complex needs of women's health. See Chapter 9 for recommendations aimed at enhancing opportunities for women's health researchers to access effective career development programs and secure grant funding. These suggestions complement other recommendations in Chapter 9 that tackle structural, policy, and program barriers to advancing WHR at NIH.

REFERENCES

AAUW (American Association of University Women). n.d.-a. *Deeper in Debt: Women & Student Loans.* https://www.aauw.org/resources/research/deeper-in-debt/ (accessed August 14, 2024).

AAUW. n.d.-b. *Fast Facts: Women & Student Debt.* https://www.aauw.org/resources/article/fast-facts-student-debt/ (accessed Ocotber 22, 2024).

Agarwal, R. K., N. Macioce, C. Hunter, and J. A. Clayton. 2023. ORWH, NIH, SCORE career enhancement core programs are shaping the future of women's health and sex and gender research training. *Journal of Women's Health* 32(8):838–839.

Albany Med Health System. n.d. *Albany Medical Center Prize in Medicine and Biomedical Research.* https://www.albanymed.org/albany-prize/ (accessed October 22, 2024).

Albert and Mary Lasker Foundation. n.d. *All Awards and Winners.* https://laskerfoundation.org/all-awards-winners/ (accessed October 22, 2024).

Arenson, K. W. 2005. Little advance is seen in Ivies' hiring of minorities and women. *The New York Times.* https://www.nytimes.com/2005/03/01/education/little-advance-is-seen-in-ivies-hiring-of-minorities-and-women.html (accessed August 14, 2024).

Bates, C. R., D. M. Bakula, A. H. Egbert, C. A. Gerhardt, A. M. Davis, and A. M. Psihogios. 2023. Addressing barriers to career development awards for early career women in pediatric psychology. *Journal of Pediatric Psychology* 48(4):320–329.

Bennett, W. L., A. L. McRae-Clark, and M. M. B. Morrow. 2023. Mechanisms of career enhancement at specialized centers of research excellence (SCORE) on sex differences. *Journal of Women's Health* 32(8):840–842.

Berge, J. M., K. Macheledt, C. Bakker, S. Allen, B. Thyagarajan, and J. F. Wyman. 2022. Bibliometric approach to evaluating the impact of a building interdisciplinary research careers in women's health K12 research career development program. *Journal of Women's Health* 31(10):1422–1431.

Biernat, M., M. Carnes, A. Filut, and A. Kaatz. 2020. Gender, race, and grant reviews: Translating and responding to research feedback. *Personality and Social Psychology Bulletin* 46(1):140–154.

Breakthrough Prize Foundation. n.d. *Life Sciences Breakthrough Prize: Laureates.* https://breakthroughprize.org/Laureates/2 (accessed October 22, 2024).

Catherino, W. 2024. *Women's Health Research Career Development Programs and Workforce Needs. Presentation to the NASEM Committee on the Assessment of NIH Research on Women's Health, Meeting 5, Part 1 (May 20, 2024).* https://www.nationalacademies.org/documents/embed/link/LF2255DA3DD1C41C0A42D3BEF0989ACAECE3053A6A9B/file/DA0D9C1A29E7A2B7872C7BF5B1374224DC59E77F7974?noSaveAs=1 (accessed August 13, 2024).

Cebotari, E., and N. Praskievicz. 2024. *NIH's Research, Condition, and Disease Categorization (RCDC) System. Presentation to the NASEM Committee on the Assessment of NIH Research on Women's Health, Meeting 2 (January 25, 2024).* https://www.nationalacademies.org/event/docs/D0195AEF81CCEAE1E0BEA79C3AA37C7D6EE52D5DFAF3?noSaveAs=1 (accessed February 26, 2024).

Choo, E., S. Mathis, T. Harrod, K. E. Hartmann, K. M. Freund, M. Krousel-Wood, T. E. Curry, and J.-M. Guise. 2020. Contributors to independent research funding success from the perspective of K12 BIRCWH program directors. *American Journal of the Medical Sciences* 360(5):596–603.

Coffman, K., M. P. Ugalde Araya, and B. Zafar. 2024. A (dynamic) investigation of stereotypes, belief-updating, and behavior. *Economic Inquiry* 62(3):957–983.

Coutifaris, C. 2024. *NIH/NICHD Career Development Awards for OB/GYN's: The Women's Reproductive Health Research (WRHR) Program. Presentation to the NASEM Committee on the Assessment of NIH Research on Women's Health, Meeting 5, Part 1 (May 20, 2024).* https://www.nationalacademies.org/documents/embed/link/LF2255DA3DD1C-41C0A42D3BEF0989ACAECE3053A6A9B/file/D83A0567EF32BDB62E46D92BD6F5 7100B35674643CEE?noSaveAs=1 (accessed May 20, 2024).

CSR (Center for Scientific Review). 2022. *Center for Scientific Review NIH 2022–2027 strategic plan.* Bethesda, MD: National Institutes of Health.

Dr. Paul Janssen Award. n.d. *Meet Our Past Winners.* https://www.pauljanssenaward.com/winners?page=0%2C0 (accessed October 22, 2024).

Education Data Initiative. n.d.-a. *Average Medical School Debt.* https://educationdata.org/average-medical-school-debt (accessed August 14, 2024).

Education Data Initiative. n.d.-b. *Student Loan Debt by Gender.* https://educationdata.org/student-loan-debt-by-gender (accessed August 14, 2024).

Fry, R., B. Kennedy, and C. Funk. 2021. *STEM jobs see uneven progress in increasing gender, racial and ethnic diversity.* Washington, DC: PEW Research Center.

Gairdner Foundation. n.d. *Canada Gairdner Award Winners.* https://www.gairdner.org/winners (accessed October 22, 2024).

GAO (Government Accountability Office). 2018. *NIH research: Action needed to ensure workforce diversity strategic goals are achieved.* Washington, DC: Government Accountability Office.

Ginther, D. K., W. T. Schaffer, J. Schnell, B. Masimore, F. Liu, L. L. Haak, and R. Kington. 2011. Race, ethnicity, and NIH research awards. *Science* 333(6045):1015–1019.

Ginther, D. K., J. Basner, U. Jensen, J. Schnell, R. Kington, and W. T. Schaffer. 2018. Publications as predictors of racial and ethnic differences in NIH research awards. *PLoS One* 13(11):e0205929.

Glazerman, S. and N. Seftor. 2005. *The NIH intramural research loan repayment program: Career outcomes of participants and nonparticipants final report.* Princeton, NJ: Mathematica Policy Research, Inc.

Guise, J. M., J. D. Nagel, and J. G. Regensteiner. 2012. Best practices and pearls in interdisciplinary mentoring from building interdisciplinary research careers in women's health directors. *Journal of Women's Health* 21(11):1114–1127.

Guise, J. M., S. Geller, J. G. Regensteiner, N. Raymond, and J. Nagel. 2017. Team mentoring for interdisciplinary team science: Lessons from K12 scholars and directors. *Academic Medicine* 92(2):214–221.

Hamberg, K. 2008. Gender bias in medicine. *Women's Health* 4(3):237–243.

Hardy, S. M., K. L. McGillen, and B. L. Hausman. 2021. Dr. Mom's added burden. *Journal of the American College of Radiology* 18(1 Pt A):103–107.

Harker, J. 2024. President Biden requests $12b for research on women's health NIH is poised to perform. *NIH Catalyst* 32(3). https://irp.nih.gov/catalyst/32/3/president-biden-requests-12b-for-research-on-womens-health (accessed August 14, 2024).

Headen, I. 2024. *Structural Changes to Support Structural Determinants Research in Women's Health: Presentation to the NASEM Committee on the Assessment of NIH Research on Women's Health, Meeting 4 (April 11, 2024).* https://www.nationalacademies.org/documents/embed/link/LF2255DA3DD1C41C0A42D3BEF0989ACAECE3053A6A9B/file/DA81A7014AD0D94CBE0B576E4271A1563640B19949CF?noSaveAs=1 (accessed August 27, 2024).

Heggeness, M. L., L. Evans, J. R. Pohlhaus, and S. L. Mills. 2016. Measuring diversity of the National Institutes of Health-funded workforce. *Academic Medicine* 91(8):1164–1172.

HHS (Department of Health and Human Services). 2018. *Specialized Centers of Research Excellence (SCORE) on Sex Differences (U54 Clinical Trial Optional): Reissue of RFA-OD-11-003.* https://grants.nih.gov/grants/guide/rfa-files/RFA-OD-18–004.html (accessed August 11, 2024).

HHS. 2024. *Building Interdisciplinary Research Careers in Women's Health (BIRCWH) (K12 Clinical Trial Optional): RFA-OD-24-013.* https://grants.nih.gov/grants/guide/rfa-files/RFA-OD-24–013.html (accessed August 11, 2024).

Hoppe, T. A., A. Litovitz, K. A. Willis, R. A. Meseroll, M. J. Perkins, B. I. Hutchins, A. F. Davis, M. S. Lauer, H. A. Valantine, J. M. Anderson, and G. M. Santangelo. 2019. Topic choice contributes to the lower rate of NIH awards to African-American/Black scientists. *Science Advances* 5(10):eaaw7238.

Jagsi, R., K. A. Griffith, R. D. Jones, A. Stewart, and P. A. Ubel. 2017. Factors associated with success of clinician-researchers receiving career development awards from the National Institutes of Health: A longitudinal cohort study. *Academic Medicine* 92(10):1429–1439.

Kaiser, J. 2023. *Women, Black Researchers Less Likely to Hold Multiple NIH Grants.* https://www.science.org/content/article/women-black-researchers-less-likely-hold-multiple-nih-grants (accessed August 23, 2024).

Kalantari, R., X. Tigno, S. Colombini-Hatch, J. Kiley, and N. Aggarwal. 2021. Impact of the National Heart, Lung, and Blood Institute's loan repayment program funding on retention of the National Institutes of Health biomedical workforce. *ATS Scholar* 2(3):415–431.

Koning, R., S. Samila, and J.-P. Ferguson. 2021. Who do we invent for? Patents by women focus more on women's health, but few women get to invent. *Science* 372(6548):1345–1348.

Lauer, M. 2019. *Outcomes for NIH Loan Repayment Program Awardees: A Preliminary Look.* https://nexus.od.nih.gov/all/2019/05/21/outcomes-for-nih-loan-repayment-program-awardees-a-preliminary-look/ (accessed August 11, 2024).

Lauer, M. 2024. *FY 2023 by the Numbers: Extramural Grant Investments in Research.* https://nexus.od.nih.gov/all/2024/02/21/fy-2023-by-the-numbers-extramural-grant-investments-in-research/ (accessed August 11, 2024).

Lauer, M., and D. Roychowdhury. 2024. *Mentored career development application (K) funding rates by race-ethnicity FY2010–FY2023.* Bethesda, MD: NIH.

Libby, A. M., H. G. McGinnes, and J. G. Regensteiner. 2020. Educating the scientific workforce on sex and gender considerations in research: A national scan of the literature and building interdisciplinary research careers in women's health programs. *Journal of Women's Health* 29(6):876–885.

Lo, J. O., E. R. Boniface, A. Heflin, A. K. Stanic-Kostic, K. C. Fuh, and D. J. Schust. 2023. Reproductive scientist development program: Bridging the gap to the physician scientist career. *Reproductive Science* 30(9):2615–2622.

Malcom, S. M., P. Q. Hall, and J. W. Brown. 1976. *The double bind: The price of being a minority woman in science.* Washington, DC: American Association for the Advancement of Science.

McCoy, E. E., R. Katz, D. K. N. Louden, E. Oshima, A. Murtha, C. Gyamfi-Bannerman, N. Santoro, E. A. Howell, L. Halvorson, S. D. Reed, and B. A. Goff. 2023. Scholarly activity following National Institutes of Health women's reproductive health research K12 training—a cohort study. *American Journal of Obstetrics & Gynecology* 229(4): 425.e1–425.e16.

Mirin, A. A. 2021. Gender disparity in the funding of diseases by the U.S. National Institutes of Health. *Journal of Women's Health* 30(7):956–963.

Morgan, R., K. Hawkins, and J. Lundine. 2018. The foundation and consequences of gender bias in grant peer review processes. *CMAJ* 190(16):E487–E488.

Nagel, J. D., A. Koch, J. M. Guimond, S. Glavin, and S. Geller. 2013. Building the women's health research workforce: Fostering interdisciplinary research approaches in women's health. *Global Advances in Health and Medicine* 2(5):24–29.

NASEM (National Academies of Sciences, Engineering, and Medicine). 2024a. *Discussion of policies, systems, and structures for research on women's health at the National Institutes of Health: Proceedings of a workshop—in brief.* Washington, DC: The National Academies Press.

NASEM. 2024b. *Overview of research gaps for selected conditions in women's health research at the National Institutes of Health: Proceedings of a workshop—in brief.* Washington, DC: The National Academies Press.

NASEM. 2024c. *Supporting family caregivers in STEMM: A call to action.* Washington, DC: The National Academies Press.

National Institutes of Health Loan Repayment Program Evaluation Working Group. 2009. *NIH LRP evaluation extramural loan repayment programs fiscal years 2003–2007.* Bethesda, MD: NIH.

National Partnership for Women and Families. 2024. *The Wage Gap #irl (in Real Life) for Women of Color: Groceries, Child Care and Student Loans.* https://nationalpartnership. org/wp-content/uploads/2023/02/quantifying-americas-gender-wage-gap.pdf (accessed October 22, 2024).

Nature. 2024. *Nature* publishes too few papers from women researchers—that must change. *Nature*(627):7–8.

Nguyen, M., S. I. Chaudhry, M. M. Desai, K. Dzirasa, J. E. Cavazos, and D. Boatright. 2023. Gender, racial, and ethnic inequities in receipt of multiple National Institutes of Health research project grants. *JAMA Network Open* 6(2):e230855.

NICHD (*Eunice Kennedy Shriver* National Institute of Child Health and Human Development). 2023a. *Reproductive Scientist Development Program (RSDP).* https://www.nichd. nih.gov/research/supported/rsdp (accessed August 11, 2024).

NICHD. 2023b. *Women's Reproductive Health Research (WRHR) Career Development Program.* https://www.nichd.nih.gov/research/supported/wrhr (accessed August 11, 2023).

NIDDK (National Institute of Diabetes and Digestive and Kidney Diseases). 2024. *The Special Diabetes Program: 25 Years of Advancing Type 1 Diabetes Research.* https://www. niddk.nih.gov/news/archive/2024/special-diabetes-program-25-years-advancing-type-1-diabetes-research (accessed August 11, 2024).

Nielsen, M. W., J. P. Andersen, L. Schiebinger, and J. W. Schneider. 2017. One and a half million medical papers reveal a link between author gender and attention to gender and sex analysis. *Nature Human Behaviour* 1(11):791–796.

Nietzel, M. 2024. *Top 20 Universities for NIH funding; Johns Hopkins Ranks First Again.* https://www.forbes.com/sites/michaeltnietzel/2024/02/10/top-20-universities-for-nih-funding-johns-hopkins-ranks-first-again/ (accessed August 11, 2024).

NIH (National Institutes of Health). n.d.-a. *About the Office of Extramural Research (OER) at NIH.* https://grants.nih.gov/aboutoer/intro2oer.htm (accessed August 14, 2024).

NIH. n.d.-b. *Career Development Programs & Projects.* https://orwh.od.nih.gov/career-development-education#card-1161 (accessed October 22, 2024).

NIH. n.d.-c. *Clinical Research LRP for Individuals from Disadvantaged Backgrounds Expands Participation to Include All NIH Institutes and Centers.* https://www.lrp.nih.gov/ node/127 (accessed August 14, 2024).

NIH. n.d.-d. *Diversity Matters.* https://extramural-diversity.nih.gov/diversity-matters (accessed August 11, 2024).

NIH. n.d.-e. *Division of Loan Repayment—Home Page.* https://www.lrp.nih.gov/ (accessed August 11, 2024).

NIH. n.d.-f. *Eligibility & Programs.* https://www.lrp.nih.gov/eligibility-programs (accessed August 14, 2024).

NIH. n.d.-g. *Extramural Demographics.* https://report.nih.gov/nihdatabook/category/30 (accessed August 23, 2024).

NIH. n.d.-h. *Frequently Asked Questions.* https://www.lrp.nih.gov/faqs (accessed August, 2024).

NIH. n.d.-i. *Funding by Institutes & Centers.* https://report.nih.gov/nihdatabook/report/508 (accessed August 23, 2024).

NIH. n.d.-j. *Immediate Office of the Director (IMOD).* https://grants.nih.gov/aboutoer/oer_offices/imod.htm (accessed August 14, 2024).

NIH. n.d.-k. *Intramural Data Book.* https://report.nih.gov/nihdatabook/category/31 (accessed August 8, 2024).

NIH. n.d.-l. *NIH Administrative Supplement Programs Support Early-Career Biomedical Investigators.* https://orwh.od.nih.gov/career-development-education/research-continuity-retention-supplements (accessed October 22, 2024).

NIH. n.d.-m. *NIH Awards by Location & Organization.* https://report.nih.gov/award/index. cfm?fy=2010&sumcol=fun&sumdir=desc&view=stateorg (accessed August 11, 2024).

NIH. n.d.-n. *NIH Data Book Extramural Overview.* https://report.nih.gov/nihdatabook/ category/29 (accessed August 14, 2024).

NIH. n.d.-o. *NIH Division of Program Coordination, Planning, and Strategic Initiatives.* https://dpcpsi.nih.gov/ (accessed August 14, 2024).

NIH. n.d.-p. *NIH Institutes, Centers, and Offices Workforce Demographics.* https://www.edi. nih.gov/data/demographics/2023-ic-workforce-demographics#csr (accessed August 14, 2024).

NIH. n.d.-q. *NIH Total Workforce Demographics for Fiscal Year 2023 Fourth Quarter.* https:// www.edi.nih.gov/data/demographics (accessed August 14, 2024).

NIH. n.d.-r. *Office of Research Reporting and Analysis (ORRA).* https://grants.nih.gov/ aboutoer/oer_offices/orra.htm (accessed August 14, 2024).

NIH. n.d.-s. *OPA Staff.* https://dpcpsi.nih.gov/opa/staff (accessed August 14, 2024).

NIH. n.d.-t. *Organization and Leadership.* https://irp.nih.gov/about-us/organization-and-leadership (accessed August 14, 2024).

NIH. n.d.-u. *Report of the Director, National Institutes of Health: Fiscal Years 2019–2021.* https://dpcpsi.nih.gov/sites/default/files/2023–09/FY19–21%20Triennial_Report_FINAL_508C.pdf (accessed August 11, 2024).

NIH. n.d.-v. *Scientific Focus Areas.* https://irp.nih.gov/our-research/scientific-focus-areas (accessed August 14, 2024).

NIH. n.d.-w. *Specialized Centers of Research Excellence on Sex Differences (U54 Clinical Trial Optional).* https://orwh.od.nih.gov/sex-gender/orwh-mission-area-sex-gender-in-research/specialized-centers-of-research-excellence-on-sex-differences-u54-clinical-trial (accessed October 22, 2024).

NIH. n.d.-x. *Staff Listing.* https://orwh.od.nih.gov/about/staff (accessed August 14, 2024).

NIH. 1998. *Women's Reproductive Health Research Career Development Centers.* https:// grants.nih.gov/grants/guide/rfa-files/rfa-hd-98–004.html (accessed August 11, 2024).

NIH. 2017a. *Individual Fellowships (F) Kiosk.* https://researchtraining.nih.gov/programs/ fellowships (accessed August 22, 2024).

NIH. 2017b. *Institutional Training Grants (T) Kiosk.* https://researchtraining.nih.gov/ programs/training-grants (accessed August 22, 2024).

NIH. 2017c. *Research Career Development Awards (K) Kiosk.* https://researchtraining.nih. gov/programs/career-development (accessed August 22, 2024).

NIH. 2019. *Understanding Research Career Development (K) Award Specifics*. https://www.
niaid.nih.gov/grants-contracts/understanding-research-career-development-k-award-
specifics (accessed August 11, 2024).

NIH. 2020. *Notice of Intent to Publish the Reissuance of Building Interdisciplinary Research
Careers in Women's Health Program (K12 Clinical Trial Optional)*. https://grants.nih.gov/
grants/guide/notice-files/NOT-OD-21–036.html (accessed October 22, 2024).

NIH. 2022a. *About OIR*. https://oir.nih.gov/about (accessed October 22, 2024).

NIH. 2022b. *Ending Structural Racism*. https://www.nih.gov/ending-structural-racism/
developing-extramural-workforce-diversity-inclusivity-biomedical-research-ecosystem
(accessed August 11, 2024).

NIH. 2022c. *NIH-Funded Research Workforce*. https://www.nih.gov/ending-structural-racism/
nih-funded-research-workforce (accessed August 11, 2024).

NIH. 2022d. *Reproductive Scientist Development Program (RSDP) (K12 Clinical Trial Not
Allowed)*. https://grants.nih.gov/grants/guide/rfa-files/RFA-HD-23–012.html (accessed
October 2024, 2024).

NIH. 2022e. *RFA-OD-22-014: Specialized Centers of Research Excellence (SCORE) on Sex
Differences (U54 Clinical Trial Optional)*. https://grants.nih.gov/grants/guide/rfa-files/
RFA-OD-22–014.html (accessed October 14, 2024).

NIH. 2023a. *Impact of NIH Research: Direct Economic Contributions*. https://www.nih.gov/
about-nih/what-we-do/impact-nih-research/serving-society/direct-economic-contributions
(accessed August 7, 2024).

NIH. 2023b. *Personnel Demographics (End FY23)*. https://oir.nih.gov/sourcebook/personnel/
irp-demographics/intramural-research-program-personnel-demographics-end-fy23
(accessed August 22, 2024).

NIH. 2023c. *Trends in Race/Ethnicity of NIH-Supported Ph.D. Recipients, 1997–2021*.
https://report.nih.gov/nihdatabook/report/270 (accessed August 11, 2024).

NIH. 2023d. *Women's Reproductive Health Research (WRHR) Career Development Program
Overview*. https://www.nichd.nih.gov/research/supported/wrhr (accessed October 22,
2024).

NIH. 2024a. *Budget*. https://www.nih.gov/about-nih/what-we-do/budget (accessed October 22,
2024).

NIH. 2024b. *Chief Officer for Scientific Workforce Diversity*. https://diversity.nih.gov/about-us
(accessed August 11, 2024).

NIH. 2024c. *Division of Program Coordination, Planning, and Strategic Initiatives (DPCPSI)
Staff*. https://dpcpsi.nih.gov/staff (accessed October 22, 2024).

NIH. 2024d. *NHLBI R35 Outstanding Investigator Award (OIA) and Emerging Investigator
Award (EIA) Program*. https://www.nhlbi.nih.gov/grants-and-training/policies-and-guidelines/
nhlbi-r35-outstanding-investigator-award-oia-and-emerging-investigator-award-eia-program
(accessed October 22, 2024).

NIH. 2024e. *Number of NIH Principal Investigators Funded by Grant Mechanism and
Ethnicity*. https://report.nih.gov/nihdatabook/category/26 (accessed August 11, 2024).

NIH. 2024f. *RFA-HD-25-005: Women's Reproductive Health Research (WRHR) Career
Development Program (K12 Clinical Trial Optional)*. https://grants.nih.gov/grants/guide/
rfa-files/RFA-HD-25–005.html (accessed October 14, 2024).

NIH. 2024g. *RFA-OD-24-013: Building Interdisciplinary Research Careers in Women's
Health (BIRCWH) (K12 Clinical Trial Optional)*. https://grants.nih.gov/grants/guide/
rfa-files/RFA-OD-24–013.html (accessed October 14, 2024).

NIH. 2024h. *Specialized Centers of Research Excellence (SCORE) on Sex Differences 2024
Annual Meeting Keynote and Capstone Addresses*. https://orwh.od.nih.gov/about/news-
room/events/specialized-centers-of-research-excellence-score-on-sex-differences-2024-an-
nual-meeting-keynote-and (accessed October 22, 2024).

NIH. 2024i. *Success Rates: Non-Research Project Grants.* https://report.nih.gov/nihdatabook/category/11 (accessed August 11, 2024).

NIH. 2024j. *Understanding Research Career Development (K) Award Specifics.* https://www.niaid.nih.gov/grants-contracts/understanding-research-career-development-k-award-specifics (accessed October 22, 2024).

NIH. 2024k. *UNITE Progress Report 2023–2024.* https://www.nih.gov/sites/default/files/research-training/initiatives/ending-structural-racism/2023–2024-unite-progress-report.pdf (accessed August 11, 2024).

NIH. 2024l. *Women's Reproductive Health Research (WRHR) Career Development Program (K12 Clinical Trial Optional).* https://grants.nih.gov/grants/guide/rfa-files/RFA-HD-25–005.html (accessed October 22, 2024).

Nobel Foundation. 2024. *All Nobel Prizes.* https://www.nobelprize.org/prizes/lists/all-nobel-prizes/ (accessed October 22, 2024).

Okeigwe, I., C. Wang, J. A. Politch, L. J. Heffner, and W. Kuohung. 2017. Physician-scientists in obstetrics and gynecology: Predictors of success in obtaining independent research funding. *American Journal of Obstetrics and Gynecology* 217(1):84.e81–84.e88.

ORWH (Office of Research on Women's Health). n.d.-a. *Building Interdisciplinary Research Careers in Women's Health (BIRCWH).* https://orwh.od.nih.gov/our-work/building-interdisciplinary-research-careers-in-womens-health-bircwh (accessed August 11, 2024).

ORWH. n.d.-b. *Research Supplements to Promote Reentry and Reintegration into Health Related Research Careers.* https://orwh.od.nih.gov/career-development-education/research-supplements-promote-reentry-and-reintegration-health-related (accessed August 11, 2024).

ORWH. n.d.-c. *Specialized Centers of Research Excellence on Sex Differences (U54 Clinical Trial Optional).* https://orwh.od.nih.gov/sex-gender/orwh-mission-area-sex-gender-in-research/specialized-centers-of-research-excellence-on-sex-differences-u54-clinical-trial (accessed August 11, 2024).

ORWH. 2023. *Report of the Advisory Committee on Research on Women's Health, fiscal years 2021–2022: Office of Research on Women's Health and NIH support for research on women's health.* Bethesda, MD: National Institutes of Health.

Parchem, J. G., C. D. Townsel, S. A. Wernimont, and Y. Afshar. 2022. More than grit: Growing and sustaining physician-scientists in obstetrics and gynecology. *American Journal of Obstetrics & Gynecology* 226(1):1–11.

Raymond, N. C., J. F. Wyman, S. Dighe, E. M. Harwood, and M. Hang. 2018. Process evaluation for improving K12 program effectiveness: Case study of a National Institutes of Health Building Interdisciplinary Research Careers in Women's Health research career development program. *Journal of Women's Health* 27(6):775–781.

Rennels, C., S. G. Murthy, M. A. Handley, M. D. Morris, B. K. Alldredge, P. Dahiya, R. Jagsi, J. L. Kerns, and C. Mangurian. 2024. Informal caregiving among faculty at a large academic health sciences university in the United States: An opportunity for policy changes. *Academic Psychiatry* 48(4):320–328.

Reue, K., and A. P. Arnold. 2023. Inclusion of sex as a biological variable in biomedical sciences at the undergraduate level and beyond. *Journal of Women's Health* 32(8):891–896.

Rothenberg, E. 2024. *U.S. Scientists Are Leaving Academia: That's Bad News for Drug Companies.* https://www.cnn.com/2024/04/01/business/scientists-drug-companies-academia/index.html (accessed August 27, 2024).

Sadovsky, Y., A. B. Caughey, M. DiVito, M. E. D'Alton, and A. P. Murtha. 2018. Research to knowledge: Promoting the training of physician-scientists in the biology of pregnancy. *American Journal of Obstetrics and Gynecology* 218(1):B9–B13.

Schust, D. J. 2024. *The Reproductive Scientist Development Program. Presentation to the NASEM Committee on the Assessment of NIH Research on Women's Health, Meeting 5, Part 1 (May 20, 2024).* https://www.nationalacademies.org/documents/embed/link/LF2255DA3DD1C41C0A42D3BEF0989ACAECE3053A6A9B/file/D4F5FD21DE0E10CE06AC5CFB7927B7E3654629229B9D?noSaveAs=1 (accessed May 20, 2024).

Shaw Prize. n.d. *The Shaw Prize in Life Science and Medicine*. https://www.shawprize.org/prizes-and-laureates/life-science-medicine/ (accessed October 22, 2024).

Skarupski, K. A., D. L. Roth, and S. C. Durso. 2021. Prevalence of caregiving and high caregiving strain among late-career medical school faculty members: Workforce, policy, and faculty development implications. *Human Resources for Health* 19(1):36.

Twombly, D. A., S. L. Glavin, J. Guimond, S. Taymans, C. Y. Spong, and D. W. Bianchi. 2018. Association of National Institute of Child Health and Human Development career development awards with subsequent research project grant funding. *JAMA Pediatrics* 172(3):226–231.

Vassar, L. 2015. *How Medical Specialties Vary by Gender*. https://www.ama-assn.org/medical-students/specialty-profiles/how-medical-specialties-vary-gender (accessed August 11, 2024).

Wosen, J. 2023. *Exodus of Life Scientists from Academia Reaches Historic Levels, New Data Show*. https://www.statnews.com/2023/09/28/scientists-exodus-from-academia-historic-levels/ (accessed August 27, 2024).

Yank, V., C. Rennels, E. Linos, E. K. Choo, R. Jagsi, and C. Mangurian. 2019. Behavioral health and burnout among physician mothers who care for a person with a serious health problem, long-term illness, or disability. *JAMA Internal Medicine* 179(4):571–574.

Yong, C., A. Suvarna, R. Harrington, S. Gummidipundi, H. M. Krumholz, R. Mehran, and P. Heidenreich. 2023. Temporal trends in gender of principal investigators and patients in cardiovascular clinical trials. *Journal of the American College of Cardiology* 81(4):428–430.

9

Road Map to Prioritizing Women's Health Research

The vitality of women's health research (WHR) requires continuing efforts to build the cadre of talented WHR investigators, consistent investments in WHR to establish a strong scientific foundation, and effective oversight to ensure that research priorities are implemented and met. The National Institutes of Health (NIH) asked the committee to provide recommendations to improve NIH structure, systems, and review processes to optimize WHR; training and education efforts to build, support, and maintain a robust WHR workforce (i.e., those who undertake such research, not only women researchers); and the appropriate level of funding to address WHR gaps at NIH. The committee reviewed why WHR is needed (Chapter 2); the structure, policies, and programs related to women's health at NIH (Chapter 3); the level and distribution of funding for WHR at NIH (Chapter 4); biological (Chapter 5) and social (Chapter 6) factors that contribute to women's health in the United States; research gaps among diseases and conditions that are female specific, are more common among women, or affect women differently (Chapter 7); and NIH WHR workforce programs and support (Chapter 8). Based on its review, the committee concluded the approach at NIH is not meeting the scientific workforce's and, ultimately, the public's need for WHR.

Conclusion 1: A comprehensive approach is needed to develop a robust women's health research (WHR) agenda and establish a supportive infrastructure at the National Institutes of Health (NIH). Augmented funding for WHR, while crucial, needs to be complemented by enhanced accountability, rigorous oversight, prioritization, and seamless integration of women's health research across NIH Institutes, Centers, and Offices. This multifaceted approach is essential to fully capitalize on both existing and future funding and resources.

Conclusion 2: Overall, the National Institutes of Health (NIH) is underspending on research to support women's health, leading to significant scientific and clinical spending gaps on female-specific conditions and women's health conditions that do not fall within the primary expertise of existing NIH Institutes and Centers. The past 10 years' funding on women's health research have been flat and decreased as a share of overall NIH funding.

RECOMMENDATIONS OVERVIEW

In response to the sponsor's request to identify improvements to NIH structure, policies, and programs to advance WHR, the committee conducted a thorough and deliberate review of the investments and NIH structure to support WHR and recommends an integrated organizational approach to address the persistent gaps (see Recommendations 1–8). Figure 9-1 provides a high-level overview of key elements of the committee's recommendations.

The committee recommends that NIH build on and strengthen institution-wide policies that support advances in WHR. Accountability, priority setting, and oversight of women's health starts at the top of NIH with the Office of the Director (OD) but also sits squarely on the Institutes and

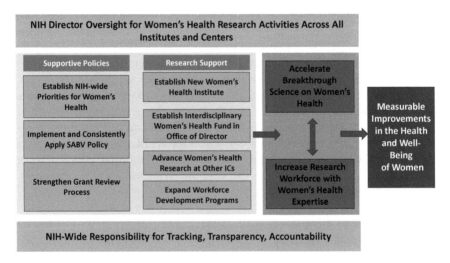

FIGURE 9-1 Recommended organization, structure, and actions to improve women's health research at the National Institutes of Health (NIH).
NOTE: ICs = Institutes and Centers; SABV = sex as a biological variable.

Centers (ICs). Without their engagement and commitment, progress will continue to lag. Needed crosscutting supportive policies include a data-driven and stakeholder-informed NIH-wide priority setting process that starts with the OD but also engages all ICs and Offices (ICOs), building on and expanding policies that support producing high-quality, impactful WHR, such as consistently implementing an enhanced sex as a biological variable (SABV) policy, and a more robust and informed grant review process that intentionally includes women's health expertise.

Creating a new WHR Institute is needed to support and build the body of research on female-specific conditions, as is creating a new interdisciplinary WHR fund, continued and increased contributions by the existing ICs, and a significant expansion in WHR training programs to support the workforce to build on the knowledge base. An infusion of new funds to conduct this research and train the workforce needs to accompany these changes, ultimately leading to major breakthroughs that would improve the health and well-being of U.S. women.

The committee identified five steps Congress and NIH should take to advance WHR:

1. Create pathways to facilitate and support innovative and transformative research for women's health;
2. Strengthen oversight, prioritization, and coordination for women's health research across NIH;
3. Expand, train, support, and retain the women's health research workforce;
4. Optimize NIH programs and policies to support women's health research; and
5. Increase NIH investment in women's health research.

The committee notes the tension between the support needed to build women's health and common needs for other areas of study. However, WHR represents an acute problem that requires immediate attention to address a long-standing gap and make needed breakthroughs. In addition, several of the committee's recommendations could be expanded to strengthen other areas of study (e.g., recommendations on tracking NIH investments, priority setting, and retention of the workforce).

CREATE PATHWAYS TO FACILITATE AND SUPPORT INNOVATIVE AND TRANSFORMATIVE WHR

NIH Organizational Structure

NIH's structure results from "a set of complex evolving social and political negotiations among a variety of constituencies, including Congress, the administration, the scientific community, the health advocacy community, and others interested in research, research training, and public policy related to health" (IOM and NRC, 2003, p.26). The evolution of NIH to the institution it is today is not the result of an intentional approach but rather an organic process responding to developments in knowledge, national health needs, and advocacy. NIH's structure does not adequately integrate or support women's health researchers or WHR and greatly limits its ability to ensure women's health is comprehensively addressed.

There is a lack of accountability within NIH to address women's health, and major constraints on the Office of Research on Women's Health (ORWH) hinder its ability to incentivize and persuade ICs to fund more priority women's health and sex differences research. In addition, many women's health conditions and women-specific life stages, such as gynecological issues other than cancer related and menopause, do not align with the priorities of the ICs. In its analysis, the committee found that WHR only accounted for 8.8 percent of NIH research spending from 2013 to 2023. This low rate of proportionate funding has decreased over time, with 9.7 percent of total NIH funding granted in fiscal year (FY) 2013 and 7.9 percent in FY 2023 (see Figure 4-2 in Chapter 4). Funding for several conditions, such as diabetes, pregnancy-related conditions, and perimenopause and menopause, appeared to derive from multiple IC sources. This indicates that these areas of research have not been consistently identified within the purview of any single IC. The relatively scant funding for most conditions relevant to women's health suggests these areas of research have also lacked a consistent IC source of funding or, sometimes, any IC funding at all (see Chapter 4).

An analysis of the challenges to supporting high-quality and innovative WHR needs to consider the broader structural and social barriers of gender bias and sexism within the United States—these biased systems informed NIH's founding and initial guiding frameworks focused primarily on cisgender men and their health (see Chapters 2 and 3 for examples of male-centered research as a foundation to NIH). Over the past several decades, NIH has launched major efforts to address these concerns, and despite progress, persistent gaps remain (see Chapter 8). To overcome the barriers described in this report, oversight for WHR is needed at NIH by an entity that can oversee strategic planning and implementation of processes and policies to expand WHR funding and ensure accountability (see Chapter 3 for an overview of the NIH structure and its limitations for WHR).

An option the committee considered is to maintain the NIH structure that designates ORWH as the main responsible entity. However, the committee concluded that the status quo has proven insufficient to address the research gaps and fulfill the NIH goal of fostering "fundamental creative discoveries, innovative research strategies, and their applications as a basis for ultimately protecting and improving health" for the nation (NIH, 2017).

As Chapter 3 described, ORWH is the hub for WHR at NIH. Despite many successes, it is a small, inadequately funded Office without the authority to require ICs to conduct WHR or oversee compliance with the NIH SABV policy. This has left a considerable gap in the attention to and investment in WHR across NIH. Without the ability to hold ICs accountable or power that comes with a large budget to support grants, the structure leaves WHR underfunded and understudied. ORWH lacks the needed authority, visibility, funding, and infrastructure to advance WHR.

> Conclusion 3: The current organizational structure of the National Institutes of Health limits its ability to address gaps in women's health research. There is inadequate oversight to ensure that women's health is studied comprehensively. There is limited ability for the Office of Research on Women's Health to incentivize Institutes and Centers (ICs) to prioritize research on women's health and sex differences. Furthermore, many women's health conditions and women-specific life stages do not easily align within the purview of the 27 existing ICs despite the millions of women who experience the burdens of these conditions.

The committee considered several structural solutions to improve WHR at NIH. It assessed these solutions for their potential to facilitate the study of female-specific conditions not prioritized by or under the purview of an NIH IC and to advance sex differences research; coordinate and implement NIH-wide strategic planning for WHR across the life-span; oversee strategic development of the WHR workforce; increase funding for WHR; and provide oversight and accountability for policies related to women's health and identified WHR priorities.

Potential Structural Changes at NIH to Ensure a Robust WHR Agenda

Keep the current organization but significantly increase funding for ORWH
One weakness of ORWH is its limited budget, which is too small to provide grants independently, forcing it to rely on partnering with other ICOs that might be interested in funding a topic that it identifies as a priority. For perspective, the National Institute of Deafness and Other Communication Disorders is one of the smaller ICs. It supports studies on hearing, taste, smell, and some communication problems. While these are important problems, its budget was $534 million in 2023—7 times that of ORWH 2023 budget ($76 million), which represents almost 51 percent of the U.S. population (Census Bureau, n.d.; Sekar, 2024).

Providing ORWH with significantly more funding would make it easier for it to invest in WHR priorities that the ICs are not fulfilling. However, without a major infusion of funds, it could not build the needed infrastructure—including staff and physical workspaces—to provide grants without partnering with another IC. It also would not have an intramural research program. The committee recognized that with sufficient funds, ORWH capacity could expand, enabling it to provide additional funds to the ICs for WHR, similar to the model the Office of AIDS Research uses, and increasing the chances that it could work with ICs to fill WHR gaps. However, the ICs will still need to prioritize WHR within their domains, and no mechanism would yet exist by which ORWH could incentivize other ICs and hold them accountable for investing in WHR. With a large funding increase, it could also undertake more strategic planning for workforce development and have more funds to offer ICs to participate in those programs.

A fund for WHR

Another solution the committee considered was to create a central fund for WHR in the OD to support interdisciplinary women's health and sex differences research with a focus on innovation and accelerating biomedical discoveries. This idea builds on NIH funds and initiatives with similar goals on different topics, such as the Common Fund, Cancer Moonshot, and Brain Research through Advancing Innovative Neurotechnologies (BRAIN) Initiative, discussed later.

The 2006 NIH Reform Act[1] created a "common fund," a funding entity within NIH that supports biomedical and behavioral research programs that the Division of Program Coordination, Planning, and Strategic Initiatives would administer. One of the Common Fund's criteria for funding is collaboration between multiple ICOs (NIH, 2024a). When the fund was first announced in FY 2004, each IC contributed 1 percent of its budget to it. That first year, the fund's budget totaled $132 million, or 0.5 percent of NIH's $27.9 billion budget (Erickson, 2014). With the 2006 NIH Reform Act, the Common Fund was authorized as a line item in the NIH budget, and in FY 2007, $483 million was appropriated, accounting for 1.7 percent of the NIH budget. The act stipulated that the fund could not drop to a lower percentage and anticipated a rise to 5 percent (Collins et al., 2014). This stable funding source allows NIH to develop unique programs that traditional funding mechanisms cannot support.

The Common Fund's budget has grown steadily since its inception. The FY 2025 budget request is $722.4 million, and it has ranged from $544 million in FY 2010 to its peak of $735 million in FY 2023 (NIH, 2010, 2024b). The fund supports research ranging from basic science to clinical applications, along with the development of new scientific methods and tools. In FY 2023, it reported funding of 23 scientific programs, 544 principal investigators (PIs), including 188 high-risk, high-reward PIs, 102

---

[1] Public Law 109–482 (January 15, 2007).

of them early-career PIs.[2] It had 142 competing research project grants and 23 ICOs coleading programs (NIH, 2024b).

A central fund for WHR could be modeled after the Common Fund. The ICs would compete for funds, presenting novel areas of WHR. If similarly administered at the level of the NIH director, it would have a template, making it easier to implement. It could be staffed by experts in women's health, thereby growing NIH's internal expertise. It would encourage coordination and interdisciplinary approaches because it would prioritize applications submitted by ICs working together. Centrally situated, the fund would enable exploring a wide range of WHR topics.

Another example is the Cancer Moonshot, a comprehensive initiative the government launched in 2016 to accelerate progress in cancer research and improve prevention, detection, treatment, and care. The 21st Century Cures Act[3] authorized $1.8 billion to it from 2017 to 2023 (NCI, n.d.). The initiative represents a significant national effort to transform cancer research and care, beyond the substantial investment that NIH was already making. The research it generated has improved the understanding of cancer biology and risk factors, contributed to developing new diagnostics and treatments, and enhanced collaboration across the cancer research community (NCI, 2023).

The BRAIN Initiative, a comprehensive research effort aimed at revolutionizing understanding of the human brain, launched in 2013 and invested $680 million in FY 2023 (BRAIN Initiative, 2024a,b; White House, n.d.). Congress funds it from two streams: line items in the budgets of 10 ICs provide a base allocation and funding authorized by the 21st Century Cures Act serves as a supplement (BRAIN Initiative, 2024b). The BRAIN Initiative is a partnership between federal and nonfederal collaborators and has contributed to innovative tools and technologies and new methods for monitoring and manipulating neural activity (BRAIN Initiative, 2023, n.d.). This could also be a model for collaboration with industry to prioritize women's health and address additional gaps in the field (e.g., joint funding of projects or specific application calls for products specific to women or studies on sex differences in adverse events from medications).

A WHR fund in the OD would also help continue breaking down the research silos that inhibit WHR, incentivizing ICs to prioritize WHR and collaborate to identify the most innovative and pressing needs in a multidisciplinary manner. However, it alone would not address the need for coordination, accountability, oversight, and workforce development identified by the committee or result in a home for female-specific conditions outside

---

[2] Yearly averages for FY 2019–FY 2023.
[3] Public Law 114–255 (December 13, 2016).

the purview of existing ICs. Although some of these mechanisms could be built into fund administration, such as some aspects of coordination, the administering Office would not have the capacity to ensure a robust research agenda for female-specific conditions or oversee the work of ICs.

Create a new WHR institute

One proposed solution the committee considered is to create an institute that focuses on women's health. This would highlight the prominence of women's health at NIH, but it is a complicated solution. As discussed in previous chapters, aspects of women's health are and should be integrated into existing ICs, capitalizing on the expertise of the ICs' staff and extramural research community. However, the ICs do not comprehensively cover all pressing diseases and conditions that affect women, leaving significant research gaps.

One of the major concerns with creating a women's health institute is the potential to isolate WHR. However, creating a women's health institute does not imply that the other ICs are only about men's health, and it would not need to be chartered with the goal of addressing all of women's health at NIH. For example, the National Cancer Institute (NCI) would still need to address women's cancers, and the National Heart, Lung, and Blood Institute would still address cardiovascular disease in women, including how the condition and its treatments affect women differently. Therefore, the committee considered a new institute with a narrow mission—with the primary responsibility to lead, conduct, and support research on female physiology and chromosomal differences, reproductive milestones across the life course, and female-specific conditions that do not fall under the purview of other ICs. The institute would support clinical and public health research relevant to women and girls and also harness the relevant expertise of the other ICs, as is now done between existing ICs.

An Institute is subjected to a higher level of oversight, as Congress assesses the work of the ICs, increasing accountability. However, since other ICs would still study women's health, a high level of coordination would still be required to sustain cross-IC collaboration on WHR if a new institute were created. Thus, this solution alone would not address all the shortcomings in the organizational structure.

A women's health institute could oversee peer review for studies on women's health and establish study sections that represent the expertise needed to address women's health and sex differences research, which other ICs could also use. It would house deep expertise in such research in its staff, something ORWH cannot do because it is a small Office, such that it would be a resource to all of NIH. It would also provide a "home" and grants for conditions specific to women that are not prioritized by other ICs, such as endometriosis, fibroids, pelvic floor disorders, polycystic ovary syndrome, and vulvodynia, while also developing and funding the next generation of researchers. As Chapter 8 discussed, growing WHR requires a robust workforce, and WHR might appeal more to early-career investigators if they know a stable institute exists where they can apply for grants, another positive aspect of creating the institute.

ICs that oversee research receive more funding than NIH Offices because they are expected to fund intramural and extramural research to fulfill their mission. However, they have a range of funding levels, with NCI receiving $7.3 billion in FY 2023 and the National Center for Complementary and Alternative Medicine receiving $170 million (NIH, 2023a,b). Congress would need to fund an institute on WHR at a level commensurate with its task—that is, conducting and funding research and serving as a reservoir of experts on WHR, a resource for peer review, and a collaborator with other ICs.

One important barrier to creating a new institute is that NIH authorizing legislation, the NIH Reform Act states:[4] "In the National Institutes of Health, the number of national research institutes and national centers may not exceed a total of 27, including any such Institutes or Centers established under authority of paragraph (2) or under authority of this title as in effect on the day before the date of the act enactment of the National Institutes of Health Reform Act of 2006." The secretary of the Department of Health and Human Services (HHS) would need to eliminate one IC or merge one with another, or congressional action would be needed to expand the number of ICs allowable.[5]

The committee considered the consequences of restraining biomedical science to a prespecified organizational structure. Medical and surgical subspecialties continue to evolve as clinical practice changes based on new evidence. Modern approaches to managing most chronic illnesses involve collaborations that were uncommon just a few decades ago. As Chapter 3 discussed, NIH has made changes as research has advanced and new health priorities have evolved. For example, the National Institute on Minority Health and Health Disparities (NIMHD) was first an Office and then a Center before becoming an Institute (NIMHD, 2024a). It is worth asking how often highly competitive, forward-looking organizations are locked into a permanently fixed organizational structure. Even within NIH, ICOs regularly evaluate their internal structure in relation to evolving strategic objectives. Typically, appointing a new IC director triggers a new strategic plan that often involves internal reorganization.

Since the last NIH reorganization in 2006, there have been remarkable advances in genetics, cell biology, computer science, artificial intelligence, social epidemiology, and health care delivery. Individual research

---

[4] Public Law 109–482, 120 Stat. 3676 (January 15, 2007).
[5] Public Law 109–482 (January 15, 2007).

investigation has given way to large interdisciplinary collaborative efforts and team science. As a result, it may be appropriate to reexamine the organization of the world's most influential biomedical research enterprise.

Recently, members of Congress have shown interest in changing the structure of NIH. In 2024, Senator Bill Cassidy (R-LA), ranking member of the Senate Health, Education, Labor, and Pensions Committee, released a white paper with recommendations to modernize NIH, including that it increase its focus on maintaining a balanced portfolio so all stages of medical research and other public health priorities are funded adequately (Cassidy, 2024). In June of 2024, Representative Cathy McMorris Rodgers (R-WA-05), chair of the House Energy and Commerce Committee, released a proposal to overhaul NIH that calls for combining ICs to reduce the number from 27 to 15, concluding that the uncoordinated growth at NIH has led to research gaps and duplication of effort, stating these and other shortcomings have affected its ability to respond appropriately to new scientific and public health challenges (Rodgers, 2024) (see Chapter 1 for more information). While the idea of creating a new WHR institute seems on its face contradictory to the conclusion that uncoordinated growth is a problem at NIH, if this is implemented with appropriate oversight and accountability, such issues could be avoided while also providing the support needed for WHR. It was outside the purview of the committee to assess the pros and cons of either proposal, but it attests to the need for NIH to change as new needs surface. The committee notes, however, that neither proposal mentions women's health or sex differences research. Such proposals are unlikely to be considered by the current Congress but could form the basis for future discussion. Any such reorganization requires careful consideration by Congress on how to integrate WHR to best meet the current and evolving needs of women.

Oversight for WHR activities by the NIH director

Establishing a new institute and research fund would provide avenues for increased funding for innovative science across ICs and research on female-specific conditions that do not fall under the priorities or purview of the 27 ICs. However, these actions do not provide a mechanism of accountability for prioritizing WHR across NIH. A new institute on women's health would not have authority over other ICs; this duty could be given to the NIH director, the only person with direct authority over the ICs, who could set annual benchmarks with the ICs for WHR and provide an annual report to Congress on progress. This oversight is essential for the success of WHR at NIH.

A Path Forward

Based on its review, the committee concluded that the NIH structure for WHR is insufficient to catapult it forward to address the urgent need and persistent gaps. Rather, progress will continue to be slow and stagnant for many conditions. Given the complexity of women's health, the committee concluded that no single solution could address the support needed to develop a robust WHR enterprise. A constellation of changes is required. For example, providing ORWH with significantly more funding to partner with ICs would still leave the problems of independent administration of grants in high-need areas, coordination, authority, clout, and accountability unaddressed. Creating an institute on women's health with a broad scope and purview would duplicate the expertise in other ICs that study health conditions that impact women more or differently than men, though currently research on women is not prioritized. Creating an institute with a narrower scope would be an effective strategy but still leave women's health conditions that fall in the purview of other ICs underfunded. Each strategy alone would not ensure women's health is integrated and prioritized, and each involves tradeoffs. Therefore, the committee recommends

Recommendation 1: The National Institutes of Health (NIH) should form a new Institute to address the gaps in women's health research (WHR) and create a new interdisciplinary research fund. Furthermore, NIH leadership should expand its oversight and support for WHR across the Institutes and Centers (ICs). Congress should appropriate additional funding to adequately support these new efforts. Specifically,

1a. Congress should elevate the Office of Research on Women's Health (ORWH) to an Institute with primary responsibility to lead, conduct, and support research on female physiology and chromosomal differences, reproductive milestones across the life course, and female-specific conditions that do not fall under the purview of other ICs.

- Certain programs currently housed in ORWH, such as women's health workforce development programs, and their corresponding budget will be part of the new WHR Institute.
- The new WHR Institute should have a dedicated independent budget comparable to that of other NIH Institutes with similar scope, amounting to at least $4 billion over the first 5 years.

1b. Congress should establish a new fund for WHR in the Office of the Director to support interdisciplinary women's health and sex differences research with a focus on innovation and accelerating biomedical discoveries. The fund should have a dedicated independent budget comparable to that of other major NIH initiatives, such as the Common Fund, Cancer Moonshot, and BRAIN Initiative. The fund will ramp up over the first 2 years, achieving full funding of $3 billion in Year 3, with a total investment of $11.4 billion over the initial 5 years.

1c. The NIH director and IC directors should prioritize WHR. The NIH director should assume oversight and responsibility for the WHR portfolio across NIH with respect to funding allocations and implementation of priorities, such as sex as a biological variable, and policies relevant to women's health. IC directors should increase support for WHR that falls under their purview.

- The NIH director, in collaboration with IC directors, should set annual benchmarks in the year-to-year proportion of extramural and intramural funding to be granted for WHR, following a comprehensive analysis of research needs (see Recommendation 3).
- The NIH director should evaluate progress on addressing WHR gaps and associated funding levels across NIH and should submit an annual report to Congress and to the public on the year-to-year trends by IC. The Office of the Director should receive additional funds to support NIH-wide programmatic evaluation and increased administrative responsibilities.
- The Director of the National Institute on Minority Health and Health Disparities (NIMHD) should expand the Institute's role to include women, girls, and females among the populations that experience disparities. Congress should increase NIMHD's budget to adequately support including women's health disparities research into its portfolio and coordinate this research with other ICs.

Guidance for Creating the New WHR Institute

Implementing Recommendation 1a—creating a new WHR Institute—would require a statutory change by Congress or a reorganization of ICs, since the NIH Reform Act[6] limits ICs to 27. The new WHR Institute would work closely with other ICs. This includes, for example, the *Eunice Kennedy Shriver* National Institute of Child Health and Human Development, which would continue its focus on human reproduction and the study of pregnancy as it relates to fetal and child outcomes. Other ICs would cofund grants or cosponsor program announcements on WHR with the new Institute. Table 9-1 lists the roles and responsibilities of the new WHR Institute proposed by the committee.

The new WHR Institute should have a dedicated independent budget comparable to that of other ICs with similar scope: $4 billion over the first 5 years followed by a reassessment at 5 years to determine if the subsequent annual budget—recommended at $800 million—is sufficient to meet the need. This is commensurate with the budgets of midsize Institutes

---

[6] Public Law 109–482 (January 15, 2007).

TABLE 9-1 Roles and Responsibilities for Women's Health Research at NIH: Committee Recommendations

Existing ICs	• Existing ICs should continue to support WHR that falls under their purview/expertise but increase their investment in research for conditions that have been understudied in females and women, such as sex differences in cardiovascular and Alzheimer's disease and certain women's cancers, via
	  ○ Increasing the proportion of their budget spent on WHR, and
	  ○ Accessing new funding from the newly created WHR fund.
	• Existing ICs should support research that rigorously assesses if findings from research on conditions that affect both women and men, including conditions known to affect women differently than men, are valid for women and assess sex and gender differences.
	• NIMHD should expand its role regarding women, girls, and females as populations that experience disparities; funding for NIMHD should be increased to adequately support the inclusion of women's health disparities research into its portfolio and in its coordination of aspects of this research focused on social and structural determinants with other ICs.

New Women's Health Research Institute	• The new WHR Institute will have primary responsibility for supporting intramural and extramural research across female life stages, with a focus on female physiology and chromosomal differences and conditions that do not fall under the purview or priorities of other ICs, such as fibroids, polycystic ovary syndrome, endometriosis, vulvodynia, pelvic floor disorders, pregnancy outcomes relevant to the mother, the menopause transition, biomedical and clinical study of sex and gender diversity, and health effects of hormonal changes across gender identity groups. • The new WHR Institute will not be the primary funder of research in areas that fall within the expertise of other ICs, such as cancer, neurologic, cardiometabolic, autoimmune, mental health conditions. However, it may partner with other ICs on these topics, such as studying endometriosis and fibroids as risk factors for cancer.
New Women's Health Research Fund	• Funds will be available to all ICs, including the new WHR Institute, to support interdisciplinary research on women's health and sex differences by, for example, prioritizing multi-IC applications. There should be a focus on innovation and accelerating biomedical discoveries. • It will be housed in the OD; oversight and accountability will sit with the OD. • It will have a dedicated independent budget comparable to that of the other NIH initiatives, such as the BRAIN Initiative, Common Fund, and Cancer Moonshot.

(continued)

TABLE 9-1 Continued

ORWH	• ORWH will be elevated to become the new WHR Institute. Once the transition of elevating ORWH to a WHR Institute is complete, ORWH as a coordinating Office would no longer be needed, as the NIH director would take on this role (see "Director of NIH" section in this table). The current roles of ORWH should be divided between the new WHR Institute and the OD. The new WHR Institute will oversee workforce programs such as the Building Interdisciplinary Research Careers in Women's Health, Specialized Centers of Research Excellence on Sex Differences, and Women's Reproductive Health Research Career Development programs. The OD should oversee the implementation of the sex as a biological variable and inclusion in clinical trials policies. • During the transition to establish the new WHR Institute, ORWH will continue its current responsibilities and assist in establishing the Institute.
Director of NIH	• Has oversight and responsibility for the WHR portfolio across NIH regarding funding allocations, implementation of priorities, and policies relevant to women's health, which aligns with the director's responsibility for "providing leadership to the Institutes and for constantly identifying needs and opportunities, especially for efforts that involve multiple Institutes" (NIH, 2024f). • Sets benchmarks with each IC on the proportion of its portfolio that will focus on WHR priorities. • Reports annually to Congress on the status and progress on achieving WHR priorities.

NOTE: BRAIN = Brain Research through Advancing Innovative Neurotechnologies; IC = Institutes and Centers; NIH = National Institutes of Health; NIMHD = National Institute on Minority Health and Health Disparities; OD = Office of the Director; ORWH = Office of Research on Women's Health; WHR = women's health research.

with a similar scope, such as the National Eye Institute, National Institute of Environmental Health Sciences, and National Institute of Arthritis and Musculoskeletal and Skin Diseases (NIH, 2023a).

As the recommendation notes, the new WHR Institute would be responsible for many programs ORWH oversees, including WHR workforce programs. Increased funding for workforce programs (see Recommendation 5) and the infrastructure afforded by an Institute will allow for strategic development of the women's health workforce. Responsibilities that require oversight to ensure accountability, such as the SABV and clinical trial inclusion policies and prioritization setting, should move to the NIH director. The new WHR Institute could not oversee policies other ICs implement, since one IC cannot oversee others. As part of its work, the WHR Institute should undertake communication and dissemination responsibility for new WHR findings and discoveries. This includes translating scientific evidence into practice for the public, researchers, relevant medical associations and other organizations, policymakers, and industry.

One might ask, why not have an institute on men's health? As discussed throughout this report, the majority of research focused on men's health as the default. Diagnostic and treatment criteria based on one sex for non-sex-specific diseases has typically been based on men, leading to persistent misunderstanding and underdiagnosis of the disease in women (see Chapter 5 for examples). While NIH has made important strides toward balancing representation by sex in research, more needs to be done, including ensuring that researchers conduct sex differences analyses. Perhaps once WHR has benefited from the same dedication and resulting innovation for prevention, diagnosis, and treatment as research that has mainly focused on men, some efforts recommended for women's health will no longer be needed, and rigorous research that benefits men and women will be the norm across ICs. Unfortunately, that is not the current state.

Guidance for the New Women's Health Fund

The WHR Fund (Recommendation 1b) would operate much like the NIH Common Fund, supporting interdisciplinary women's health and sex differences research with a focus on innovation and accelerating biomedical discoveries. It would also serve as a mechanism through which the NIH director can ensure all ICs have an opportunity to contribute to WHR in collaborative and innovative ways in line with their missions. The goal of the fund is to continue supporting scientific initiatives that fall under individual ICs and provide a mechanism for collaboration with the new WHR Institute.

The fund would be used primarily to support research involving collaboration between at least two ICs to encourage interdisciplinary research and submission of grant proposals in novel areas of WHR. The ICs initiating the idea would oversee successful applications. Special emphasis panels would evaluate competing grants, unless a relevant study section has at least one WHR expert.

The new fund should have a dedicated, independent budget of $3 billion per year with an initial ramp-up of $900 million in Year 1 and $1.5 billion in Year 2. The committee estimated that rapid progress requires a 10 percent increase in funding. NIH provides approximately 60,000 grants per year (Lauer, 2023), so 10 percent amounts to 6,000 grants. Using a conservative estimate of $500,000 per grant (Lauer, 2023), a $3 billion annual investment is needed. While this amount is larger than previous initiatives, such as the Cancer Moonshot and the BRAIN Initiative, it is necessary based on the committee's assessment. This is critical given that the low rate of proportionate funding for women's health has decreased over the past decade, with 9.7 percent of total NIH funding in FY 2013 and 7.9 percent in FY 2023 (based on the committee's analysis, see Chapter 4), with an average 8.8 percent investment in FY 2013–FY 2023. Overcoming the tremendous gaps in knowledge of women's health, from understanding basic female physiology to successful prevention, diagnosis, and treatment, requires a significant investment to urgently address these gaps and offset delayed progress on improving the health of over half the U.S. population (Census Bureau, n.d.).

Role of NIMHD

NIH should increase its support of science focused specifically on health disparities among women and girls and coordinate this research with other ICs. Health disparities research furthers identification of the epidemiology and mechanisms of social and structural factors affecting disparate outcomes among women and among subgroups of women across various health conditions.

NIMHD has been a leader in increasing the scientific community's focus on nonbiological factors, such as socioeconomics, politics, discrimination, culture, and environment in relation to health disparities. As Chapter 3 discussed, it initially focused solely on racial and ethnic disparities in health but has added several other domains. Though women and girls are not a minority group in the United States, they experience well-documented discrimination, bias, and subjugation that are root causes of health disparities (see Chapter 6). NIMHD is well suited to support research and training specifically on disparities experienced as a function of the treatment of sex, gender, and the status of women, both specifically and intersectionally. To do so adequately, NIMHD would need significantly more funding to expand its portfolios under its Division of Clinical and Health Services Research[7] and Community Health and Population Science.[8] The committee was unable to develop an estimate for the increased amount, as it requires a deeper understanding of the NIMHD portfolio to do so. The committee is not proposing any new authoritative or organizational structures, but program officers with expertise in gender- and sex-related health disparities

---

[7] "Under this research interest area, NIMHD supports a comprehensive range of clinical research and health services research to generate new knowledge to improve health/clinical outcomes and quality of health care for populations that experience health and health care disparities" (NIMHD, 2024c).

[8] "The Division of Community Health and Population Science supports research on interpersonal, family, neighborhood, community and societal-level mechanisms and pathways that influence disease risk, resilience, morbidity, and mortality in populations experiencing health disparities" (NIMHD, 2024b).

would be needed if they are not already present. As the committee recommends for other ICs, this work would be coordinated by the NIH director.

Oversight of WHR by the NIH Director

Oversight and accountability within NIH, and by key external stakeholders, is essential for progress on WHR. Recommendation 1c includes routine evaluation and oversight of activities across all NIH ICs regarding funding allocations and implementation of priorities and policies relevant to women's health. The OD will require additional funds to operationalize its WHR evaluation and oversight role, but the committee did not have the needed NIH budget information to estimate the amount. Some ORWH funds might be available, but the portion of the ORWH budget supporting existing programs, such as Building Interdisciplinary Research Careers in Women's Health (BIRCWH) and Specialized Centers of Research Excellence (SCORE) on Sex Differences, should be included in the budget of the new WHR Institute.

The Office of Autoimmune Disease Research (OADR) sits in ORWH and was created in the 2022 in response to a National Academies of Sciences, Engineering, and Medicine (National Academies) report, *Enhancing NIH Research on Autoimmune Disease* (NASEM, 2022a; OADR, n.d.). Although the Office currently sits in ORWH, it should not be moved to the new WHR Institute. Many autoimmune diseases disproportionately affect women but also affect men. The 2022 report found that "autoimmune diseases are complex and share commonalities that would benefit from a coordinated, multidisciplinary research approach to better understand basic mechanisms, etiology and risk factors, and to support the development of interventions to mitigate the impact of autoimmune diseases and associated co-morbidities and complications across the lifespan" (p. 417) and that the best option for addressing these challenges and opportunities would be creating an Office of Autoimmune Disease in the OD. Therefore, this is one possible option.

Summary of Recommendation 1

Recommendation 1 is fundamental to advancing WHR at NIH. If the same structure remains, progress on WHR will continue to be slow, incremental, sporadic, and insufficiently responsive to women's urgent health needs. While the infrastructure for the new WHR Institute and Fund is being developed, ORWH should continue its role. Should a new WHR Institute not be created, the next best solution would be for ORWH to have a significant and meaningful infusion of funding, as with money comes influence, and that would allow it to partner with more ICs on identified priorities for WHR and workforce development across NIH. However, oversight is needed at a high enough level to ensure priorities are met, which would still be lacking.

STRENGTHEN OVERSIGHT, PRIORITIZATION, AND COORDINATION FOR WHR ACROSS NIH

Tracking NIH Investments in WHR

As discussed in Chapter 4, the NIH Research, Condition, and Disease Categorization (RCDC) system is unable to accurately report the proportion of the NIH budget devoted to WHR overall or for specific conditions within women's health. The committee suggests alternative accounting systems and methods to improve accuracy. Due to multiplicative counting of grants in RCDC categories, misclassifications, and other factors, the system is inadequately designed to guide budget allocations and inform Congress and the public on how much is spent in distinct research areas.

Conclusion 4: The Research, Condition, and Disease Categorization (RCDC) system—the system designed to sort National Institutes of Health (NIH)-funded projects into scientific categories for reporting to the public by conditions, diseases, and research area—does not provide accurate estimates of NIH spending on women's health research. The RCDC system, in its current form, is inadequate for guiding budget allocations; for informing Congress and the public on how much is spent in any distinct research area, by condition or disease, or by Institute or Center; or for reliably tracking changes in funding over time.

Recommendation 2: The National Institutes of Health (NIH) should reform its process for tracking and analyzing its investments in research funding to improve accuracy for reporting to Congress and the public on expenditures on women's health research (WHR).

2a. The new process should improve accuracy of grants coded as Women's Health and eliminate duplicate or multiplicative counting of grants across Research, Condition, and Disease Categorization (RCDC) categories. This may be achieved by applying proportionate accounting of grants to generate more accurate estimates for categories related to WHR.

2b. NIH should update its process for reviewing, revising, and adding new RCDC categories that pertain to WHR.

2c. NIH should make transparent and accessible the process and data used for portfolio analysis so researchers, analysts, and the public can examine and replicate NIH investments into research for women's health.

Recommendation 2, and retrospective funding analyses, should be facilitated by expanding the use of modern data analysis methods, such as large language models (LLMs; see Chapter 4 and Appendix A) that can efficiently identify and categorize content of a grant with equal or superior accuracy and reliability compared to historical systems. The committee's funding analysis could serve as a model for NIH to refine and test. The committee used LLMs because of their ability, as very large deep learning models, to process human language and derive predictions on vast amounts of similar data based on pretraining. A successful LLM algorithm can accurately identify and categorize a grant as related to women's health based on all available relevant information, just as a human should be able to confidently perform the same task after learning from experience and training what kind of title, abstract, or narrative is characteristic of such a grant. NIH is already using LLMs for some aspects of its portfolio analysis (NASEM, 2024b); further development and expansion of these approaches to more efficiently and effectively assess spending on WHR are needed. Because state-of-the-art LLMs can be especially helpful for identifying and categorizing investments in biomedical areas that are crosscutting, including WHR, newer LLM methods can also be used to accurately analyze the allocation of funding for many other research areas supported by NIH. Furthermore, updated methods may allow NIH to track a more extensive set of diseases and conditions, given their ability to quickly assess funding-related data.

Priority Setting for WHR

The significant gaps in WHR at NIH are the result of the substantial historical underrepresentation, lack of accountability, inadequate funding, and dearth of comprehensive research that have long characterized this field. Decades of insufficient focus have resulted in critical knowledge deficits and disparities in health outcomes for women. Investments in WHR need to be allocated in a targeted way to ensure it bridges these research gaps. The prioritization process is failing to establish or implement cohesive and cross-agency priorities for WHR, resulting in a lack of responsiveness to critical research gaps and perpetuating knowledge gaps (see Chapter 3). To address these issues, a comprehensive, NIH-wide prioritization process is needed.

Conclusion 5: Most National Institutes of Health (NIH) Institutes and Centers (ICs) have a strategic plan to inform their research priorities, but these plans rarely mention women's health. In addition, the strategic plans of the ICs do not include elements of the NIH-Wide Strategic Plan for Research on the Health of Women, which outlines important strategic priorities. The timing of the IC plans varies significantly, with some at the beginning, middle, or end of their respective timelines when the agency-wide plan is released. This complicates NIH's ability to set, implement, and oversee cohesive and cross-agency priorities for women's health research that are responsive to critical research gaps. Furthermore, the data and input used to inform these plans are not always clear. To address these issues, a comprehensive prioritization process is needed—one that fully uses available data and community input.

Recommendation 3: The Director of the National Institutes of Health (NIH) should develop and implement a transparent, biennial process to set priorities for women's health research (WHR). The process should be data driven and include input from the scientific and practitioner communities and the public. Priorities of the director and the Institutes and Centers (ICs) should respond to the gaps in the evidence base and evolving women's health needs. To inform research priorities for women's health, NIH should

3a. Employ data-driven methods, such as epidemiologic studies and disability or quality-adjusted life years, to assess the public health effect of conditions that are female specific, disproportionately affect women, or affect women differently. NIH should report this assessment publicly and use it, in combination with other analyses as needed (e.g., of expected return on investment), to identify research priorities and direct funding for WHR.

3b. To ensure priorities for WHR are implemented, ICs should issue Requests for Applications, Notices of Special Interest, Program Announcements, and similar mechanisms, in addition to current funding activities.

This process would allow IC directors to still have discretion to enact their strategic priorities and address emerging issues (such as during the COVID pandemic), while also being held accountable to ensure that women's health and sex differences research is prioritized.

EXPAND, TRAIN, SUPPORT, AND RETAIN THE WHR WORKFORCE

To address WHR, it is essential to have a robust and productive NIH intramural and extramural research workforce with broad expertise in biomedical research, clinical trials, and implementation science. The committee found that NIH support of the WHR workforce falls short of what is needed to address the unmet needs of women's health (see Chapter 8). Investment is needed to develop the next generation of researchers. IC program staff also need expertise in women's health for effective prioritization and coordination. Inadequate funding of WHR has led to an insufficient number of investigators and even fewer with interest and expertise in women's health at the intersection of other important social identities, including race and disability.

WHR Career Pathways

Chapter 8 underscores the need for NIH and other stakeholders to comprehensively prepare a broad-based effort to train a robust research workforce that meets the needs for WHR. Achieving this goal requires a multifaceted, coordinated approach, including substantial support for training and retaining both laboratory-based researchers and physician-scientists specializing in women's health. Addressing workforce issues throughout the research career continuum—from high school through midcareer—is crucial. This includes enhancing educational opportunities for scientists at various stages, such as clinical and doctoral training programs. Recommendations 4 and 5 highlight opportunities to build and support the WHR workforce across the entire spectrum of career development.

Conclusion 6: Establishing a robust infrastructure for intra- and extramural research in women's health and sex differences at the National Institutes of Health is critical to success. The Institute and Center program staff need a high level of expertise in women's health for effective prioritization and coordination. This infrastructure is needed to cultivate a vibrant women's health workforce, provide essential support for grantees and early-career researchers through funding and mentoring, and instill confidence in stable funding, thereby attracting researchers to women's health research topics.

Conclusion 7: Inadequate funding of women's health research (WHR) has led to an insufficient number of WHR investigators and even fewer with interest and expertise in studying women's health at the intersection of other important social identities, such as race and disability. A coordinated approach to attracting and supporting researchers across their careers to make meaningful discoveries in women's health is needed. The current grant mechanisms are inadequate to support career trajectories in WHR. Increased funding allocation and expanded numbers of career support grants for early-career investigators in WHR are needed from mentorship to conception of ideas for grant proposals, including sponsorship, mentorship, and protected time through training grants.

Conclusion 8: Mentorship and career development are vital to the development of the extramural women's health research (WHR) workforce and for maximizing research dollars spent. Many institutions do not have the needed funding to support early-career clinician-scientists, particularly in surgical subspecialties, including obstetrics and gynecology. National Institutes of Health research funding does not provide funding for mentors in many WHR training grants, which is critical for progress.

Conclusion 9: Gender-based bias and sexism persist in the United States, including in its health and research systems. For the National Institutes of Health (NIH), these biases affect the grant review and award-making processes, from the initial application and review stages to funding allocation and the accumulation of multiple grants. NIH has acknowledged these issues and has implemented initiatives to address them. However, the research suggests that significant disparities remain, and further structural changes may be necessary to achieve equity in the grant-making process.

Conclusion 10: In addition to sexism, bias related to race and ethnicity has been identified as an independent and intersectional contributor to gaps in health research generally and women's health research specifically.

Recommendation 4: The National Institutes of Health (NIH) should augment existing and develop new programs to attract researchers and support career pathways for scientists through all stages of the careers of women's health researchers.

4a. NIH should create a new subcategory within the Loan Repayment Program (LRP) for investigators conducting research in women's health or sex differences. K awardees who study women's health or sex differences should be automatically considered for an LRP grant. For every year in the program, awardees should receive loan repayment assistance up to $50,000 for up to 5 years, allowing up to $250,000 in loan repayments.

4b. NIH should create new and expand existing early-career grant mechanisms (K, T, and F grants) that specifically support growing and developing the women's health research workforce. Appropriate models for new mechanisms are the Stephen I. Katz and Grants for Early Medical/Surgical Specialists' Transition to Aging Research awards. These grants should prioritize early-career investigators with innovative approaches focused on women's health.

4c. NIH should create new and expand existing midcareer investigator awards to support and promote the midcareer women's health research workforce (e.g., K24, R35, U, P, and administrative supplement grants).

4d. NIH should allow financial support of up to 10 percent, as a line-item component, for mentors (primary or designee mentor) on all mentored grants, such as F31, K01, K99, and T32 grants, that support careers of early and midcareer investigators in women's health and sex differences research.

4e. All early-career mentored institutional K-awards should be supported up to 5 years to increase the likelihood of retaining a workforce to study women's health.

The LRP is critically important to address the lifelong bias that disadvantages women economically and could ensure appropriate diversity within the workforce (see Chapter 8 for more information).

Creating new early-career mechanisms for WHR (Recommendation 4b) can be modeled on existing mechanisms. For example, the Stephen I. Katz award is an R01 research project grant for early-stage investigators' innovative projects that are a change in the research focus and have no preliminary data; it is intended to encourage innovation and new approaches by supporting new disciplines, techniques, targets, or methodologies (NIH, 2023c,d, 2024e). The award is open to research relevant to participating ICs' missions. Another example is the Grants for Early Medical/Surgical Specialists' Transition to Aging Research (GEMSSTAR) program from the National Institute on Aging aimed at early-career dentist- and physician-scientists starting a career in aging research in their clinical specialty area (NIA, 2024). To help meet the health care needs of the aging U.S. population with complex medical issues, the program is open to scientists with medical, surgical, or dental training in any specialty whose aging-related research will improve care and treatment options for older patients. Special emphasis panels with appropriate expertise review grant applications (Eldadah, 2021). This approach could be augmented for WHR. Though not a career development award, it uses the research grant (R03) mechanism to support the research project but also requires a professional development plan supported by non-R03 funding sources that includes activities concurrent with the R03 award that provide training and mentorship in aging science (NIA, 2024). GEMSSTAR awards can be a solid basis for competitive K applications (Eldadah, 2021). The new grants should target researchers interested in changing their field of study to involve a new or a more deliberate focus on women's health, including those from fields other than medicine, such as engineering, looking to use their skills to support WHR. It is also essential to ensure opportunities for midcareer investigators to further refine their skills and allow them to support early-career investigators (see Recommendation 4e). For example, the K24, R35, U, P, administrative supplement,[9] and similar grant mechanisms could be expanded (not all ICs offer these) and/or new mechanisms developed.

Another important consideration for the WHR workforce is the impact of caregiving on an individual's ability to fully participate in the NIH community, whether that be applying for grants or participating on NIH study sections or meetings. The 2024 National Academies report *Supporting Family Caregivers in STEMM: A Call to Action* has actionable recommendations to shift structural and policy solutions to increase women's and other primary caregivers' ability to participate in science (see Chapter 8 for more on this topic and the 2024 report [NASEM, 2024c]).

Expand WHR Workforce Development Programs

Several WHR workforce development programs the committee reviewed have been effective at launching and supporting researchers' careers. Increased funding and expansion of successful programs—BIRCWH, SCORE, Women's Reproductive Health Research (WRHR) Career Development Program, and Research Scientist Development Program (RSDP)—are vital to support and sustain these efforts. By addressing these critical issues and leveraging proven programs, NIH can help build a robust research workforce capable of addressing the complex needs of women's health (see Chapter 8).

> **Recommendation 5: The National Institutes of Health (NIH) should augment existing and develop new grant programs specifically designed to promote interdisciplinary science and career development in areas related to women's health. NIH should prioritize and promote participation of women and investigators from underrepresented communities.**
>
> **5a. NIH should double the Building Interdisciplinary Research Careers in Women's Health (BIRCWH) program to achieve a total of 40 centers, with 6 new centers awarded in the next fiscal year and 5 centers each of the following 3 fiscal years. NIH should augment funding for each center to $1.5 million annually, amounting to a total of $60 million per year for the enhanced BIRCWH program.**
>
> **5b. NIH should expand the Specialized Centers of Research Excellence (SCORE) on Sex Differences program by engaging Institutes and**

---

[9] See, for example: Notice of Special Interest (NOSI) NOT-OD-24-001: Administrative Supplements to Recognize Excellence in Diversity, Equity, Inclusion, and Accessibility (DEIA) Mentorship (https://diversity.nih.gov/act/DEIA-mentorship-supplements; accessed September 30, 2024).

Centers (ICs) to add 5 additional centers to achieve a total of 17 centers over the next 3 to 5 fiscal years. At least three of these centers should reside in the new Women's Health Research Institute (see Recommendation 1). The NIH director should provide incentives for other ICs to participate in this program, which could include the provision of matching funds from the Office of the Director. NIH should augment funding for each SCORE to $2.5 million annually, amounting to a total of $42.5 million annually for the enhanced SCORE program, with long-term commitment of funds to renew SCORE programs that meet their goals.

5c. NIH should fund additional multi-project program grants, with or without built-in training components, that focus on women's health research (e.g., P and U grants) to both expand research on these topics and to support researchers studying women's health across the career spectrum.

5d. NIH should expand the Women's Reproductive Health Research (WRHR) program to include 5 additional centers to achieve a total of 20 centers over the next 2 fiscal years. Existing centers that have demonstrated successful metrics should receive funding to host additional scholars. The funding for each center should be augmented to $500,000 annually, amounting to a total of $10 million annually for the enhanced WRHR program.

5e. NIH should expand the Research Scientist Development Program (RSDP) to support 10 scholars with full support, including salary, supplies, and travel, for a total of 5 years, amounting to $1.25 million annually for the enhanced RSDP program.

Any expansion should include additional funding to ensure that existing research budgets are not reduced. These programs should be distributed across the country, and grantee institutions should collaborate with other disciplines within their organization to offer mentees a comprehensive and multidisciplinary research experience. The expansion of these programs should be coupled with NIH IC programmatic staff support.

Regarding 5b, SCORE operates differently than the other workforce programs in that funding depends on an IC's interest in and capacity for it.[10] The structure constrains the number of possible topics, since SCORE relies on IC participation. To incentivize participation, NIH could change the structure of SCORE grants such that there is cost-sharing with substantial or matching funds from the OD or from the new WHR Fund (see Recommendation 1). Ideally, each IC would support at least one SCORE to

---

[10] For example, the 2024 SCORE Request for Applications (RFA) only included eight Institutes (NIH, 2022).

expand the impact of the program, as it builds both the evidence base for WHR and careers across the spectrum of career development. Implementation of Recommendation 5c would also support researchers who focus on women's health across the career spectrum. As the WHR workforce grows, implementing Recommendations 4c and 5c will become increasingly important to assure resources are available to support midcareer and senior faculty and ensure a solid career trajectory in WHR. These recommendations will also increase opportunities to fund innovative WHR, which could be funded in part by the WHR Fund.

Metrics to track success of these programs for workforce development include if those participating receive additional NIH funding, including R01 or equivalent grants, stay in academia, or participate as reviewers in special emphasis panels or study sections. See later in this chapter for a discussion on metrics.

The augmented funding for each program allows for different needs, including a line item to cover mentor time, funding to cover travel and supplies, and additional protected time for grantees to engage in clinical research. For example, funding for BIRCWH has been sparse. For example, the 2024 RFA set a maximum of $840,000 per year per center in direct costs (NIH, 2024d). This typically does not allow for support for mentors. Thus, the increase will almost the double funding per center and double the number of centers to broaden geographic diversity and expand overall impact.

Funding for SCORE has been lean, at a maximum of $1.5 million per year per center in total costs, with up to about $1 million in direct costs per year in the most recent RFA. This typically does not allow for full potential program development or any support for mentors contributing to the career enhancement core. The recommendation is to substantially increase funding per center and the total number of centers to broaden geographic diversity and expand overall impact. Similarly, adding five centers to the WRHR program will expand its reach, and increasing funding from approximately $315 to $500 million in direct costs per center will allow for more mentorship and protected time for research (NIH, 2024c). The RSDP program suffered cuts in recent years and can only partially cover its scholars using NIH funds (see Chapter 8 for more details on how RSDP is structured) (Schust, 2024). Increasing funding for each scholar from about $110,000 to $125,000 per year will allow for covering travel and supply costs. Adding three additional scholars will help grow the workforce of obstetricians and gynecologists who are most likely to address female-specific diseases, such as gynecologic cancers, fibroids, endometriosis, vulvodynia, and obstetric-related conditions.

OPTIMIZE NIH PROGRAMS AND POLICIES TO SUPPORT WHR

Peer Review

The peer review process is complex, with the Center for Scientific Review (CSR) overseeing tens of thousands of grants each year through a rigorous and thorough process on varied topics and areas (CSR, 2024). While progress has been made in many aspects of the peer review process, and concerted efforts by CSR continue, efforts to increase expertise on women's health in the process will continue to be essential moving forward. (See Chapter 3 for a discussion of a variety of proposals from academia and others to improve the peer review process and actions already underway by CSR).

Conclusion 11: Representation of women's health expertise is essential during the National Institutes of Health (NIH) peer review process— including expertise of staff in the Center for Scientific Review, Institute and Center program officers and council members, and peer reviewers. Despite NIH efforts to expand the cadre of reviewers with women's health research (WHR) expertise, a large proportion of WHR–related grants are evaluated by special emphasis panels, not standing study sections, indicating that standing study sections do not yet have the required expertise to review WHR grants.

Recommendation 6: The National Institutes of Health (NIH) should continue and strengthen its efforts to ensure balanced representation and appropriate expertise when evaluating grant proposals pertaining to women's health and sex differences research in the peer review process.

6a. NIH should sustain and broaden its efforts to systematically employ data science methods to identify experts, use professional networks, and recruit recently funded investigators.

6b. The NIH Center for Scientific Review (CSR) should expand the Early-Career Reviewer program to enroll qualified individuals from underrepresented areas of expertise in women's health and include women's health, sex differences, and sex as a biological variable training for participants.

6c. CSR should work with NIH-funded institutions to identify qualified individuals with expertise in women's health. Institutions would provide rosters of trained reviewers to CSR to enrich the pool of reviewers.

6d. In the immediate term, special emphasis panels should be used more often to ensure that applications for women's health and sex differences research receive expert and appropriate reviews.

SABV Policy

The NIH SABV policy, implemented in 2016, is designed to recognize the importance of sex in research and address the persistent exclusion or underrepresentation of females in preclinical and clinical research (Arnegard et al., 2020; Miller et al., 2017; ORWH, 2023) (see Chapter 3). Despite efforts by NIH to implement SABV policies across investigator-initiated scientific projects, uptake and application in practice has been suboptimal (Arnegard et al., 2020; White et al., 2021), hindering the potential generation of knowledge that could help to address sex disparities and improve women's health. ORWH has developed resources and training materials on the SABV policy and on sex and gender research for the research community, but the training has room for improvement—particularly in tailoring education for scientists conducting research in certain fields and using certain methodologies wherein SABV considerations may not be intuitive (see Chapter 3 for more information). There are opportunities to improve implementation of the SABV policy in NIH-funded research in part by incentivizing or requiring researchers to be accountable for proposing and conducting sex-specific analyses.

Conclusion 12: Addressing the persistent and extensive gaps in knowledge about how conditions disproportionately affect, present in, and progress differently in women requires that sex as a biological variable be meaningfully factored into research designs, analyses, and reporting in vertebrate animal and human studies.

Conclusion 13: The National Institutes of Health (NIH) sex as a biological variable (SABV) policy was an important advancement, and the number of grants addressing SABV has increased since the policy was implemented. However, overall uptake and application of SABV in practice has not been optimal. This is in part due to a lack of practical, field-specific SABV knowledge and experience among investigators as well as limited NIH oversight and assurance of implementation.

Conclusion 14: Although guidance and trainings on the National Institutes of Health sex as a biological variable (SABV) policy outline distinctions between sex and gender and indicate in some ways that studies of gender satisfy adherence to the policy, the current policy's language and implementation is not clearly geared toward studies of gender, gender identity, and intersex status. Explicit guidance on addressing intersex status and conditions and gender identity across its continuum within the SABV policy is needed.

Conclusion 15: There remains no cross-agency mechanism at the National Institutes of Health for assessing how sex as a biological variable (SABV) in grants is evaluated or for tracking appropriateness and completeness of SABV implementation in the conduct of research. Furthermore, there are no consequences for grantees if they do not implement the plans for SABV included in their grant proposals, and there are no incentives to do so.

Recommendation 7: The National Institutes of Health (NIH) should revise how it supports and implements its sex as a biological variable (SABV) policy to ensure it fulfills the intended goals. For its intramural and extramural review processes, where applicable:

7a. NIH should expand education and training resources for investigators on how to implement SABV, with separate programs that are more effectively tailored for scientists in distinct fields (e.g., basic, preclinical, clinical, translational, and population research).

7b. NIH should ensure that SABV is consistently and systematically reviewed. Reviewers should be required to undergo training to enable them to assess SABV in proposals and grant applications.

7c. The NIH Center for Scientific Review should, as part of the competitive renewal applications process, include an evaluation of grantee efforts and publications relating to previously proposed studies of SABV as it applies to the project funded in the last cycle, as well as that proposed in the current renewal application.

7d. To strengthen and foster research designed to rigorously examine sex, gender, or gender identity differences aimed at providing new insights into women's health, that research should

• Be protected from across-the-board budget cuts to protect the sample sizes and analyses needed to study sex differences.

• Have access to administrative supplements to ensure sex, gender, and gender identity differences can be studied rigorously and with adequate sample size.

• Have priority for funding when such projects fall in the discretionary range of the payline.

• Undergo a streamlined process for requesting higher budgets than those allowed by the program announcement or request for proposal.

7e. NIH should expand the SABV policy in human studies to explicitly factor the effect of biological sex, gender, and gender identity in research designs, analyses, and reporting to promote research on sex and gender diversity, including intersex status, gender expression, and nonbinary-identified populations. This expansion may involve adapting the policy language.[11]

Although Recommendation 7d would afford a status to grants that focus on SABV that is not available to all grants, the committee believes these actions are needed to incentivize and support investigators intending to address SABV meaningfully and support them in doing so. Research on sex differences benefits the entire population because, when sex is completely accounted for in study designs and analyses, the resulting discoveries have importance and impact for both sexes. After the study of sex differences becomes more consistently incorporated into NIH-funded research, these protections can be revisited. In addition, women-only cohorts should not be at a disadvantage based on the SABV requirement, given the lack of research on female-specific conditions.

INCREASE NIH INVESTMENT IN WHR

The committee was asked to "determine the *appropriate* level of funding that is needed to address gaps in women's health research at NIH" and recommend "the allocation of funding needed to address gaps in women's health research at NIH."

Defining the appropriate amount of funding is an ambiguous task, with many ways to conceptualize it. However, the committee interpreted this as a request to identify the level of funding necessary to catapult new efforts and bolster existing investments in NIH-supported WHR over the next 5 years and into the future.

Researchers are only beginning to understand the complexities of sex differences in health. Research on many female-specific conditions as well as research on the impact of gender and society on women's health has been neglected. To close this knowledge gap—compared to conditions that have benefited from extensive scientific understanding in prevention, diagnosis, and treatment—significant funding is essential. Even with adequate support, it will take decades to address these issues. Additionally, as research needs and gaps evolve, NIH needs to commit to sustaining efforts for WHR.

For example, a 2023 analysis found that $2.7 billion was spent globally on breast cancer research from 2016 to 2020, which was 11.2 percent of the total $24.5 billion invested in cancer research (McIntosh et al., 2023). NCI estimates show it spent approximately $2.7 billion during that time period (NCI, 2024). Of course, NIH research on breast cancer

---

[11] Recommendation 7 was changed after release of the report to clarify that it applies to both extramural and intramural research.

started much earlier—Congress appropriated $25 million for it in 1991 in the Army's Research, Development, Test, and Evaluation Program, laying the groundwork for decades of successful research (IOM, 1997). Other organizations have funded breast cancer research as well, synergistically building the knowledge base, but this has taken decades of investment, and effective grassroots advocacy made breast cancer a national research priority (Osuch et al., 2012). But, as Chapter 7 noted, despite significant progress, important research gaps still remain for breast cancer. Considering the nascent state of research on numerous female-specific conditions, along with the gaps in understanding differences in health effects between sexes, the substantial investment dedicated solely to breast cancer for early detection and effective treatment underscores the vast resources that would be required to achieve comparable advancements across all women's health conditions.

If making progress on WHR is a priority for NIH, the committee concluded that more than an increase in funding is needed. Augmented funding needs to be supported by enhanced accountability, rigorous oversight, prioritization, and seamless, sustained integration of women's health across all NIH structures and processes. The committee notes in its recommendations and surrounding text where increased funding will be needed to advance WHR and increase the workforce and expertise in women's health.

Table 9-2 summarizes where funds are needed based on the committee's recommendations to address research gaps. Sometimes, the information to estimate the amount to implement a recommendation was not available. NIH will need to assess those instances, as it requires more detailed knowledge of operational costs and capacity than is publicly available.

The committee recommends $15.71 billion in new funding be appropriated to invest in women's health and sex differences research and workforce development over the next 5 years. This includes an initial ramp-up of the new women's health fund—$900 million in Year 1 and $1.5 billion in Year 2—and therefore an estimated annualized investment of approximately $3.87 billion in new funding in Years 4–5 to implement the recommended actions by the committee. Over the 5-year period, this would approximately double the average NIH yearly investment in WHR (which was $3.41 billion on average over the past 5 years based on the committee funding analysis). However, as noted, additional funds will be needed to cover operational costs, increased oversight by the NIH director, and increased funding for NIMHD. The level of funding recommended by the committee aligns with recommendations by other groups or organizations in recent years. For example, the White House called for a $12 billion investment in new funding for WHR at NIH, and Women's Health Access Matters called for doubling the WHR budget based on 2021 analyses (Baird et al., 2021; White House, 2024) (see Chapter 1 for more information).

TABLE 9-2 New Funding Needed to Accelerate Progress to Fill the Women's Health Research Knowledge Gap

Action	New Funding (in Millions of Dollars)					Total 5-Year Funding (New)	Total 5-Year Funding (New and Existing)
	Year 1	Year 2	Year 3	Year 4	Year 5		
New Institute	$800.000	$800.000	$800.000	$800.000	$800.000	$4,000.000	$4,000.000
New Fund	$900.000	$1,500.000	$3,000.000	$3,000.000	$3,000.000	$11,400.000	$11,400.000
Expanded Workforce Programs*	$42.770	$56.795	$66.795	$74.295	$74.295	$314.950	$314.950
Total New Funding	**$1,742.770**	**$2,356.795**	**$3,866.795**	**$3,874.295**	**$3,874.295**	**$15,714.950**	**$15,714.950**
Existing Research Funding for WHR^	$3,405.000	$3,405.000	$3,405.000	$3,405.000	$3,405.000	-	$17,025.000
Total Funding	**$5,147.770**	**$5,761.795**	**$7,271.795**	**$7,279.295**	**$7,279.295**	**$15,714.950**	**$32,739.950**

NOTES: *Expanded workforce programs are: BIRCWH, RSDP, SCORE, WRHR. ^Existing research funding is the estimated average spending on WHR 2019–2023 based on the committee's funding analysis and includes the historical workforce investments; assumes no change in years 1 to 5, although this number should increase each year as NIH Institutes and Centers prioritize WHR. New funding calculations are based on Recommendation 5 in this report, with initial ramp-up of BIRCWH in years 1–4, SCORE in years 1–3, and WRHR in years 1 and 2. Current funding for workforce programs was subtracted from the total recommended amount in years 1–5 to calculate expanded workforce program funding. BIRCWH = Building Interdisciplinary Research Careers in Women's Health; RSDP = Reproductive Scientist Development Program; SCORE = Specialized Centers of Research Excellence on Sex Differences; WHR = women's health research; WRHR = Women's Reproductive Health Research Career Development Program.
SOURCES: Existing funding data for BIRCWH, RSDP, SCORE, and WRHR used for these calculations from NIH, 2022, 2024c,d; Schust, 2024; other calculations are based on funding levels in Recommendation 5 in this report.

These investments are only a first step. Moving the United States on a path to improve quality of life and decrease morbidity and mortality resulting from conditions that are female specific, disproportionately affect women, or affect women differently than men requires sustained commitment, additional funding, and accountability. In an ideal world, far greater than this amount would be invested in the short term, as the need is urgent and the weight of neglecting research on women's health falls not only on half of the population, but society as a whole.

TRACKING AND ACCOUNTABILITY

Monitoring and assessing progress on investments in research on the health of women is a complex and challenging undertaking requiring a wide range of data inputs and tools to meet the needs of NIH, Congress, and the public. Ultimately, the outcomes of taxpayer investments in WHR should be measurable scientific advances leading to demonstrated improvements in the health and well-being of women and girls across the nation, including those who have been marginalized and disenfranchised by society. Preventing and treating disease and promoting women's health requires the research enterprise to prioritize studies across the basic science to translational research spectrum. Assessing success of various NIH efforts to increase and improve WHR, both what it has implemented and what this committee recommends, involves examining accurate and transparent data reflecting what research NIH funds, whom NIH funds, the workforce composition, and how much women's health care and health outcomes change at the population level as a function of improved science.

A standardized and transparent approach to collecting and reporting data on WHR over time is fundamental to establishing metrics for tracking the success of financial and workforce investments. The committee provides several options that would assist policy makers, researchers, and the public in establishing success metrics and tracking NIH performance. They span from tracking short-term outcomes, such as the size and composition of the workforce or ICs' spending allocations, to longer-term outcomes that can measure the effect of scientific advances related to women's health. The following section highlights data inputs already collected and monitored but not assessed systematically or collectively to track WHR and not all uniformly publicly reported. The following section also identifies new, needed sources of data. The committee provides key measures for tracking progress, which may need to be adjusted as progress in WHR advances. Regardless of which key metrics NIH ultimately reports on, the measures should not be burdensome to the agency and the research community to collect and analyze, clearly and concisely reported to Congress, and directly meaningful to WHR.

Funding Allocation Trends

A core necessity is an accurate accounting of spending on WHR. Existing issues with the system make it difficult to develop a clear picture of what NIH is spending on WHR arising from counting grant funds in multiple RCDC categories with the full grant allocation, difficulties in accurately identifying grants on WHR, and lack of consistency in categorization over time (see Chapter 4 and Recommendation 2). One area presenting a challenge that needs to be addressed is how to allocate studies involving pregnant people that focus on fetal or child outcomes and whether they should be counted directly as WHR. The committee suggests NIH should track this funding separately but report it alongside WHR (see Chapter 4).

Since the RCDC categories are limited (see Recommendation 2), NIH should consider an alternative approach, perhaps the comparative analysis LLM model strategy this study used or tailoring new approaches that assess a larger number of conditions and categories and provide users with options to investigate new topics and assessments as issues arise. NIH should continue track the WHR funding in multiple ways: over time as an aggregate amount, as a percentage of NIH funding overall, by IC, by condition, and in relation to disease burden. The committee understands this will not be a straightforward task initially, but it is needed to adequately establish metrics and use data to track success. A system that can track these metrics for WHR will also likely enable a wide range of stakeholders to understand investments across other NIH programs and priority areas.

Accurately tracking NIH investments is a valuable tool as a proxy for progress on WHR at NIH, but it is also important to track the balance of research in the NIH portfolio. A valuable approach would be to update and continue an analysis, such as the 2021 study that illustrated gender disparities in NIH allocation of funds across diseases by assessing disease burden, of which gender is a major factor, and funding level (Mirin, 2021). NIH's portfolio should also balance the range of methodologies, health conditions, and issues. It is important that NIH track what proportions of WHR are conducted within translational, disparities, behavioral, clinical, and basic research methodological frameworks.

Suggested Metrics for Funding/Investment

- Accurately count spending on intramural and extramural WHR as an absolute amount and as a percentage of all NIH grant funding in a consistent and unduplicated manner.
  - Report funding as absolute spending and percent of NIH grant funding by IC.
  - Report spending on the range of conditions that are female specific, are more common in women, or affect women differently.

- o Include funding for grants that are focused in part on maternal health but are more focused on fetal and child outcomes, but note the proportion of funding in this maternal-child health category separately from other WHR categories.
- Measure sex and gender disparities in NIH allocation of funds across diseases.

Women's Health Workforce Trends

It is imperative to develop the scientific workforce across disciplines and research settings to increase its capacity to address unmet needs in WHR and biases against women and gender minorities. NIH should track funding for workforce training and development at NIH overall and across ICs, relative to the total investment in workforce pathways and programs.

Tracking the effect of investing in workforce grants and programs that support women's health researchers will be essential to ensure the workforce is growing to meet the challenge of addressing the immense gaps in WHR. This could be done by tracking the NIH-funded early-career investigators who continue to publish and procure NIH grants. While NIH already tracks publications in general,[12] it should add WHR specifically across all funding mechanisms. NIH already collects data on grants awarded by recipient sex, race, and ethnicity but does not regularly assess the intersections of these categories. NIH should regularly report on the intersection of sex with race and ethnicity in WHR grants and look at these measures by career stage, number of grants, and retention. These metrics are needed to ensure that growth in the workforce is equitable.

In addition, NIH should track the types of expertise these training programs support to identify where gaps exist and help tailor outreach and efforts to broaden the workforce and ensure grantees and scholars from different fields and subspecialties are being supported and trained. Ultimately, it would be ideal to track the types of expertise that all WHR grants support to understand the disciplines or specialties where NIH is funding the WHR workforce and where gaps exist. One possibility would be to include this information in grant applications, and, if funded, for NIH RePORTER to list it. The measurement goal of such tracking is to identify whether the range of disciplines needed to optimize scientific innovation are represented.

One example that may help track workforce-related measures is CareerTrac, a "production-level, outward-facing, Web-based system serving multiple ICs" (NIEHS, 2024). This application collects trainee data and information using existing systems such as xTrain, IMPACII, and PubMed, as well as entries from the principal investigator or directly from the trainee

---

[12] For example, see https://dpcpsi.nih.gov/opa/Publications (accessed October 13, 2024).

through the Trainee Portal, though participation is optional, and only a few ICs participate (NIEHS, 2024, n.d.). However, this system or a similar approach would need to be recalibrated to assess the specific metrics mentioned here and used across ICs.

Data on existing NIH expertise, both internally and among those serving NIH through scientific review processes, are needed to assess whether it is adequate to support this committee's recommended increase in WHR research. No publicly available data or internally examined reports indicate the foci and expertise of NIH staff—both at the program level, such as in program officers at ICs that oversee grants or among staff at CSR who oversee peer review, and among intramural researchers—that would help assess possible substantive gaps in the workforce to support current and future efforts in WHR. Furthermore, tracking the proportion of these researchers represented in study sections is needed to evaluate progress in this area. Their expertise is required to ensure the grant review process reflects these research and funding priorities and that knowledge gaps regarding women's health are recognized and addressed.

Suggested Tracking Metrics for Workforce

- Amount of funding to women's health training grants relative to total training grant funding.
- Composition of the WHR workforce including the discipline, types of research expertise, specialty and subspecialties, and demographic characteristics of individuals supported by these WHR workforce development grants.
- Retention of grantees in academic, industry, and government research.
- Amount of funding to women's health mid/late career awards relative to the total of such funding, including at the intersection of sex, gender identity, race, and ethnicity.
- Areas of WHR expertise of NIH staff—both for program staff and intramural researchers.
- Proportion of women's health and sex differences researchers represented in study sections.

Research Process, Output, and Impact

A key issue in building the evidence base on the health of women and girls is accurately assessing where research has not considered it, whether because of underrepresentation in study samples or the failure to assess whether or how the findings differed by sex and gender. Simply expanding research to include women, who account for half the U.S. population, has not and will not correct for using diagnostic criteria based on disease presentation and trajectories in men. Fully prioritizing investment in the health of women and girls requires understanding not only what proportion of research funding examines their health but also the size and nature of the gaps in an evidence base built on the study of cisgender men, including their presentation of diseases and conditions, diagnosis, incidence, and prevalence, and treatment and outcomes.

NIH needs several additional forms of tracking it does not support, such as comprehensively tracking how well grants fulfilled the SABV policy by not only enrolling females in studies but also assessing for sex and gender differences in study results and reporting these findings. This would strengthen the implementation of SABV by supporting advances in understanding where and how sex and gender differences affect prevention, diagnosis, treatment, and outcomes and accelerate a shift in the scientific culture regarding the conduct and reporting of sex and gender analyses. NIH should consider systematic and periodic reviews of funded studies to report whether they assessed sex and gender differences. These reviews need to distinguish between whether studies found no sex differences or whether they did not assess sex differences. This distinction is crucial, as failing to assess sex differences does not imply evidence of their nonexistence or nonsignificance. To better assess gender differences, the enrollment tables required in grants that include male/female boxes could be updated to be inclusive of gender minorities. In addition, many of the gaps in sexual and gender minority (SGM)-related work are related to a lack of measurement and data. To assess this, NIH-supported research would need to include SGM-specific variables (see *Measuring Sex, Gender Identification, and Sexual Orientation* for more information) (NASEM, 2022b).

Unfortunately, relying on external investigators invested in documenting the WHR landscape or artificial intelligence approaches for scans of the published literature is likely not enough to address the decades of research that overlooked women, dismissed the scientific study of sex and gender differences in disease course, and failed to assess whether and how study results differ for women. The committee recognizes that simple counts of publications are limited as an evaluative metric, but the public does not benefit from funding research when the results are not made public. NIH itself needs to monitor and track the published literature or require post-award reporting from investigators on their publications related to WHR to assess how well SABV is implemented throughout the research process, not just at the point of application, and assess the collective findings of those efforts.

Ultimately, the aim of public investment in biomedical and public health science is to improve the health and well-being of the population. A core marker of success of NIH's investment in WHR and science is evidence of improved health care services and practice and ultimately improvement in women and girls' health at the population level. Another set of important metrics would be cataloging and tracking whether and how NIH-funded WHR results in published best practices or evidence-based interventions and scientific patents and new technologies. This could include developing a database for WHR similar to the Evidence-Based Intervention compendium developed by the Centers for Disease Control and Prevention (CDC) for HIV interventions (CDC, 2024). It would allow for searching and tracking the range of services, technologies, and interventions rigorously developed for women and girls and also facilitate designing effective approaches to disseminating findings to key stakeholders beyond journal readership and inform dissemination strategies and the evaluation of remaining barriers to advancing evidence-based health care for women. NIH could work with the Agency for Healthcare Research and Quality (AHRQ) and CDC to assure such research discoveries reach the public.

In the interest of tracking movement in women and girls' health, more coordination among entities within HHS is needed to develop data sources that assess core areas. This includes strengthening federally collected public health surveys, including the National Health Interview Survey, National Survey of Family Growth, Medical Expenditure Panel Survey, and National Health and Nutrition Examination Survey to include data on often ignored and emerging relevant issues. NIH should collaborate with its counterpart agencies—CDC, National Center for Health Statistics, AHRQ, and the Substance Abuse and Mental Health Services Administration—to develop a strategy to use national surveys to monitor changes in the health of women and girls. These surveys may also offer the opportunity to add, leverage, or improve data on gender minorities and people with intersex conditions under the framework of WHR, addressing another long-standing information gap.

Suggested Metrics for Research Outcomes, Processes, and Impact

- Track the extent to which grants fulfilled the NIH SABV policy, by not only enrolling females in studies but also assessing sex and gender differences in study results and reporting these findings and identified trends.
- Track whether NIH-funded research in women's health results in published best practices or evidence-based interventions; track research productivity by monitoring peer reviewed publications, article citations, and popular media coverage of research studies.
- Catalogue scientific patents and new technologies developed through WHR grants.
- Monitor long-term outcomes by tracking to what extent women's health care and health outcomes change at the population level,

including by race and ethnicity and geographic location, as a function of improved science.

Summary of Tracking and Accountability

Data to support many of the suggested metrics the committee identified are already collected but could be improved. It may also be necessary to develop other types of measures and methods for collecting these metrics. In both cases, the data need to be monitored with oversight by the NIH director and used to set NIH-wide and IC-specific priorities for WHR and assess their effect.

WHR PRIORITIES: LOOKING FORWARD

There are exciting opportunities to advance WHR, with substantial opportunities to apply new science and discovery to improve the lives of not only women but, in the case of sex differences research, the health of all. Significant knowledge gaps remain in prevention, diagnosis, and treatment for WHR. However, by cultivating a well-trained and adequately supported workforce, along with supportive policies, careful prioritization, and accountability for progress, the potential for meaningful progress in women's health is considerable.

Given the breadth of conditions that are female specific, are more prominent in women, and progress differently in women, and the need to support innovation into new lines of inquiry over time, the committee does not provide specific priority conditions to be studied. Instead, it describes types of research needed along the translational science continuum from basic science to preclinical, clinical, implementation science, and population-based research.

The committee based these priority areas on a combination of its review (see Chapters 2, 5, 6, and 7), public input (see Chapter 1), and recent National Academies reports (NASEM, 2022a, 2024a). Of particular relevance is the research agenda laid out in the 2024 report *Advancing Research on Chronic Conditions in Women*, which should also be used as a guide for women's health researchers (NASEM, 2024a). Progress in these research areas will advance the field's understanding of the etiology of multiple conditions (Sciarra et al., 2023). For example, studies have shown that many conditions relevant to women's health share similar inflammatory pathways. In addition, diseases often have sex differences in clinical presentation, which can be related to these inflammatory processes (NASEM, 2024a; Overstreet et al., 2023). Studying these conditions will improve health in the long term for women, and understanding sex differences and how they contribute to risk and pathogenesis of disease will also lead to important findings for improving the health of the entire population.

Research on the role of sex, gender, gender identity, and sex beyond the binary within each type of research will improve health across the population by improving an understanding of the mechanisms through which these factors play a role in disease prevention, development of health conditions, and treatment outcomes. Within these areas, funding should be allocated by a process like that described in Recommendation 3.

> Recommendation 8: The National Institutes of Health should prioritize research that includes but is not limited to the following:
> 1. Basic science research:
>   a. Research that rigorously assesses hormonal profiles and basic female physiology to understand the mechanisms of biological sex differences in risk factors, disease prevalence, pathology, and progression, such as studies to improve the understanding of sex steroid hormones and how they integrate with the nervous and immune systems to influence disease.
>   b. Research to increase the understanding of sex chromosome influence on lifetime sex differences in health and disease.
>   c. Research that explores variability in hormone signaling within biological sexes (animal and human models) and gender (human models) groupings, including assessing the impact of physical and social environments on behavioral and physiological endpoints.
>   d. Research that reveals the physiology and pathophysiology of pregnancy, including mechanisms for normal and abnormal labor, and how pregnancy may increase risk for future disease.
>   e. Research that includes human and animal studies to enhance bidirectional translation of findings that will lead to a mechanistic understanding of adaptive and maladaptive brain responses to stress and ovarian hormone changes across the life-span.
> 2. Preclinical research:
>   a. Research to understand basic etiology of female-specific and gynecologic chronic conditions.
>   b. Research to improve understanding of the lifetime effects of stress and trauma on the function and structure of the brain and female hormonal response.
>   c. Research to understand how the hormonal changes and variation across the female life course, such as puberty, menstruation, pregnancy, and the menopause transition, affect physical and mental health outcomes and clinical manifestations and treatment efficacy.

3. Clinical research:
   a. Treatment studies that collect and analyze data separately for women and men to identify any differences in efficacy, side effects, and overall effects with attention to hormonal, genetic, and metabolic factors that might influence pharmacokinetics, pharmacodynamics, and efficacy of drugs and biologic therapies as well as behavioral interventions.
   b. Well-powered, clinical trial research focused on the management of peri- and postmenopause symptoms with existing medications, supplements, and alternative treatments. For example, although depression is the leading cause of menopause-related impairment, no randomized controlled trials have examined the comparative effectiveness of existing treatments for perimenopause-onset depression.
   c. Large-scale, randomized, controlled trials to disentangle the effects of hormonal treatments for the menopause transition from the effects of aging (e.g., cardiovascular, cognitive, immune, metabolic) and other risk factors and to examine their synergistic effects on both risk and resilience.
   d. Large-scale studies to disentangle the effects of hormonal fluctuations during pubertal onset among girls and gender minorities with uteruses on cognition, mental health, and well-being from the effects of social and other risk factors.
   e. Studies to improve diagnosis, reduce misclassification, and improve treatment of female-specific conditions and those more common in women, such as endometriosis, polycystic ovary syndrome (PCOS), vulvodynia, fibroids, chronic pain, multiple chronic conditions, and autoimmune diseases.
   f. Large randomized controlled trials to test the effectiveness of interventions for the leading causes of maternal morbidity and mortality, including mental health disorders, cardiac disease, preeclampsia, and postpartum hemorrhage, and social factors, such as food insecurity, lack of transportation, intimate partner violence, and racism.
4. Population-based research:
   a. Research that leverages community input to reduce health inequities by recognizing and managing structural and interpersonal discrimination, recognizing the importance of health, and engaging community resources to address social determinants and advocacy to address structural determinants.
   b. Research that investigates how health-promoting lifestyle behaviors influence health conditions in women, the extent to which these behaviors have uniform effect across subgroups of

women, and mechanisms to address the structural and social determinants that affect individuals' ability to engage in such behaviors.

c. Research that studies the mechanisms by which structural and social determinants, such as poverty, discrimination (racism; sexism; bias against lesbian, gay, bisexual, transgender, queer or questioning, intersex, and asexual [LGBTQIA+] people), gender-based violence, and workforce conditions impact women's health, affect health care access and treatment outcomes, and identifies how to mitigate harms and improve outcomes.

d. Research that investigates the role of structural and social determinants, such as criminalization systems and social, health, and reproductive policies, on health and health care access and assesses interventions that prevent and mitigate their impact.

e. Research that studies how policies at the system, payor, local, state, and national levels affect women's health and whether there is disparate effect of these policies on women at greater risk for marginalization and poorer health outcomes, such as racially and ethnically minoritized women, women with disabilities, women living in rural and geographically isolated communities, sexual and gender minority populations, and those who are low income.

5. Across the research spectrum:

a. Research that prioritizes conditions that impact a women's quality of life (such as depressive disorder, endometriosis, fibroids, irritable bowel syndrome, osteoarthritis, osteoporosis, PCOS, sleep disturbance/disorders, and substance use disorders) to reduce the amount of time women live with painful or debilitating conditions, as well as conditions that cause early mortality, including cardiovascular disease and female-specific cancers.

b. Studies of the interaction of sex and gender in the design and analysis of preclinical and clinical studies.

c. Research that prioritizes studying women from minoritized groups to address the enhanced marginalization of being both a woman and a part of other groups experiencing discrimination, such as being racially and ethnically minoritized or having LGBTQIA+ status, disability status, or higher weight.

d. Expanded research focused on pregnancy that is centered on women and those capable of pregnancy, before, during, and after pregnancy, as well as nulliparity and improving basic understanding of hormonal effects, including factors that contribute to differences in health and adverse pregnancy outcomes among subgroups who have been historically marginalized or who have disproportionately faced discrimination, as well as clinical and systemic interventions to eliminate these disparities.

e. Research that advances and improves sexual and reproductive health. This includes the development of more effective interventions to prevent and address undesired pregnancies, support desired pregnancies, and identify and implement innovative approaches to facilitate access to the full range of reproductive and sexual health care services, including abortion, family formation and fertility assistance, avoidance of sexually transmitted diseases, and contraceptive care. Research that documents the disparate impact on health and well-being when access to these services is denied is also needed, particularly among groups that otherwise experience discrimination and marginalization.

f. Investigations into why diseases manifest differently in women and men and why women are more or less prone to certain diseases. Consideration should be given to variability in disease manifestation within and across subgroups of women and girls, which may be related to chromosomes, hormones, environment, or epigenetics.

g. Studies of the interaction of gender and epigenetics and how the environment women live in throughout their life-span (such as exposure to adverse childhood experiences, hormonal axes, epigenetics, substance use, toxins, violence, and discrimination) affects the development and manifestation of illness and leads to diseases later in life.

h. Within-group analyses should also be recognized as a gold standard in research methodologies instead of the traditional epidemiological approach that often involves comparing outcomes between racially and ethnically minoritized women and White women. In addition, it is essential to emphasize the importance of adequately powering studies to include and represent groups experiencing discrimination.

6. Implementation science research:

a. Research that fills the gap between scientific advances in understanding women's health and successful implementation of evidence-based health promotion interventions across traditional and community settings.

b. Research that develops and tests strategies for community engagement for delivery of preventive and innovative health care services, particularly those that include and focus on communities experiencing health disparities.

These lines of inquiry will uncover new pathways to enhance women's health and generate the essential knowledge required to empower women to make informed decisions about their health, enable clinicians to deliver more precise and effective care, and provide policy makers with evidence-based insights for crafting informed and equitable health policies.

CONCLUDING OBSERVATIONS

Girls, women, families, society, and the economy all pay a price for the gaps in knowledge about women's health. In this report, the committee provides salient examples of critical deficiencies in the research enterprise's response to the needs of women and girls. It underscores the failure to address fundamental questions about female physiology, the lack of research into numerous debilitating conditions that disproportionately affect women, and the gaps in understanding how prevention, diagnosis, and treatments—often studied primarily in men—apply to women. Its analysis found that just 8.8 percent of NIH research dollars are spent on WHR, but even using NIH's estimate of 10 percent (Clayton, 2023; ORWH, 2023), this is not proportionate to the burden of disease. Most of the NIH WHR investment funds research on breast cancer, HIV/AIDs, and reproduction and pregnancy, areas that are all important, but the strategy has left behind many other pressing women's health conditions. The analysis also shows low levels of funding for many such conditions, including endometriosis, fibroids, pelvic floor disorders, PCOS, postpartum depression, uterine cancer, and vulvodynia, and trend analysis shows many of these conditions have had flat amounts of funding for the past decade. Addressing these needs will require more than increased funding for WHR; it will require dedicated action, careful prioritization, and oversight to ensure objectives are achieved. The committee's recommendations present the critical, transformative actions required to elevate WHR to a level that adequately supports the health needs of half the nation's population and benefits our total society.

REFERENCES

Arnegard, M. E., L. A. Whitten, C. Hunter, and J. A. Clayton. 2020. Sex as a biological variable: A 5-year progress report and call to action. *Journal of Women's Health* 29(6): 858–864.

Baird, M. D., M. A. Zaber, A. Chen, A. W. Dick, C. E. Bird, M. Waymouth, G. Gahlon, D. D. Quigley, H. Al-Ibrahim, and L. Frank. 2021. *The WHAM report: The case to fund women's health research: An economic and societal impact analysis.* Santa Monica, CA: RAND Corporation.

BRAIN (Brain Research through Advancing Innovative Neurotechnologies) Initiative. n.d. *The Brain Initiative scientific accomplishments.* Bethesda, MD: National Institutes of Health.

BRAIN Initiative. 2023. *Brain Partners.* https://braininitiative.nih.gov/about/brain-partners (accessed October 14, 2024).

BRAIN Initiative. 2024a. *Overview.* https://braininitiative.nih.gov/about/overview (accessed October 14, 2024).

BRAIN Initiative. 2024b. *Understanding the Brain Initiative Budget.* https://braininitiative.nih.gov/funding/understanding-brain-initiative-budget (accessed October 14, 2024).

Cassidy, B. 2024. *NIH in the 21st century: Ensuring transparency and American biomedical leadership.* Washington, DC: Senate Committee on Health, Education, Labor, and Pensions.

CDC (Centers for Disease Control and Prevention). 2024. *Compendium of Evidence-Based Interventions and Best Practices for HIV Prevention.* https://www.cdc.gov/hiv/research/interventionresearch/compendium/index.html (accessed September 11, 2024).

Census Bureau. n.d. *Quickfacts: United States.* https://www.census.gov/quickfacts/fact/table/US/PST045219 (accessed August 8, 2024).

Clayton, J. A. 2023. *NASEM Committee on the Assessment of NIH Research on Women's Health.* Presentation to NASEM Committee on the Assessment of NIH Research on Women's Health, Meeting 1 (December 14, 2023). https://www.nationalacademies.org/event/41452_12-2023_assessment-of-nih-research-on-womens-health-meeting-1-part-3 (accessed August 22, 2024).

Collins, F. S., E. L. Wilder, and E. Zerhouni. 2014. NIH roadmap/Common Fund at 10 years. *Science* 345(6194):274–276.

CSR (Center for Scientific Review). 2024. *CSR Data and Evaluations: CSR Overview.* https://public.csr.nih.gov/AboutCSR/Evaluations (accessed October 14, 2024).

Eldadah, B. 2021. *GEMSSTAR: NIA's Pioneering Program for Early-Career Physicians in Aging Research.* https://www.nia.nih.gov/research/blog/2021/08/gemsstar-nias-pioneering-program-early-career-physicians-aging-research (accessed August 23, 2024).

Erickson, B. E. 2014. *NIH's Common Fund at 10: Alternative Funding Mechanism Stimulates Innovation, But Ongoing Support for Some Efforts Is Uncertain.* https://cen.acs.org/articles/92/i27/NIHs-Common-Fund-10.html (accessed August 23, 2024).

IOM (Institute of Medicine). 1997. *A review of the Department of Defense's program for breast cancer research.* Washington, DC: National Academy Press.

IOM and NRC (National Research Council). 2003. *Enhancing the vitality of the National Institutes of Health: Organizational change to meet new challenges.* Washington, DC: The National Academies Press.

Lauer, M. 2023. *FY 2022 by the Numbers: Extramural Grant Investments in Research.* https://nexus.od.nih.gov/all/2023/03/01/fy-2022-by-the-numbers-extramural-grant-investments-in-research/ (accessed October 14, 2024).

McIntosh, S. A., F. Alam, L. Adams, I. S. Boon, J. Callaghan, I. Conti, E. Copson, V. Carson, M. Davidson, H. Fitzgerald, A. Gautam, C. M. Jones, S. Kargbo, G. Lakshmipathy, H. Maguire, K. McFerran, A. Mirandari, N. Moore, R. Moore, A. Murray, L. Newman, S. D. Robinson, A. Segaran, C. N. Soong, A. Walker, K. Wijayaweera, R. Atun, R. I. Cutress, and M. G. Head. 2023. Global funding for cancer research between 2016 and 2020: A content analysis of public and philanthropic investments. *Lancet Oncology* 24(6):636–645.

Miller, L. R., C. Marks, J. B. Becker, P. D. Hurn, W. J. Chen, T. Woodruff, M. M. McCarthy, F. Sohrabji, L. Schiebinger, C. L. Wetherington, S. Makris, A. P. Arnold, G. Einstein, V. M. Miller, K. Sandberg, S. Maier, T. L. Cornelison, and J. A. Clayton. 2017. Considering sex as a biological variable in preclinical research. *FASEB Journal* 31(1):29–34.

Mirin, A. A. 2021. Gender disparity in the funding of diseases by the U.S. National Institutes of Health. *Journal of Women's Health* 30(7):956–963.

NASEM (National Academies of Sciences, Engineering, and Medicine). 2022a. *Enhancing NIH research on autoimmune disease.* Washington, DC: The National Academies Press.

NASEM. 2022b. *Measuring sex, gender identity, and sexual orientation.* Washington, DC: The National Academies Press.

NASEM. 2024a. *Advancing research on chronic conditions in women.* Washington, DC: The National Academies Press.

NASEM. 2024b. *Discussion of policies, systems, and structures for research on women's health at the National Institutes of Health: Proceedings of a workshop—in brief.* Washington, DC: The National Academies Press.

NASEM. 2024c. *Supporting family caregivers in STEMM: A call to action.* Washington, DC: The National Academies Press.

NCI (National Cancer Institute). n.d. *Cancer Moonshot—Recent Fiscal Year Funding.* https://www.cancer.gov/about-nci/budget/fact-book/cancer-moonshot (accessed August 23, 2024).

NCI. 2023. *About the Cancer Moonshot.* https://www.cancer.gov/research/key-initiatives/moonshot-cancer-initiative/about (accessed October 14, 2024).

NCI. 2024. *Funding for Research Areas.* https://www.cancer.gov/about-nci/budget/fact-book/data/research-funding (accessed August 14, 2024).

NIA (National Institute on Aging). 2024. *Grants for Early Medical/Surgical Specialists' Transition to Aging Research (GEMSSTAR).* https://www.nia.nih.gov/research/dcg/grants-early-medical-surgical-specialists-transition-aging-research-gemsstar (accessed August 23, 2024).

NIEHS (National Institute of Environmental Health Sciences). n.d. *About CareerTrac.* https://careertrac.niehs.nih.gov/public/staticPage/about (accessed August 23, 2024).

NIEHS. 2024. *CareerTrac Overview One Pager.* https://careertrac.niehs.nih.gov/public/CareerTrac%20Overview.pdf (accessed August 23, 2024).

NIH (National Institutes of Health). 2010. *Common Fund: Congressional justification FY 2011.* Bethesda, MD: National Institutes of Health.

NIH. 2017. *Mission and Goals.* https://www.nih.gov/about-nih/what-we-do/mission-goals (accessed August 20, 2024).

NIH. 2022. *RFA-OD-22-014: Specialized Centers of Research Excellence (SCORE) on Sex Differences (U54 Clinical Trial Optional).* https://grants.nih.gov/grants/guide/rfa-files/RFA-OD-22-014.html (accessed October 14, 2024).

NIH. 2023a. *Appropriations (Section 1).* https://www.nih.gov/about-nih/what-we-do/nih-almanac/appropriations-section-1 (accessed August 23, 2024).

NIH. 2023b. *Appropriations (Section 2).* https://www.nih.gov/about-nih/what-we-do/nih-almanac/appropriations-section-2 (accessed August 23, 2024).

NIH. 2023c. *PAR-24-075: Stephen I. Katz Early Stage Investigator Research Project Grant (R01 Clinical Trial Not Allowed).* https://grants.nih.gov/grants/guide/pa-files/PAR-24-075.html (accessed August 23, 2024).

NIH. 2023d. *PAR-24-076: Stephen I. Katz Early Stage Investigator Research Project Grant (R01 Basic Experimental Studies with Human Required).* https://grants.nih.gov/grants/guide/pa-files/PAR-24-076.html (accessed August 23, 2024).

NIH. 2024a. *The Common Fund: Who We Are and What We Do.* https://commonfund.nih.gov/about (accessed October 14, 2024).

NIH. 2024b. *NIH Common Fund: Congressional justification FY 2025.* Bethesda, MD: National Institutes of Health.

NIH. 2024c. *RFA-HD-25-005: Women's Reproductive Health Research (WRHR) Career Development Program (K12 Clinical Trial Optional).* https://grants.nih.gov/grants/guide/rfa-files/RFA-HD-25-005.html (accessed October 14, 2024).

NIH. 2024d. *RFA-OD-24-013: Building Interdisciplinary Research Careers in Women's Health (BIRCWH) (K12 Clinical Trial Optional).* https://grants.nih.gov/grants/guide/rfa-files/RFA-OD-24-013.html (accessed October 14, 2024).

NIH. 2024e. *Stephen I. Katz Early Stage Investigator Research Project Grant.* https://grants.nih.gov/funding/katz-esi-r01.htm (accessed August 23, 2024).

NIH. 2024f. *Who We Are: NIH Leadership.* https://www.nih.gov/about-nih/who-we-are/nih-leadership (accessed August 23, 2024).

NIMHD (National Institute on Minority Health and Health Disparities). 2024a. *About NIMHD.* https://www.nimhd.nih.gov/about/ (accessed September 10, 2024).

NIMHD. 2024b. *Community Health and Population Science.* https://www.nimhd.nih.gov/programs/extramural/research-areas/community-science.html (accessed August 23, 2024).

NIMHD. 2024c. *Division of Clinical and Health Services Research.* https://www.nimhd.nih.gov/programs/extramural/research-areas/clinical-research.html (accessed October 14, 2024).

OADR (Office of Autoimmune Disease Research). n.d. *About the Office of Autoimmune Disease Research (OADR-ORWH).* https://orwh.od.nih.gov/OADR-ORWH (accessed August 23, 2024).

ORWH (Office of Research on Women's Health). 2023. *Report of the Advisory Committee on Research on Women's Health, fiscal years 2021–2022: Office of Research on Women's Health and NIH support for research on women's health.* Bethesda, MD: National Institutes of Health.

Osuch, J. R., K. Silk, C. Price, J. Barlow, K. Miller, A. Hernick, and A. Fonfa. 2012. A historical perspective on breast cancer activism in the United States: From education and support to partnership in scientific research. *Journal of Women's Health* 21(3):355–362.

Overstreet, D. S., L. J. Strath, M. Jordan, I. A. Jordan, J. M. Hobson, M. A. Owens, A. C. Williams, R. R. Edwards, and S. M. Meints. 2023. A brief overview: Sex differences in prevalent chronic musculoskeletal conditions. *International Journal of Environmental Research and Public Health* 20(5).

Rodgers, C. M. 2024. *Reforming the National Institutes of Health: Framework for discussion.* Washington, DC: House Committee on Energy and Commerce.

Schust, D. J. 2024. *The Reproductive Scientist Development Program. Presentation to the NASEM Committee on the Assessment of NIH Research on Women's Health, Meeting 5, Part 1 (May 20, 2024).* https://www.nationalacademies.org/documents/embed/link/LF2255DA3DD1C41C0A42D3BEF0989ACAECE3053A6A9B/file/D4F5FD21DE0E10CE06AC5CFB7927B7E3654629229B9D?noSaveAs=1 (accessed May 20, 2024).

Sciarra, F., F. Campolo, E. Franceschini, F. Carlomagno, and M. A. Venneri. 2023. Gender-specific impact of sex hormones on the immune system. *International Journal of Molecular Sciences* 24(7).

Sekar, K. 2024. *CRS report R43341: National Institutes of Health (NIH) funding: FY1996–FY2025.* Washington, DC: Congressional Research Service.

White, J., C. Tannenbaum, I. Klinge, L. Schiebinger, and J. Clayton. 2021. The integration of sex and gender considerations into biomedical research: Lessons from international funding agencies. *Journal of Clinical Endocrinology and Metabolism* 106(10):3034–3048.

White House. n.d. *The Brain Initative.* https://obamawhitehouse.archives.gov/BRAIN (accessed October 14, 2024).

White House. 2024. *Fact Sheet: President Biden Issues Executive Order and Announces New Actions to Advance Women's Health Research and Innovation.* https://www.whitehouse.gov/briefing-room/statements-releases/2024/03/18/fact-sheet-president-biden-issues-executive-order-and-announces-new-actions-to-advance-womens-health-research-and-innovation/ (accessed March 25, 2024).

Appendix A

Committee Analysis of National Institutes of Health Grant Funding for Women's Health Research: Methodology

Authors: Hamad Al-Ibrahim,[1] Susan Cheng,[2] Nancy Sun,[2] Julianne Kwong,[2] and Wasay Warsi[2]

INTRODUCTION

Congress tasked the Committee on the Assessment of National Institutes of Health (NIH) Research on Women's Health to conduct an analysis of the proportion of NIH-funded research on women's health, including conditions that are female specific, are more common in women, or differentially affect women via sex differences. The committee used a multimethod and multistaged approach for a comprehensive analysis of NIH funding on women's health research (WHR). This analysis focused on the last 11 full fiscal years (FYs) of funding, FY 2013–FY 2023, to discern trends over time, while accounting for expected deviations in funding allocation resulting from known events, such as the COVID-19 pandemic. The committee obtained the data analyzed for each FY on April 25, 2024, through the publicly available NIH ExPORTER[3] online tool, which includes all data in NIH RePORTER (811,599 grants).[4] The data available for each grant included the grant title and number, name of the principal investigator(s), dates of funding, amounts of funding (total costs without direct and indirect cost breakdown), abstract text (also known as the "summary"), and public health relevance statement (also known as the "narrative"). These data, compiled across the study period, composed the study dataset. Additional data

[1] Policy Tech Innovation LLC; Social and Economic Survey Research Institute, Qatar University.

[2] Department of Cardiology, Smidt Heart Institute, Cedars-Sinai Medical Center.

[3] See https://reporter.nih.gov/exporter (accessed April 25, 2024).

[4] See https://reporter.nih.gov/ (accessed April 25, 2024).

pertaining to each grant, such as the actual contents of each grant proposal or submitted progress reports, were not available for analysis (see limitations section). The committee's analysis of results and findings are in Chapter 4.

TRAINING SET

Anticipating the need to develop an algorithm to identify from the dataset the funded grants related to WHR, the committee developed a training set of grants. After cleaning grant abstract text, including removing stop words, removing punctuation, and stemming words, the committee applied unsupervised k-means clustering method to identify up to five clusters of grants per FY. The committee did so using the similarity of words provided in the abstract, such that certain clusters were more likely to be enriched with words including or related to topics that may have had time-specific relevance. For example, COVID-19 was predominant among grants funded in FY 2020, FY 2021, and FY 2022. For each FY, the committee then identified an equal number of grants within each cluster that did or did not contain the key term "women." The committee randomly sampled a total of 80 grants per FY, including 20 grants (four from each cluster) containing the key term "women" and 60 grants (from each cluster) without it for a total of 800 grants representing the breadth of grants that were funded over a 10-year period.

Two teams of trained researchers separately adjudicated the data in NIH RePORTER for each of these 800 grants, using both a binary and an ordinal scoring system. The binary scoring system consisted of a simple "yes" or "no" for "probably women's health related." The five-level ordinal scoring system range included 1 for "not related," 2 for "minimally related," 3 for "moderately related," 4 for "largely related," and 5 for "definitely or completely related." After each team separately adjudicated all 800 grants, a third-party reviewer with multidisciplinary expertise on research both related and unrelated to women's health reviewed the teams' results, including any details regarding discrepancies, which accounted for approximately 8 percent of the total. All identified discrepancies were then resolved by third-party review with feedback provided to the two primary teams and full consensus reached, resulting in the final adjudicated dataset that comprised the training set for analyses.

EMPIRICAL ANALYSIS

The initial stage of analyses involved evaluating an empirical approach to identifying women's health–related research from the larger grant dataset. The committee generated a list of over 430 key terms representing conditions, diseases, concepts, treatments, and methodologies either specific to or related to women's health. The committee reviewed each term to include all possible forms, such as "sex biased" versus "sex-biased," and assigned a priority score out of 100 to represent its relevance to women's health. For conditions and diseases, the committee included only those with at least two-thirds prevalence in women documented using the most up-to-date published data, as reported in epidemiology studies available in PubMed, on prevalence rate for women compared to men, and this was used to assign the priority score. For conditions and diseases, an alternate approach could involve weighting relevance based on disability-adjusted life years (DALYs) instead of prevalence, although DALY data are not as readily available for all conditions and diseases included in the analyses.

The committee developed an algorithm to calculate a relevance score based on a search script to identify terms listed within three locations for any given grant: the abstract (summary), public health relevance statement (narrative), and grant title. The score was calculated as:

Relevance score =
1 * ([frequency factor * priority score] for any term(s) appearing in the summary)
+ 5 * ([frequency factor * priority score] for any term(s) appearing in the narrative)
+ 10 * ([frequency factor * priority score] for any term(s) appearing in the title)
Frequency factor = (the number of times a term appeared in a section of text) / (the total number of words in that text).

The committee applied this algorithm to a pilot test of 40 grants, and performance was suboptimal: a sizable proportion of WHR research grants were misclassified or miscategorized when results were compared to the adjudicated women's health relevance score. Fine-tuning the weightings used in the relevance score calculation did not substantially change these findings. For this reason, the committee developed a natural language processing–based algorithm instead.

Natural Language Processing–Based Analysis

The committee used large language models (LLMs) for the analysis given their ability, as large, deep learning models, to process human language text, such as in a grant title, abstract, or narrative, and derive predictions on vast amounts of similar data based on pretraining. In effect, a successful LLM algorithm can accurately identify and categorize a grant as related to women's health based on all available relevant information, just as a human should be able to confidently perform the same task after learning from experience and training what kind of title, abstract, or narrative is characteristic of a grant focused on research relevant to women's health.

First, the committee conducted a comparative analysis of various available LLMs, recognizing the breadth and complexity of the task; women's health spans multiple conditions, diseases, and domains of biomedical science. These LLMs included GPT-3.5 Turbo, GPT-4o, Claude Sonnet, and Claude Opus, with the committee selecting the flagship model from each provider—GPT-4o and Opus—and comparing each on a random set of 100 samples against a source of truth (the human-adjudicated dataset). GPT-4o outperformed Claude Opus with an overall accuracy of 93.19 percent but lagged in true negatives (see Figure A-1). Additional LLMs may be tested in the future, including Llama3, Google Gemini, Anthropic Claude, and Falcon. Future analyses may also consider applying multiple algorithms in parallel as part of efforts to further enhance the quality and consistency of results.

After selecting GPT-4o, the committee repeated a manual review of the training set of WHR-related grants to ensure that sample grants with high relevance scores were truly highly relevant and those with low relevance scores were less or not relevant. A sample set of 426 grants was finalized for an initial algorithm run, which produced some discrepancies; some grants manually assigned low relevance scores were found on re-review to be relevant, and some grants manually assigned high relevance scores were found on re-review to be less or not relevant. A careful examination of each sample grant that produced conflicting results revealed that ambiguity tended to arise for grants related to maternal-child health, where women are involved in the research but at least some or more focus is on child or fetal health outcomes, such as research on risks of pregnant women acquiring Zika virus. Following detailed rereview of grants that tended to result in ambiguous classification, the committee decided to remove grants that

Training Set				
OUTPUT \ TARGET	Truth	False	SUM	
Truth	58 13.62%	40 9.39%	98 59.18% 40.82%	
False	3 0.70%	325 76.29%	328 99.09% 0.91%	
SUM	61 95.08% 4.92%	365 89.04% 10.96%	383 / 426 89.91% 10.09%	

Claude Opus

Training Set				
OUTPUT \ TARGET	Truth	False	SUM	
Truth	56 13.15%	24 5.63%	80 70.00% 30.00%	
False	5 1.17%	341 80.05%	346 98.55% 1.45%	
SUM	61 91.80% 8.20%	365 93.42% 6.58%	397 / 426 93.19% 6.81%	

GPT-4o

FIGURE A-1 Iterative evaluation of multiple available large language models available for implementation to conduct the funding analysis task identified GPT-4o as superior in performance.

exclusively focused on child or infant health outcomes and retain grants that described plans to assess outcomes in both mothers and children or infants.

The iterative review to identify potential sources of ambiguity and discrepancy in categorization significantly enhanced the model's accuracy. To address these discrepancies, the committee identified samples where the model's predictions conflicted with the true positive and true negative classifications. The committee carefully examined each conflicted sample and manually corrected the labels in the new dataset. This meticulous process enabled efficient refinement of the data and improvement of its overall quality. After running the model again and manually analyzing these classifications, the overall accuracy of the model improved to approximately 97 percent. The accuracy of detecting true positives increased from 76 to 86 percent without changing any item in the prompts. There was a slight tradeoff in detecting true negatives, which did not affect the overall trend, as the negatives were filtered with a high accuracy of 98.5 percent in the first step.[5] To further assure the quality of the final generated dataset, additional versions of the prompts were tested to clarify identified areas of ambiguity (e.g., classification of a grant related to maternal-child health but focused primarily on child versus maternal health outcomes or a grant related to a disease affecting two sexes and including or not a focus on sex differences or sex-specific outcomes). This additional testing revealed less than 1 percent variation in results generated by different versions of the prompts used. Although several iterations of prompts were used for the analysis, Box A-1 shows a representative version of the main prompt.

Data Extraction

After evaluating and optimizing accuracy of the model and the prompt, the committee extracted data for the analysis. A summary of each major step of the extraction process is listed. Between each one, the committee performed a random sampling of its output before passing it on to the next step. If the accuracy was low during a stage of manual checking, the prior step(s) was repeated with modifications in the prompt to achieve and maintain high accuracy.

First Step: Binary Classification Whether the grant was related to women's health was identified. These statements defined women's health studies:

- The study topic directly affects women's health;
- The subject of the study is another preclinical model species, such as mice, but has potential translation to human women's health;

---

[5] Data and additional data tables from this analysis are available in the project's public access file; materials can be requested from PARO@nas.edu.

BOX A-1
Representative Version of Main Prompt Used for
Committee Analysis

Task: Determine Relevance to Women's Health

Instructions: You are an expert in women's health. Your task is to analyze a given text and determine if it is strictly related to women's health.

Step 1: Carefully read the provided summary text.
Criteria for Categorization as relevant to women's health:
- The study is on a female-specific condition or disease.
- The study is directly related to women's health.
- The study involves a non-human species, but the results are especially pertinent to or affect the health of women.
- The study is about or includes both women and men, but is focused on a condition or disease that predominantly affects women.
- The study is about sex differences or sex-specific outcomes for a condition or disease that affects both women and men, with a focus on health outcomes in women.
- The study is about or includes pregnant women and is focused on the health outcomes of women, not only on outcomes of the fetus, infant, or child.

Step 2: Output Your Decision
- If the text is relevant to women's health, output "YES".
- If the text is irrelevant to women's health, output "NO".

Response Format:
- YES/NO

Example Responses:
- "YES"
- "NO"

- The study is about both men and women, but it predominantly affects women's health; or,
- The study is about maternal health and has a greater effect on women's health than child health.

Second Step: Categorization The grants were further categorized as either related or not to maternal health, wherein maternal health was defined as related to studies affecting pregnant and postpartum women and their health, including prenatal care, pregnancy complications, and conditions related to pregnancy.

Third Step: Identification of Diseases and Conditions The disease or condition in the grant was identified next. Grants could be focused on a specific disease or condition, such as endometriosis or chronic pain; a group of diseases, such as off-target effects of immunotherapy treatment of cancers in women, or conditions, such as interventions to improve sleep disorders in women; or a life stage, such as menopause or advanced aging.

Fourth Step: Disease Classification Given that some grants focused on general disease categories, such as cancer, whereas others focused on very specific subtypes of diseases, such as triple-negative breast cancer, two levels of disease classification were created:

- Level 1: A broad classification based on a broadly used name of the disease.
- Level 2: A specific classification based on a specific disease name extracted from the grant abstract.

Fifth Step: Classification of Specific Diseases of Interest In Step 4, granular-level results were produced with the categories generated by the model. The committee also wanted to be able to report on a somewhat broader level of conditions with all related disorders/diseases included, such as on the broader category of eating disorders versus grants on bulimia, anorexia, and other related conditions individually. Instead of using a model-generated list of diseases and conditions drawn from the database of all grants, in Step 5, a list of prespecified diseases and conditions was given to the model. Terms for this analysis were drawn from the list of women's health-related terms the NIH Office of Research on Women's Health analyzed in its biennial report (ORWH, 2023) (see Chapter 4), the committee DALY analysis (see Chapter 7), and committee expertise, with a total of 67 diseases, conditions, and terms (see Appendix Table A-3).

The final data with all generated categorizations were then compiled and underwent several stages of validation by multiple investigators and research staff, iteratively using the NIH RePORTER tool to carefully review all available grant data and verify number, types, and categorizations of grants as identified by the algorithm. These data were used for analyses, including graphical visualizations of funding trends.

The committee used funding Institute or Center (IC), rather than administrative IC, data in this analysis and combined data for ICs that were redesignated within the analysis period (i.e., the National Center on Minority Health and Health Disparities was redesignated to the National Institute on

Minority Health and Health Disparities in 2010 and the National Center for Complementary and Alternative Medicine was redesignated as the National Center for Complementary and Integrative Health in 2014) (NIH, 2023a,b).

Limitations

Several limitations merit consideration. The final algorithm applied to identify grants related to women's health is not expected to have achieved perfect accuracy for many reasons, including lack of access to the contents of the full grant and, in turn, limited ability to discern if the information in the abstract contained terms or concepts pertaining to women's health in or out of proportion to the proposed work detailed in the specific aims or research strategy. Additionally, regarding the clustering method applied to produce the analyses' training set, a larger number of clusters could have yielded variation in the types of grants selected as part of the sampling strategy. This number was limited to five to accommodate year-to-year shifts in the types of grants being funded (e.g., before compared to during and then after the COVID-19 pandemic). The sampling size was limited to 800 grants, given the time and resources available for analyses; a larger sampling size could have generated greater variation in the types of grants analyzed. The adjudication process was limited to review of data available on NIH RePORTER, including the grant title, summary, and public health relevance statement, given lack of access to the full contents of the grants themselves.

Many grants were not specific to women's health but included a focus that was at least partially relevant to women's health, and so these grants were counted in their entirety as opposed to having their funding allocation divided. For example, a cancer center grant that received funding to study mechanisms underlying multiple cancers, including breast and prostate cancer, was identified as relevant to women's health without any attempt to divide the allocated funding, given insufficient information available to determine the most appropriate proportions. This issue also applied to grants to study diseases or conditions that affect both women and men and those related to maternal-child health funded to study the health outcomes of both mothers and infants or children. Thus, the overall funding allocated to WHR is likely overestimated by some amount.

In addition, analyses of funding allocated for certain individual diseases and conditions were also limited by the available text content of each grant abstract and, thus, are not considered perfectly accurate. Additionally, in a comprehensive analysis of WHR funding allocation, it would be ideal to understand the geographic and regional distribution (e.g., across states or between rural versus urban communities). This type of analysis was not possible given the lack of access to the full contents of each funded grant. Many NIH-funded grants awarded to a single primary institution will have portions of the total funding reallocated through subcontracts to other institutions that may be located elsewhere within or even outside of the country. Furthermore, funds allocated to any given institution may be spent to operationalize research in a region or locale that is different from where the institution is located. Thus, future investigations, ideally involving access to additional grant details, are needed to understand geographic and regional distributions of WHR funding allocations. Moreover, because of the absence of an established benchmark for comparison during the validation phase and the limitations of the Research, Condition, and Disease Categorization system and RePORTER search functionality (see Chapter 4), data may not serve as a dependable reference for comparing results and are additional challenges.

SUPPLEMENTAL DATA

See Chapter 4 for more information on the committee's results from the funding analysis; supplemental data to the committee's findings are presented here.

TABLE A-1 National Institutes of Health (NIH) Grant Funding and Number of Research Grants Overall and for Women's Health Research (WHR) by Fiscal Year

Fiscal Year	WHR Spending (Dollars)	WHR as Percentage of Total Spending	Total Spending (Dollars)	Number of WHR Grants	WHR as Percentage of Total Grants	Total Grants
2013	2,551,041,179	9.69	26,322,140,168	6,319	9.33	67,693
2014	2,606,329,910	9.59	27,179,627,138	6,330	9.48	66,795
2015	2,477,623,280	9.09	27,270,999,613	6,135	9.15	67,059
2016	2,590,605,120	8.87	29,215,998,129	6,221	9.11	68,304
2017	2,804,458,353	9.12	30,750,611,354	6,370	9.09	70,092
2018	2,962,977,736	9.00	32,913,199,571	6,876	8.88	77,438
2019	3,180,563,172	8.96	35,515,754,029	7,068	9.31	75,895
2020	3,087,492,113	7.77	39,748,192,231	6,966	8.90	78,265
2021	3,548,306,504	8.59	41,306,576,608	7,484	9.47	79,070
2022	3,779,350,407	8.94	42,292,623,824	7,730	9.65	80,112
2023	3,430,004,435	7.85	43,674,286,203	7,043	8.71	80,876

TABLE A-2 National Institutes of Health (NIH) Grant Spending for Women's Health Research (WHR) and Other Fiscal Year 2013–2023

Institute, Center, or Office	WHR Spending (Dollars)	Other Spending (Dollars)	Total Spending (Dollars)	Percentage of Total Spending for WHR
NCI	9,182,200,162	48,709,667,749	57,891,867,911	15.86
NIAID	4,135,534,926	51,386,145,635	55,521,680,561	7.45
NHLBI	1,952,137,016	32,011,069,773	33,963,206,789	5.75
NIGMS	873,642,214	28,027,917,693	28,901,559,907	3.02
NIA	1,367,788,117	25,728,310,478	27,096,098,595	5.05
NINDS	600,814,709	20,534,221,838	21,135,036,547	2.84
NIDDK	1,288,024,755	19,833,559,093	21,121,583,848	6.10
OD	1,491,406,854	18,684,719,009	20,176,125,863	7.39
NIMH	1,475,560,092	16,515,804,872	17,991,364,964	8.20
NICHD	5,270,342,607	9,124,361,815	14,394,704,422	36.61
NIDA	1,018,554,209	11,844,527,785	12,863,081,994	7.92
NIEHS	1,409,201,246	6,739,308,773	8,148,510,019	17.29
NCATS	83,769,184	7,779,706,623	7,863,475,807	1.07
NEI	80,562,927	7,698,808,092	7,779,371,019	1.04
NIAMS	588,356,192	5,285,813,177	5,874,169,369	10.02
NHGRI	173,384,662	5,465,946,660	5,639,331,322	3.07
NIAAA	486,382,453	4,519,041,970	5,005,424,423	9.72
NIDCD	62,698,746	4,527,141,338	4,589,840,084	1.37
NLM	34,088,293	4,422,001,832	4,456,090,125	0.76
NIDCR	242,622,513	4,190,339,076	4,432,961,589	5.47

NIBIB	263,202,816	4,045,480,301	4,308,683,117	6.11
NIMHD	518,831,659	3,425,201,726	3,944,033,385	13.15
NINR	223,758,399	1,285,125,793	1,508,884,192	14.83
NCCIH	91,687,619	1,186,497,279	1,278,184,898	7.17
FIC	98,959,585	579,474,031	678,433,616	14.59
RMOD	81,465	148,006,143	148,087,608	0.06
CIT	5,951,248	109,201,405	115,152,653	5.17

NOTE: CIT = Center for Information Technology; FIC = Fogarty International Center; NCATS = National Center for Advancing Translational Sciences; NCCIH = National Center for Complementary and Integrative Health; NCI = National Cancer Institute; NEI = National Eye Institute; NHGRI = National Human Genome Research Institute; NHLBI = National Heart, Lung, and Blood Institute; NIAAA = National Institute on Alcohol Abuse and Alcoholism; NIA = National Institute on Aging; NIAID = National Institute of Allergy and Infectious Diseases; NIAMS = National Institute of Arthritis and Musculoskeletal and Skin Diseases; NIBIB = National Institute of Biomedical Imaging and Bioengineering; NICHD = *Eunice Kennedy Shriver* National Institute of Child Health and Human Development; NIDA = National Institute on Drug Abuse; NIDCD = National Institute on Deafness and Other Communication Disorders; NIDCR = National Institute of Dental and Craniofacial Research; NIDDK = National Institute of Diabetes and Digestive and Kidney Diseases; NIEHS = National Institute of Environmental Health Sciences; NIGMS = National Institute of General Medical Sciences; NIMH = National Institute of Mental Health; NIMHD = National Institute on Minority Health and Health Disparities; NINDS = National Institute of Neurological Disorders and Stroke; NINR = National Institute of Nursing Research; NLM = National Library of Medicine; OD = Office of the Director; RMOD = Road Map/Common Fund.

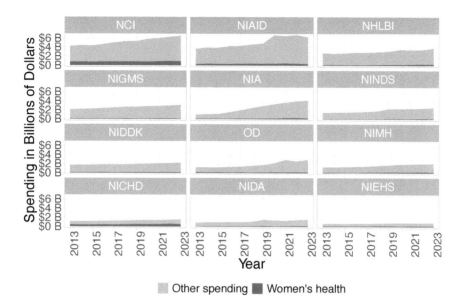

FIGURE A-2 National Institutes of Health grant funding for women's health research fiscal year 2013–2023 for each of the 12 Institutes and Offices with the largest women's health research portfolio.

NOTE: NCI = National Cancer Institute; NHLBI = National Heart, Lung, and Blood Institute; NIA = National Institute on Aging; NIAID = National Institute of Allergy and Infectious Diseases; NICHD = *Eunice Kennedy Shriver* National Institute of Child Health and Human Development; NIDA = National Institute on Drug Abuse; NIDDK = National Institute of Diabetes and Digestive and Kidney Diseases; NIEHS = National Institute of Environmental Health Sciences; NIGMS = National Institute of General Medical Sciences; NIMH = National Institute of Mental Health; NINDS = National Institute of Neurological Disorders and Stroke; OD = Office of the Director.

TABLE A-3 Conditions, Diseases, and Terms Used in Step 5 of the Committee's Funding Analysis to Classify Specific Conditions and Diseases of Interest

Abortion	Depressive disorders	Lupus	Rheumatoid arthritis
Alzheimer's disease and related dementias	Diabetes	Menopause and perimenopause	Scleroderma
Amenorrhea	Dysmenorrhea	Migraines	Sexually transmitted infections
Anemia	Dyspareunia	Multiple sclerosis	Sjogren's syndrome
Anxiety disorder	Eating disorders	Myalgic encephalomyelitis/ chronic fatigue syndrome	Substance misuse disorders
Asthma	Endometrial cancer	Osteoarthritis	Temporomandibular joint disorder
Autism spectrum disorder	Endometriosis	Osteoporosis	Thyroid cancer
Bacterial vaginosis	Female sexual dysfunction	Ovarian cancer	Turner syndrome
Breast cancer	Fibroids	Parathyroid cancer	Uterine cancer
Breastfeeding and lactation	Fibromyalgia	Pelvic floor disorders	Vaginal cancer
Candidiasis	Heart failure	Pelvic inflammatory disease	Violence against women
Caregiving research	HIV/AIDS	Polycystic ovary syndrome	Vulvar cancer
Carpal tunnel syndrome	Hyperthyroid disorders	Postpartum depression	Vulvodynia
Cerebrovascular disease	Hypothyroid disorders	Pregnancy	
Cervical cancer	Infertility	Premature ovarian failure	
Contraception	Interstitial cystitis	Premenstrual syndrome	
Coronary heart disease	Irritable bowel syndrome	Pulmonary hypertension	
Cystocele	Lung cancer	Rett syndrome	

REFERENCES

NIH (National Institutes of Health). 2023a. *NIH Almanac: National Center for Complementary and Integrative Health (NCCIH)*. https://www.nih.gov/about-nih/what-we-do/nih-almanac/national-center-complementary-integrative-health-nccih#events (accessed October 17, 2024).

NIH. 2023b. *NIH Almanac: National Institute on Minority Health and Health Disparities (NIMHD)*. https://www.nih.gov/about-nih/what-we-do/nih-almanac/national-institute-minority-health-health-disparities-nimhd (accessed October 17, 2024).

ORWH (Office of Research on Women's Health). 2023. *Report of the Advisory Committee on Research on Women's Health, fiscal years 2021–2022: Office of Research on Women's Health and NIH support for research on women's health*. Bethesda, MD: National Institutes of Health.

Appendix B

National Institutes of Health Research Career Development Awards (K Awards)

TABLE B-1 Types of National Institutes of Health (NIH) Research Career Development Awards (K Awards)

Type	Name	Purpose
K01	Mentored Research Scientist Career Development Award	The purpose of this program is to provide support and protected time for an intensive, supervised career development experience in the biomedical, behavioral, or clinical sciences leading to research independence. Some NIH Institutes use the K01 to enhance workforce diversity, or for individuals who propose to train in a new field, or for individuals who have had a hiatus in their research career.
K02	Independent Research Scientist Development Award	The purpose of this program is to foster the development of newly independent, outstanding scientists who can demonstrate the need for a period of intensive research, to enable them to expand their potential to make significant contributions to their field of research.
K05	Senior Research Scientist Award	The purpose of this program is to provide protected time to established researchers to devote effort to basic or clinical research and to act as research mentors to early-stage investigators. Candidates for this award should have independent, peer-reviewed, research support at the time of award and possess a demonstrated record of mentoring.

(continued)

449

TABLE B-1 Continued

Type	Name	Purpose
K07	Academic Career Development Award	The purpose of this program is to provide support for academic researchers and to enhance the educational or research capacity at the sponsoring institution. The K07 supports both development awards for more junior candidates, and leadership awards for more senior individuals with acknowledged scientific expertise and leadership skills.
K08	Mentored Clinical Scientist Research Career Development Award	The purpose of this program is to prepare clinically trained individuals for careers that have a significant impact on the health-related research needs of the Nation. This program provides support and protected time for an intensive, supervised research career development experience in the fields of biomedical, behavioral, or clinical research, including translational research.
K12	Clinical Scientist Institutional Career Development Program Award	The purpose of this program is to support institutional career development awards designed to prepare newly trained clinicians who have made a commitment to independent research careers, and to facilitate their transition to more advanced support mechanisms, e.g., K08 and K23.
K18	Research Career Enhancement Award for Established Investigators	This program provides either full-time or part-time support for experienced scientists to augment or redirect their research programs through the acquisition of new research skills or to make changes in their research careers by acquiring new research skills or knowledge.
K22	Career Transition Award	The goal of this program is to facilitate the transition of investigators to independent, productive research careers. One or two phase award; an initial period of mentored research, followed by a period of independent research at an extramural institution.
K23	Mentored Patient-Oriented Research Career Development Award	The purpose of this program is to support the career development of individuals with a clinical doctoral degree who have the potential to develop into productive, clinical investigators, and who have made a commitment to focus their research endeavors on patient-oriented research.
K24	Midcareer Investigator Award in Patient-Oriented Research	The purpose of this program is to provide support to mid-career health-professional doctorates or equivalent who are typically at the Associate Professor level for protected time to devote to patient-oriented research and to act as research mentors primarily for clinical residents, clinical fellows and/or junior clinical faculty.

TABLE B-1 Continued

Type	Name	Purpose
K25	Mentored Quantitative Research Career Development Award	The purpose of this award is to attract to NIH-relevant research those investigators whose quantitative science and engineering research has thus far not been focused primarily on questions of health and disease. The K25 supports productive professionals with quantitative (e.g., statistics, economics, computer science, physics, chemistry) and engineering backgrounds to integrate their expertise with NIH-relevant research.
K26	Midcareer Investigator Award in Biomedical and Behavioral Research	The purpose of this award is to support biomedical and behavioral scientists to allow them protected time to devote to their research and mentoring. The goal of this program is to support established, outstanding investigators by providing protected time for research and mentoring.
K43	Emerging Global Leader Award	The purpose of the Fogarty Emerging Global Leader Award is to provide research support and protected time to a research scientist from a low- or middle-income country (LMIC) with a junior faculty position at an LMIC academic or research institution leading to an independently funded research career.
K76	Emerging Leaders Career Development Award	The purpose of this program is to develop a cadre of talented scientists prepared and willing to take an active leadership role in transformative change that will lead to improved health care outcomes.
K99/ R00	Pathway to Independence Award	The purpose of this program is to increase and maintain a strong cohort of new and talented, NIH-supported, independent investigators. This program is designed to facilitate a timely transition of outstanding postdoctoral researchers or clinician-scientists from mentored research positions to independent, tenure-track or equivalent faculty positions, and to provide independent NIH research support during the transition that will help these individuals launch competitive, independent research careers.

SOURCE: Excerpts from NIH, 2017.

REFERENCES

NIH (National Institutes of Health). 2017. *Research Career Development Awards (K) Kiosk.* https://researchtraining.nih.gov/programs/career-development (accessed August 22, 2024).

Appendix C

Public Meeting Agendas

December 14, 2023

Virtual Meeting

4:00 pm ET Welcome
Sheila Burke and Alina Salganicoff, Committee Cochairs

4:05–4:35 **Presentation of the Statement of Task and Background**
Janine Austin Clayton, M.D., FARVO
Associate Director, Research on Women's Health
Director, Office of Research on Women's Health
National Institutes of Health

4:35–5:00 **Discussion/Q&A with Committee Members**
Janine Austin Clayton, M.D., FARVO
Associate Director, Research on Women's Health
Director, Office of Research on Women's Health
National Institutes of Health

Vivian Ota Wong, Ph.D., FACMG, CGC
Deputy Director, Office of Research on Women's Health
National Institutes of Health

Sarah Temkin, M.D.
Associate Director for Clinical Research, Office of Research
   on Women's Health
National Institutes of Health

5:00   Adjourn

SECOND PUBLIC MEETING

January 25, 2024

Hybrid Meeting

Washington, DC

9:00 am ET Welcome
Sheila Burke and Alina Salganicoff, Committee Cochairs

9:05–9:45   **Structural Determinants of Health at the Intersection of
    Race, Gender, and Sexuality & Discussion**
Madina Agénor (*virtual*)
Associate Professor
Departments of Behavioral and Social Sciences and Epidemiology
Center for Health Promotion and Health Equity
Brown University School of Public Health

9:45–10:30 **Research Gaps in Women's Health & Discussion**

Society for Women's Health Research
Lindsey Miltenberger
Chief Advocacy Officer
Society for Women's Health Research

Women First Research Coalition
Irina Burd (*virtual*)
Sylvan Frieman, MD Endowed Professor of Obstetrics,
   Gynecology & Reproductive Sciences
Chair
Department of Obstetrics, Gynecology and Reproductive
   Sciences University of Maryland

Lisa Barroilhet *(virtual)*
Associate Professor
Department of Obstetrics and Gynecology
University of Wisconsin School of Medicine and Public
  Health

Women's Health Access Matters (WHAM)
Lori Frank
Incoming President
WHAM

10:30–10:45 Break

10:45–11:35 Overview of Portfolio Analysis and Review at NIH &
  Discussion
Marina Volkov *(virtual)*
Director
Office of Evaluation, Performance, and Reporting
NIH

George Santangelo
Director
Office of Portfolio Analysis
NIH

11:35–
12:05 pm Research Capacity Building at NIH & Discussion
Michele McGuirl *(virtual)*
Acting Director
Division for Research Capacity Building
National Institute of General Medical Sciences
NIH

12:05–1:00 Lunch

1:00–1:50 Disease Categorization and Analysis at NIH & Discussion
Evelina Cebotari
Lead Scientific Information Analyst
Division of Scientific Categorization and Analysis
Office of Extramural Research
NIH

Nancy Praskievicz
Lead Scientific Information Analyst
Division of Scientific Categorization and Analysis
Office of Extramural Research
NIH

Discussant
Jake Scholl
Lead Scientific Information Analyst
Division of Scientific Categorization and Analysis
Office of Extramural Research
NIH

1:50–2:20   **NIH Center for Scientific Review Policies and Procedures &**
              Discussion
              Kristin Kramer
              Director
              Office of Communications and Outreach
              Center for Scientific Review
              NIH

2:20–2:35   **Break**

2:35–3:45   **Stakeholder Perspectives**
              Please see note at end of this agenda to with information to
              sign up

3:45–4:30   **Overview of National Institute on Minority Health and**
              Health Disparities
              Overview of Sexual & Gender Minority Research Office

              Joint Discussion
              Eliseo J. Pérez-Stable (*virtual*)
              Director
              National Institute on Minority Health and Health Disparities
              NIH

              Karen L. Parker (*virtual*)
              Director
              Sexual & Gender Minority Research Office
              NIH

4:30   **Adjourn**

THIRD PUBLIC MEETING

March 7, 2024

Hybrid Meeting

Washington, DC

9:00 am ET Welcome
Sheila Burke and Alina Salganicoff, Committee Cochairs

9:10–10:05 **Science of Sex Differences & Discussion**
Margaret M. McCarthy
James and Carolyn Frenkil Dean's Professor and Chair,
Department of Pharmacology, University of Maryland
School of Medicine;
Director, University of Maryland—Medicine Institute of
Neuroscience Discovery

Karen Reue
Distinguished Professor and Vice Chair, Department of
Human Genetics, David Geffen School of Medicine at
UCLA;
Associate Director, UCLA/Caltech Medical Scientist
Training Program

10:05–11:05 **Perspectives on Women's Reproductive and Gynecologic
Health Research Needs & Discussion**

American College of Obstetricians and Gynecologists
Christopher M. Zahn
Interim CEO and Chief, Clinical Practice and Health Equity
and Quality, American College of Obstetricians and
Gynecologists

Coalition to Expand Contraceptive Access
Jamie Hart (*virtual*)
Executive Director, Coalition to Expand Contraceptive
Access

Society of Family Planning
Amanda Dennis (*virtual*)
Executive Director, Society of Family Planning

Black Mamas Matter Alliance
Angela Doyinsola Aina (*virtual*)
Cofounder and Executive Director, Black Mamas Matter
    Alliance
Ayanna Robinson (*virtual*)
Director, Research and Evaluation, Black Mamas Matter
    Alliance

11:05–11:20 Break

11:20–   Research on Women's Mental and Behavioral Health &
12:20 pm   Discussion

Tory Eisenlohr-Moul (*virtual*)
Director, CLEAR Lab;
Associate Professor, Department of Psychiatry;
Associate Director, Medical Scientist Training Program,
    University of Illinois at Chicago College of Medicine

Kristina M. Deligiannidis (*virtual*)
Director, Women's Behavioral Health, Zucker Hillside
    Hospital, Northwell Health;
Medical Director, Reproductive Psychiatry, Project TEACH,
    New York State Office of Mental Health;
Professor of Psychiatry, Molecular Medicine, and Obstetrics
    and Gynecology, Donald and Barbara Zucker School of
    Medicine at Hofstra/Northwell;
Professor, Feinstein Institutes for Medical Research,
    Northwell Health;
Adjunct Professor of Psychiatry, University of Massachusetts
    Chan Medical School

C. Neill Epperson (*virtual*)
Robert Freedman Endowed Professor and Chair,
    Department of Psychiatry;
Professor, Department of Family Medicine, University of
    Colorado School of Medicine

12:20–1:20 Lunch Break
*Lunch will not be provided. There is a small market in
the cafeteria on the lower level and restaurants near
the Foggy Bottom-GWU metro stop, including Western
Market Foodhall (~15-minute walk).*

1:20–2:35   Research on Women's Cancers & Discussion

1:20–1:45   *Lessons from Breast Cancer Research and Remaining Gaps*
             Reshma Jagsi *(virtual)*
             Lawrence W. Davis Professor and Chair, Department
                 of Radiation Oncology, Emory University School of
                 Medicine

1:45–2:35   *Lessons from Gynecologic Cancer Research and
                 Remaining Gaps*
             Beth Y. Karlan *(virtual)*
             Nancy Marks Endowed Chair in Women's Health Research;
             Vice Chair and Professor, Department of Obstetrics and
                 Gynecology, David Geffen School of Medicine at UCLA;
             Director, Cancer Population Genetics, UCLA Jonsson
                 Comprehensive Cancer Center

             Victoria L. Bae-Jump *(virtual)*
             Professor and Associate Division Director of Gynecologic
                 Oncology;
             Director, Lineberger Endometrial Cancer Center of
                 Excellence;
             Medical Director, Lineberger Clinical Trials Office,
                 University of North Carolina at Chapel Hill School of
                 Medicine

2:35–3:35   Research on Non-Malignant Gynecologic Conditions &
                 Discussion
             Erica E. Marsh
             Vice Chair, Department of Obstetrics and Gynecology;
             Chief, Division of Reproductive Endocrinology and
                 Infertility;
             S. Jan Behrman Collegiate Professor of Reproductive
                 Medicine, University of Michigan Medical School;
             University Diversity and Social Transformation Professor;
             Professor, Department of Women's and Gender Studies,
                 College of Literature, Science and the Arts, University of
                 Michigan;
             Associate Director, Michigan Institute for Clinical Health
                 Research

Steven Young
Professor and Division Chief, Reproductive Endocrinology
and Infertility, Duke University School of Medicine

Carolyn W. Swenson *(virtual)*
Associate Professor, Department of Obstetrics and
Gynecology;
Division Chief, Urogynecology and Reconstructive Pelvic
Surgery, University of Utah Health

3:35–3:45   **Break**

3:45–5:00   **Public Comment**
*Please see note at end of this agenda to with information to
sign up.*

5:00   **Adjourn**

FOURTH PUBLIC MEETING

April 11, 2024

Hybrid Meeting

Washington, DC

1:30 pm ET   **Welcome**
Sheila Burke and Alina Salganicoff, Committee Cochairs

1:40–2:20   **Tara Schwetz**
Deputy Director for Program Coordination, Planning, and
Strategic Initiatives, National Institutes of Health

2:20–2:50   **Carolyn Mazure**
Chair, White House Initiative on Women's Health Research

2:50–3:10   **Break**

3:10–3:50   **Irene Headen**
Assistant Professor of Black Health, Department of
Community Health and Prevention, Dornsife School of
Public Health, Drexel University

3:50–5:00   Stakeholder Input

5:00   Adjourn

FIFTH PUBLIC MEETING

May 20, 2024

Virtual Meeting

2:00 pm ET Welcome
            Alina Salganicoff, Committee Cochair

2:05–2:40   **History of NIH Office of Research on Women's Health**
            Vivian Pinn
            Former Director (Retired), Office of Research on Women's
                Health, NIH; Former Senior Scientist Emerita, Fogarty
                International Center, NIH

2:40–3:55   **Women's Health Research Career Development Programs
            and Workforce Needs**
            Christos Coutifaris
            Celso-Ramon Garcia Professor, Perelman School of
                Medicine, University of Pennsylvania

            Danny J. Schust
            Edwin Crowell Hamblen Distinguished Professor of
                Reproductive Biology and Family Planning, Duke
                University

            William Catherino
            American Association of Obstetricians and Gynecologists
                Foundation Scholar Committee

            Karen Freund
            Physician in Chief, Tufts Medical Center; Sheldon M. Wolff
                Professor and Chair, Department of Medicine, Tufts
                University School of Medicine; Harry and Elsa Jiler
                Clinical Research Professor, American Cancer Society

3:55–4:00   **Closing and Adjourn**

Appendix D

Committee Member and
Staff Biosketches

Sheila P. Burke, M.P.A., R.N., FAAN (Cochair), is an adjunct lecturer at the J. F. Kennedy School of Government at Harvard University, where she previously served as executive dean. She is also the senior public policy advisor and chair of the Government Relations and Policy Group at Baker Donelson. Ms. Burke is the vice chair of the Commonwealth Fund board of directors and a member of the board of directors of Abt Associates and Ascension Health Care. She was chief of staff to Senate Majority Leader Bob Dole and served as deputy staff director of the Senate Committee on Finance and the Secretary of the Senate, the chief administrative officer of the body. She was a commissioner on the Medicare Payment Advisory Commission and chair of the Kaiser Foundation Board. Early in her career, she was a staff nurse in California. Ms. Burke is a member of the National Academy of Medicine, where she previously served as a member of its council and received the David Rall Award. She is also a fellow of the American Academy of Nursing and member of the National Academy of Public Administration. Ms. Burke graduated from the University of San Francisco and Harvard University and has honorary degrees from Marymount University and the Uniformed Services University of the Health Sciences. She has served on several National Academies committees, most recently as cochair of the Committee on the Review of Federal Policies That Contribute to Racial and Ethnic Health Inequities.

Alina Salganicoff, Ph.D. (Cochair), is a senior vice president and the director of Women's Health Policy at KFF, where her work focuses on health policies of importance to women throughout their life-span with an emphasis on coverage and access challenges facing underserved and marginalized women. Dr. Salganicoff has written and lectured extensively on the financing of and access to health services for women on topics ranging from sexual and reproductive health to long-term care. She has served on numerous federal, state, and nonprofit advisory committees. She is also on the advisory panel of the American College of Obstetricians and Gynecologists' Women's Preventive Services Initiative and Public Policy Advisory Group of Power to Decide and an associate editor of the peer-reviewed journal *Women's Health Issues*. Born in Argentina, she is a native Spanish speaker. She holds a B.S. from Pennsylvania State University and a Ph.D. in health policy from Johns Hopkins Bloomberg School of Public Health. Dr. Salganicoff is a member of the National Academies of Sciences, Engineering, and Medicine (National Academies) Standing Committee on Reproductive Health Equity and Society. She served on the Institute of Medicine committee that issued recommendations for preventive services for women now covered under the Affordable Care Act and National Academies committees on abortion safety and quality, the control and prevention of sexually transmitted infections, and women's health research.

Neelum T. Aggarwal, M.D., FAMWA, is a professor in the Department of Neurological Sciences at the National Institute on Aging–funded Rush Alzheimer's Disease Center (Rush University Medical Center) and the center's senior cognitive neurologist. She is also research director for the Rush Heart Center for Women and steering committee member for the Alzheimer's Clinical Trial Consortium. Her recent clinical and research interests lie in the diagnosis and clinical management of cognitive change and dementia prevention by identifying how risk factors for cardiovascular disease and stroke—including genetics and blood and neuroimaging biomarkers—vary by race/ethnicity and sex and gender. She has served in numerous leadership roles throughout her career. She is the chief diversity and inclusion officer for the American Medical Women's Association (AMWA), AMWA Delegate to the American Medical Association (AMA), past chair of the AMA—Women's Physician Section, and recipient of the 2022 Rush Excellence in Research Award and the 2016 AMWA Women in Science Award. She has also served as the cochair for the Alzheimer's Association—International Society to Advance Alzheimer's Research and Treatment Sex Differences and Diversity special interest group and was a member of the Society of Women's Health Research Alzheimer's Disease Interdisciplinary Network. Dr. Aggarwal completed her M.D. at Chicago Medical School, residency in neurology at Henry Ford Hospital, and aging and neurodegenerative disorders fellowship at the Rush Alzheimer's Disease Center.

Veronica Barcelona, Ph.D., M.S.N., P.H.N.A.-B.C., R.N., is a public health nurse, perinatal epidemiologist, and assistant professor at Columbia University School of Nursing. Her research centers on how racism and discrimination underlie mechanisms and risk factors for adverse pregnancy and birth outcomes; the goal is to achieve healthy and safe birth outcomes for all. Her research is funded by the *Eunice Kennedy Shriver* National Institute of Child Health and Human Development, Betty Irene Moore Nurse Leader Fellowship, and Data Science Institute at Columbia University. She has been recognized for excellence in research by the Friends of the National Institute of Nursing Research Protégé Award, Johns Hopkins University School of Nursing Dean's Award, International Society for Nurses in Genetics Founders Award, and Connecticut Nurses Association Virginia Henderson award. Dr. Barcelona earned degrees from the University of Michigan (B.S.N.), Johns Hopkins University (M.S.N./M.P.H.), and Tulane University School of Public Health and Tropical Medicine (Ph.D.). She completed postdoctoral studies in epigenomics and a K01 project funded by the National Institute of Nursing Research at Yale University School of Nursing.

Alyssa M. Bilinski, Ph.D., M.Sc., A.M., is the Peterson Family Assistant Professor of Health Policy at Brown University School of Public Health in the Departments of Health Services, Policy, & Practice and Biostatistics. Her research lies at the intersection of policy evaluation and modeling: developing novel methods to support decision making and applying these to identify interventions that can most efficiently improve population health and well-being. She has published extensively in peer-reviewed medical, science, policy, and methods journals, including *Journal of the American Medical Association, Annals of Internal Medicine, Proceedings of the National Academy of Sciences, Health Affairs, Journal of Econometrics*, and *Value in Health*, and collaborated with state, local, and federal public health officials to help translate her research into practice. Her current work related to women's health quantifies the population health effects of excluding pregnant people from clinical trials and defines priorities for addressing gaps in clinical evidence. Dr. Bilinski received a Ph.D. in health policy (evaluative science and statistics) and an A.M. in statistics from Harvard University, an M.Sc. in medical statistics from the London School of Hygiene and Tropical Medicine as a Marshall Scholar, and a B.A. from Yale College.

Chloe E. Bird, Ph.D., M.A., is the director of the Center for Health Equity Research at Tufts Medical Center, Sara Murray Jordan Professor of Medicine at Tufts University School of Medicine, a senior sociologist at RAND, and professor of policy analysis at Pardee RAND Graduate School. She is a medical sociologist and national expert in women's health and health disparities, determinants of sex and gender differences in health and health care, gaps in the evidence base on women's health, and the social and economic impact of increasing investments in research on women's health. Dr. Bird has served as a senior advisor in the National Institutes of Health Office of Research on Women's Health and editor of the journal *Women's Health Issues*. She received the 2021 Distinguished Career Award in the Practice of Sociology from the American Sociological Association. She is a fellow of the American Association for the Advancement of Science and the American Academy of Health Behavior and a member of Women of Impact in Healthcare. She earned her Ph.D. and M.A. in sociology from the University of Illinois at Urbana-Champaign and her B.A. from Oberlin College.

Susan Cheng, M.D., M.M.Sc., M.P.H., is the Erika J. Glazer Chair in Women's Cardiovascular Health and Population Science, director of the Institute for Research on Healthy Aging, director of public health research, and professor and vice chair of research in cardiology in the Smidt Heart Institute at Cedars-Sinai. She is a clinician-scientist who leads research programs aimed at uncovering the drivers of cardiovascular aging in women and men. Dr. Cheng consults with companies on off-target cardiac effects of medications. She has authored over 400 research manuscripts, and her work has been supported by continuous National Institutes of Health funding. Dr. Cheng has served on the editorial boards of major cardiovascular journals and leadership committees for the American Heart Association and American College of Cardiology. She is an elected member of the Association of University Cardiologists and elected councilor for the American Society for Clinical Investigation. Dr. Cheng received her A.B. from Harvard University, M.D. from McMaster University, M.M.Sc. from Massachusetts Institute of Technology, and M.P.H. from Harvard School of Public Health. She completed internal medicine training at Johns Hopkins Hospital and cardiology fellowship training at Brigham and Women's Hospital.

Felina Cordova-Marks, Dr.P.H., M.P.H., M.Sc. (Hopi), is an assistant professor at the University of Arizona Zuckerman College of Public Health in the department of Health Promotion Sciences, executive committee member of the Hopi Education Endowment Fund Board, and associate editor for the American Association for Cancer Research's journal *Cancer Research Communications*. She is a published author on topics such as cancer, cardiology, informal health caregiving, mental health, health disparities, and American Indian health. She provides ad hoc consulting on appropriate mechanisms for tribal consultation and culturally responsive training with Indigenous populations. Dr. Cordova-Marks has recently been named a "Health Hero" by the National Indian Health Board, receiving the Regional/Local impact award for her wellness program IndigiWellbeing©. She was also named a Diversity and Inclusion Leader for Arizona and is an American Psychosocial Oncology Society Health Equity Scholar. Her awards and recognition include being named Tucson's Woman of the Year—40 Under 40 by the Tucson Hispanic Chamber of Commerce, Ben's Bells Honoree, an National Institutes of Health Health Disparities Research Institute Fellow, a Tribal Researchers Cancer Control Fellow, National Native American 40 Under 40, and University of Arizona Centennial Award recipient. Dr. Cordova-Marks earned her M.P.H., M.Sc., and Dr.P.H. from the University of Arizona.

Sherita H. Golden, M.D., M.H.S., is the Hugh P. McCormick Family Professor of Endocrinology and Metabolism at Johns Hopkins University School of Medicine. An internationally recognized physician-scientist, she has used epidemiology and health services research to identify biological and systems contributors to disparities in Type 2 diabetes and its outcomes. She served as vice president and chief diversity officer for Johns Hopkins Medicine (JHM) 2019–2024; she oversaw diversity, inclusion, and health equity strategy and operations for the School of Medicine and Johns Hopkins Health System. She executed implementation of Culturally and Linguistically Appropriate Services Standards; staff training for accurate collection of self-identified patient demographic data; system-wide policies prohibiting patient discrimination and discriminatory aggression toward employees and trainees and allowing for chosen names on identification badges; system-wide in-person and online unconscious bias and antioppression education programs; and a system-wide Disability and Accessibility Workgroup. In partnership with JHM human resources, she helped launched the Levi Watkins, Jr. Mentorship Program, which is designed as part of a talent management strategy focused on identifying and developing high-potential leaders from underrepresented groups. During the COVID-19 pandemic, she facilitated mobile community testing and education for the marginalized in Baltimore City and equitable vaccine distribution to nonclinical, minoritized frontline staff across JHM. Dr. Golden is a leader in the national discussion advancing health equity, including supporting Maryland legislators in drafting and testifying in support of state-level health equity policy. She is an elected member of the National Academy of Medicine, Association of American Physicians, and American Society of Clinical Investigation. She is a member of the Maryland Prescription Drug Affordability Stakeholder Council and was a member of the Data Subcommittee of the Maryland Commission on Health Equity (2022–2024) and cochair of the Health Equity Advisory Committee for the Maryland Hospital Association (2020–2024). In May 2024, Dr. Golden became a member of the North America Medical Advisory Board for Abbott Diabetes Care. She received her M.D. from the University of Virginia and completed her residency in internal medicine and fellowship in endocrinology, diabetes, and metabolism at Johns Hopkins Hospital. She received her M.H.S. in clinical epidemiology from the Johns Hopkins Bloomberg School of Public Health. Dr. Golden served as a member on the National Academies Committee on Living Well with Chronic Disease.

Holly A. Ingraham, Ph.D., is a professor of cellular and molecular pharmacology and the Herzstein Endowed Professor of Molecular Physiology at the University of California, San Francisco (UCSF) School of Medicine. She also directs the UCSF National Institute of General Medical Sciences–funded Institutional Research and Academic Career Development Award Program to create opportunities for postdoctoral scholars and build diversity in the nation's biomedical workforce and faculty. Dr. Ingraham's research focuses on sex differences and hormone-responsive nodes in the brain and peripheral tissues that maintain metabolic, skeletal, and gut physiology in females to address the significant gaps in women's health. Through question-driven basic science, Dr. Ingraham aims to elucidate the molecular underpinnings of adaptive responses in female physiology across the life-span to understand better the effects of how hormonal fluctuations during the reproductive and postreproductive periods impact females. She has made fundamental contributions to the field of hormone signaling and sex-dependent physiological regulatory mechanisms. Her most recent high-impact studies have been highlighted in the *New York Times* Science Section (10/26/21) and the *NIH Director's Blog* (8/1/24). Dr. Ingraham has chaired and served on scores of National Institutes of Health and other scientific review panels. She is also on several scientific advisory boards and a founder of a new biotech venture to improve women's health. In addition to numerous scientific awards, she is an elected fellow of the American Association for the Advancement of Science and a member of the National Academy of Sciences and the American Academy of Arts and Science. She earned her Ph.D. from the University of California, San Diego.

Robert M. Kaplan, Ph.D., M.A., is a senior scholar at the Stanford School of Medicine Clinical Excellence Research Center and directs the Stanford-Athena Institute Fund for Behavioral Immunology in Women's Wellness. He is also a Distinguished Research Professor of Health Policy and Management at the University of California, Los Angeles (UCLA). He served as chief science officer at the Agency for Healthcare Research and Quality (AHRQ) and as associate director of the National Institutes of Health, where he led the behavioral and social sciences programs. He led the UCLA/ RAND AHRQ health services training program and the UCLA/RAND Prevention Research Center at the Centers for Disease Control and Prevention. He was chair of the Department of Health Services (2004–2009). From 1997 to 2004, he was professor and chair of the Department of Family and Preventive Medicine at the University of California, San Diego. He is a past president of five national or international professional organizations and has served as editor in chief for *Health Psychology* and *Annals of Behavioral Medicine*. His 21 books and over 600 articles or chapters have been cited more than 76,000 times (*h*-index >120), and Google Scholar includes him in the list of the most cited authors in science. In 2019, Dr. Kaplan took on a new role as an opinion editorialist, contributing pieces on about a monthly basis. His work has appeared in *The Wall Street Journal*, *USA Today*, *Los Angeles Times*, *The Boston Globe*, *The Mercury News*, *San Francisco Chronicle*, *STAT News*, *RealClear Politics*, *MedPage*, *Health Affairs*, *The Hill*, and a variety of other newspapers. Dr. Kaplan was elected to the National Academy of Medicine in 2005. He received his A.B. in psychology from San Diego State University and M.A. and Ph.D. from the University of California, Riverside. He has served on numerous National Academies activities, most recently as a member of the Roundtable on Population Health Improvement.

Nancy E. Lane, M.D., is a distinguished professor of medicine and rheumatology at the University of California Davis School of Medicine and an adjunct professor of immunology and rheumatology at Stanford School of Medicine. Dr. Lane is an internationally recognized expert in research related to musculoskeletal diseases of aging, including osteoarthritis and osteoporosis. She has performed foundational studies to reverse osteoporosis in individuals on chronic glucocorticoids and investigated mechanisms that foster peak bone mass and, on the other end of the life-span, how the skeleton weakens with age. Dr. Lane has also studied osteoarthritis (OA). When, early in her career, she determined that exercise (jogging) did not accelerate the degeneration of knee joints in older runners without known OA, she continued to follow them, finding that exercise of any form increased both the quality of life and life-span. As a translational scientist, Dr. Lane has investigated genetic association with OA of the hip and knee. Dr. Lane has also dedicated her professional career to training the next generation of researchers in musculoskeletal diseases and championed an effort for over 18 years, through the U.S. Bone and Joint Decade/Initiative and National Institutes of Health, to train young investigators to obtain research grants. This has resulted in over 300 new investigators receiving NIH grants. Dr. Lane has also been instrumental in training junior faculty to perform research in women's health through training grants awarded to the University of California, Davis. In the past, she has consulted with a pharmaceutical company on osteoporosis. Dr. Lane's accomplishments have been recognized with election to the National Academy of Medicine, National Academy of Inventors, and Association of American Physicians. Dr. Lane received her M.D. from University of California, San Francisco School of Medicine and B.S. from University of California, Davis.

Jane E. Salmon, M.D., is the Collette Kean Research Professor and Director of the Lupus and Antiphospholipid Center of Excellence at Hospital for Special Surgery. She is professor of medicine and obstetrics and gynecology and associate dean of faculty affairs at Weill Cornell College of Medicine. Dr. Salmon's research has focused on elucidating mechanisms of tissue injury in lupus and other autoimmune diseases. Her basic, translational, and clinical studies have led to a paradigm shift in the understanding of mechanisms of pregnancy loss, cardiovascular disease, and end-organ damage in patients with lupus. Groundbreaking laboratory discoveries about causes of pregnancy loss and preeclampsia, and subsequent observational studies in women with lupus and antiphospholipid syndrome, have allowed her to identify new targets to reduce damage and improve outcomes in patients with autoimmune illness. She is leading the first trial of a biologic therapy to prevent complications in high-risk pregnancies. In recognition of her contributions, she was awarded the Carol Nachman international prize in rheumatology, Virginia Kneeland Frantz '22 Distinguished Women in Medicine Award from the Columbia P&S Alumni Association, and Evelyn V. Hess Award from the Lupus Foundation of America. She has been recognized as a Master of the American College of Rheumatology and elected to the American Association of Physicians and National Academy of Medicine. She also serves on the board of scientific counselors for the National Institute of Arthritis and Musculoskeletal and Skin Diseases and board of directors of the New York Community Trust. She has previously served on scientific advisory boards for a pharmaceutical company manufacturing autoimmunity medications. Dr. Salmon graduated magna cum laude from New York University and earned her M.D. in 1978 from the College of Physicians and Surgeons of Columbia University, where she was the first woman enrolled in its Medical Scientist Training Program. She completed training in internal medicine at the New York Hospital and in rheumatology at Hospital for Special Surgery.

Crystal Edler Schiller, Ph.D., is a licensed clinical psychologist and tenured associate professor of psychiatry at the University of North Carolina (UNC) at Chapel Hill. She serves as associate director of the UNC Center for Women's Mood Disorders and director of the UNC School of Medicine Clinical Psychology Internship Program. She conducts a National Institutes of Health–funded research program that focuses on sex steroid regulation of neural circuits and mood in women across the reproductive life-span. Her research also aims to identify novel ways to expand access to evidence-based psychotherapy. Dr. Schiller completed predoctoral training in clinical psychology at the University of Iowa, T32-funded postdoctoral training in reproductive hormone–related mood disorders and affective neuroscience at UNC Chapel Hill, and a K23 career development award focused on the effects of estrogen on the neural reward system in perimenopause.

Angeles Alvarez Secord, M.D., M.H.Sc., is a professor in the Division of Gynecologic Oncology, Department of Obstetrics & Gynecology, in the Duke University Health System. She is the director of Gynecologic Oncology Clinical Trials, associate director of Clinical Research, Gynecologic Oncology, and NRG Oncology principal investigator (PI) at the Duke Cancer Institute. She is the site PI for numerous clinical trials related to female-specific cancers. Dr. Secord served as a board member for the GOG Foundation, Foundation for Women's Cancer, Society of Gynecologic Oncology, and American Association Obstetricians and Gynecologists Foundation. She participated in scientific advisory meetings for GSK on endometrial cancer and AbbVie relating to ovarian cancer in 2024; she served on other advisory boards and clinical trial steering committees for pharmaceutical companies prior to serving on this National Academies committee. She also participated in educational meetings related to gynecologic malignancies for which she reviewed honoraria. She is committed to mentoring the next generation of clinical trialists with expertise in translational research and serves as the NRG Oncology New Investigator Committee vice chair and GOG Foundation Education and Mentoring chair. Her research interests include novel therapeutics and biomarker development to direct treatment for patients with gynecologic cancer. She has received National Institutes of Health and Department of Defense funding and numerous institutional, regional, and national awards for her research. Dr. Secord is a fellow of the American College of Obstetricians and Gynecologists and an active member of American Society of Clinical Oncology, American Gynecological & Obstetrical Society, and International Gynecologic Cancer Society. She received her undergraduate degree with honors from Carroll College and graduated Alpha Omega Alpha with honors from the University of Washington School of Medicine. Dr. Secord completed her residency in obstetrics and gynecology and fellowship in gynecologic oncology at the Duke University Medical Center.

Methodius G. Tuuli, M.D., M.B.A., M.P.H., is the Chace-Joukowsky Professor and chair of the Department of Obstetrics and Gynecology at the Warren Alpert Medical School of Brown University and Chief of Obstetrics and Gynecology at Women & Infants Hospital. His top priority is to improve the quality of maternal care and eliminate disparities in perinatal outcomes. A board-certified maternal-fetal medicine physician, he focuses on predicting and preventing adverse obstetric outcomes, including preventing surgical site infection after cesarean delivery, managing labor, and optimizing management of medical complications in pregnancy. He leads three R01s for ongoing multicenter trials on treating postpartum hemorrhage, managing anemia in pregnancy, and optimizing glycemic control in overweight and obese women with gestational diabetes. He also leads a Department of Health and Human Services grant to develop a participatory model for integrating community-based maternal support services into perinatal care to address care coordination and social determinants of health and test the impact on perinatal health equity. Dr. Tuuli is an elected member of the National Academy of Medicine. He earned his M.D. from the University of Ghana Medical School in 2001 and M.P.H. from the University of California, Berkeley with concentration in maternal and child health in 2003. He completed residency training in obstetrics and gynecology at Emory University in 2008 and fellowship training in maternal-fetal medicine at Washington University in 2011. Dr. Tuuli completed the Business of Medicine Physician M.B.A. program at the Kelley School of Business at Indiana University in 2020.

Bianca D. M. Wilson, Ph.D., is an associate professor in the Department of Social Welfare and affiliate faculty member of the California Center for Population Research at the University of California, Los Angeles (UCLA). She was a Senior Scholar of Public Policy at the Williams Institute on Sexual Orientation and Gender Identity Law and Public Policy at UCLA School of Law. Her research explores the relationships between culture, oppression, and health. Dr. Wilson examines lesbian, gay, bisexual, transgender, and queer (LGBTQ) economic instabilities and involvement with systems of care and criminalization, with a focus on how racialization, sexual orientation, gender identity, and gender expression play a role in creating disproportionality and disparities. Notably, she was the lead investigator on the first study to establish population estimates of how many LGBTQ youth are in foster care and has led similar work in juvenile criminalization. Similarly, she has led the largest qualitative study of the life and needs of LGBTQ people experiencing economic insecurity. Acknowledging the impact of this work, she was awarded the Distinguished Contribution to Public Policy Award by the American Psychological Association Division 44 (Society for the Psychology of Sexual Orientation and Gender Diversity). Underlying her substantive work on LGBTQ health, system involvement, and economic security is her attention to sexual orientation, gender identity, and gender expression data collection and data policy; she has conducted this measurement research among youth and adults and continues to work with local, state, and federal government efforts on increasing and improving LGBTQ-inclusive data collection. She served on the National Academy of Sciences, Engineering, and Medicine Consensus Panel on the Measurement of Sex, Gender, and Sexual Orientation. Dr. Wilson earned her Ph.D. in psychology from the Community and Prevention Research program at the University of Illinois at Chicago with a minor in statistics, methods, and measurement and received postdoctoral training at the University of California, San Francisco (UCSF) Institute for Health Policy Studies and the UCSF Lesbian Health and Research Center through an AHRQ postdoctoral fellowship. She served on the National Academies Panel on Measuring Sex, Gender Identity, and Sexual Orientation for the National Institutes of Health.

National Academy of Medicine Fellows

2023–2025 Gant/American Board of Obstetrics and Gynecology Fellow
Michelle P. Debbink, M.D., Ph.D., is a maternal-fetal medicine specialist and assistant professor at the University of Utah in the Department of Obstetrics and Gynecology. She also serves as the departmental vice chair for Equity, Diversity, and Inclusion for the Obstetrics and Gynecology Department. Her clinical interests include complex maternal and fetal care, with a particular emphasis on high-quality, responsive care for structurally and historically marginalized people with high-risk pregnancies. She has focused her clinical, professional, and investigational efforts on the structural and community factors that contribute to racial and geographic health equity in pregnancy outcomes. As a Reproductive Scientist Development Program scholar, she conducts community-engaged mixed-methods research with Native Hawaiian and Pacific Islander and Native American/Indigenous mothers to understand community risk and resilience related to maternal morbidity and perinatal health. These collaborations have resulted in multiple funded awards to develop, implement, and test culturally responsive interventions for perinatal mental health, substance use disorders, and respectful care. She also has expertise in geographic information science as applied to population health and social epidemiology analyses that inform and bolster qualitative and community-led research. She serves as a committee member for the Utah Perinatal Mortality Review Committee. Dr. Debbink earned her M.D. and Ph.D. in health services organization and policy at the University of Michigan. She completed her obstetrics and gynecology residency at the University of Michigan and maternal-fetal medicine fellowship at the University of Utah.

2021–2023 American Board of Emergency Medicine Fellow
Tracy Madsen, M.D., Ph.D., FAHA, FACEP, is an associate professor of emergency medicine and epidemiology at Brown University, the vice chair of research in the Department of Emergency Medicine, and interim director of the Division of Sex and Gender in Emergency Medicine. She has expertise in sex and gender-based medicine, women's health, acute cerebrovascular disease, stroke epidemiology and prevention, and disparities in the health care system. Dr. Madsen's research is funded by the National Heart, Lung, and Blood Institute, the American Heart Association, and the Agency for Healthcare Research and Quality. She has over 110 peer-reviewed publications and speaks nationally and internationally on topics including stroke in women, health inequities in stroke, and disparities in the academic medicine workforce. She is regarded as an expert in the fields of cerebrovascular and cardiometabolic disease in women. Dr. Madsen is an active investigator in the Women's Health Initiative Study, where she leads the stroke/venous

thromboembolism working group and serves as a consultant for both the Fred Hutchinson Cancer Center and Western Regional Coordinating Center at Stanford University. Dr. Madsen received her M.D. from Boston University School of Medicine and completed a residency, with her last year as chief resident, at Brown University before completing a research fellowship in the Division of Sex and Gender Medicine at Brown University. She then completed an M.S. in clinical and translational research and a Ph.D. in epidemiology, both at the Brown University School of Public Health. She is also a 2021 National Academy of Medicine Fellow in Emergency Medicine.

STAFF

Amy Geller, M.P.H., is a senior program officer in the Health and Medicine Division (HMD) on the Board on Population Health and Public Health Practice. During her 20 years at the National Academies, she has staffed committees spanning many topics, including advancing health equity, prevention of sexually transmitted infections, reducing alcohol-impaired driving fatalities, workforce resilience, vaccine safety, reducing tobacco use, drug safety, and treating post-traumatic stress disorder. She was and is the study director, respectively, for the recently released HMD report *Federal Policy to Advance Racial, Ethnic, and Tribal Health* and the HMD Committee on the Assessment of NIH Research on Women's Health. She also directs the DC Public Health Case Challenge, a joint activity of HMD and NAM that aims to promote interdisciplinary, problem-based learning for college students at universities in the DC area.

Aimee Mead, M.P.H., is a program officer in the Health and Medicine Division and on the Board on Population Health and Public Health Practice. She has supported National Academies consensus studies on a range of public health challenges, including eliminating hepatitis B and C in the United States, reducing alcohol-impaired driving, reviewing the health consequences of e-cigarettes, preventing sexually transmitted infections, evaluating the health effects and patterns of use of premium cigars, and reviewing federal policies that contribute to racial and ethnic health inequities. Earlier, she worked at the National Heart, Lung, and Blood Institute. She holds an M.P.H. from the Yale School of Public Health (epidemiology) and B.S. (biology) from Cornell University.

L. Brielle Dojer, M.P.H., is a research associate in the Health and Medicine Division and on the Board on Population Health and Public Health Practice. She holds an M.P.H. from the Icahn School of Medicine at Mount Sinai and a B.A. in biology from Boston University. Earlier, she worked on health equity issues as an intern with the Access Challenge, a 501(c)(3) nonprofit, and as a volunteer with the student-founded organization ContraCOVID NYC. She also worked in research laboratories at NYU Langone and Mount Sinai Hospital before pursuing a career in public health.

Maggie Anderson, M.P.H., is an HMD research assistant and on the Board on Population Health and Public Health Practice. Earlier, she worked at Program Savvy Consulting as an independent contractor and as an intern with the Food Policy Council of Buffalo and Erie County. She received a B.A. in biology with a minor in environmental studies from Mount Holyoke College and her M.P.H. from George Mason University.

Rachel Riley Sorrell was a senior program assistant in HMD on the Board on Population Health and Public Health Practice. She received her B.S. in public health and politics and international affairs from Furman University. Earlier, she worked at different health advocacy nonprofits in South Carolina and Washington, DC as a health policy/law intern.

Rose Marie Martinez, Sc.D., has been the director of the Health and Medicine Division (formerly the Institute of Medicine) Board on Population Health and Public Health Practice since 1999. Dr. Martinez was a senior health researcher at Mathematica Policy Research (1995–1999), where she conducted research on the impact of health system change on the public health infrastructure, access to care for vulnerable populations, managed care, and the health care workforce. She is a former assistant director for Health Financing and Policy with the Government Accountability Office and served for 6 years directing research studies for the Regional Health Ministry of Madrid, Spain.

Y. Crysti Park is a program coordinator in the Health and Medicine Division on the Board on Population Health and Public Health Practice. Earlier, she was in marketing and sales management for over 15 years, working on creating catalogs, merchandising, and production in the garment industry. She attended the Fashion Institute of Technology and Cornell University.